COLOR ATLAS AND SYNOPSIS OF HEART FAILURE

COLOR ATLAS AND SYNOPSIS OF HEART FAILURE

EDITOR

R. R. Baliga, MD, MBA, FACP, FRCP (Edin), FACC

Director, Cardio-Oncology Center of Excellence
Associate Director
Division of Cardiovascular Medicine
Professor of Internal Medicine
The Ohio State University Wexner Medical Center
Columbus, Ohio

SERIES EDITOR

William T. Abraham, MD, FACP, FACC, FAHA, FESC

Professor of Medicine, Physiology, and Cell Biology
Chair of Excellence in Cardiovascular Medicine
Director, Division of Cardiovascular Medicine
Deputy Director, Davis Heart and Lung Research Institute
The Ohio State University
Columbus, Ohio

New York   Chicago   San Francisco   Athens   London   Madrid   Mexico City
Milan   New Delhi   Singapore   Sydney   Toronto

Color Atlas and Synopsis of Heart Failure

Copyright © 2019 by McGraw-Hill Education. All rights reserved. Printed in China. Except as permitted under the United States Copyright Act of 1976, no part of this publication may be reproduced or distributed in any form or by any means, or stored in a data base or retrieval system, without the prior written permission of the publisher.

1 2 3 4 5 6 7 8 9   DSS   23 22 21 20 19 18

ISBN 978-0-07-174938-1
MHID 0-07-174938-1

This book was set in Arno pro by Cenveo® Publisher Services.
The editors were Karen G. Edmonson, Cindy Yoo, and Robert Pancotti.
The production supervisor was Richard Ruzycka.
Project management was provided by Revathi Viswanathan, Cenveo Publisher Services.

Library of Congress Cataloging-in-Publication Data

Names: Baliga, R. R., editor.
  Title: Color atlas and synopsis of heart failure / editor, Ragavendra Baliga.
  Description: New York : McGraw-Hill Education, [2019] | Includes
    bibliographical references.
  Identifiers: LCCN 2018009892| ISBN 9780071749381 (hardcover) | ISBN
    0071749381 (hardcover)
  Subjects: LCSH: Heart failure--Atlases. | Heart failure--Case studies.
  Classification: LCC RC685.C53 C615 2019 | DDC 616.1/29--dc23
  LC record available at https://lccn.loc.gov/2018009892

McGraw-Hill Education books are available at special quantity discounts to use as premiums and sales promotions or for use in corporate training programs. To contact a representative, please visit the Contact Us pages at www.mhprofessional.com.

DEDICATION

To my mentor

Dr. P. Ranganath Nayak, MD, DM
Senior Cardiologist
Vikram Hospital
Bengaluru

for his friendship and for providing superior medical care gratis for my extended family for more than three decades.

CONTENTS

Videos for Chapter 21 can be found at www.BaligaHeartFailureCh21.com

Abeer Almasary, MD (Chapter 19)
Research Coordinator
Emergency Department
Baylor College of Medicine
Ben Taub General Hospital
Houston, Texas

Emmanuel A. Amulraj, MD (Chapter 41)
Cardiothoracic Surgery
Baylor Scott and White
Temple, Texas

JoAnne Arcand, PhD, RD (Chapter 25)
Assistant Professor, Faculty of Health Sciences
University of Ontario Institute of Technology
Oshawa, Ontario, Canada

Ross Arena, PhD, PT (Chapter 45)
Professor and Head, Department of Physical Therapy
College of Applied Health Sciences
University of Illinois at Chicago
Chicago, Illinois

R. R. Baliga, MD, MBA, FACP, FRCP (Edin), FACC (Chapter 12)
Director, Cardio-Oncology Center of Excellence
Associate Director, Division of Cardiovascular Medicine
Professor of Internal Medicine
The Ohio State University Wexner Medical Center
Columbus, Ohio

Todd A. Barrett, MD (Chapter 44)
The Ohio State University Wexner Medical Center
Columbus, Ohio

Cecilia Berardi, MD (Chapter 20)
La Sapienza University of Rome
Rome, Italy

Philip F. Binkley, MD, MPH (Chapter 8)
James W. Overstreet Chair in Cardiology; Professor of Medicine
The Ohio State University Department of Internal Medicine;
Professor of Epidemiology, The Ohio State University College of Public Health
The Ohio State University
Columbus, Ohio

Sam Bond, MS (Chapter 45)
Visiting Clinical Assistant Professor
Department of Physical Therapy
Department of Biomedical and Health Information Sciences
University of Illinois at Chicago
Chicago, Illinois

Elisa Bradley, MD (Chapter 17)
Assistant Professor of Medicine
The Ohio State University & Nationwide Children's Hospital
Columbus, Ohio

Darshan H. Brahmbhatt, MB BChir, MA, MPhil, MRCP (Chapter 10)
Specialist Registrar in Cardiology, Department of Cardiology
Royal Papworth Hospital NHS Foundation Trust
Cambridge, United Kingdom

Khadijah Breathett, MD, MS, FACC (Chapter 12)
Assistant Professor of Medicine
Division of Cardiology
Sarver Heart Center
University of Arizona
Tucson, Arizona

Quinn Capers IV, MD, FACC, FSCAI (Chapter 12)
Associate Dean of Admissions
The Ohio State University School of Medicine
Columbus, Ohio

Scipione Carerj, MD, FESC (Chapter 37)
Associate Professor of Cardiology, Department of Clinical and Experimental Medicine–Section of Cardiology
University of Messina
Messina, Italy

Rahul Chaudhary, MD (Chapter 13)
Academic Hospitalist
Johns Hopkins University/Sinai Hospital of Baltimore
Baltimore, Maryland

Eloisa Colin-Ramirez, BSc, MSc, PhD (Chapter 25)
Researcher, National Council of Science and Technology (CONACYT), and National Institute of Cardiology
Ignacio Chavez
Mexico City, Mexico

Maria Rosa Costanzo, MD, FAHA, FACC, FESC (Chapter 33)
Medical Director, Heart Failure Research
Advocate Heart Institute
Medical Director, Edward Hospital Center for Advanced Heart Failure
Naperville, Illinois

Karla M. Daniels, MS (Chapter 45)
Clinical Exercise Physiologist, Shapiro Heart and Vascular Care Center
Brigham and Women's Hospital
Boston, Massachusetts

Steven M. Dean, DO, FSVM, RPVI (Chapter 18)
Clinical Professor of Internal Medicine
Division of Cardiovascular Medicine
Ohio State University Wexner Medical Center
Columbus, Ohio

Anita Deswal, MD, MPH (Chapter 28)
Professor of Medicine
Section of Cardiology, Department of Medicine
Baylor College of Medicine
Chief of Cardiology
Michael E. DeBakey Veterans Affairs Medical Center
Houston, Texas

CONTRIBUTORS

Kumar Dharmarajan, MD, MBA (Chapter 14)
Section of Cardiovascular Medicine
Department of Internal Medicine
Yale University School of Medicine
Yale-New Haven Hospital Center for
Outcomes Research and Evaluation
New Haven, Connecticut

Sitaramesh Emani, MD (Chapters 33 and 39)
Director of Heart Failure Clinical Research, Advanced Heart
Failure & Cardiac Transplant Section
The Ohio State University Wexner Medical Center
Columbus, Ohio

Jerry Estep, MD (Chapter 38)
Department of Cardiovascular Medicine
Cleveland Clinic, Cleveland, Ohio;
and the Heart and Vascular Institute
Kaufman Center for Heart Failure
Cleveland Clinic, Cleveland, Ohio

Justin A. Ezekowitz, MBBCh, MSc (Chapter 25)
Professor, Division of Cardiology, Department of Medicine, and
Canadian VIGOUR Centre
University of Alberta
Edmonton, Alberta, Canada

Sutton Fox, MPH (Chapter 20)
University of California San Diego School of Medicine
University of California San Diego
San Diego, California

Heba R. Gaber, MD (Chapter 19)
Research Fellow
Emergency Department
Baylor College of Medicine
Ben Taub General Hospital
Houston, Texas

Jalaj Garg, MD, FESC (Chapter 13)
Division of Cardiology, Lehigh Valley Health Network
Allentown, Pennsylvania

Morie A. Gertz, MD (Chapter 11)
Chair Emeritus, Department of Internal Medicine and Consultant
Hematologist
Mayo Clinic
Rochester, Minnesota

Randal Goldberg, MD (Chapter 34)
Fellow in Cardiovascular Disease, Leon H. Charney Division of
Cardiology
New York University School of Medicine
New York, New York

Zachary D. Goldberger, MD, FACC, FAHA, FHRS (Chapter 26)
Associate Professor of Medicine
Division of Cardiovascular Medicine
University of Wisconsin School of Medicine and Public Health
Madison, Wisconsin

Ashrith Guha, MD, MPH, FACC (Chapter 38)
Division of Heart Failure & Heart Transplant, Methodist DeBakey
Heart & Vascular Center, Cardiology Department
Houston Methodist Hospital
Houston, Texas

Jillian L. Gustin, MD, FAAHPM (Chapter 44)
The Ohio State University Wexner Medical Center
Columbus, Ohio

Garrie J. Haas, MD (Chapter 27)
Professor of Medicine
Advanced HF Program
The Ohio State University Wexner Medical Center
Columbus, Ohio

Mariko W. Harper, MD, MS (Chapter 26)
Staff Cardiologist
Virginia Mason Medical Center
Seattle, Washington

Ayesha Hasan, MD, FACC (Chapter 40)
Professor of Clinical Internal Medicine; Medical Director, Cardiac
Transplant Program; Director, Advanced Heart Failure and
Cardiac Transplantation Fellowship Program
The Ohio State University Wexner Medical Center
Columbus, Ohio

Lauren J. Hassen, MD, MPH (Chapter 17)
Resident, Internal Medicine & Pediatrics
The Ohio State University & Nationwide Children's Hospital
Columbus, Ohio

Ray Hershberger, MD (Chapter 5)
Divisions of Human Genetics and Cardiovascular Medicine
Department of Internal Medicine, Dorothy M. Davis Heart and
Lung Research Institute
The Ohio State University Wexner Medical Center
Columbus, Ohio

Ha Mieu Ho, BS (Chapter 20)
Director of Investigator-Initiated Studies
University of California, San Diego
La Jolla, California

Christopher M. Hritz, MD (Chapter 44)
The Ohio State University Wexner Medical Center
Columbus, Ohio

Zeina Ibrahim, MD, FASE, FACC, FAHA (Chapter 15)
Advanced Imaging Cardiologist
Department of Medicine, Division of Cardiology
Mount Sinai Hospital
Chicago, Illinois

Abiodun Ishola, MD (Chapter 21)
St. Elizabeth Healthcare
Heart and Vascular Institute
Edgewood, Kentucky

Renuka Jain, MD (Chapter 37)
Aurora Cardiovascular Services
Aurora Sinai/Aurora St. Luke's Medical Centers
Milwaukee, Wisconsin

Rami Kahwash, MD (Chapters 30 and 31)
Assistant Professor of Medicine, Section of Heart Failure/
Transplant, Davis Heart and Lung Research Institute
Ross Heart Hospital, Wexner Medical Center
The Ohio State University
Columbus, Ohio

Mahwash Kassi, MD (Chapter 38)
Methodist DeBakey Cardiology Associates
JC Walter Transplant Center
Houston Methodist Hospital
Houston, Texas

Waleed Kayani, MD (Chapter 28)
Section of Cardiology, Department of Medicine
Baylor College of Medicine
Houston, Texas

**David Kaye, MBBS, PhD, FRACP, FACC,
FESC (Chapter 6)**
Director, Department of Cardiology
Alfred Hospital
Head, Heart Failure Research Laboratory
Baker Heart and Diabetes Institute
Melbourne, Victoria, Australia

Ashley K. Keates, BHSc (PH) (Chapter 1)
Centre of Research Excellence in Health Service Research to
Reduce Inequality in Heart Disease
Australian Catholic University
Melbourne, Victoria, Australia

Asaad Khan, MD (Chapter 9)
Cardiology Department
Massachusetts General Hospital
Boston, Massachusetts

**Bijoy K. Khandheria, MD, FACP, FESC,
FASE, FACC (Chapter 37)**
Aurora Cardiovascular Services
Aurora Sinai/Aurora St. Luke's Medical Centers
Milwaukee, Wisconsin

Ahmet Kilic, MD, FACS (Chapters 36 and 42)
Division of Cardiac Surgery
The Johns Hopkins Hospital
Baltimore, Maryland

Arman Kilic, MD (Chapter 36)
Assistant Professor of Cardiothoracic Surgery
University of Pittsburgh Medical Center
Pittsburgh, Pennsylvania

**Christopher J. Kramer, BA, ACS, RDCS,
FASE (Chapter 37)**
Echocardiography Education Program Director
Advanced Cardiac Sonography
Aurora Cardiovascular Services
Aurora Sinai/Aurora St. Luke's Medical Centers
Milwaukee, Wisconsin

Brent C. Lampert, DO (Chapter 24)
Associate Professor of Clinical Medicine, Division of
Cardiovascular Medicine
The Ohio State University Wexner Medical Center
Columbus, Ohio

Gregg M. Lanier, MD, FACC (Chapter 13)
Division of Cardiology, Westchester Medical Center and
New York Medical College
Valhalla, New York

**Peter H. U. Lee, MD, PhD, MPH, FACC,
FACS (Chapter 35)**
Assistant Professor of Surgery
The Ohio State University
Columbus, Ohio

Srihari K. Lella, MD (Chapter 41)
Department of Vascular Surgery
Masachusetts General Hospital
Boston, Massachusetts

Daniel Lenihan, MD, FACC (Chapter 16)
Professor of Medicine
Director, Cardio-Oncology Center of Excellence
Advanced Heart Failure
Clinical Research
Cardiovascular Division
Washington University in St. Louis
St. Louis, Missouri

Scott M. Lilly, MD, PhD (Chapter 32)
Associate Professor, Division of Cardiovascular Medicine
The Ohio State University Wexner Medical Center
Columbus, Ohio

Luca Longobardo, MD (Chapter 37)
Department of Clinical and Experimental Medicine
Section of Cardiology
University of Messina
Messina, Italy

Alan S. Maisel, MD (Chapter 20)
Professor of Medicine Emeritus
University of California San Diego
San Diego, California

Mahim Malik, MD (Chapter 42)
Assistant Professor
Department of Surgery
Aga Khan University
Karachi, Pakistan

CONTRIBUTORS

William H. Marshall V, MD (Chapter 17)
Resident, Internal Medicine & Pediatrics
The Ohio State University & Nationwide Children's Hospital
Columbus, Ohio

Claire Mayeur, MD (Chapter 43)
Department of Anesthesiology and Intensive Care
Lariboisière University Hospital
Paris, France

Peter A. McCullough, MD, MPH (Chapter 7)
Baylor Heart and Vascular Institute
Baylor University Medical Center
Dallas, Texas

Alexandre Mebazaa, MD, PhD (Chapter 43)
Department of Anesthesiology and Intensive Care
Lariboisière University Hospital
Paris, France

Nishaki Mehta, MD (Chapter 2)
Assistant Professor
Division of Cardiovascular Medicine (Electrophysiology) and
Biomedical Engineering
University of Virginia School of Medicine
Charlottesville, Virginia

James Monaco, MD (Chapter 27)
Division of Cardiovascular Medicine, The Ohio State University
Wexner Medical Center, Columbus, Ohio

Shane Nanayakkara, MBBS, FRACP (Chapter 6)
Cardiologist, Department of Cardiology
Alfred Hospital
Melbourne, Victoria, Australia

Cemal Ozemek, PhD, CEP (Chapter 45)
Clinical Assistant Professor, Department of Physical Therapy
University of Illinois at Chicago
Chicago, Illinois

Katherine Panettiere-Kennedy, BS, MD (Candidate 2021) (Chapter 7)
MD candidate
University of Texas Southwestern Medical Center
Dallas, Texas
MPH candidate
University of Texas Health Science Center at Houston School of
Public Health
Houston, Texas

W. Frank Peacock, MD, FACEP, FACC (Chapter 19)
Associate Chair and Research Director
Emergency Department
Baylor College of Medicine
Ben Taub General Hospital
Houston, Texas

Mohammed Quader, MD (Chapter 41)
Virginia Commonwealth University School of Medicine
Cardiothoracic Surgeon, McGuire Veterans Medical Center
Richmond, Virginia

Shaline Rao, MD (Chapter 34)
Assistant Professor of Medicine, Leon H. Charney Division of
Cardiology
New York University School of Medicine
New York, New York

Yazhini Ravi, MD (Chapter 41)
Research Associate, Division of Cardiothoracic Surgery
Baylor Scott and White
Temple, Texas

Alexander Reyentovich, MD (Chapter 34)
Associate Professor of Medicine, Leon H. Charney
Division of Cardiology
New York University School of Medicine
New York, New York

Michael W. Rich, MD (Chapter 14)
Cardiovascular Division, Department of Internal Medicine
Washington University School of Medicine
St. Louis, Missouri

Vera H. Rigolin, MD, FASE, FACC, FAHA (Chapter 15)
Professor of Medicine
Northwestern University Feinberg School of Medicine
Medical Director, Echocardiography Laboratory
Northwestern Memorial Hospital
Chicago, Illinois

Emily A. Ruden, MD (Chapter 23)
Cardiovascular Disease
St. Vincent Medical Group
Noblesville, Indiana

Lucy Safi, DO (Chapter 9)
Cardiology Department
Massachusetts General Hospital
Boston, Massachusetts

Chittoor B. Sai-Sudhakar, MD (Chapter 41)
Division Director, Division of Cardiothoracic Surgery
Baylor Scott and White Medical Center
Temple, Texas

Kavita Sharma, MD (Chapter 2)
Ohio Health Heart and Vascular Physicians
Delaware, Ohio

Mark J. Shen, MD (Chapter 29)
Division of Cardiology
McGaw Medical Center
Northwestern University
Feinberg School of Medicine
Chicago, Illinois

Taimur Sher, MD (Chapter 11)
Consultant Hematologist
Mayo Clinic
Jacksonville, Florida

Jai Singh, MD (Chapter 16)
Sanger Heart & Vascular Institute
Atrium Health
Charlotte, North Carolina

Gbemiga G. Sofowora, MBChB, FACC (Chapter 21)
Division of Cardiovascular Diseases, Davis Heart and Lung Research Center
The Ohio State University Wexner Medical Center
Columbus, Ohio

Simon Stewart, PhD (Chapter 1)
Visiting Professor, Hatter Institute for Cardiovascular Research in Africa
University of Cape Town
Cape Town, South Africa

Amy C. Sturm, MS, LCGC (Chapter 5)
Genomic Medicine Institute
Geisinger
Danville, Pennsylvania

Katharine Tweed, MB BS, BMedSci, FRCR (Chapter 10)
Consultant Radiologist, Department of Radiology
Royal Papworth Hospital NHS Foundation Trust
Cambridge, United Kingdom

Matt Umland, ACS, RDCS, FASE (Chapter 37)
Echocardiography System Coordinator, Advanced Cardiac Sonographer
Aurora Cardiovascular Services
Aurora Sinai/Aurora St. Luke's Medical Centers
Milwaukee, Wisconsin

Christopher W. Valentine, MD (Chapter 3)
Ohio Kidney Consultants
Columbus, Ohio

Amanda R. Vest, MBBS, MPH (Chapter 4)
Assistant Professor of Medicine
Division of Cardiology
Tufts Medical Center
Tufts University
Boston, Massachusetts

Akira Wada, MD (Chapters 2 and 32)
Heart and Vascular Physicians
Ohio Health
Columbus, Ohio

Bryan A. Whitson, MD, PhD, FACS (Chapters 36 and 42)
Associate Professor of Surgery
Interim Director, Division of Cardiac Surgery
Director, Thoracic Transplantation and Mechanical Circulatory Support
Co-Director, COPPER Laboratory
Department of Surgery, Division of Cardiac Surgery
The Ohio State University
Columbus, Ohio

Lynne K. Williams, MBBCh, FRCP, PhD (Chapter 10)
Consultant Cardiologist, Department of Cardiology
Royal Papworth Hospital NHS Foundation Trust
Cambridge, United Kingdom

Shannon Willis, MD (Chapter 12)
Hospitalist, Memorial Medical Center
Savannah, Georgia
Department of Internal Medicine, Gwinnett Medical Center
Lawrenceville, Georgia

Eugene E. Wolfel, MD (Chapter 22)
Professor of Medicine, Section of Advanced Heart Failure and Transplant Cardiology, Division of Cardiology
University of Colorado School of Medicine
Aurora, Colorado

Malissa Wood, MD (Chapter 9)
Cardiology Department
Massachusetts General Hospital
Boston, Massachusetts

Karolina M. Zareba, MD (Chapter 23)
Assistant Professor, Division of Cardiovascular Medicine
Associate Program Director, Cardiovascular Diagnostics Training Program
Wexner Medical Center, The Ohio State University
Columbus, Ohio

Douglas P. Zipes, MD (Chapter 29)
Krannert Institute of Cardiology, Department of Medicine
Indiana University School of Medicine
Indianapolis, Indiana

Concetta Zito, MD, PhD (Chapter 37)
Assistant Professor, Department of Clinical and Experimental Medicine, Section of Cardiology
University of Messina
Messina, Italy

As the burden of heart failure continues to grow, it is predicted that 1 in every 33 Americans will be affected by heart failure in the next decade. In addition, it is anticipated that the cost of managing heart failure will be approximately $70 billion in 2030. Currently, heart failure results in more than 1 million hospitalizations every year. With the estimated 5-year mortality at approximately 50%, treatments that will improve survival and alleviate the economic burden of this condition are urgently needed. With all of this in mind, this *Color Atlas and Synopsis of Heart Failure* has been put together. This book is intended for medical students, postgraduate trainees, practicing cardiologists, physician assistants, internal medicine physicians, and general practitioners so that they can rapidly assimilate information on a wide variety of topics related to heart failure.

This book contains 45 chapters; it is illustrated generously with color photographs and includes a substantial amount of clinically oriented material. The hope is that this book not only will help practitioners to provide better care for their heart failure patients but also will provide a stimulus for further research in this area.

R. R. Baliga, MD, MBA, FACP, FRCP (Edin), FACC

1 ECONOMICS OF HEART FAILURE

Simon Stewart, PhD
Ashley K. Keates, BHSc (PH)

PATIENT CASE

A 72-year-old man with a history of coronary artery disease is admitted with acute pulmonary edema secondary to acute coronary syndrome (confirmed by 12-lead ECG and a positive high-sensitivity troponin test). Following initial emergency management with intravenous loop diuretics, nitrate therapy, and continuous-positive airway pressure support, he is admitted to the hospital's coronary care unit for 2 days and then spends a further 5 days in a general medical unit. A coronary angiogram shows that a previous drug-eluting stent in the right coronary artery remains patent, but there is evidence of progressive diffuse disease in the left anterior descending and circumflex artery. Echocardiography reveals morphological and functional changes indicative of ischemic cardiomyopathy with left ventricular systolic dysfunction (left ventricular ejection fraction of 38%). Discharged to home on gold-standard medical therapy with follow-up by an outpatient heart failure management team, he is diagnosed with chronic heart failure (NYHA class II-III but clinically stable) requiring ongoing surveillance and treatment.

This de novo, heart failure–related event did not occur in isolation. Nor does it prove to be the last time this patient's quality of life and prognosis are influenced by a costly syndrome that is as malignant as many forms of cancer.[1]

ECONOMIC ASPECTS OF HEART FAILURE

In the United States and Europe alone, there are currently more than 20 million people affected by heart failure.[2] Heart failure is routinely ascribed to be the number one cause of hospitalizations in those aged >65 years; hospital care traditionally consumes more than two-thirds of health care costs.[3]

As shown in Figure 1-1, the genesis of this particular case of heart failure began almost 20 years ago when, as a middle-aged man, the patient's increasingly sedentary lifestyle and diet contributed to the development of metabolic syndrome and undiagnosed and untreated hypertension. The sequence of events highlights the key economic aspects of heart failure.

PRIMARY AND SECONDARY CARE

Heart failure patients experience regular visits with primary care personnel and are mainly cared for by their primary care physician by requesting clinic appointments. Secondary care presents when the heart failure patient is admitted into hospital.

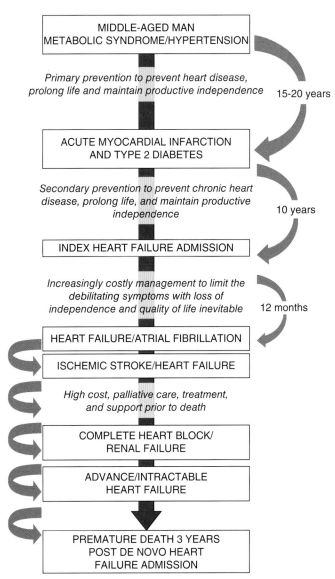

FIGURE 1-1 Cascade of increasingly costly (at the individual to society level) cardiac events in a 72-year-old man who initially presents with acute heart failure and dies 3 years later from advanced heart failure and multimorbidity.

TREATMENT AND MANAGEMENT

Once established, the syndrome of heart failure (usually presenting as acute decompensation requiring hospitalization) is typically characterized by progressive cardiac dysfunction, multimorbidity (including concurrent cerebrovascular and renal disease), and costly inpatient and outpatient management and treatment prior to death. Additionally, treatment and management options are rarely curative, but target achieving clinical stability (by reducing costly rehospitalization) and prolonged life.[4]

EFFECTS OF HEART FAILURE

For the affected individual, activities of daily living (including employment if appropriate) and quality of life are progressively impaired leading to loss of independence and residential care placement. Therefore, palliative management for those with advanced intractable heart failure is becoming an increasing and additionally costly feature of the syndrome.

KEY COMPONENTS OF HEART FAILURE COSTS

As reflected in contemporary guidelines,[4] there are a myriad of increasingly expensive health care costs associated with the diagnosis and treatment of acute and chronic forms of heart failure, as well as the complex multimorbid conditions that typically contribute to poor and very costly health outcomes; isolated heart failure being rare (<10% of cases). Despite a plethora of cost-effective analyses to support reimbursement for individual therapeutic strategies, there is no definitive analysis of the cost-effectiveness of multifaceted management of the syndrome. The widely accepted threshold for proving cost-effectiveness (and therefore willingness to pay for that health improvement) is $50,000 per quality-adjusted life-year gained. Given variable health systems, reimbursement mechanisms, and health insurance plans, there is no definitive source for health care costs associated with heart failure. Indicative costs (mainly derived from 2 key sources[2,5]) in this section are for the United States only, represent the lower price range, and are presented in U.S. dollars.

DIRECT COSTS

The direct cost of heart failure typically comprises any investigations typically directed toward determining an individual's cardiac function (eg, echocardiography and brain natriuretic peptide levels), the treatment of that individual (pharmacological and non-pharmacological), and health care contacts and activity specifically related to an acute heart failure event or its ongoing management. The most obvious, and often most costly, component of management is a primary hospital admission (where heart failure is the principal diagnosis) for the syndrome.

Initial Screening and Diagnosis

The initial screening process of heart failure involves clinical profiling (Figure 1-2), plasma concentrations of natriuretic peptides (>$50 per assay), 12-lead ECG (>$200 per test, Figure 1-3), and transthoracic echocardiography (>$1000 per test) that require

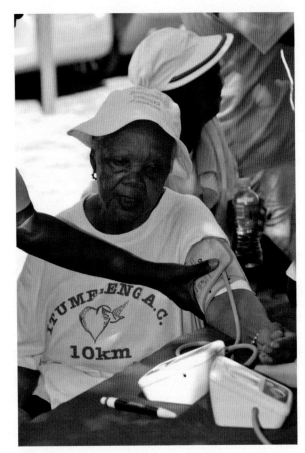

FIGURE 1-2 Clinical assessment.

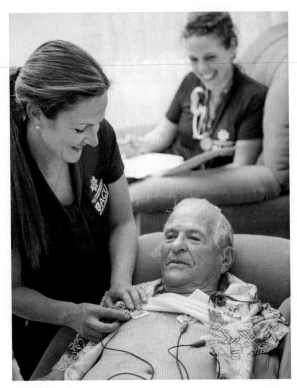

FIGURE 1-3 Twelve-lead ECG.

both trained technicians and expert cardiology review to determine the extent and type of cardiac dysfunction present (Figure 1-4).[4]

Other imaging modalities of increasing cost include chest x-ray ($200), stress echocardiography (>$2500), cardiac magnetic resonance imaging (>$2500), positron emission tomography (>$5000), coronary angiography (>$5000), and cardiac computed tomography (>$500).[4]

Pharmacological Treatment

A combination of angiotensin-converting enzyme inhibitors (noting the potential substitution with angiotensin receptor neprilysin inhibitor) and beta blockers supplemented by loop diuretics, mineralocorticoid (aldosterone) receptor antagonists, and I_r channel inhibitor, forms the basis for the primary treatment of heart failure with reduced ejection fraction[4] at a cost of >$1000 per person/annum for the simplest of drug regimes.

Nonsurgical Devices

Two major device-based therapies are now routinely applied to prevent sudden cardiac death and improve cardiac function in selected high-risk patients.[4] These two devices are (1) implantable cardiac defibrillators (>$25,000 for insertion, Figure 1-5); and (2) cardiac resynchronization therapy (>$25,000). Both require ongoing maintenance and surveillance from specialist cardiology teams.

Surgical Procedures

Depending on the underlying etiology (ie, coronary artery disease and/or valvular heart disease), there are a number of surgical options to prevent or delay progressive cardiac dysfunction. These include the most common revascularization procedures such as noninvasive, percutaneous angioplasty with placement of a drug-eluting stent (>$30,000), and coronary artery bypass surgery (>$100,000); as well as the valvular correction procedures such as transcatheter aortic valve replacement (>$80,000) and mitral valve replacement (>$150,000). In a minority of cases, heart transplantation (>$800,000) may be indicated and, considering the difficulties in tissue-typing and organ availability, bridging strategies such as left ventricular assist devices (Figure 1-6) for mechanical circulatory support (>$200,000) are often applied in this setting.[4]

Management

The ongoing management of heart failure is characterized by long periods of community-based care coordinated by primary care physicians punctuated by periods of acute (and inherently costly) hospital care followed by outpatient care.[3] Per diem hospital care costs >$650 with the average length of stay (in the United States) 5 days per episode (>$3000) with each cardiology outpatient visit costing >$1200. For acute decompensated heart failure, many individuals require specialist intensive coronary care with the application of advanced support (eg, hemodialysis/filtration and/or intra-aortic balloon pump) and pharmacotherapy (inotropic agents) that dramatically increase costs. These costs do not include the nonsurgical and surgical procedures outlined above.

In the immediate post discharge period, multidisciplinary management programs (predominantly nurse-led) are recommended.[4] These programs often combine community visits, allied health support, exercise programs, and ongoing surveillance with brain natriuretic peptide

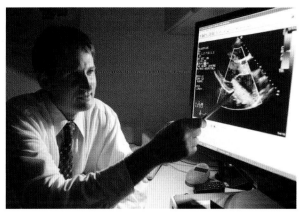

FIGURE 1-4 Expert review of echocardiography essential to the diagnosis of heart failure.

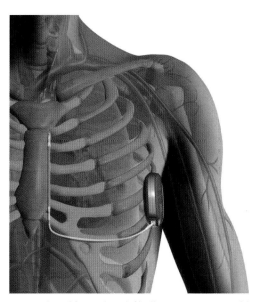

FIGURE 1-5 Implantable cardiac defibrillator to prevent sudden cardiac death in heart failure.

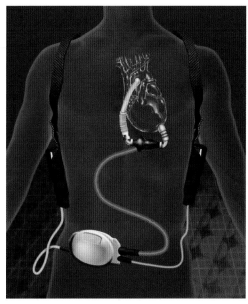

FIGURE 1-6 Implantable ventricular assist device to bridge the gap to heart transplantation.

levels (>$1000 per patient). Increasingly, these programs are being supplemented by structured telephone support and telemonitoring devices and surveillance (the latter involving implantable devices with physiological monitoring capabilities) that dramatically increase costs without necessarily reducing health care costs overall.

INDIRECT COSTS

The indirect cost of heart failure is less well defined but can be broken into three principal categories:

Societal costs: Loss of income and productivity, premature life-years lost, and quality-adjusted life-years lost due to heart failure and the societal level are also difficult to quantify. Whole-population data from Sweden at least suggest that, on this basis, the wider societal impact of heart failure is greater than the most common forms of cancer for both men and women.[1]

Additional health system costs: Hospital admissions where heart failure is listed as a closely linked (and often causative) secondary diagnosis are becoming an increasingly commonly and costly phenomenon[3] in the setting of heart failure and multimorbidity.[6] This increasing component of expenditure typically costs more than primary admissions for heart failure.[3] One of the other major, indirect consequences of heart failure is the loss of independence (physically and mentally), often following an acute hospitalization, that requires high-level, supportive care (>$200 per day in a nursing home or skilled nursing facility). In the United Kingdom alone in 2000, this additional component of expenditure was estimated to be equivalent to more than 15% of direct health care expenditure.[3] Hospice care for the palliative management of advanced cases costs a minimum of $10,000 per episode.

Individual costs: Depending on the health care system and socioeconomic profile of the affected individual, the costs of health insurance, transport to clinic visits, loss of employment/income, and the expense of caring for someone debilitated by the syndrome may be highly prohibitive. These costs are often not calculated. This aspect of the economic impact of heart failure is particularly important when considering affected individuals in low- to middle-income countries who are of working age and support their family and wider community.

ECONOMIC BURDEN OF HEART FAILURE

The total economic burden of heart failure, as a complex syndrome, is not easy to calculate or compare from country to country due to variable definitions of the syndrome, cost calculations, and the cost dynamics of health care expenditure.[2,3] However, a global estimate of the economic burden of heart failure in 2012[7] with country-by-country comparisons revealed:

- The total annual cost of heart failure is close to $110 billion around the globe.
- Sixty percent of costs are directly attributable to heart failure ($65 billion per annum).
- On a proportional basis, heart failure typically consumes 1.5% to 2.0% of total health care expenditure.
- The cost dynamics of heart failure are markedly different for high-income countries (Figure 1-7) compared to low- to middle-income countries (Figure 1-8).

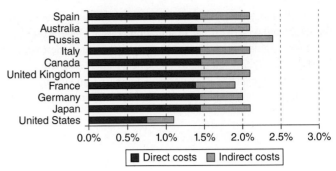

FIGURE 1-7 Economic cost of heart failure as a proportion of health care expenditure in the 10 highest-spending, high-income countries.

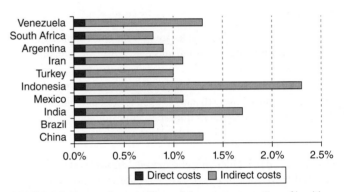

FIGURE 1-8 Economic cost of heart failure as a proportion of health care expenditure in the 10 highest-spending, low- to middle-income countries.

The United States represents an outlier in respect to proportion of total health care expenditure directed toward heart failure and these data contrast with an equivalent estimate of 3.2% for that country.[2]

A LOW- TO MIDDLE-INCOME COUNTRY PERSPECTIVE

The preponderance of robust and reliable epidemiological and subsequently economic data on heart failure is derived from high-income countries. As shown in Figure 1-9, these countries are not immune to the economic impact that indirect costs have on heart failure patients, posing as the greatest component of expenditure.[7] The International Congestive Heart Failure (INTER-CHF) study[8] describes significant regional variability in socioeconomic and clinical factors, etiologies, and treatments in patients with heart failure from Africa, Asia, the Middle East, and South America, with marked differences in the natural history and pattern of morbidity and mortality relative to cases of heart failure in Europe and North America.

Unique health economic data from the largest populations in sub-Saharan Africa (eg, Nigeria) provide a specific counter-perspective to the profile and economic burden of heart failure in high-income countries[9]:

- Hypertensive heart failure is predominant.
- Patients are a near equitable balance of men and women.
- In most cases, patients are aged <60 years. Any loss of income and productivity due to disability or death is more impactful to the patient's family.
- Total inpatient/hospital care (direct costs) account for <50% of total health care costs.
- Mean cost of care per annum is ~$2000 per patient (approximately one-tenth of the cost in high-income countries).

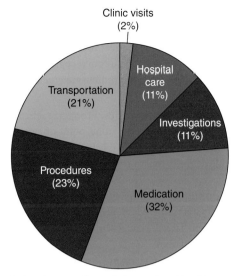

FIGURE 1-9 Distribution of heart failure–related health care costs in Nigeria.

COST PRESSURES IN HEART FAILURE

Already affecting 1% to 2% of most populations, depending on the definition being used, the overall prevalence and economic foot-print of heart failure is likely to rise for the foreseeable future due to the following dynamics:

Population dynamics: In most high-income countries, the absolute number and proportion of individuals in the high-risk age group (following the Baby Boomer phenomenon after World War II) is increasing.

Residually high-risk factors: Untreated, poorly controlled hypertension, particularly among older women, along with historically high levels of physical inactivity and metabolic syndromes and obesity are growing risk factors of heart failure.

Surviving acute coronary events: Survival rates from previously fatal cardiac events (most notably acute myocardial infarction) continue to increase.

Expanded definition: Beyond heart failure with reduced ejection fraction, the definition and formal recognition of heart failure has been expanded to incorporate heart failure with pre-served ejection fraction.

Greater awareness/surveillance: Increasing efforts to diagnose heart failure earlier via symptom recognition and screening with brain natriuretic peptide profiling are crucial in the reduction of heart failure.

Increasingly costly therapeutics: From magnetic resonance imaging to replace echocardiography, point-of-care machines for biomarker surveillance (notably brain natriuretic peptides), implantable defibrillators to combat high levels of sudden cardiac death, cardiac resynchronization therapy to improve cardiac function and output, and implantable devices linked to remote monitoring systems, there is an increasing appetite for device-based therapies that will change the cost dynamics (increasingly upward) of heart failure.

Prolonged survival in heart failure: There are inherent cost pressures from an increasingly larger cohort of heart failure patients in whom effective treatment options prolong survival without cure with the potential adverse trade-off toward increased risk of recurrent and costly hospitalization in the longer term.

Multimorbidity in heart failure: An increasing burden of multimorbidity (including renal dysfunction and diabetes) in the setting of heart failure will contribute to increased rates of rehospitalization (with heart failure typically listed as a secondary diagnosis).

Emergence of heart failure in low- to middle-income countries: Driven by profound economic change and population shifts from rural to urban communities and traditional to Western lifestyles, an increasing proportion of relatively young individuals in these developing countries is developing nonischemic (predominantly hypertension) heart failure.

HEART FAILURE'S FUTURE FOOTPRINT

No matter which population has been studied (Figure 1-10 shows the future burden of heart failure in Australia as an example), the future burden and cost of heart failure is predicted to rise. In the United States alone, it is predicted that between 2010 and 2030:

- The population prevalence will increase 2.8% to 3.5%
- Prevalent cases will increase by 3 million to a historical high of 15 million affected individuals.
- Indirect and productivity costs will rise from $9.7 to $17.4 billion.
- Direct health care costs will rise from $24.7 to $77.7 billion.[10]

PATIENT AND PROVIDER RESOURCES

Irish Heart Foundation: https://www.irishheart.ie

CostHelper (What People Are Paying): http://www.costhelper.com

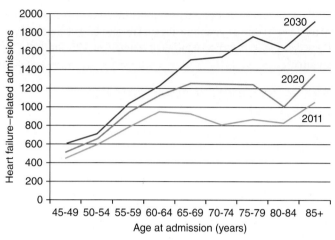

FIGURE 1-10 Projected increase in all heart failure–related admissions in Australia (2010-2030).

British Heart Foundation: https://www.bhf.org.uk/publications/healthcare-and-innovations/an-integrated-approach-to-managing-heart-failure-in-the-community

National Institute for Health and Care Excellence (NICE): https://www.nice.org.uk

REFERENCES

1. Stewart S, Ekman I, Ekman T, Oden A, Rosengren A. Population impact of heart failure and the most common forms of cancer: a study of 1,162,309 hospital cases in Sweden (1988 to 2004). *Circ Cardiovasc Qual Outcomes.* 2010;3(6):573-580.

2. Voigt J, John S, Taylor A, et al. A reevaluation of the costs of heart failure and its implications for allocation of health resources in the United States. *Clin Cardiol.* 2014;37(5):312-321.

3. Stewart S, Jenkins A, Buchan S, et al. The current cost of heart failure to the National Health Service in the UK. *Eur J Heart Fail.* 2002;4:361-371.

4. Acute and chronic heart failure (ESC Clinical Practice Guidelines). https://www.escardio.org/Guidelines/Clinical-Practice-Guidelines/Acute-and-Chronic-Heart-Failure/. Accessed May 2018.

5. Costhelper health. http://www.costhelper.com. Accessed May 2018.

6. Stewart S, Riegel B, Boyd C, et al. Establishing a pragmatic framework to optimise health outcomes in heart failure and multimorbidity (ARISE-HF): a multidisciplinary position statement. *Int J Cardiol.* 2016;212:1-10.

7. Cook C, Cole G, Asaria P, et al. The annual global economic burden of heart failure. *Int J Cardiol.* 2014;171:368-376.

8. Dokainish H, Teo K, Zhu J, et al. Heart Failure in Africa, Asia, the Middle East and South America: the INTER-CHF study. *Int J Cardiol.* 2016;204:133-141.

9. Ogah OS, Stewart S, Onwujekwe OE, et al. Economic burden of heart failure: investigating outpatient and inpatient costs in Abeokuta, southwest Nigeria. *PLoS One.* 2014;9(11):e113032.

10. Heidenreich PA, Albert NM, Allen LA, et al. Forecasting the impact of heart failure in the United States: a policy statement from the American Heart Association. *Circ Heart Fail.* 2013;6(3):606-619.

2 STAGE A HEART FAILURE: DYSLIPIDEMIA

Akira Wada, MD
Nishaki Mehta, MD
Kavita Sharma, MD

PATHOPHYSIOLOGY

Along with proteins and carbohydrates, lipids play an integral role in maintaining cell function and sustaining life. Lipids are a family of water-insoluble organic compounds that includes fats, oils, sterols, and triglycerides. Cholesterols and phospholipids are the building blocks for the cell wall and the plasma membrane, respectively. Triglycerides are made of fatty acids, which can be utilized for energy production.

Given that the human body is primarily aqueous and lipids are water-insoluble, lipids are transported via a unique lipoprotein family. This consists of a water-soluble outer coat with nonpolar lipid coat. Apolipoproteins are proteins that help in this transport system (Figure 2-1).

Briefly, there are two major sources for lipids in the body: diet and hepatic production. The chylomicrons deliver lipids from dietary fat to the plasma, and the very low-density lipoproteins (VLDLs) transport lipids from the hepatic production of lipids to the body (Figure 2-2). Lipoprotein lipase breaks down the VLDL to low-density lipoprotein (LDL), which is internalized by the cells to provide fatty acid for cell function and energy (Figure 2-3). Cholesteryl ester transfer protein (CETP) permits exchange of triglycerides and cholesteryl esters from VLDL to high-density lipoprotein (HDL), allowing for reverse cholesterol transport via the HDL system (Figure 2-4).

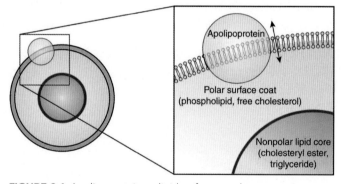

FIGURE 2-1 Apolipoprotein on lipid surface membrane.

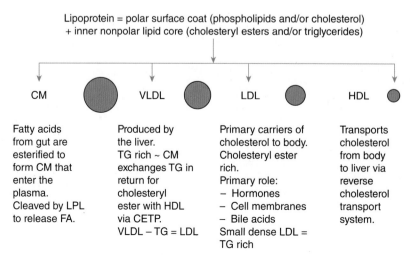

FIGURE 2-2 Lipid subtypes. The circles indicate the relative size of these lipid particles. Abbreviations: CM: chylomicrons; FA, fatty acids; HDL: high-density lipoprotein; LDL: low-density lipoprotein; LPL: lipoprotein lipase; TG: triglycerides; VLDL; very low-density lipoprotein.

LIPID DISORDERS

Hyperlipidemia is a condition in which there are abnormally elevated levels of lipids or lipoproteins in the blood. They can be divided into primary or secondary causes. Primary hyperlipidemia is typically due to a genetic cause, whereas secondary hyperlipidemia usually occurs as a result of a systemic disorder, such as diabetes mellitus. The types of familial hyperlipidemia are categorized by the Fredrickson classification (Table 2-1).

Type IIa familial hyperlipidemia is due to mutations in the gene encoding the LDL receptor, which is essential for the transport and metabolism of cholesterol. The human LDL receptor gene is located on chromosome 19 and there are more than 900 known mutations. Those who are heterozygous tend to have a 2- to 3-fold increase in plasma cholesterol whereas those who are homozygous will have a 5- to 6-fold elevation.

Common findings include xanthomas, xanthelasmas, corneal arcus, and premature atherosclerosis. In all types of type IIa familial hyperlipidemia, there is a decrease of clearance of LDL, which in turn causes a larger proportion of plasma LDL. Patients with familial hyperlipidemia have been shown to be associated with increased atherosclerotic coronary artery disease and premature death.

Mutations in the apolipoprotein B-100 (APOB) gene and the gene encoding for proprotein convertase subtilisin/kexin type 9 (PCSK9) can cause a clinical familial hyperlipidemia phenotype.

Secondary causes of hyperlipidemia include diabetes, hypothyroidism, nephrotic syndrome, hepatitis, and HIV. In diabetes, insulin resistance and subsequent hyperinsulinemia cause a characteristic

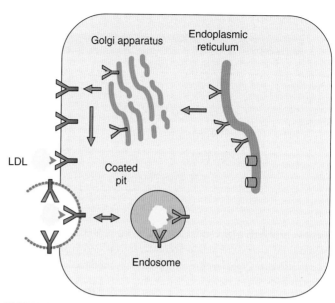

FIGURE 2-3 Internalization of LDL.

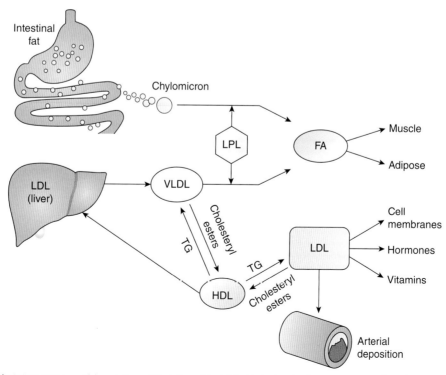

FIGURE 2-4 Lipids and their interactions. Abbreviations: FA: fatty acids; HDL: high-density lipoprotein; LDL: low-density lipoprotein; LPL: lipoprotein lipase; TG: triglycerides; VLDL: very low-density lipoprotein.

Table 2-1 Frederickson Classification System

Type	Lipoprotein Abnormality	Triglycerides	Name
I	↑ Chylomicron	Markedly elevated	Familial chylomicron syndrome
IIa	↑ LDL	Normal	Familial hypercholesterolemia
IIb	↑ LDL and VLDL	Elevated	
III	↑ Remnants	Elevated	Familial dysbetalipoproteinemia
IV	↑ VLDL	Elevated	
V	↑ VLDL and chylomicron	Markedly elevated	Familial hypertriglyceridemia

increase in plasma triglycerides and a lowering of HDL. Certain medications such as steroids, oral contraceptives, and thiazide diuretics can also affect lipid levels. Some potentially modifiable causes of hypercholesterolemia are excessive alcohol consumption, cigarette smoking, and obesity.

MANAGEMENT

The revised 2013 ACC/AHA guidelines on lipid management have changed the landscape of lipid management.[1] Firstly, risk calculators that are gender- and race-specific have been proposed (Table 2-2). Secondly, the guidelines focus on statins as the mainstay for treatment. Statins have been classified as moderate- and high-intensity statins (Figure 2-5). Four groups of patients have been identified to benefit from treatment (Figure 2-6). Although the major criticism is overestimation of risk, there have been ongoing efforts to validate this scoring system.

STATINS

Mechanism of Action

Statins inhibit HMG-CoA reductase, the rate-limiting step in the synthesis of cholesterol (Table 2-3). Reduction in the intrahepatic production of cholesterol leads to an increase in LDL receptor turnover, which leads to lowering of LDL levels.

Therapeutic Effects

LDL: Falls by 30% to 63%

HDL: Rises by 5%

Triglycerides: Falls by 20% to 40%

Statin Monitoring

Per the new guidelines, there have been 2 major changes for monitoring side effects and target goals as below.

1. Patients should be initiated on high- or moderate-intensity statins (Figure 2-5).

2. There is no role for treating to target LDL cholesterol levels; rather, fasting lipid profiles should be tested to assess for adherence to lifestyle and medications.

Table 2-2 Atherosclerotic Cardiovascular Disease Risk Calculator Variables

Gender	Male
	Female
Race	White
	African-American
	Other
Systolic blood pressure	
Diabetes	
Age	
Total cholesterol	
HDL-cholesterol	
Treatment for hypertension	
Smoker	

Adapted from 2013 ACC/AHA Cardiovascular Risk Guideline.

High intensity	Moderate intensity
Atorvastatin 40-80 mg Rosuvastatin 20-40 mg	Atorvastatin 10-20 mg Rosuvastatin 5-10 mg Simvastatin 20-40 mg Pravastatin 40-80 mg Lovastatin 40 mg Fluvastatin 80 mg Fluvastatin 40 mg bid Pitavastatin 2-4 mg

FIGURE 2-5 Classification of statins per 2013 guidelines. (Data from Stone NJ, Robinson J, et al. 2013 ACC/AHA guideline on the treatment of blood cholesterol to reduce atherosclerotic cardiovascular risk in adults: a report of the American College of Cardiology/American Heart Association task force on practice guidelines. *J Am Coll Cardiol.* 2014 Jul 1;63[25 Pt B]:2889-2934.)

Side Effects

Side effects include myopathy (0.3-3/100,000 person years) and hepatic dysfunction (0.5-1/100,000 person years).[2]

Best TIme to Take Statins

Because the intrahepatic production of lipids primarily occurs at night, the short-acting statins are best taken in the evening to allow maximal body concentration at night. In contrast, long-acting statins can be taken at any hour (Figure 2-7).

Statin Interactions

Fluvastatin and pravastatin are the water-soluble statins. They are uniquely metabolized as well—fluvastatin is metabolized by CYP2C9 and pravastatin is excreted unchanged in the urine. Because these are not metabolized by CYPA3A4, they pose the least concern for interaction with drugs. Additionally, they are associated with the lowest risk of myopathy.

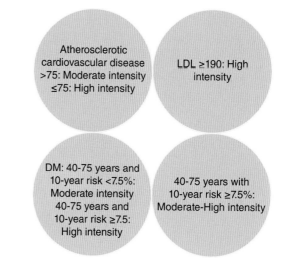

FIGURE 2-6 Four groups of patients who should be on statin therapy. (Data from Stone NJ, Robinson J, et al. 2013 ACC/AHA guideline on the treatment of blood cholesterol to reduce atherosclerotic cardiovascular risk in adults: a report of the American College of Cardiology/American Heart Association task force on practice guidelines. *J Am Coll Cardiol.* 2014 Jul 1;63[25 Pt B]:2889-2934.)

Table 2-3 Lipid-Lowering Medications

Medication	Mechanism of Action	Cholesterol Effects	Side Effects
HMG-CoA reductase inhibitors	Inhibit HMG-CoA reductase	Decrease LDL 30%-60% / Increase HDL 5% / Decrease TG 20%-40%	Hepatic dysfunction / Myopathy
Bile acid resins	Interrupt enterohepatic circulation, increasing bile acid production, which increases LDL clearance, and decreases plasma LDL levels	Decrease LDL 28% / Increase HDL 4%-5% / Can increase TG	Constipation / Diarrhea / Gas / Impairment of fat-soluble vitamins
Ezetimibe	Cholesterol absorption inhibitor	Decrease LDL 18% / Increase HDL 1% / Decrease TG 2%	
Fibrates	Activate PPAR-alpha 1. Increases LPL activity, thereby increasing TG catabolism in VLDL and chylomicrons 2. Increases HDL 3. Decrease VLDL 4. Decrease Apo CIII	Decrease TG 20%-70% / Increase or decrease LDL (in hypertriglyceridemic patients, can increase LDL)	GI upset / Can interact with statins to increase risk of rhabdomyolysis
Niacin	1. Decrease free fatty acid mobilization, leading to a decrease in VLDL 2. Decrease Apo B production 3. Increase HDL	Decrease LDL up to 40% / Decrease TG 20%-25% / Increase HDL 25%-50%	Flushing / Hepatotoxicity
Omega-3 fatty acids		Decrease TG / Increase LDL in hypertriglyceridemic patients	

OTHER LIPID-REGULATING DRUGS

Bile Acid-Binding

Agents in this group include the resins cholestyramine and colestipol and the polymer colesevelam (refer to Table 2-3). These drugs are positively charged molecules that bind to bile acids that are negatively charged. The bile acids are unable to be reabsorbed in the intestine and subsequently more hepatic cholesterol is converted to form new bile acids. There is typically a 15% to 30% reduction in plasma LDL with these agents and they may also cause an increase in triglyceride levels due to augmented VLDL production.

Cholesterol Absorption Inhibitors

This class of compounds, which includes ezetimibe, prevents the uptake of cholesterol from the brush border of epithelial cells in the small intestine. With the inhibition of cholesterol absorption, these agents reduce chylomicron production and subsequently reduce the delivery of cholesterol to the liver. When used as standalone agents, cholesterol absorption inhibitors can reduce LDL levels by 15% to 30%, but when combined with statin therapy, a synergistic effect may be observed with a marked lowering of LDL by up to 60%.

Fibrates

Gemfibrozil and fenofibrate are fibric acid derivates that have several mechanisms of action but have the primary effect of lowering triglyceride levels via their interaction with peroxisome proliferator-activated receptor alpha. These agents have the largest effect on decreasing triglycerides by as much as 50% as well as modestly increasing HDL levels.

Niacin

Niacin has favorable effects on all circulating lipid elements. It is the most effective agent for raising HDL cholesterol with modest LDL lowering by 20% to 25%. Niacin also reduces circulating levels of lipoprotein(a), which carries an independent risk of cardiovascular disease. The major downside to niacin is the cutaneous flushing, nausea, and abdominal pain some may experience, which is prostaglandin-mediated.

PCSK9 Inhibitors

Recently, several monoclonal antibodies to the PCSK9 enzyme, which is involved in LDL receptor degradation, have been developed and are currently in clinical trial. These agents interrupt the interaction between the enzyme PCSK9 and the LDL receptor, which in turn decreases receptor degradation.

LIPIDS IN HEART FAILURE

Trials focusing on the benefits of statins in the heart failure population have been negative. In the CORONA trial, patients with New York Heart Association (NYHA) class II, III, or IV ischemic heart failure and an ejection fraction of no more than 40% were assigned to receive 10 mg of rosuvastatin or placebo, and rosuvastatin did not reduce the primary outcome of death from cardiovascular causes, nonfatal myocardial infarction, or nonfatal stroke, or the secondary outcome of number of deaths from any cause.[3] In the GISSI-HF trial, patients

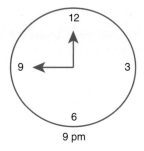

9 pm

To be taken in the evening:
Simvastatin
Lovastatin
Fluvastatin

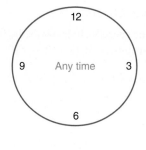

To be taken at any time:
Pravastatin
Atorvastatin
Rosuvastatin

FIGURE 2-7 Best time to take statins.

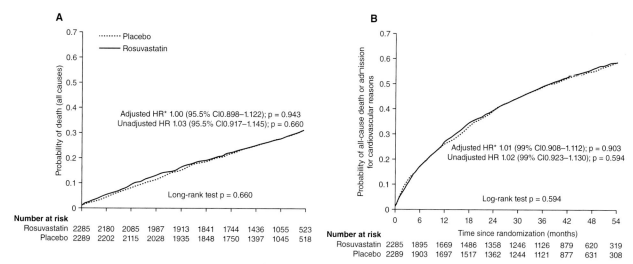

FIGURE 2-8 Rosuvastatin vs. Placebo in the NYHA Class II-IV CHF (GISSI-HF trial). (Reprinted with permission. Tavazzi L, Maggioni AP, et al. Effect of rosuvastatin in patients with chronic heart failure (the GISSI-HF trial): a randomized, double-blind, placebo-controlled trial. *Lancet.* 2008:372[9645]:1231-1239.)

with chronic NYHA class II to class IV heart failure of any cause or ejection fraction were assigned to rosuvastatin 10 mg daily or placebo. Rosuvastatin 10 mg daily did not affect the clinical outcomes of death or admission to the hospital for cardiovascular reasons. Therefore in the 2013 ACC/AHA lipid guidelines, no recommendation is made regarding the initiation or discontinuation of statins in patients with NYHA class II to class IV heart failure (Figure 2-8).[4]

REFERENCES

1. Stone NJ, Robinson J, Lichtenstein AH, et al; American College of Cardiology/American Heart Association Task Force on Practice Guidelines. 2013 ACC/AHA guideline on the treatment of blood cholesterol to reduce atherosclerotic cardiovascular risk in adults: a report of the American College of Cardiology/American Heart Association task force on practice guidelines. *J Am Coll Cardiol.* 2014 Jul 1;63(25 Pt B):2889-2934.

2. Law M, Rudnicka AR. Statin safety: a systematic review. *Am J Cardiol.* 2006;97(8A):52C-60C.

3. Kjekshus J, Apetrei E, Barrios V, et al. Rosuvastatin in older patients with systolic heart failure. *N Engl J Med.* 2007;357(22):2248-2261.

4. Tavazzi L, Maggioni AP, Marchioli R, et al; GISSI-HF Investigators. Effect of rosuvastatin in patients with chronic heart failure (the GISSI-HF trial): a randomised, double-blind, placebo-controlled trial. *Lancet.* 2008;372(9645):1231-1239.

3 HYPERTENSIVE HEART DISEASE

Christopher W. Valentine, MD

PATIENT CASE

A 52-year-old Caucasian man presents for an annual physical examinaion. He complains of fatigue and daytime sleepiness. He has a sedentary job and a long daily commute. He eats fast food once a day. He drinks 2 to 3 bottles of beer most nights. His past medical history is significant for essential hypertension and hypercholesterolemia. His medications include lisinopril 10 mg daily, hydrochlorothiazide 25 mg daily, and atorvastatin 40 mg daily. His cardiovascular review of systems is negative.

His body mass index is 33. He has a pulse rate of 82 and a seated blood pressure of 148/92 mm Hg. Neck size is 18 inches. His cardiac and pulmonary examinations are normal and he has no pitting edema in the lower extremities.

1. What lifestyle modification issues should be discussed?

2. What additional diagnostic information is needed?

3. Are changes to his medications indicated at this time?

EPIDEMIOLOGY

Hypertension (HTN) is defined as systolic blood pressure ≥140 mm Hg or diastolic blood pressure ≥90 mm Hg. Hypertensive heart disease is the response of the heart to elevated arterial pressure and peripheral vascular resistance. There is an increase in afterload on the left ventricle. There are several cardiac manifestations of this, including left ventricular hypertrophy (LVH), cardiac dysrhythmias, ischemic heart disease, and congestive heart failure (CHF).

The prevalence of HTN in the United States is estimated to be 29%. The prevalence among Americans older than age 60 years is 65%. HTN is more common in non-Hispanic black adults, who are 40% to 50% more likely to have HTN. There is no difference in prevalence between women and men. The rate of control of diagnosed HTN in the United States has been improving. The rate of control was 31.5% in the year 2000 and is now 54%. The Healthy People 2020 target is 61.2% controlled by the year 2020.[1]

Resistant HTN is defined as a blood pressure above goal in spite of concurrent use of 3 antihypertensive medications of different classes. One of those medications should be a diuretic, and all should be at optimal doses. If a patient's blood pressure is controlled on 4 or more medications, then that patient is still considered to have treatment-resistant HTN. Some patient factors associated with resistant HTN are older age, obesity, excessive dietary sodium intake, chronic kidney disease, diabetes mellitus, black race, and female sex.

ETIOLOGY AND PATHOPHYSIOLOGY

$$\text{Blood pressure} = \text{Cardiac output} \times \text{Peripheral resistance}$$

Blood pressure is a function of cardiac output and peripheral resistance. An increasing cardiac output or an increase in peripheral resistance will lead to an increase in blood pressure. The pathogenesis of essential HTN is multifactorial and complex. Excessive dietary sodium or renal sodium retention results in increased intravascular fluid volume and elevated blood pressure. An increase in sympathetic nervous system activity will increase cardiac output and by that mechanism increase blood pressure. Activation of the renin angiotensin system would be expected to cause an increase in peripheral resistance and therefore increase blood pressure. Obesity, hyperinsulinemia, and endothelial factors can also lead to increased peripheral resistance and therefore increase blood pressure. More than 20 gene polymorphisms have been reported in HTN.

In the clinical evaluation of HTN, there are several important things to consider. Adherence to prescribed medications must be reviewed with each patient. Failure to take medications as prescribed is the most common cause of poorly controlled HTN. Furthermore, medications prescribed for other conditions might increase blood pressure.

The possibility of white-coat HTN must also be considered. Blood pressure measurements obtained at home at various times of day should be requested and then compared to office blood pressures. Lifestyle factors are also important. Dietary factors such as excessive sodium intake and excessive alcohol intake may increase blood pressure. Lack of physical activity and obesity may also increase blood pressure.

In approximately 10% of patients with HTN, there is a secondary cause. If HTN is sudden in onset, occurs at a young age, is associated with hypokalemia, or is treatment-resistant, then secondary causes should be considered.

Hypertensive heart disease refers to a variety of abnormalities ranging from asymptomatic LVH to systolic dysfunction to diastolic dysfunction to arrhythmias. In the setting of chronically elevated blood pressure, the left ventricular wall may thicken or dilate in order to minimize wall stress. Ultimately clinical heart failure (HF) develops with either preserved or reduced left ventricular ejection fraction. When there is wall thickening, the LVH is classified concentric. When there is chamber dilation but no increase in wall thickness, the LVH is eccentric. The response of the left ventricle to high blood pressure varies among individuals. Black patients with HTN have greater risk for LVH and concentric geometry than white patients (Figure 3-1).[2]

LVH is associated with microvascular disease, which results in reduced coronary blood flow and increased myocardial oxygen demand. In addition, HTN leads to acceleration of atherosclerotic coronary artery disease (Figure 3-2). Plaque rupture is more common in patients who have LVH.[3]

DIAGNOSIS

Normal blood pressure is <120/80 mm Hg. Stage 1 HTN is defined by blood pressure of 142 to 159/90 to 99 mm Hg. Stage 2 HTN is ≥160 over ≥100. Hypertensive crisis is defined by a blood pressure >180/>110 mm Hg.

For office measurement of blood pressure, the patient should be seated quietly for 5 minutes with the arm bare and supported at the level of the heart. The blood pressure cuff should circle at least 80% of the circumference of the arm. Blood pressure should be measured in both arms. Three sets of readings at least 1 week apart should be obtained to make a diagnosis of HTN.

Automated office blood pressure measurement has been demonstrated to reduce the white-coat response. Automated office blood pressure is also superior to manual office blood pressures in terms of correlation with ambulatory blood pressure monitoring.[4]

There is a normal decrease or "dip" in blood pressure at night related to sleep and decrease in physical activity. A patient who does not have this decrease is a "nondipper." Several studies have shown that nondippers have worse cardiovascular outcomes including strokes, cardiac hypertrophy, diastolic dysfunction, and arrhythmias. A typical nocturnal decrease in blood pressure is 15%.

White-coat HTN is defined as a blood pressure measured by a physician or nurse persistently ≥140 mm Hg systolic or ≥90 mm Hg diastolic when out-of-office blood pressure is <130 systolic and <80 diastolic for 24-hour blood pressure and <135/85 mm Hg for a home blood pressure. The estimated prevalence of white-coat HTN is 30% to 40% of the population with an elevated office blood pressure.

Masked HTN is a condition in which clinic blood pressure is below 140/90 mm Hg, but home blood pressure or 24-hour blood pressure is above normal. Available data indicate that 10% of the general population has masked HTN. The cardiovascular risk associated with masked HTN is nearly the same as the risk with true HTN.

Ambulatory blood pressure monitoring is better than conventional office-based blood pressure measurement in the prediction of cardiovascular outcomes. This was demonstrated in a prospective study published in 1983 by Perloff and later confirmed by other investigators. Blood pressures at night and ambulatory systolic blood pressures have been the strongest predictors for cardiac death. The use of a 24-hour ambulatory blood pressure monitor for

Table 3-1 AHA/ACC/ASH Statement 2015

Group	Blood Pressure Goal
Secondary prevention with coronary artery disease	<140/90 mm Hg, but 130/80 mm Hg in some if prior myocardial infarction (MI), transient ischemic attack, cerebrovascular accident
Coronary artery disease and stable angina	<140/90 mm Hg, but 130/80 mm Hg in some if prior cerebrovascular accident or transient ischemic attack
Acute coronary syndrome	<140/90 mm Hg but 130/80 mm Hg by hospital discharge
Ischemic heart failure	<140/90 mm Hg but consider 130/80 mm Hg; if octogenarian check orthostatics

Table 3-2 Evaluation of Hypertension

- Medication adherence
- White-coat HTN? Need home or ambulatory blood pressure
- Lifestyle: Obesity, inactivity, alcohol >1-2 drinks/day, sodium
- Adverse effects of other medications
- If none of above is true, look for secondary causes.

Table 3-3 Medications That May Elevate Blood Pressure

- Nonsteroidal anti-inflammatory drugs (NSAIDs)
- Aspirin (ASA)
- COX-2 inhibitors
- Sympathomimetics—decongestants, cocaine, diet pills
- Stimulants—amphetamines, methylphenidate
- Alcohol
- Oral contraceptives
- Cyclosporine
- Erythropoietin
- Natural licorice
- Ephedra, ma huang

all patients with HTN is limited due to the cost and convenience for the patient. Self-monitoring of blood pressure may be used in order to identify a subset of patients who would benefit from wearing a 24-hour monitor. If there is a large disparity between clinic and home measurements, then a formal 24-hour assessment might be helpful. Measurement of home blood pressures twice daily in the morning and evening for 1 to 2 weeks is a simple and low-cost method.

MANAGEMENT

BLOOD PRESSURE GOALS

The Eighth Joint National Committee (JNC-8) guidelines published in December 2013 were controversial and not widely accepted. They called for a tolerance of higher blood pressure in multiple different groups of patients. For adults older than 60 years of age, the goal was 150/90; for adults younger than 60 years of age, the goal was 140/90. However, the panel of experts charged with writing these guidelines was not able to reach unanimity on the recommendations and some were in favor of a lower blood pressure target.[5]

In January 2014, the American Society of Hypertension and International Society of Hypertension published clinical practice guidelines for the management of HTN in the community. They suggested a goal of 150/90 for patients over age 80 but a goal of 140/90 or lower if tolerated in adults age 18 to 55. For patients with diabetes or chronic kidney disease they recommended a blood pressure target of 140/90. For the special circumstance of chronic kidney disease with albuminuria, some experts suggest a lower goal of 130/80 if tolerated.[6]

In 2015, the American Heart Association, the American College of Cardiology, and the American Society of Hypertension released a joint statement regarding treatment of HTN in patients with coronary artery disease.[7] Their recommendations for blood pressure goals are summarized in Table 3-1.

DIETARY SODIUM

A typical American diet includes 4 to 6 g of sodium per day. The majority of the sodium in the American diet is in processed foods. It is estimated that 75% of total daily intake is from processed foods. Table salt is 40% sodium so every 1000 mg of table salt contains 400 mg of sodium. American food labels use 2400 mg per day of sodium as a recommended value.

The DASH (dietary approaches to stop HTN) trial[8] was a comprehensive diet-intervention study. The DASH diet is rich in fruits and vegetables and low in saturated fat. The DASH diet and subsequently the reduced-sodium DASH diet have been proven to reduce blood pressure, allow people to take less blood pressure medication, and prevent the age-associated increase in blood pressure. The DASH diet also lowers cholesterol because it includes restriction of red meat and animal fat. The DASH-I diet contains 2800 mg of sodium per day. Even with 2800 mg of sodium per day, this diet resulted in improvement in blood pressure. For patients with blood pressure >140/90 at baseline, the blood pressure

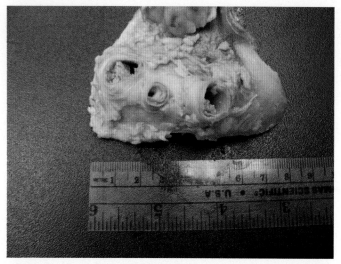

FIGURE 3-1 Atherosclerosis of vessels on aortic arch. (Image used with permission from Dr. C. Eric Freitag.)

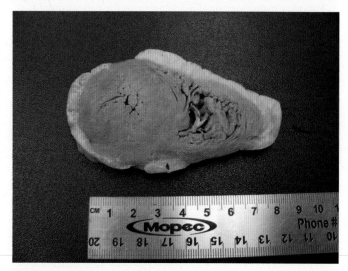

FIGURE 3-2 Concentric LVH. (Image used with permission from Dr. C. Eric Freitag.)

Table 3-4 Secondary Causes of Hypertension

- 12.7% of patients over age 50 referred to an HTN clinic had a secondary cause.

- Common causes

  - Primary aldosteronism: 11% in those referred to a specialized HTN clinic

  - Obstructive sleep apnea: 83% prevalence in resistant-HTN females, and 96% in resistant-HTN males

  - Renal artery stenosis

  - Chronic kidney disease

improved by 11/5 mm Hg. For all patients in the study, the average decrease in blood pressure was 5.5/3 mm Hg. For African-American patients, the DASH diet was associated with a decrease in blood pressure of 6.9/3.3 mm Hg. It has been suggested that the increased intake of potassium, calcium, and magnesium were at least partially responsible for the improvement in blood pressure. The DASH diet also lowered cholesterol compared to the control diet. Total cholesterol was reduced by 13.7 mg/dL and low-density lipoprotein (LDL) was reduced by 10.7 mg/dL. The DASH-II diet is the reduced-sodium version, and contains 1520 mg of sodium per day. For patients with HTN at baseline, the low-sodium DASH diet reduced systolic blood pressure by 12 mm Hg.

ALCOHOL

Moderate alcohol consumption, meaning 1 to 2 portions per day, has been demonstrated to have a protective effect on cardiovascular diseases. One portion is 360 mL (12 fl oz) of beer, 120 mL (4 fl oz) of wine, or 45 mL (1.5 fl oz) of liquor. Some studies have shown that wine is more protective than beer or whiskey, but that may be confounded by healthier lifestyle habits of wine drinkers. Alcohol intake at higher levels is known to increase blood pressure. For the management of HTN, it is recommended that women consume no more than 1 drink per day and men consume no more than 2 drinks per day.

MEDICAL MANAGEMENT

ADHERENCE

The most common cause of uncontrolled HTN is poor adherence with medical therapy. Jung et al reported in the *Journal of Hypertension* in April 2013 on 375 patients referred for uncontrolled HTN despite being prescribed 4 medications.[9] They performed urine liquid chromatography and mass spectrometry to test for the presence of the antihypertensive medications and their metabolites. Of study patients, 53% were proven to be nonadherent with medications. Among those who were nonadherent, 30% had complete nonadherence and 70% had partial nonadherence.

DIURETICS

Diuretics are a cornerstone of therapy for HTN. Among the thiazides and related compounds, chlorthalidone should be used as first line. Major clinical trials including SHEP and ALLHAT were done with chlorthalidone. Chlorthalidone has a half-life of 40 hours, which is much longer than the 5- to 15-hour half-life of hydrochlorothiazide. For patients who have a glomerular filtration rate below 30 mL per minute, no thiazide is likely to be effective, and loop diuretics should be used. Diuretic resistance is common, and may be a result of excessive sodium intake or NSAID use.

RAAS SYSTEM BLOCKADE

The renin angiotensin aldosterone system is a critical component of blood pressure regulation. Angiotensin-converting enzyme (ACE) inhibitors block the conversion of angiotensin I to the potent vasoconstrictor angiotensin II. ACE inhibitors also decrease

Table 3-5 Hypertension Treatment: Lifestyle

- A weight loss of 10 kg is associated with a 6/4.6 mm Hg decrease in blood pressure.
- Salt restriction can reduce blood pressure by 5-10/2-6 mm Hg.
- Limit alcohol to 1 to 2 drinks per day.
- The DASH diet can improve blood pressure by 11/5.5 mm Hg. The DASH diet is rich in fruits and vegetables and includes high-fiber, low-fat foods, and low-fat dairy products.

Table 3-6 Medical Therapy of HTN: General Principles

- Long-acting drugs are preferred.
- Use agents with different mechanisms of action.
- Maximize diuretic regimen.
- Use loop diuretic rather than thiazide if glomerular filtration rate is <30 or using minoxidil.
- If treatment-resistant add a melanocortin (MC) receptor antagonist such as spironolactone.

aldosterone secretion and inhibit the breakdown of bradykinin. ACE inhibitors have been proven to be effective in regression of LVH and myocardial fibrosis. They reduce mortality after acute myocardial infarction (MI). They are effective in both acute chronic CHF via their effect on remodeling and afterload. Except for captopril, which is very short-acting, most ACE inhibitors have a long duration of action and can be used once a day.

Angiotensin II receptor blockers (ARBs) displace AII from its AT1 receptor, and cause a fall in peripheral resistance. ARBs also induce regression of LVH. One key clinical trial relevant to hypertensive heart disease is the LIFE study.[10] In this trial of more than 9000 patients with HTN who already had LVH, losartan was superior to atenolol in terms of regression of LVH and mortality. The losartan group had significantly fewer strokes (HR 0.75) and less new-onset diabetes (HR 0.75). Although losartan was the first angiotensin receptor blocker approved in the United States, it is the least potent drug in its class for lowering blood pressure.

ALDOSTERONE ANTAGONISTS

The Randomized ALdactone Evaluation (RALES) study[11] was a double-blind study of 1663 patients with class III or IV HF and an average left ventricular ejection fraction of 25%. Patients were treated with an ACE inhibitor and a loop diuretic. They were then randomly assigned to receive 25 mg of spironolactone daily or placebo. The study was discontinued early due to a 30% reduction in risk of death in the spironolactone group. This was attributed to decreased risk of progressive HF as well as sudden cardiac death. There was also a 35% reduction in hospitalization for worsening HF. Gynecomastia or breast pain occurred in 10% of men on spironolactone. A dose of 12.5 to 25 mg of spironolactone daily is effective in blocking aldosterone receptors. Serum potassium and creatinine must be monitored during treatment with any aldosterone antagonist.

The selective aldosterone receptor antagonist eplerenone is also available and has less risk of gynecomastia. The Eplerenone Post-Acute Myocardial Infarction Heart Failure Efficacy and Survival (EPHESUS) study[12] was a double-blind placebo-controlled study of eplerenone on morbidity and mortality in more than 6000 patients with acute MI complicated by left ventricular dysfunction and HF. Patients received standard therapies for HF including ACE inhibitors or angiotensin receptor blockers, beta blockers, and diuretics. The relative risk of death in the eplerenone group was 0.85. The rate of serious hyperkalemia defined as potassium >6 mmol/L was 5.5% in the eplerenone group and 3.9% in the placebo group. Among patients with a baseline creatinine clearance of less than 50 mL per minute, serious hyperkalemia occurred in 10% of the eplerenone group and 5.9% of the placebo group.

The male gynecomastia rate with eplerenone use was only 0.5% and similar to placebo. The improvement in cardiovascular mortality with eplerenone was largely due to a reduction in the rate of sudden cardiac death. The authors concluded that the addition of eplerenone to optimal medical therapy contributes to improvement in survival and hospitalization rates for patients with acute MI complicated by left ventricular dysfunction and HF.

CALCIUM CHANNEL BLOCKERS

Calcium blockers were originally used as antianginal drugs in the 1970s. In the 1980s they began to be used for blood pressure. Diltiazem and verapamil are effective for slowing heart rate and also induce vasodilation. The dihydropyridine calcium channel blockers such as nifedipine and amlodipine have a larger effect on vascular dilation and are more potent for lowering blood pressure. It has been demonstrated that black patients respond better to calcium channel blockers than to ace inhibitors or beta blockers. In addition, patients with chronic kidney disease generally have a good blood pressure response to calcium channel blocker therapy.

BETA BLOCKERS

Beta blockers are indicated for patients with coronary artery disease. They cause a decrease in cardiac output. In terms of effect on blood pressure, the beta blockers that also have an alpha blocking effect, such as carvedilol and labetalol, are more potent for blood pressure. It is known that black patients and the elderly have less significant response to beta blockers for blood pressure.

DIRECT VASODILATORS

Direct vasodilators such as hydralazine and minoxidil should be third- or fourth-line therapies for HTN. Hydralazine has a number of unpleasant adverse effects and it causes sympathetic activation. It can cause headaches, flushing, and tachycardia. It is also known to induce a lupuslike reaction. Minoxidil is a highly potent vasodilator and should be reserved for cases in which other classes of drugs have not been effective. Minoxidil use results in tachycardia and sodium and fluid retention. For this reason, it should be used in combination with a beta blocker and a diuretic. Minoxidil is also known to cause hirsutism.

IMPACT OF CPAP FOR OBSTRUCTIVE SLEEP APNEA

For most patients with HTN who also have obstructive sleep apnea, treatment with continuous positive airway pressure (CPAP) will have only a modest impact on their blood pressure. A typical reduction is in the range of 2 to 3 mm Hg in systolic blood pressure. However, among patients who have treatment-resistant HTN, meaning that they were not controlled with 3 medications, improvement in systolic blood pressure is greater. The mean net change in ambulatory blood pressure from 4 randomized controlled trials was −6.74 in systolic blood pressure and −5.94 in diastolic blood pressure with CPAP use.[13]

RENAL ARTERY STENOSIS

For atherosclerotic renal artery stenosis there is no evidence that angioplasty or stenting is superior to medical therapy. Three randomized trials failed to show a benefit from renal artery stenting. Most recently in January 2014 the CORAL study[14] results showed no significant difference between renal artery stenting and medical therapy on the composite endpoint of death from cardiovascular or renal cause, MI, stroke, hospitalization for HF, progressive renal insufficiency, or the need for renal replacement therapy. For the fibromuscular dysplasia of the renal arteries, which is usually seen in young women, renal artery angioplasty is indicated.

PATIENT EDUCATION RESOURCES

American Heart Association: http://www.heart.org/
HEARTORG/Conditions/HighBloodPressure/High-Blood-
Pressure-or-Hypertension_UCM_002020_SubHomePage.jsp

National Heart, Lung, and Blood Institute: https://www.
nhlbi.nih.gov/health/health-topics/topics/dash

FOLLOW-UP

The patient described at the beginning of the chapter should be
advised to limit sodium intake to 2000 mg per day or less and to
decrease his alcohol intake. In addition gradual increase in physical activity and weight loss would be beneficial. He should have
testing including electrolytes and kidney function at a minimum.
He should be questioned regarding symptoms of sleep apnea and
he might benefit from a sleep study. Prior to making medication
changes, he should monitor blood pressure at home and discuss
those results with his physician.

REFERENCES

1. Yoon SS, Carroll MD, Fryar CD. Hypertension prevalence and
   control among adults: United States, 2011-2014. *NCHS Data
   Brief.* 2015 Nov;(220):1-8.

2. Kizer JR1, Arnett DK, Bella JN, et al. Differences in left ventricular structure between black and white hypertensive adults:
   the Hypertension Genetic Epidemiology Network Study.
   Hypertens. 2004;43(6):1182-1188.

3. Frohlich ED, Apstein C, Chobanian AV, et al. The heart in
   hypertension. *N Engl J Med.* 1992;327:998-1008.

4. Myers MG, Godwin M, Dawes M, et al. Conventional versus
   automated measurement of blood pressure in primary care
   patients with systolic hypertension: randomized parallel design
   controlled trial. *BMJ.* 2011;342:d286.

5. James PA, Oparil S, Carter BL, et al. 2014 evidence-based
   guideline for the management of high blood pressure in adults
   report from the panel members appointed to the Eighth Joint
   National Committee (JNC 8). *JAMA.* 2014;311:507-520.

6. Weber MA, Schiffrin EL, White WB, et al. Clinical practice
   guidelines for the management of hypertension in the community: a statement by the American Society of Hypertension and
   the International Society of Hypertension. *J Clin Hypertens.*
   2014;16:14-26.

7. Rosendorff C, Lackland DT, Allison M, et al. Treatment
   of hypertension in patients with coronary artery disease: a
   scientific statement from the American Heart Association,
   American College of Cardiology, and American Society of
   Hypertension. *J Am Soc Hypertens.* 2015;1-46.

8. Sacks FM, Svetkey LP, Vollmer WM, et al; DASH-Sodium
   Collaborative Research Group. Effects on blood pressure of
   reduced dietary sodium and the dietary approaches to stop
   hypertension (DASH) diet. *N Engl J Med.* 2001;344:3-10.

9. Jung O, Gechter JL, Wunder C, Paulke A, Bartel C, Geiger H,
   et al. Resistant hypertension? Assessment of adherence by
   toxicological urine analysis. *J Hypertens.* 2013;31(4):766-774.

10. Dahlof B, Devereux RB, Kjeldsen SE, et al; LIFE Study
    Group. Cardiovascular morbidity and mortality in the
    Losartan intervention for endpoint reduction in hyperten-
    sion study (LIFE): a randomized trial against atenolol. *Lancet.*
    2002;359:995-1003.

11. Pitt B, Zannad F, Remme WJ, et al. The effect of spironolac-
    tone on morbidity and mortality in patients with severe heart
    failure. Randomized Aldactone Evaluation Study Investigators.
    N Engl J Med. 1999;341:709-717.

12. Pitt B, Remme W, Zannad F, et al; Eplerenone Post-Acute
    Myocardial Infarction Heart Failure Efficacy and Survival
    Study Investigators. Eplerenone, a selective aldosterone
    blocker in patients with left ventricular dysfunction after myo-
    cardial infarction. *N Engl J Med.* 2003;348:1309-1321.

13. Iftikhar IH, Valentine CW, Bittencourt LR, et al. Effects of con-
    tinuous positive airway pressure on blood pressure in patients
    with resistant hypertension and obstructive sleep apnea: a
    meta-analysis. *J Hypertens.* 2014 Dec;32(12):2341-2350.

14. Cooper CJ, Murphy TP, Cutlip DE, et al; CORAL Investiga-
    tors. Stenting and medical therapy for atherosclerotic renal
    artery stenosis. *N Engl J Med.* 2014;370:13-22.

4   OBESITY AND THE OBESITY PARADOX

Amanda R. Vest, MBBS, MPH

PATIENT CASE

A 48-year-old man with nonischemic cardiomyopathy (left ventricular ejection fraction [LVEF] 20%) presents for subspecialty heart failure evaluation. He has a history of multiple decompensated heart failure hospitalizations (4 within the past year), episodes of ventricular tachycardia, hypertension, hyperlipidemia, hypothyroidism, a thromboembolic stroke with no residual neurological deficit, atrial fibrillation, sleep apnea, and deep vein thrombosis. His weight at the time of evaluation is 162 kg (358 lb); he is volume overloaded in clinic, but after inpatient diuresis his dry weight is established at 156 kg, giving a body mass index (BMI) of 46.8 kg/m^2. He is receiving full doses of guideline-directed medial therapy and is anticoagulated. What is the potential impact of obesity on his clinical cardiovascular course and what recommendations should the clinician make regarding weight management for this patient?

INTRODUCTION

Obesity is a key determinant of health status and has the potential to affect multiple organ systems (Figure 4-1). The overweight and obese states are commonly defined by BMI, with overweightness diagnosed in the BMI range of 25 to 30 kg/m^2 and obesity ≥30 kg/m^2 (Table 4-1). The prevalence of obesity has grown rapidly since the 1960s, with over one-third of adults and 17% of youth in the United States now classified as obese.[1] Obesity has long been known to pose a major threat to cardiovascular population health.[2] Higher BMI, and other anthropometric measures of obesity such as waist circumference, are independent risk factors for the development of coronary heart disease and heart failure (HF),[3,4] particularly heart failure with preserved ejection fraction (HFpEF),[5] as well as for cardiovascular death.[6] There are probably contributions from multiple pathways including the development of hyperlipidemia, insulin resistance, low-level inflammation, and left ventricular hypertrophy, with a potential pathogenic role for the adipokine and gut hormone signaling to the myocardium.

Lifestyle interventions including dietary changes and exercise can help to reduce weight and may improve cardiovascular health.[7] Bariatric surgery is indicated for treatment of obesity after unsuccessful dietary and exercise interventions in patients with BMI ≥40 kg/m^2 or BMI ≥35 kg/m^2 with comorbidities such as type 2 diabetes mellitus or hypertension.[8,9] Bariatric procedures can achieve marked weight loss and remission of diabetes, dyslipidemia, and hypertension.[10] There is growing interest in bariatric surgery for managing severe obesity in patients with coronary artery disease (CAD) and evidence for a reduction in cardiovascular events after bariatric surgery,[11] but the role of surgical weight loss in HF remains controversial.[12,13]

There are several areas of controversy surrounding obesity in the context of cardiovascular health. One is the recognition that the cardiometabolic impact of excess adipose tissue may be dependent on its location, with visceral adiposity portending worse cardiovascular outcomes than subcutaneous fat deposits, as well as the ratio of brown to white fat.[14-17] Brown fat is rich in mitochondria and predominantly generates body heat, whereas white fat, which predominates in adults, appears to generate the negative metabolic signals leading to obesity-associated diseases. Beige adipocytes have recently been identified, which may promote metabolic health.[18] None of these complexities is adequately captured in the crude measurement of BMI, potentially obscuring the true relationship between differing patterns of adiposity and future cardiovascular risk. Hence the relationship between excessive weight and an abnormal metabolic profile is not absolute; obesity does not always cause a clinical metabolic disease, and not all patients with insulin resistance, hypertension, and hypertriglyceridemia are obese. An additional complicating factor is the so-called obesity paradox observed in some cohorts with established HF, casting doubts upon obesity management recommendations for HF patients.[19]

OBESITY AND THE CARDIOVASCULAR SYSTEM

The obese state is proinflammatory, prothrombotic, and proinsulin-resistant. This metabolic milieu promotes endothelial dysfunction and atherosclerotic plaque formation and instability, which are key mechanisms for cardiovascular events such as myocardial infarctions (MI) and strokes. In addition to being an independent predictor of cardiovascular events, obesity is closely associated with other key risk factors such as hypertension, diabetes, hypercholesterolemia, and sleep-disordered breathing.[20] In a large standardized case-control study of acute MI in 52 countries, incorporating 15,152 cases and 14,820 controls, abdominal obesity was independently associated with MIs, with a population attributable risk of 20.1% (95% confidence interval, CI; 15.3, 26.0%) for the top 2 tertiles versus the lowest tertile of abdominal obesity, as measured by waist-hip ratios.[21] Excess weight was an independent predictor of CAD and cardiovascular death over 26 years of follow-up of Framingham Heart Study participants.[22]

Obesity is associated with several hemodynamic alterations, including an increased circulating volume, increased cardiac output (mostly through augmented stroke volume rather than increased heart rate), reduced systemic vascular resistance, and a greater degree of sympathetic activation, but a lower maximal oxygen uptake (peak VO$_2$).[23,24] Various pathophysiological mechanisms have been postulated to explain the relationship between obesity and incident HF, such as increased blood volume or chronically

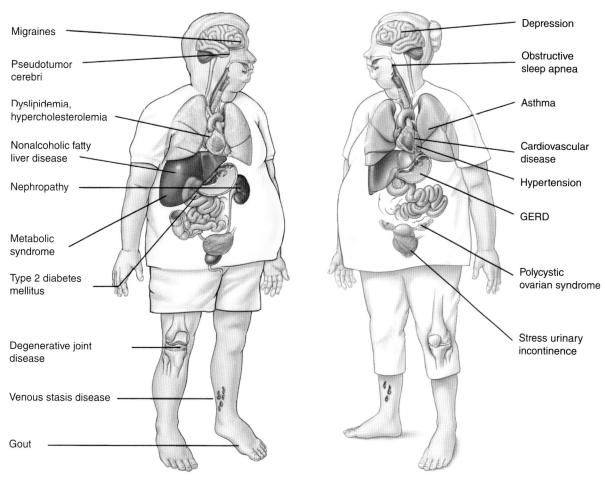

Migraines

Pseudotumor
cerebri

Dyslipidemia,
hypercholesterolemia

Nonalcoholic fatty
liver disease

Nephropathy

Metabolic
syndrome

Type 2 diabetes
mellitus

Degenerative joint
disease

Venous stasis disease

Gout

Depression

Obstructive
sleep apnea

Asthma

Cardiovascular
disease

Hypertension

GERD

Polycystic
ovarian syndrome

Stress urinary
incontinence

FIGURE 4-1 The impact of obesity on the body. (Reproduced, with permission, from Cleveland Clinic Center for Medical Art & Photography ©
2005-2017. All rights reserved.)

elevated intrathoracic pressure leading to chamber dilatation,
hypertension causing left ventricular hypertrophy, the presence
of epicardial fat (Figure 4-2) and myocardial fatty infiltration, or a
direct cardiotoxic effect of adipose tissue mediated by hormones
and inflammatory proteins.[25] Elevated BMI, waist circumference,
and waist-hip ratio are each associated with incident HF.[26-28] Obese
individuals with greater metabolic abnormalities appear to have
the greatest risk of HF development.[29,30] Among 59,178 adults
followed for mean 18.4 years, the adjusted hazard ratios for HF
incidence at BMIs <25, 25 to 29.9, and ≥30 kg/m^2 were 1.00, 1.25,
and 1.99 (p<0.001) for men and 1.00, 1.33, and 2.06 (p<0.001) for
women.[31]

The pediatric literature provides some of the clearest evidence
for a direct association between obesity and myocardial dysfunction. Obese children have a low prevalence of intermediaries such
as diabetes, hypertension, and CAD and so the isolated effect of
obesity on myocardial function may be easier to detect in younger
individuals. A number of studies have demonstrated that excess
adiposity in childhood is strongly associated with increased left ventricular mass both in childhood and into adulthood, independent of
the effect of hypertension.[32-34] Abnormal diastolic function has also
been reported in obese children, as has abnormal left ventricular
circumferential strain imaging.[35-37] These pediatric findings support

Table 4-1 Body Mass Index Chart

Height (inches)	Normal						Overweight					Obese (Body Weight, pounds)										Extreme Obesity															
BMI	19	20	21	22	23	24	25	26	27	28	29	30	31	32	33	34	35	36	37	38	39	40	41	42	43	44	45	46	47	48	49	50	51	52	53	54
58	91	96	100	105	110	115	119	124	129	134	138	143	148	153	158	162	167	172	177	181	186	191	196	201	205	210	215	220	224	229	234	239	244	248	253	258
59	94	99	104	109	114	119	124	128	133	138	143	148	153	158	163	168	173	178	183	188	193	198	203	208	212	217	222	227	232	237	242	247	252	257	262	267
60	97	102	107	112	118	123	128	133	138	143	148	153	158	163	168	174	179	184	189	194	199	204	209	215	220	225	230	235	240	245	250	255	261	266	271	276
61	100	106	111	116	122	127	132	137	143	148	153	158	164	169	174	180	185	190	195	201	206	211	217	222	227	232	238	243	248	254	259	264	269	275	280	285
62	104	109	115	120	126	131	136	142	147	153	158	164	169	175	180	186	191	196	202	207	213	218	224	229	235	240	246	251	256	262	267	273	278	284	289	295
63	107	113	118	124	130	135	141	146	152	158	163	169	175	180	186	191	197	203	208	214	220	225	231	237	242	248	254	259	265	270	278	282	287	293	299	304
64	110	116	122	128	134	140	145	151	157	163	169	174	180	186	192	197	204	209	215	221	227	232	238	244	250	256	262	267	273	279	285	291	296	302	308	314
65	114	120	126	132	138	144	150	156	162	168	174	180	186	192	198	204	210	216	222	228	234	240	246	252	258	264	270	276	282	288	294	300	306	312	318	324
66	118	124	130	136	142	148	155	161	167	173	179	186	192	198	204	210	216	223	229	235	241	247	253	260	266	272	278	284	291	297	303	309	315	322	328	334
67	121	127	134	140	146	153	159	166	172	178	185	191	198	204	211	217	223	230	236	242	249	255	261	268	274	280	287	293	299	306	312	319	325	331	338	344
68	125	131	138	144	151	158	164	171	177	184	190	197	203	210	216	223	230	236	243	249	256	262	269	276	282	289	295	302	308	315	322	328	335	341	348	354
69	128	135	142	149	155	162	169	176	182	189	196	203	209	216	223	230	236	243	250	257	263	270	277	284	291	297	304	311	318	324	331	338	345	351	358	365
70	132	139	146	153	160	167	174	181	188	195	202	209	216	222	229	236	243	250	257	264	271	278	285	292	299	306	313	320	327	334	341	348	355	362	369	376
71	136	143	150	157	165	172	179	186	193	200	208	215	222	229	236	243	250	257	265	272	279	286	293	301	308	315	322	329	338	343	351	358	365	372	379	386
72	140	147	154	162	169	177	184	191	199	206	213	221	228	235	242	250	258	265	272	279	287	294	302	309	316	324	331	338	346	353	361	368	375	383	390	397
73	144	151	159	166	174	182	189	197	204	212	219	227	235	242	250	257	265	272	280	288	295	302	310	318	325	333	340	348	355	363	371	378	386	393	401	408
74	148	155	163	171	179	186	194	202	210	218	225	233	241	249	256	264	272	280	287	295	303	311	319	326	334	342	350	358	365	373	381	389	396	404	412	420
75	152	160	168	176	184	192	200	208	216	224	232	240	248	256	264	272	279	287	295	303	311	319	327	335	343	351	359	367	375	383	391	399	407	415	423	431
76	156	164	172	180	189	197	205	213	221	230	238	246	254	263	271	279	287	295	304	312	320	328	336	344	353	361	369	377	385	394	402	410	418	426	435	443

Adapted from Clinical Guidelines on the Identification, Evaluation, and Treatment of Overweight and Obesity in Adults: The Evidence Report. National Heart, Lung, and Blood Institute. National Institutes of Health, 1998. Bethesda, MD.

the hypothesis that there may be a period of left ventricular hypertrophy and increasing diastolic dysfunction, with or without subclinical systolic dysfunction, which precedes the expression of symptomatic HF with either preserved or reduced ejection fraction. Fortunately there is also some evidence that these childhood abnormalities of cardiac structure and function may be reversible with substantial weight loss.[38,39]

In obese adults, the relationship between obesity and HF is not only confounded by intermediates such as diabetes, hypertension, and CAD, but also by the impact of obesity on many of our tools for HF diagnosis. Symptoms such as dyspnea, lower extremity edema, orthopnea, and reduced exercise capacity are features of both severe obesity and HF. Physical examination signs of HF may be harder to discern in obese individuals and furthermore the diagnostic markers brain natriuretic peptide (BNP) and N-terminal pro-B natriuretic peptide (NT-proBNP) are affected by the obese state. Multiple investigators have demonstrated an inverse association between BNP/NT-proBNP and BMI.[3,5,28,31,40,41] The primary imaging tool for determining left ventricular dysfunction, the transthoracic echocardiogram, also has reduced sensitivity in obese patients and access to cardiac magnetic resonance imaging may be limited by equipment weight restrictions. In addition, excess fluid from decompensated HF cannot be distinguished from excess adiposity in the calculation of BMI and so may misrepresent the degree of obesity in HF patients. Through a combination of all these limitations, a clear diagnosis of HF—especially HFpEF—can become challenging among adults with obesity.

Recent research has revealed the role of adipose tissue as an endocrine organ with widespread homeostatic influences, mediated by adipokines, and the potential to adversely affect cardiovascular health (Figure 4-3). The term *adiposopathy* was adopted to describe the anatomical and functional abnormalities of adipose tissue promoted by positive caloric balance in genetically and

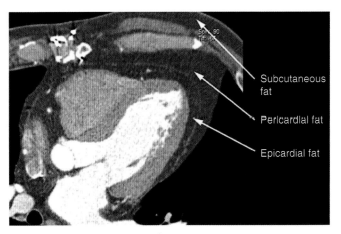

FIGURE 4-2 Excess epicardial adipose tissue on computed tomography imaging. (Reproduced, with permission, from Cosyns B, Plein S, Nihoyanopoulos P, et al. European Association of Cardiovascular Imaging (EACVI) position paper: multimodality imaging in pericardial disease. *Euro Heart J—Cardiovascular Imaging.* Oxford University Press. 2015;16(1):12-31.)

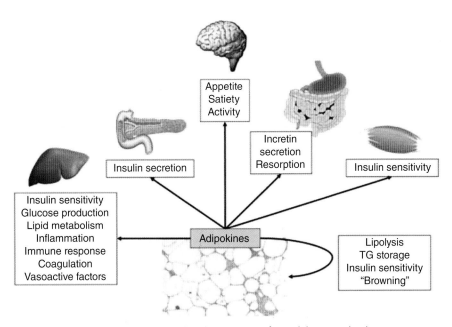

FIGURE 4-3 Endocrine activities of adipose tissue. (Reproduced, with permission, from Blüher M. Adipokines—removing road blocks to obesity and diabetes therapy. *Molecular Metabolism.* Elsevier. 2014;3(3):230-240.)

environmentally susceptible individuals. These abnormalities of adipose tissue result in adverse endocrine and immune responses that can directly and indirectly contribute to metabolic disease and cardiovascular disease (CVD) risk.[42] Of particular relevance to the cardiovascular system are the secretion of adiponectin, resistin, leptin, chemerin, visfatin, apelin, and omentin, as well as the inflammatory mediators tumor necrosis factor alpha (TNF-α), interleukin-6 (IL-6), angiotensinogen, and plasminogen activator inhibitor-1 (PAI-1) from adipose tissue.[43,44]

The adipokines can exert both negative and positive effects on the cardiovascular system, depending upon the balance of substances secreted. For example, adiponectin, which is produced both by adipocytes and myocytes, promotes insulin sensitivity, fatty acid breakdown, and normal endothelial function, and is anti-inflammatory and antiatherogenic.[45,46] Furthermore, adiponectin affects myocyte signaling and prevents the negative consequences of myocardial pressure overload and ischemia-reperfusion injury. Adiponectin levels are usually reduced in obesity. In CVD, levels may be elevated with evidence of functional adiponectin resistance at the level of the skeletal muscles.[47]

Conversely, leptin is potentially proinflammatory, atherogenic, thrombotic, and angiogenic and may contribute to the pathogenesis of type 2 diabetes mellitus, hypertension, atherosclerosis, left ventricular hypertrophy, and HF.[48-51] Deficiency caused by leptin gene mutations causes insulin resistance and obesity, but in obese states not associated with this rare gene mutation, circulating leptin levels are high because of leptin resistance.[52] In a prospective study of 4080 older men, higher circulating leptin was significantly associated with the risk of incident HF in men without preexisting coronary heart disease, independent of BMI and potential mediators, although no association was seen in those with preexisting coronary heart disease.[53] Despite the predominantly negative cardiovascular effects of leptin, it may afford some protection against ischemia-reperfusion injury.[54]

The gut hormones may also contribute to the relationship between obesity and HF. The appetite-stimulating hormone ghrelin has been experimentally used as an intravenous HF therapy in 2 small trials, with encouraging results on left ventricular function.[55,56] The incretins, including glucagon-like peptide 1 (GLP-1) and gastric inhibitory polypeptide (GIP), are a family of gut hormones that stimulate postprandial insulin release, inhibit glucagon, slow gastric emptying rate, and promote weight loss. GLP-1 analogs are used to treat type 2 diabetes mellitus and have attracted attention regarding potentially favorable cardiovascular effects (Figure 4-4). GLP-1 receptors are found on cardiomyocytes, and initial pilot studies indicated positive effects of GLP-1 infusions on left ventricular function for subjects with MI and HF.[57-59] Recognizing that the myocardium becomes increasingly insulin-resistant as HF progresses and that myocardial glucose uptake might be increased by GLP-1 administration, the Functional Impact of GLP-1 for Heart Failure Treatment (FIGHT) study was conceived,[60] although liraglutide was ultimately found to have no positive effects on HF outcomes. Regardless, there remain biologically plausible endocrine mechanisms linking adiposopathy to abnormalities in ventricular mass and contractility that could contribute to the development of obesity-associated myocardial dysfunction.

Likewise, paracrine signaling from epicardial and perivascular adipose tissue fat may influence local myocardial and coronary function. Epicardial adipose tissue is a normal finding, but fat volume is often increased in obese individuals (Figure 4-2).[61] Epicardial fat has high rates of both lipogenesis and lipolysis and may accommodate local fat storage for the rapid provision of free fatty acids at times of high myocardial substrate demand. Perivascular adipose tissue follows the course of the coronary arteries, and is concentrated in the acute marginal atrioventricular and interventricular sulci. Periventricular adipose tissue secretes mainly beneficial adipokines, predominantly adiponectin.[62] Despite these putative benefits, epicardial adipose tissue—like visceral adipose tissue—is susceptible to dysfunction in obese individuals and a causative role in local inflammation and cardiovascular pathology has been proposed.[63] Epicardial adipose tissue in patients with CAD has shown higher inflammatory cytokine mRNA and protein levels than paired subcutaneous adipose tissue, accompanied by a dense inflammatory infiltrate in the epicardial adipose tissue.[64] Similarly, higher inflammatory cytokine mRNA and fatty acid levels were observed in the epicardial adipose tissue, compared with paired subcutaneous adipose tissue, in patients with systolic HF.[65] However, there are some contradictory data in this field and the existing CVD outcomes evidence does not show additive prognostic information for epicardial adipose tissue volume over visceral adipose tissue volume.[66,67]

THE OBESITY SURVIVAL PARADOX IN HEART FAILURE

Despite the association between excess adiposity and an elevated risk of incident HF, multiple epidemiology studies suggest that obese subjects with established HF have either no increased mortality risk compared with normal-weight counterparts, or even a lower mortality risk (Figure 4-5).[68-75] This survival paradox has been the source of much uncertainty and debate in the HF literature. For example, all-cause mortality in the Digitalis Investigation Group (DIG) trial decreased in a near linear fashion through increasing BMI groups, from 45.0% in the underweight group to 28.4% in the obese group (p for trend <0.001).[76] After risk adjustment, overweight and obese subjects maintained a lower mortality than the normal-weight subjects: overweight hazard ratio (HR) 0.88, 95% CI 0.80 to 0.96; obese HR, 0.81, 95% CI 0.72 to 0.92. The highest hazard for mortality was in the underweight group: HR 1.21, 95% CI 0.95 to 1.53. A similar pattern was observed in the Acute Decompensated Heart Failure National Registry (ADHERE) of acute HF hospitalizations across 263 hospitals in the United States. Among 108,927 decompensated HF patients, each incremental 5 kg/m^2 increase in BMI was associated with a 10% reduction in mortality during the index hospitalization.[77] A meta-analysis of 28,209 patients across 9 studies, mainly ad hoc analyses of HF therapy trials, compared subjects with normal BMI to those with overweight or obese BMI ranges. The overweight and obese states were both associated with a lower risk of all-cause mortality (adjusted HR 0.88; 95% CI 0.83-0.93 and adjusted HR 0.93; 95% CI 0.89-0.97, respectively) at mean follow-up 2.7 years, which was also consistently seen through the component studies.

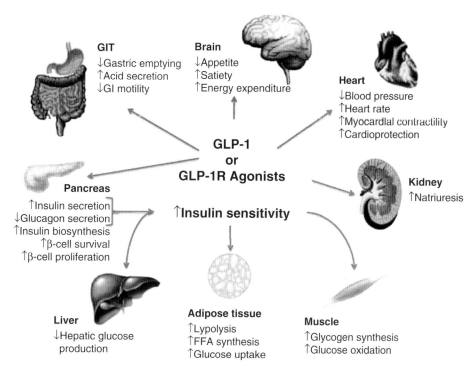

FIGURE 4-4 Organ effects of GLP-1 signaling. (Reproduced, with permission, from Futter JE, Cleland JGF, Clark AL. Body mass indices and outcome in patients with chronic heart failure. *Eur J Heart Fail*. 2011;13(2):207-213.)

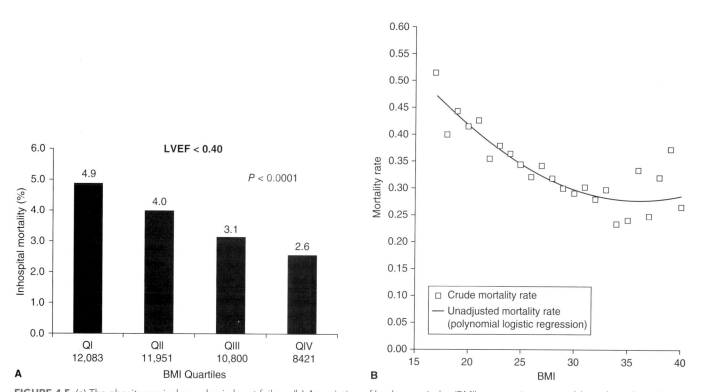

FIGURE 4-5 (a) The obesity survival paradox in heart failure. (b) Association of body mass index (BMI) as a continuous variable and unadjusted all-cause mortality using polynomial logistic regression. Each point represents the mortality rate associated with a BMI integer. (Reproduced, with permission, from Fonarow GC, Srikanthan P, Costanzo MR, Cintron GB, Lopatin M. An obesity paradox in acute heart failure: analysis of body mass index and inhospital mortality for 108,927 patients in the Acute Decompensated Heart Failure National Registry. *Am Heart J*. 2007;153(1):74-81.)

The underweight ($<18.5 \, \text{kg/m}^2$) and low-normal weight ($<23 \, \text{kg/m}^2$) subjects had a higher hazard of mortality than normal-weight subjects (adjusted HR 1.11; 95% CI 1.01-1.23). The HF obesity paradox appears to persist when BMI is substituted for anthropometric measurements of obesity, such as waist circumference.[78]

A survival paradox is not universally seen in HF studies, and in some studies the relationship is U-shaped rather than linear. However, even in cohorts without a paradox, investigators have not described as much excess mortality associated with obesity as might be expected from the potential harmful effects that can accompany excess adiposity.[78,79] The paradox does not appear to be unique to HF with reduced ejection fraction (HFrEF) or HFpEF cohorts,[75,80] but among HFrEF patients the phenomenon may be strongest in patients with a nonischemic cardiomyopathy etiology.[81] The paradox does not appear to be restricted to the United States either, with a global analysis of the relationship between BMI and mortality in acutely decompensated HF showing an association between higher BMI and decreased 30-day and 1-year mortality (11% decrease at 30 days; 9% decrease at 1 year per $5 \, \text{kg/m}^2$; $p<0.05$), after adjustment for baseline risk.[82] The risk of HF rehospitalization may also be lower in obese patients.[83]

Obesity has also been associated with superior short-term, medium-term, and long-term survival in several large cohorts after acute MI,[84-86] and also after coronary artery bypass or valve surgeries.[87] A similar finding was reported in a large outpatient cohort of patients with hypertension and CAD.[88] However, the obesity paradox is not universal—1 acute MI cohort showed no independent prediction of mortality by either BMI or waist circumference.[89] An obesity/overweight paradox has also been observed in the general population without established CVD, for example in a meta-analysis of 97 studies providing a combined sample size of more than 2.88 million individuals. All-cause mortality hazard ratios relative to normal weight (BMI 18.5 to $<25 \, \text{kg/m}^2$) were 0.94 (95% CI 0.91-0.96) for overweight, 1.18 (95% CI 1.12-1.25) for obesity (all grades combined), 0.95 (95% CI 0.88-1.01) for grade 1 obesity, and 1.29 (95% CI 1.18-1.41) for grades 2 and 3 obesity.[90] These findings caused controversy in their suggestion that even among the general population, modest excess adiposity could be associated with a survival advantage.

POTENTIAL EPIDEMIOLOGICAL EXPLANATIONS FOR THE HEART FAILURE OBESITY SURVIVAL PARADOX

Several methodological considerations may explain the survival paradox, especially given that most data described above were derived from ad hoc analyses of HF medication trials or retrospective cohorts that were not assembled with the intention of analyzing the impact of obesity on survival. Potential epidemiology explanations for erroneously concluding a paradox exists when it does not could include lead-time bias, a healthy survivor effect, or inadequate risk adjustment between obese and nonobese cohorts.[91,92] Lead-time bias describes the scenario where obese patients may present earlier and be diagnosed with HF at a lesser stage of severity than their normal-weight counterparts because of the functional limitations imposed by the obesity. This could then bias the obese cohort toward a milder phenotype of HF

with a correspondingly lower mortality risk. A healthy survivor effect describes a situation where the early mortality rate in obese individuals is higher than for normal-weight individuals; thus by the time that the population begins to develop HF with significant frequency, the obese subgroup is biased toward the most healthy individuals who have survived to middle or older age. Also of note the follow-up periods are relatively short in many of these obesity paradox studies, and it is possible that a factor such as obesity may give a short-term advantage but have a detrimental effect over longer periods of exposure.

Inadequate risk adjustment between obese and nonobese cohorts can be challenging to guard against or to prove. For example, changes in cigarette smoking status after baseline data collection or undiagnosed systemic illness could unexpectedly increase the mortality hazard in lower BMI subjects—so-called reverse causality. Neurohumoral medication doses may be higher in the obese subgroups because of higher blood pressures—although medications are adjusted for in some of these studies, individual doses are not. The opposite is also possible, where intermediary factors on a biological pathway from obesity to HF mortality are entered into a multivariable model, nullifying a relationship between higher BMI and higher mortality.

A recent review from McGill University examined many of these potential methodological issues with careful epidemiological analyses.[93] The principle of collider stratification bias, a form of selection bias, was particularly investigated. This bias can arise when both the exposure (obesity) and outcome (mortality in HF) both affect inclusion into the analytic cohort; in this case, cohort inclusion is conditioned upon having established HF at baseline. It has been previously established that conditioning on a "collider" (HF diagnosis) that is affected by both the exposure and outcome can introduce a spurious association between exposure and outcome and even reverse the direction of association, making a negative exposure appear beneficial.[94] Bias analysis methodology is presented in this review to show how the magnitude of such a bias can be assessed to determine the obesity-mortality relationship in a cohort with established HF versus the obesity-mortality relationship in the general population. These analyses enable calculation of a selection bias factor; when this factor exceeds the proportion of the population affected by the collider, then the bias can be of sufficient magnitude to reverse the direction of the relationship under examination.

POTENTIAL PATHOPHYSIOLOGICAL EXPLANATIONS FOR THE HEART FAILURE OBESITY SURVIVAL PARADOX

Beyond the methodological concerns, it is also possible that a genuinely protective role of obesity exists for patients with established HF. Potential pathophysiological explanations may rest upon a greater metabolic reserve to help avoid cardiac cachexia development, or may be caused by net positive myocardial effects of the adipokines and gut hormones upregulated in obesity as outlined above. Malnutrition is a predictor of lengths of stay, readmission, and mortality in HF.[95,96] An analysis of change in weight over 6 months among 6933 patients in the Candesartan in Heart failure: Reduction in Mortality and Morbidity (CHARM) clinical trial demonstrated the negative impact of weight loss on survival over a median of 32.9 months' follow-up.[97] Subjects with ≥5% weight loss over 6 months had a >50% increase in the hazard of mortality, compared with those whose weight remained stable. Weight loss was particularly harmful in subjects who had a lower weight at study enrollment. Thus, the presence of excess adiposity may serve as a buffer to protect an individual's energy reserves when challenged by the catabolic cytokines that promote cardiac cachexia in advanced HF. However this explanation has also been contested by an analysis from the Atherosclerosis Risk in Communities (ARIC) study. Over a 10-year follow-up of 1487 subjects with incident HF, baseline BMI in the overweight or obese range was associated with more favorable survival than normal-weight BMI (HR for overweight 0.72, 95% CI 0.58-0.90, p=0.004; HR for obesity 0.70, 95% CI 0.56-0.87, p=0.001).[98] This suggests that individuals who were overweight/obese before HF development still have lower mortality after HF diagnosis, regardless of their weight after HF diagnosis, meaning that cachexia in advanced HF may not fully explain the positive effect of a higher BMI in established HF.

Another interesting pathophysiological consideration is the impact of cardiorespiratory fitness on the obesity survival paradox in HF. In several cohorts the obesity paradox has been noted to lie only among the subgroup with low cardiorespiratory fitness, for example as defined by peak VO_2 of <14 mL/kg/min.[91,99] The implication of this observation is that for patients with better cardiorespiratory fitness and hence a better HF prognosis, there is no apparent protective effect of obesity. These findings that improved functional capacity can attenuate the obesity paradox may support a pathophysiological basis for the obesity paradox observations. Another finding that may support a pathophysiological basis for the obesity paradox is the observation that the benefits of excess adiposity are stronger in overweight women than men.[92]

WEIGHT LOSS STRATEGIES IN HEART FAILURE

Despite the uncertainties regarding potential epidemiological and pathophysiological mechanisms for an obesity survival paradox in patients with HF, there remain a number of potential benefits for weight loss in such patients: improved glycemic control, improved sleep-disordered breathing, improved depression and quality of life, greater functional capacity, and improved candidacy for heart transplantation in patients with advanced HF. The sustained loss of as little as 5% to 10% of body weight can positively impact cardiovascular risk factors, metabolic dysfunction, and the degree of left ventricular hypertrophy.[100-102] Therefore, weight loss is often recommended for obese HF patients, although patients may find meaningful and sustained weight loss from diet and exercise elusive, especially if functionally limited by comorbidities. This reality was illustrated by 5-year follow-up of patients who had undergone a 10-week weight loss program; the average participant gained 12 lb after treatment termination and was ultimately 1.5 lb heavier than at study initiation.[103] A systematic review of dietary and physical activity interventions across 3910 participants concluded there was no firm evidence for sustainable weight loss.[104] Thus weight loss recommendations must be tailored to individuals with their strengths and limitations in mind.

DIET AND EXERCISE STRATEGIES

Dietary and physical activity choices must always be addressed, regardless of any additional weight loss therapies. Potential strategies to promote dietary and physical activity changes for cardiovascular risk reduction are outlined in a Scientific Statement from the American Heart Association.[105] The Look AHEAD (Action for Health in Diabetes) study was a key primary CVD prevention trial, which compared an education-only group with an intensive lifestyle therapy group among patients with overweight/obesity and type 2 diabetes mellitus.[106] The intensive therapy group achieved greater weight loss and had lower hemoglobin A1c levels and lesser diabetes medication requirements. However, despite the weight loss, increased exercise, and improvement in metabolic diseases, the subsequent incidence of CVD was unaltered. Several prospective clinical trials have demonstrated a favorable impact of a low-fat, an Indo-Mediterranean, or low-carbohydrate strategy on progression of atherosclerosis.[107-110] The impact of polyunsaturated fat intake on CVD outcomes has been an area of uncertainty.[111-113] A recent comprehensive review addresses many of these controversies and resolves disparate dietary recommendations with an updated meta-analysis on the impact of food choices on CVD.[114] Fruits, nuts, fish, vegetables, vegetable oils, whole grains, beans, and yogurts are most associated with cardiovascular health; refined grains, starches, sugars, processed meats, high-sodium foods, and industrial trans fats have the strongest associations with cardiovascular harm (Figure 4-6).

Sodium restriction has dominated the HF-specific dietary literature, with only a small number of nutritional intervention trials addressing caloric intake or nutritional supplementation in HF. Cardiac cachexia, sarcopenia, low serum cholesterol, and low albumin are all predictors of poor prognosis in HF.[115-119] Individuals with HF often have poor dietary quality and in particular may be deficient in micronutrients.[120-123] There may be a specific role for n-3 polyunsaturated fatty acid supplementation in systolic HF.[124-126] A pilot study of dietary and exercise modifications in obese patients with HF enrolled 20 patients with systolic HF and metabolic syndrome. Subjects were randomized to standard medical therapy versus medical therapy and lifestyle modification, which involved a walking program and a reduced calorie diet with 2 SlimFast® meal replacements daily.[127] At 3 months, 5 patients in each group had lost weight, although the overall weight change was marginal at −0.84 ± 3.82 and −0.50 ± 3.64 kg (p=0.85) in the control versus lifestyle groups, respectively. There were no significant differences in the defined endpoints on physical examination, laboratory values, quality of life questionnaire, 6-minute walk, or brachial ultrasound. More encouraging results were presented from a trial of a high-protein diet, versus a standard-protein diet, versus a conventional diet. Fourteen subjects with HF, NYHA class II-III, and BMI >27 kg/m² were enrolled for 3 months.[128] Subjects receiving the high-protein diet demonstrated significantly greater reductions in weight (p=0.005) and percent body fat (p=0.036), and greater improvements in 6-minute walk (p=0.010) and peak VO_2 (p=0.003), compared with those on standard-protein and conventional diets.

Lifestyle interventions have also targeted the HFpEF population, where pharmacological HF therapies are limited. For example, ≥2%

weight loss during a 3-month diet and exercise intervention among 40 patients with HFpEF was associated with improved peak VO_2 and diastolic echocardiographic parameters, and a greater freedom from rehospitalization as compared with individuals whose weight loss was <2%.[129] Another HFpEF study randomized 26 obese participants to exercise, 24 to diet, 25 to exercise plus diet, and 25 to control. Body weight decreased by 7% (7 kg) in the diet group, 3% (4 kg) in the exercise group, 10% (11 kg) in the exercise plus diet group, and 1% (1 kg) in the control group. Peak VO_2 was increased significantly by either exercise (1.2 mL/kg body mass/min [95% CI 0.7-1.7], p<0.001) or diet (1.3 mL/kg body mass/min [95% CI 0.8-1.8], p<0.001).[130] The most comprehensive exercise intervention in systolic HF was the HF-ACTION randomized trial, in which 49% of participants were obese.[131] The structured aerobic exercise program was associated with improved quality of life in all BMI categories,[132] with greater benefits for subjects with higher BMIs.[71] Exercise was also associated with nonsignificant trends toward reduced all-cause mortality and hospitalization in each BMI category. Of note, participation in an exercise program is currently the only intervention for weight loss that is recommended in the ACC/AHA/HFSA heart failure guidelines for patients with systolic HF.[133]

PHARMACOTHERAPY STRATEGIES

Pharmacotherapy has a clear role in supporting weight loss in appropriately selected obese patients, although placebo-adjusted weight losses remain modest, lying in the 2 to 6 kg range.[134] However, when used in combination with lifestyle modifications, effects can be synergistic.[135] Pharmacological therapy is suggested as an adjunct to lifestyle interventions for patients with BMI ≥30 kg/m² or ≥27 kg/m² and at least 1 obesity-associated comorbidity.[136] Although options have evolved over recent years, many agents with current FDA approval are at least relatively contraindicated in patients with established HF. With the withdrawal of sibutramine, the remaining anorectic sympathomimetics on the U.S. market—phentermine, diethylpropion, benzphetamine, and phendimetrazine—are approved for short-term use only, generally interpreted as 12 weeks maximum.[137] Adverse effects include hypertension, tachycardia, palpitations, and dizziness; their tendency to elevate blood pressure and heart rate make them poor choices for cardiac patients.[134]

Orlistat is an inhibitor of pancreatic lipase that is taken 3 times daily and causes an increase in the proportion of dietary fat that is incompletely hydrolyzed and fecally excreted. Orlistat achieved a 2.9 kg (95% CI 2.5-3.2 kg) mean weight reduction, beyond placebo, at 1 year in a meta-analysis of 15 studies.[138] The loss appears maintainable: at 4 years, mean weight loss was 5.8 kg with orlistat versus 3.0 kg with placebo, p<0.001, although conclusions were limited by loss to follow-up.[139] Orlistat is currently marketed under the trade name Xenical (120 mg) in most countries, or over-the-counter as the 60 mg Alli in the United Kingdom and United States. In obese individuals with diabetes, orlistat also has shown the potential to improve glycemic control.[140] Orlistat arguably has the most appropriate side-effect profile of the currently approved weight loss drugs for HF patients, and a small pilot suggested efficacy and safety in this population.[141] Several of the diabetes medications, including the GLP-1 agonists, are associated with weight loss and may also be appropriate options

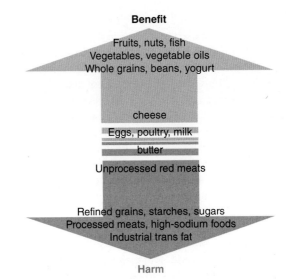

FIGURE 4-6 Evidence-based dietary priorities for cardiometabolic health. (Reproduced, with permission from Mozaffarian D. Dietary and policy priorities for cardiovascular disease, diabetes, and obesity: a comprehensive review. *Circulation.* 2016;133(2). WoltersKluwer Health, Inc.)

in patients with HF. Liraglutide 3 mg once daily subcutaneously has a separate indication for weight loss under the trade name Saxenda.

Lorcaserin, a selective 5-HT$_{2C}$ receptor agonist, was developed to promote satiety in obese or overweight adults and is currently marketed as Belviq.[142] Due to the possibility of 5-HT$_{2B}$-receptor upregulation during HF, caution is advised when considering lorcaserin use in patients with HF.[143] In the BLOSSOM trial, subjects were randomized to lorcaserin 10 mg twice daily, lorcaserin 10 mg once daily, or placebo. Subjects receiving lorcaserin 10 mg once or twice daily lost at least 5% of baseline body weight (47.2% and 40.2%, respectively), compared with placebo (25.0%, p<0.001 versus lorcaserin twice daily).[144]

An extended-release combination of phentermine and topiramate has also been approved for weight loss as Qsymia, although contraindications include unstable cardiac disease within the prior 6 months.[145] CONQUER recruited a high-risk cohort with BMI 27 to 45 kg/m^2 and 2 or more comorbidities, randomized to placebo, once-daily phentermine 7.5 mg plus topiramate 46 mg, or once-daily phentermine 15 mg plus topiramate 92 mg in a 2:1:2 ratio.[145] There was a slight rise in heart rate with the active medication, but blood pressure and lipids were significantly improved in the high-dose treatment group. EQUIP recruited a more obese population and incorporated a lower dose preparation.[146] Notably 45% of the lowest dosage group (3.75/23 mg) attained the ≥5% weight loss threshold. The resting heart rate was minimally elevated in the 15/92 mg group at 1.2 bpm above the baseline value of 73.2 bpm, and unaltered from placebo in the 3.75/23 mg group. Coupled with reduced blood pressure, the overall rate-pressure product with phentermine/topiramate was actually lower than placebo.

Contrave, a fixed-dose sustained-release combination of naltrexone and bupropion, has demonstrated greater weight loss than naltrexone alone, bupropion alone, or placebo.[147] A transient increase of around 1.5 mm Hg in mean systolic and diastolic blood pressure was followed by a reduction of around 1 mm Hg below baseline in the naltrexone-bupropion groups, but the blood pressure still remained in excess of the placebo group. Heart rate was 1.5 to 2.5 bpm higher than baseline values in active treatment subjects. COR-II showed significantly greater weight loss in the naltrexone-bupropion 32/360 mg group than placebo at 28 weeks (−6.5% versus −1.9%) and 56 weeks (−6.4% versus −1.2%).[148] More subjects in the active treatment group achieved ≥5% weight loss at week 56 (50.5% versus 17.1%) as well as greater improvements in cardiometabolic risk markers and quality of life, but the cardiovascular safety remains undefined.[149]

BARIATRIC SURGERY

Bariatric surgery is now established as one of the most efficacious and durable interventions for obesity. Restrictive procedures such as gastric banding and sleeve gastrectomy promote satiety and encourage decreased food intake, whereas malabsorptive operations such as biliopancreatic diversion decrease nutrition absorption; Roux-en-Y gastric bypass (RYGB) combines restrictive and malabsorptive features (Figure 4-7).[9] Bariatric procedures typically result in an excess weight loss of around 50%, meaning that half of the initial weight that exceeded ideal weight for height has been lost.[150] Profound effects on cardiovascular risk factors and metabolism are also observed.[10] A 22,000-patient meta-analysis

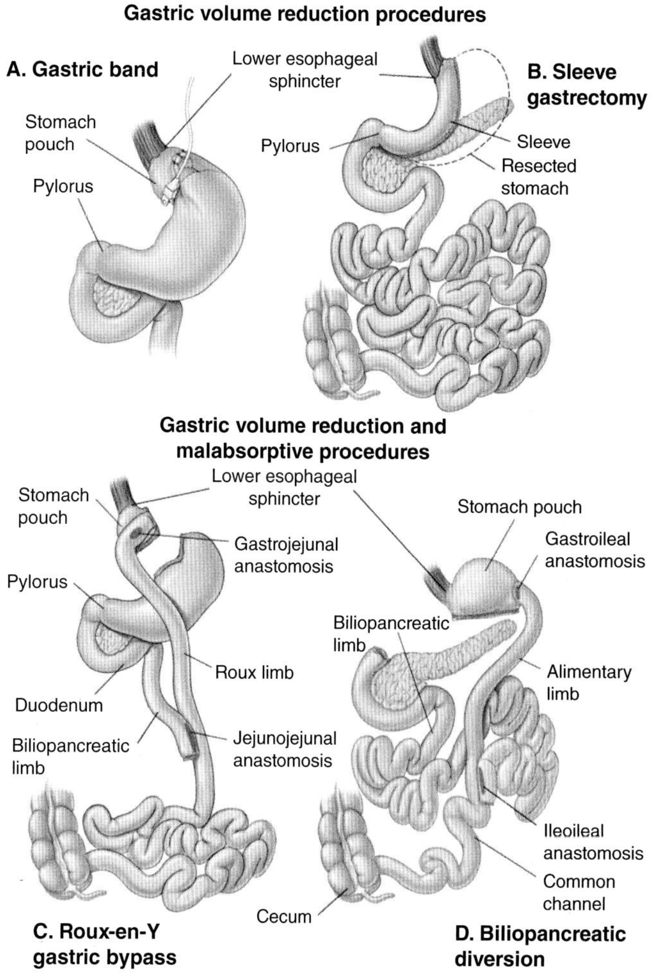

FIGURE 4-7 Anatomic modifications as created in the most common bariatric surgery procedures. (Reproduced, with permission, from Vest AR, Heneghan HM, Schauer PR, et al. Surgical management of obesity and the relationship to cardiovascular disease. *Circulation*. 2013;127(8). WoltersKluwer Health, Inc.)

demonstrated that an average postoperative excess weight loss of 61% was accompanied by significant improvements in type 2 diabetes mellitus, hypertension, dyslipidemia, and obstructive sleep apnea.[150] The STAMPEDE trial subsequently underlined the scope of bariatric surgery in the management of obese patients with type 2 diabetes.[151] The primary end point of HbA1c <6.0% at 1 year was achieved by 12% of the optimal medical therapy group, versus 42% of the gastric bypass surgical group and 37% of the sleeve gastrectomy surgical group (both p<0.01 compared with medical therapy alone). There is also nonrandomized evidence to suggest reduced cardiovascular events and mortality after bariatric surgery, with the largest and most convincing outcomes studies coming from Flum and Dellinger,[152] Adams,[153] Busetto,[154] and Sjostrom,[11] over follow-up periods of 4.4 to 14.7 years.

Significant changes in the key adipokines and gut hormones are seen in the weeks and months after RYGB or sleeve gastrectomy. Circulating levels of CRP and IL-6 fall in parallel with the improved insulin sensitivity that emerges almost immediately postoperatively.[155] Adiponectin, leptin, and GLP-1 circulating levels rapidly move toward normal and may also promote normalization of insulin sensitivity. Biochemical changes long precede the nadir of weight loss and appear independent of caloric restriction.[156,157] Changes in cardiac structure and function are also seen in the months and years after either dietary or surgical weight loss, principally with reductions in left ventricular mass that may be independent of blood pressure reductions.[102,158-162] Leptin has been proposed as a mediator of this regression of hypertrophy.[48] Postoperative improvements in diastolic function and subclinical systolic function have been reported too.[163-167]

All individuals with obesity can be considered to be ACC/AHA stage A for HF, and 3 recently-published large studies demonstrated a continuum of HF prevention efficacy across lifestyle and bariatric surgery strategies for weight loss. In the first, 1724 RYGB surgery patients were closely matched to a contemporaneous cohort of non-surgical controls. Patients were followed for a median of 6.3 years for CVD events and HF incidence. Seventy-nine patients developed HF, with an adjusted hazard ratio of 0.38 (95% confidence interval, 0.22-0.64) for the development of HF in the RYGB group, as compared to the control group.[168] A second study analysed 47,859 Swedish adults with obesity as a primary diagnosis, with 47% receiving bariatric surgery at a mean age of 41 years.[169] Over a mean of 3.7 years 1033 patients developed HF, with those who received bariatric surgery having a far lower risk of incident HF compared with nonsurgical patients, with an adjusted hazard ratio of 0.37 (95% confidence interval, 0.30–0.46). Thirdly, the incidence of HF was compared between the Scandinavian Obesity Surgery Registry and a registry of obese patients managed with a structured intensive lifestyle program. The 25,804 RYGB patients lost 22.6 kg more after 2 years than the 13,701 lifestyle modification patients.[170] The RYGB group had a significantly lower HF incidence than the lifestyle group, with a propensity-matched hazard ratio of 0.54 (95% confidence interval, 0.36-0.82), at a median of 4.1 years follow-up.

There is also a growing literature regarding bariatric surgery in obese patients with preoperative left ventricular dysfunction and HF. Initial reports of systolic dysfunction recovery after bariatric weight loss generally reported extremely obese, relatively young individuals, who may not be representative of the general obese HF population, and many did not utilize nonsurgical control groups or blinded echocardiographic readers.[171-180] More recently, data from the Cleveland Clinic compared 42 patients with LVEF <50% who underwent bariatric surgery with 2588 patients without known systolic dysfunction, and demonstrated good efficacy and safety in the systolic dysfunction group.[181] The systolic dysfunction patients had greater baseline prevalence of comorbidities and showed a slight excess of early postoperative HF and MI. However, the left ventricular systolic dysfunction group achieved good weight loss efficacy (mean decrease 22.6%) with no excess in mortality at 1 year. Dual blinded echocardiographic readers reported on 38 systolic dysfunction patients with both preoperative and postoperative echocardiographic images available. These 38 surgical patients were matched with 38 obese nonsurgical controls on age, sex, initial LVEF, and interval between echocardiograms. There was a significant mean preoperative to postoperative LVEF improvement of +5.1% ±8.3 (p=0.0005) for surgical subjects, but not for controls (+3.4% ±10.5, p=0.056). Among surgical subjects, 11 patients had an LVEF improvement of >10% postoperatively, whereas only 6 improved by >10% among nonsurgical controls; history of MI appeared to decrease the likelihood of LVEF improvement after bariatric surgery. These data suggest that bariatric surgery may be a safe and useful procedure for obese HF patients at experienced centers, although the degree of any LVEF improvement postoperatively may be small.

Furthermore, a recent analysis of an administrative database suggested that patients with a preoperative diagnosis of HF may experience reduced HF hospitalizations after bariatric surgery. A self-controlled case series study of obese patients with HF who underwent bariatric surgery identified 524 patients with HF who received surgery within 3 catchment states. During the reference period, 16.2% of patients had an emergency department visit or hospitalization for HF exacerbation. This rate was significantly lower in the subsequent 13 to 24 months after bariatric surgery (9.9%; adjusted odds ratio: 0.57; p=0.003).[182] Given the public health burdens of both obesity and HF, the possibility of remission of the HF syndrome with surgical weight loss provides an important clinical message, even if the impact on future mortality in the HF population remains uncertain thus far.

INDIVIDUALIZING OBESITY MANAGEMENT IN HEART FAILURE

In conclusion, the impact of obesity on the development of incident HF appears to be reasonably straightforward, but the impact of obesity on survival in established HF becomes more complex. The observed obesity survival paradox presents some clinical uncertainties: when counseling an HF patient such as in the case above, should we advise him to start on a weight loss program or just to stay at his current weight? As reviewed above, for HF patients with BMI ≥40 kg/m², severely depressed systolic function, and NYHA class III-IV symptoms, weight loss may provide benefits in terms of functional capacity, HF hospitalizations, future advanced therapies candidacy, and possibly even LVEF improvement. Bariatric surgery may be an appropriate option for patients with a large amount of weight to lose, who are sufficiently stable for a noncardiac surgery. Further studies are required for patients with established HF to determine the safest and most effective strategies for weight loss, as well as the impact of weight loss on future survival and quality of life. Such data will enable clinicians to better individualize recommendations for the prevention and treatment of obesity and make meaningful long-term improvements in patients' cardiovascular health.

REFERENCES

1. Ogden CL, Carroll MD, Kit BK, Flegal KM. Prevalence of childhood and adult obesity in the United States, 2011-2012. *JAMA.* 2014;311:806-814.

2. Eckel RH, Krauss RM. American Heart Association call to action: obesity as a major risk factor for coronary heart disease. AHA Nutrition Committee. *Circulation.* 1998;97:2099-2100.

3. Kenchaiah S, Evans JC, Levy D, et al. Obesity and the risk of heart failure. *N Engl J Med.* 2002;347:305-313.

4. Levitan EB, Yang AZ, Wolk A, Mittleman MA. Adiposity and incidence of heart failure hospitalization and mortality: a population-based prospective study. *Circulation: Heart Failure.* 2009;2:202-208.

5. Ho JE, Lyass A, Lee DS, et al. Predictors of new-onset heart failure: differences in preserved versus reduced ejection fraction. *Circulation: Heart Failure.* 2013;6:279-286.

6. de Koning L, Merchant AT, Pogue J, Anand SS. Waist circumference and waist-to-hip ratio as predictors of cardiovascular events: meta-regression analysis of prospective studies. *Eur Heart J.* 2007;28:850-856.

7. Eckel RH, Jakicic JM, Ard JD, et al. 2013 AHA/ACC guideline on lifestyle management to reduce cardiovascular risk: a report of the American College of Cardiology/American Heart Association Task Force on Practice Guidelines. *Circulation.* 2014;129:S76-99.

8. NIH conference. Gastrointestinal surgery for severe obesity. Consensus Development Conference Panel. 1991. p. 956-961.

9. Vest AR, Heneghan HM, Schauer PR, Young JB. Surgical management of obesity and the relationship to cardiovascular disease. *Circulation.* 2013;127:945-959.

10. Vest AR, Heneghan HM, Agarwal S, Schauer PR, Young JB. Bariatric surgery and cardiovascular outcomes: a systematic review. *Heart.* 2012;98:1763-1777.

11. Sjöström L, Peltonen M, Jacobson P, et al. Bariatric surgery and long-term cardiovascular events. *JAMA.* 2012;307:56-65.

12. Vest AR, Young JB. Should we target obesity in advanced heart failure? *Curr Treat Options Cardio Med.* 2014;16:284.

13. Lavie CJ, Alpert MA, Arena R, Mehra MR, Milani RV, Ventura HO. Impact of obesity and the obesity paradox on prevalence and prognosis in heart failure. *JACC Heart Fail.* 2013;1:93-102.

14. Larsson B, Svärdsudd K, Welin L, Wilhelmsen L, Björntorp P, Tibblin G. Abdominal adipose tissue distribution, obesity, and risk of cardiovascular disease and death: 13 year follow up of participants in the study of men born in 1913. *Br Med J (Clin Res Ed).* 1984;288:1401-1404.

15. Després J-P. Body fat distribution and risk of cardiovascular disease: an update. *Circulation.* 2012;126:1301-1313.

16. Tam CS, Lecoultre V, Ravussin E. Brown adipose tissue: mechanisms and potential therapeutic targets. *Circulation.* 2012;125:2782-2791.

17. Kiefer FW, Cohen P, Plutzky J. Fifty shades of brown: perivascular fat, thermogenesis, and atherosclerosis. *Circulation.* 2012;126:1012-1015.

18. Harms M, Seale P. Brown and beige fat: development, function and therapeutic potential. *Nat Med.* 2013;19:1252-1263.

19. Lavie CJ, McAuley PA, Church TS, Milani RV, Blair SN. Obesity and cardiovascular diseases—implications regarding fitness, fatness and severity in the obesity paradox. *J Am Coll Cardiol.* 2014;63:1345-1354.

20. Poirier P. Obesity and cardiovascular disease: pathophysiology, evaluation, and effect of weight loss: an update of the 1997 AHA scientific statement on obesity and heart disease. *Circulation.* 2006;113:898-918.

21. Yusuf S, Hawken S, Ôunpuu S, et al. Effect of potentially modifiable risk factors associated with myocardial infarction in 52 countries (the INTERHEART study): case-control study. *Lancet.* 2004;364:937-952.

22. Hubert HB, Feinleib M, McNamara PM, Castelli WP. Obesity as an independent risk factor for cardiovascular disease: a 26-year follow-up of participants in the Framingham Heart Study. *Circulation.* 1983;67:968-977.

23. Kasper EK, Hruban RH, Baughman KL. Cardiomyopathy of obesity: a clinicopathologic evaluation of 43 obese patients with heart failure. *Am J Cardiol.* 1992;70:921-924.

24. Alpert MA. Obesity cardiomyopathy: pathophysiology and evolution of the clinical syndrome. *Am J Med Sci.* 2001;321:225-236.

25. Lavie CJ, Milani RV, Ventura HO. Obesity and cardiovascular disease: risk factor, paradox, and impact of weight loss. *J Am Coll Cardiol.* 2009;53:1925-1932.

26. Djoussé L, Bartz TM, Ix JH, et al. Adiposity and incident heart failure in older adults: the cardiovascular health study. *Obesity (Silver Spring).* 2011;20:1936-1941.

27. Kenchaiah S, Sesso HD, Gaziano JM. Body mass index and vigorous physical activity and the risk of heart failure among men. *Circulation.* 2009;119:44-52.

28. Loehr LR, Rosamond WD, Poole C, et al. Association of multiple anthropometrics of overweight and obesity with incident heart failure. *Circulation: Heart Failure.* 2009;2:18-24.

29. Vardeny O, Gupta DK, Claggett B, et al. Insulin resistance and incident heart failure: the ARIC study (atherosclerosis risk in communities). *JACC Heart Fail.* 2013;1:531-536.

30. Voulgari C, Tentolouris N, Dilaveris P, Tousoulis D, Katsilambros N, Stefanadis C. Increased heart failure risk in normal-weight people with metabolic syndrome compared with metabolically healthy obese individuals. *J Am Coll Cardiol.* 2011;58:1343-1350.

31. Hu G, Jousilahti P, Antikainen R, Katzmarzyk PT, Tuomile-hto J. Joint effects of physical activity, body mass index, waist circumference, and waist-to-hip ratio on the risk of heart failure. *Circulation.* 2010;121:237-244.

32. Li X, Li S, Ulusoy E, Chen W, Srinivasan SR, Berenson GS. Child-hood adiposity as a predictor of cardiac mass in adulthood: the Bogalusa Heart Study. *Circulation.* 2004;110:3488-3492.

33. van Putte-Katier N, Rooman RP, Haas L, Verhulst SL, Desager KN, Ramet J, et al. Early cardiac abnormalities in obese children: importance of obesity per se versus associated cardiovascular risk factors. *Pediatr Res.* 2008;64:205-209.

34. Mehta S, Holliday C, Hayduk L, Wiersma L, Ricahrds N, Younoszai A. Comparison of myocardial function in children with body mass indexes ≥25 versus those <25 kg/m^2. *Am J Cardiol.* 2004;93:1567-1569.

35. Chinali M, de Simone G, Roman MJ, et al. Impact of obesity on cardiac geometry and function in a population of adoles-cents. *J Am Coll Cardiol.* 2006;47:2267-2273.

36. Saltijeral A, Isla LP de, Pérez-Rodríguez O, et al. Early myocardial deformation changes associated to isolated obesity: a study based on 3D-wall motion tracking analysis. *Obesity.* 2011;19:2268-2273.

37. Cozzolino D, Grandone A, Cittadini A, et al. Subclinical myo-cardial dysfunction and cardiac autonomic dysregulation are closely associated in obese children and adolescents: the poten-tial role of insulin resistance. *PLoS ONE.* 2015;10:e0123916.

38. Ippisch HM, Inge TH, Daniels SR, et al. Reversibility of cardiac abnormalities in morbidly obese adolescents. *J Am Coll Cardiol.* 2008;51:1342-1348.

39. Michalsky MP, Raman SV, Teich S, Schuster DP, Bauer JA. Car-diovascular recovery following bariatric surgery in extremely obese adolescents: preliminary results using Cardiac Magnetic Resonance (CMR) Imaging. *J Pediatr Surg.* 2013;48:170-177.

40. Mehra MR, Uber PA, Park MH, et al. Obesity and suppressed B-type natriuretic peptide levels in heart failure. *J Am Coll Cardiol.* 2004;43:1590-1595.

41. St Peter JV, Hartley GG, Murakami MM, Apple FS. B-type natriuretic peptide (BNP) and N-terminal pro-BNP in obese patients without heart failure: relationship to body mass index and gastric bypass surgery. *Clin Chem.* 2006;52:680-685.

42. Bays HE. Adiposopathy. *J Am Coll Cardiol.* 2011;57:2461-2473.

43. Mattu HS, Randeva HS. Role of adipokines in cardiovascular disease. *J Endocrinol.* 2013;216:T17-T36.

44. Blüher M. Adipokines—removing road blocks to obesity and diabetes therapy. *Mol Metab.* 2014;3:230-240.

45. Ukkola O, Santaniemi M. Adiponectin: a link between excess adiposity and associated comorbidities? *J Mol Med.* 2002;80:696-702.

46. Han SH, Quon MJ, Kim J-A, Koh KK. Adiponectin and cardi-ovascular disease: response to therapeutic interventions. *J Am Coll Cardiol.* 2007;49:531-538.

47. Van Berendoncks AM, Garnier A, Beckers P, et al. Functional adiponectin resistance at the level of the skeletal muscle in mild to moderate chronic heart failure. *Circulation: Heart Failure.* 2010;3:185-194.

48. Perego L, Pizzocri P, Corradi D, et al. Circulating leptin cor-relates with left ventricular mass in morbid (grade III) obesity before and after weight loss induced by bariatric surgery: a potential role for leptin in mediating human left ventricular hypertrophy. *J Clin Endocrinol Metab.* 2005;90:4087-4093.

49. Konstantinides S, Schafer K, Loskutoff DJ. The prothrom-botic effects of leptin possible implications for the risk of cardiovascular disease in obesity. *Ann N Y Acad Sci.* 2001;947:134-141; discussion 141-142.

50. Tretjakovs P, Jurka A, Bormane I, et al. Relation of inflamma-tory chemokines to insulin resistance and hypoadiponectine-mia in coronary artery disease patients. *Eur J Intern Med.* 2009;20:712-717.

51. Schulze PC, Kratzsch J, Linke A, et al. Elevated serum levels of leptin and soluble leptin receptor in patients with advanced chronic heart failure. *Eur J Heart Fail.* 2003;5:33-40.

52. Martin SS, Qasim A, Reilly MP. Leptin resistance: a possible interface of inflammation and metabolism in obesity-related cardiovascular disease. *J Am Coll Cardiol.* 2008;52:1201-1210.

53. Wannamethee SG, Shaper AG, Whincup PH, Lennon L, Sat-tar N. Obesity and risk of incident heart failure in older men with and without pre-existing coronary heart disease: does leptin have a role? *J Am Coll Cardiol.* 2011;58:1870-1877.

54. Smith CCT, Dixon RA, Wynne AM, et al. Leptin-induced cardioprotection involves JAK/STAT signaling that may be linked to the mitochondrial permeability transition pore. *AJP: Heart and Circulatory Physiology.* 2010;299:H1265-1270.

55. Nagaya N, Uematsu M, Kojima M, et al. Chronic adminis-tration of ghrelin improves left ventricular dysfunction and attenuates development of cardiac cachexia in rats with heart failure. *Circulation.* 2001;104:1430-1435.

56. Nagaya N, Moriya J, Yasumura Y, et al. Effects of ghrelin administration on left ventricular function, exercise capac-ity, and muscle wasting in patients with chronic heart failure. *Circulation.* 2004;110:3674-3679.

57. Nikolaidis LA, Mankad S, Sokos GG, et al. Effects of glucagon-like peptide-1 in patients with acute myocardial infarction and left ventricular dysfunction after successful reperfusion. *Circulation.* 2004;109:962-965.

58. Sokos GG, Nikolaidis LA, Mankad S, Elahi D, Shannon RP. Glucagon-like peptide-1 infusion improves left ventricu-lar ejection fraction and functional status in patients with chronic heart failure. *J Card Fail.* 2006;12:694-699.

59. Nathanson D, Ullman B, Löfström U, Hedman A, Frick M, Sjöholm A, Nyström T. Effects of intravenous exenatide in type 2 diabetic patients with congestive heart failure: a double-blind, randomised controlled clinical trial of efficacy and safety. *Diabetologia.* 2012;55:926-935.

60. Margulies KB, Anstrom KJ, Hernandez AF, et al. GLP-1 agonist therapy for advanced heart failure with reduced ejection fraction. *Circulation: Heart Failure.* 2014;7:673-679.

61. Iacobellis G. Echocardiographic epicardial adipose tissue is related to anthropometric and clinical parameters of metabolic syndrome: a new indicator of cardiovascular risk. *J Clin Endocrinol Metab.* 2003;88:5163-5168.

62. Iacobellis G, di Gioia CRT, Cotesta D, et al. Epicardial adipose tissue adiponectin expression is related to intracoronary adiponectin levels. *Horm Metab Res.* 2009;41:227-231.

63. Fitzgibbons TP, Czech MP. Epicardial and perivascular adipose tissues and their influence on cardiovascular disease: basic mechanisms and clinical associations. *J Am Heart Assoc.* 2014;3:1-15.

64. Mazurek T. Human epicardial adipose tissue is a source of inflammatory mediators. *Circulation.* 2003;108:2460-2466.

65. Fosshaug LE, Dahl CP, Risnes I, et al. Altered levels of fatty acids and inflammatory and metabolic mediators in epicardial adipose tissue in patients with systolic heart failure. *J Card Fail.* 2015;21:916-923.

66. Greif M, Becker A, Ziegler von F, et al. Pericardial adipose tissue determined by dual source CT is a risk factor for coronary atherosclerosis. *Arterioscler Thromb Vasc Biol.* 2009;29:781-786.

67. Britton KA, Massaro JM, Murabito JM, Kreger BE, Hoffmann U, Fox CS. Body fat distribution, incident cardiovascular disease, cancer, and all-cause mortality. *J Am Coll Cardiol.* 2013;62:921-925.

68. Horwich TB, Fonarow GC, Hamilton MA, MacLellan WR, Woo MA, Tillisch JH. The relationship between obesity and mortality in patients with heart failure. *J Am Coll Cardiol.* 2001;38:789-795.

69. Güder G, Frantz S, Bauersachs J, et al. Reverse epidemiology in systolic and nonsystolic heart failure: cumulative prognostic benefit of classical cardiovascular risk factors. *Circulation: Heart Failure.* 2009;2:563-571.

70. Futter JE, Cleland JGF, Clark AL. Body mass indices and outcome in patients with chronic heart failure. *Eur J Heart Fail.* 2011;13:207-213.

71. Horwich TB, Broderick S, Chen L, et al. Relation among body mass index, exercise training, and outcomes in chronic systolic heart failure. *Am J Cardiol.* 2011;108:1754-1759.

72. Clark AL, Fonarow GC, Horwich TB. Obesity and the obesity paradox in heart failure. *Prog Cardiovasc Dis.* 2014;56:409-414.

73. Oreopoulos A, Ezekowitz JA, McAlister FA, et al. Association between direct measures of body composition and prognostic factors in chronic heart failure. *Mayo Clin Proc.* 2010;85:609-617.

74. Lavie CJ, Osman AF, Milani RV, Mehra MR. Body composition and prognosis in chronic systolic heart failure: the obesity paradox. *Am J Cardiol.* 2003;91:891-894.

75. Kapoor JR, Heidenreich PA. Obesity and survival in patients with heart failure and preserved systolic function: a U-shaped relationship. *Am Heart J.* 2010;159:75-80.

76. Curtis JP, Selter JG, Wang Y, et al. The obesity paradox: body mass index and outcomes in patients with heart failure. *Arch Intern Med.* 2005;165:55-61.

77. Fonarow GC, Srikanthan P, Costanzo MR, Cintron GB, Lopatin M. An obesity paradox in acute heart failure: analysis of body mass index and inhospital mortality for 108,927 patients in the Acute Decompensated Heart Failure National Registry. *Am Heart J.* 2007;153:74-81.

78. Clark AL, Fonarow GC, Horwich TB. Waist circumference, body mass index, and survival in systolic heart failure: the obesity paradox revisited. *J Card Fail.* 2011;17:374-380.

79. Adamopoulos C, Meyer P, Desai RV, et al. Absence of obesity paradox in patients with chronic heart failure and diabetes mellitus: a propensity-matched study. *Eur J Heart Fail.* 2011;13:200-206.

80. Ather S, Chan W, Bozkurt B, et al. Impact of noncardiac comorbidities on morbidity and mortality in a predominantly male population with heart failure and preserved versus reduced ejection fraction. *J Am Coll Cardiol.* 2012;59:998-1005.

81. Zamora E, Lupón J, de Antonio M, et al. The obesity paradox in heart failure: is etiology a key factor? *Int J Cardiol.* 2013;166:601-605.

82. Shah R, Gayat E, Januzzi JL, et al; GREAT (Global Research on Acute Conditions Team) Network. Body mass index and mortality in acutely decompensated heart failure across the world: a global obesity paradox. *J Am Coll Cardiol.* 2014;63:778-785.

83. Zapatero A, Barba R, González N, et al. Influence of obesity and malnutrition on acute heart failure. *Rev Esp Cardiol (Engl Ed).* 2012;65:421-426.

84. Bucholz EM, Rathore SS, Reid KJ, et al. Body mass index and mortality in acute myocardial infarction patients. *Am J Med.* 2012;125:796-803.

85. Bucholz EM, Beckman AL, Krumholz HA, Krumholz HM, Dr. Bucholz was affiliated with the Yale School of Medicine and Yale School of Public Health during the time that the work was conducted. Excess weight and life expectancy after acute myocardial infarction: The obesity paradox reexamined. *Am Heart J.* 2016;172:173-181.

86. Wang L, Liu W, He X, et al. Association of overweight and obesity with patient mortality after acute myocardial infarction: a meta-analysis of prospective studies. *Int J Obes Relat Metab Disord.* 2016;40:220-228.

87. Stamou SC, Nussbaum M, Stiegel RM, et al. Effect of body mass index on outcomes after cardiac surgery: is there an obesity paradox? *Ann Thorac Surg.* 2011;91:42-47.

88. Uretsky S, Messerli FH, Bangalore S, et al. Obesity paradox in patients with hypertension and coronary artery disease. *Am J Med.* 2007;120:863-870.

89. Zeller M, Steg PG, Ravisy J, et al; RICO Survey Working Group. Relation between body mass index, waist circumference, and death after acute myocardial infarction. *Circulation.* 2008;118:482-490.

90. Flegal KM, Kit BK, Orpana H, Graubard BI. Association of all-cause mortality with overweight and obesity using standard body mass index categories: a systematic review and meta-analysis. *JAMA.* 2013;309:71-82.

91. Lavie CJ, Cahalin LP, Chase P, et al. Impact of cardiorespiratory fitness on the obesity paradox in patients with heart failure. *Mayo Clin Proc.* 2013;88:251-258.

92. Vest AR, Wu Y, Hachamovitch R, Young JB, Cho LS. The heart failure overweight/obesity survival paradox. *JACC Heart Fail.* 2015;3:917-926.

93. Banack HR, Kaufman JS. The obesity paradox: understanding the effect of obesity on mortality among individuals with cardiovascular disease. *Prev Med.* 2014;62:96-102.

94. Cole SR, Platt RW, Schisterman EF, et al. Illustrating bias due to conditioning on a collider. *Int J Epidemiol.* 2010;39:417-420.

95. Aziz EF, Javed F, Pratap B, et al. Malnutrition as assessed by nutritional risk index is associated with worse outcome in patients admitted with acute decompensated heart failure: an ACAP-HF data analysis. *Heart Int.* 2011;6:e2.

96. Kaneko H, Suzuki S, Goto M, et al. Geriatric nutritional risk index in hospitalized heart failure patients. *Int J Cardiol.* 2015;181:213-215.

97. Pocock SJ, McMurray JJV, Dobson J, et al. Weight loss and mortality risk in patients with chronic heart failure in the candesartan in heart failure: assessment of reduction in mortality and morbidity (CHARM) programme. *Eur Heart J.* 2008;29:2641-2650.

98. Khalid U, Ather S, Bavishi C, et al. Pre-morbid body mass index and mortality after incident heart failure: the ARIC Study. *J Am Coll Cardiol.* 2014;64:2743-2749.

99. Clark AL, Fonarow GC, Horwich TB. Impact of cardiorespiratory fitness on the obesity paradox in patients with systolic heart failure. *Am J Cardiol.* 2015;115:209-213.

100. Wing RR, Lang W, Wadden TA, et al; Look AHEAD Research Group. Benefits of modest weight loss in improving cardiovascular risk factors in overweight and obese individuals with type 2 diabetes. *Diabetes Care.* 2011;34:1481-1486.

101. Douketis JD, Macie C, Thabane L, Williamson DF. Systematic review of long-term weight loss studies in obese adults: clinical significance and applicability to clinical practice. *Int J Obes Relat Metab Disord.* 2005;29:1153-1167.

102. Rider OJ, Francis JM, Ali MK, et al. Beneficial cardiovascular effects of bariatric surgical and dietary weight loss in obesity. *J Am Coll Cardiol.* 2009;54:718-726.

103. Stalonas PM, Perri MG, Kerzner AB. Do behavioral treatments of obesity last? A five-year follow-up investigation. *Addict Behav.* 1984;9:175-183.

104. Tuah NA, Amiel C, Qureshi S, Car J, Kaur B, Majeed A. Transtheoretical model for dietary and physical exercise modification in weight loss management for overweight and obese adults. *Cochrane Database Syst Rev.* 2011:CD008066.

105. Artinian NT, Fletcher GF, Mozaffarian D, et al; American Heart Association Prevention Committee of the Council on Cardiovascular Nursing. Interventions to promote physical activity and dietary lifestyle changes for cardiovascular risk factor reduction in adults: a scientific statement from the American Heart Association. *Circulation.* 2010;122:406-441.

106. The Look AHEAD Research Group. Cardiovascular effects of intensive lifestyle intervention in type 2 diabetes. *N Engl J Med.* 2013;369:145-154.

107. Watts GF, Lewis B, Brunt JN, et al. Effects on coronary artery disease of lipid-lowering diet, or diet plus cholestyramine, in the St Thomas' Atherosclerosis Regression Study (STARS). *Lancet.* 1992;339:563-569.

108. Haskell WL, Alderman EL, Fair JM, et al. Effects of intensive multiple risk factor reduction on coronary atherosclerosis and clinical cardiac events in men and women with coronary artery disease. The Stanford Coronary Risk Intervention Project (SCRIP). *Circulation.* 1994;89:975-990.

109. Singh RB, Dubnov G, Niaz MA, et al. Effect of an Indo-Mediterranean diet on progression of coronary artery disease in high risk patients (Indo-Mediterranean Diet Heart Study): a randomised single-blind trial. *Lancet.* 2002;360:1455-1461.

110. Shai I, Spence JD, Schwarzfuchs D, et al; DIRECT Group. Dietary intervention to reverse carotid atherosclerosis. *Circulation.* 2010;121:1200-1208.

111. Harris WS, Mozaffarian D, Rimm E, et al. Omega-6 fatty acids and risk for cardiovascular disease: a science advisory from the American Heart Association Nutrition Subcommittee of the Council on Nutrition, Physical Activity, and Metabolism; Council on Cardiovascular Nursing; and Council on Epidemiology and Prevention. *Circulation.* 2009;119:902-907.

112. Ramsden CE, Zamora D, Leelarthaepin B, et al. Use of dietary linoleic acid for secondary prevention of coronary heart disease and death: evaluation of recovered data from the Sydney Diet Heart Study and updated meta-analysis. *BMJ.* 2013;346:e8707.

113. Mozaffarian D, Micha R, Wallace S. Effects on coronary heart disease of increasing polyunsaturated fat in place of saturated fat: a systematic review and meta-analysis of randomized controlled trials. *PLoS Med.* 2010;7:e1000252.

114. Mozaffarian D. Dietary and policy priorities for cardiovascular disease, diabetes, and obesity: a comprehensive review. *Circulation.* 2016;133:187-225.

115. Anker SD, Ponikowski P, Varney S, et al. Wasting as independent risk factor for mortality in chronic heart failure. *Lancet.* 1997;349:1050-1053.

116. Fülster S, Tacke M, Sandek A, et al. Muscle wasting in patients with chronic heart failure: results from the studies investigating co-morbidities aggravating heart failure (SICA-HF). *Eur Heart J.* 2013;34:512-519.

117. Afsarmanesh N, Horwich TB, Fonarow GC. Total cholesterol levels and mortality risk in nonischemic systolic heart failure. *Am Heart J.* 2006;152:1077-1083.

118. Greene SJ, Vaduganathan M, Lupi L, et al; EVEREST Trial Investigators. Prognostic significance of serum total cholesterol and triglyceride levels in patients hospitalized for heart failure with reduced ejection fraction (from the EVEREST Trial). *Am J Cardiol.* 2013;111:574-581.

119. Horwich TB, Kalantar-Zadeh K, MacLellan RW, Fonarow GC. Albumin levels predict survival in patients with systolic heart failure. *Am Heart J.* 2008;155:883-889.

120. Lemon SC, Olendzki B, Magner R, et al. The dietary quality of persons with heart failure in NHANES 1999-2006. *J Gen Intern Med.* 2010;25:135-140.

121. Witte KKA, Nikitin NP, Parker AC, et al. The effect of micronutrient supplementation on quality-of-life and left ventricular function in elderly patients with chronic heart failure. *Eur Heart J.* 2005;26:2238-2244.

122. Abshire M, Xu J, Baptiste D, et al. Nutritional interventions in heart failure: a systematic review of the literature. *J Card Fail.* 2015;21:989-999.

123. McKeag NA, McKinley MC, Harbinson MT, et al. The effect of multiple micronutrient supplementation on left ventricular ejection fraction in patients with chronic stable heart failure: a randomized, placebo-controlled trial. *JACC Heart Fail.* 2014;2:308-317.

124. GISSI-HF Investigators; Tavazzi L, Maggioni AP, Marchioli R, et al. Effect of n-3 polyunsaturated fatty acids in patients with chronic heart failure (the GISSI-HF trial): a randomised, double-blind, placebo-controlled trial. *Lancet.* 2008;372:1223-1230.

125. Lennie TA, Chung ML, Habash DL, Moser DK. Dietary fat intake and proinflammatory cytokine levels in patients with heart failure. *J Card Fail.* 2005;11:613-618.

126. Colin-Ramirez E, Castillo-Martinez L, Orea-Tejeda A, Zheng Y, Westerhout CM, Ezekowitz JA. Dietary fatty acids intake and mortality in patients with heart failure. *Nutrition.* 2014;30:1366-1371.

127. Pritchett AM, Deswal A, Aguilar D, et al. Lifestyle modification with diet and exercise in obese patients with heart failure—a pilot study. *J Obes Weight Loss Ther.* 2012;2:1-8.

128. Evangelista LS, Heber D, Li Z, Bowerman S, Hamilton MA, Fonarow GC. Reduced body weight and adiposity with a high-protein diet improves functional status, lipid profiles, glycemic control, and quality of life in patients with heart failure: a feasibility study. *J Cardiovasc Nurs.* 2009;24:207.

129. Ritzel A, Otto F, Bell M, Sabin G, Wieneke H. Impact of lifestyle modification on left ventricular function and cardiopulmonary exercise capacity in patients with heart failure with normal ejection fraction and cardiometabolic syndrome: a prospective interventional study. *Acta Cardiol.* 2015;70:43-50.

130. Kitzman DW, Brubaker P, Morgan T, et al. Effect of caloric restriction or aerobic exercise training on peak oxygen consumption and quality of life in obese older patients with heart failure with preserved ejection fraction: a randomized clinical trial. *JAMA.* 2016;315:36-46.

131. O'Connor CM, Whellan DJ, Lee KL, et al; Investigators FTH-A. Efficacy and safety of exercise training in patients with chronic heart failure: HF-action randomized controlled trial. *JAMA.* 2009;301:1439-1450.

132. Flynn KE, Piña IL, Whellan DJ, et al; HF-ACTION Investigators. Effects of exercise training on health status in patients with chronic heart failure: HF-action randomized controlled trial. *JAMA.* 2009;301:1451-1459.

133. Yancy CW, Jessup M, Bozkurt B, et al. 2013 ACCF/AHA guideline for the management of heart failure: a report of the American College of Cardiology Foundation/American Heart Association task force on practice guidelines. *Circulation.* 2013;128:e240-e327.

134. Li Z, Maglione M, Tu W, et al. Meta-analysis: pharmacologic treatment of obesity. *Ann Intern Med.* 2005;142:532-546.

135. Wadden TA, Berkowitz RI, Womble LG, et al. Randomized trial of lifestyle modification and pharmacotherapy for obesity. *N Engl J Med.* 2005;353:2111-2120.

136. Apovian CM, Aronne LJ, Bessesen DH, et al. Pharmacological management of obesity: an endocrine society clinical practice guideline. *J Clin Endocrinol Metab.* 2015;100:342-362.

137. Bray GA, Ryan DH. Medical therapy for the patient with obesity. *Circulation.* 2012;125:1695-1703.

138. Rucker D, Padwal R, Li S, Curioni C, Lau DCW. Long term pharmacotherapy for obesity and overweight: updated meta-analysis. *BMJ.* 2007;335:1194-1199.

139. Torgerson JS, Hauptman J, Boldrin MN, Sjöström L. XENical in the prevention of diabetes in obese subjects (XENDOS) study: a randomized study of orlistat as an adjunct to lifestyle changes for the prevention of type 2 diabetes in obese patients. *Diabetes Care.* 2004;27:155-161.

140. Miles JM, Leiter L, Hollander P, et al. Effect of orlistat in overweight and obese patients with type 2 diabetes treated with metformin. *Diabetes Care.* 2002;25:1123-1128.

141. Beck-da-Silva L, Higginson L, Fraser M, Williams K, Haddad H. Effect of orlistat in obese patients with heart failure: a pilot study. *Congest Heart Fail.* 2005;11:118-123.

142. Smith SR, Weissman NJ, Anderson CM, et al. Multicenter, placebo-controlled trial of lorcaserin for weight management. *N Engl J Med.* 2010;363:245-256.

143. Bays HE. Lorcaserin and adiposopathy: 5-HT2c agonism as a treatment for "sick fat" and metabolic disease. *Expert Rev Cardiovasc Ther.* 2009;7:1429-1445.

144. Fidler MC, Sanchez M, Raether B, et al; BLOSSOM Clinical Trial Group. A one-year randomized trial of lorcaserin for weight loss in obese and overweight adults: the BLOSSOM trial. *J Clin Endocrinol Metab.* 2011;96:3067-3077.

145. Gadde KM, Allison DB, Ryan DH, et al. Effects of low-dose, controlled-release, phentermine plus topiramate combination

on weight and associated comorbidities in overweight and obese adults (CONQUER): a randomised, placebo-controlled, phase 3 trial. *Lancet.* 2011;377:1341-1352.

146. Allison DB, Gadde KM, Garvey WT, et al. Controlled-release phentermine/topiramate in severely obese adults: a randomized controlled trial (EQUIP). *Obesity.* 2012;20:330-342.

147. Greenway FL, Dunayevich E, Tollefson G, et al; NB-201 Study Group. Comparison of combined bupropion and naltrexone therapy for obesity with monotherapy and placebo. *J Clin Endocrinol Metab.* 2009;94:4898-4906.

148. Apovian CM, Aronne L, Rubino D, et al; COR-II Study Group. A randomized, phase 3 trial of naltrexone SR/bupropion SR on weight and obesity-related risk factors (COR-II). *Obesity.* 2013;21:935-943.

149. Nissen SE, Wolski KE, Prcela L, et al. Effect of naltrexone-bupropion on major adverse cardiovascular events in overweight and obese patients with cardiovascular risk factors. *JAMA Intern Med.* 2016;315:990-1004.

150. Buchwald H, Avidor Y, Braunwald E, et al. Bariatric surgery. *JAMA.* 2004;292:1724-1737.

151. Schauer PR, Kashyap SR, Wolski K, et al. Bariatric surgery versus intensive medical therapy in obese patients with diabetes. *N Engl J Med.* 2012;366:1577-1585.

152. Flum DR, Dellinger EP. Impact of gastric bypass operation on survival: a population-based analysis. *J Am Coll Surg.* 2004;199:543-551.

153. Adams TD, Gress RE, Smith SC, et al. Long-term mortality after gastric bypass surgery. *N Engl J Med.* 2007;357:753-761.

154. Busetto L, Sergi G, Enzi G, et al. Short-term effects of weight loss on the cardiovascular risk factors in morbidly obese patients. *Obesity.* 2004;12:1256-1263.

155. Kopp HP. Impact of weight loss on inflammatory proteins and their association with the insulin resistance syndrome in morbidly obese patients. *Arterioscl Throm Vas.* 2003;23:1042-1047.

156. Luaces M, Cachofeiro V, García-Muñoz-Najar A, et al. Anatomical and functional alterations of the heart in morbid obesity. Changes after bariatric surgery. *Rev Esp Cardiol.* 2012;65:14-21.

157. Woelnerhanssen B, Peterli R, Steinert RE, Peters T, Borbély Y, Beglinger C. Effects of postbariatric surgery weight loss on adipokines and metabolic parameters: comparison of laparoscopic Roux-en-Y gastric bypass and laparoscopic sleeve gastrectomy—a prospective randomized trial. *Surg Obes Relat Dis.* 2011;7:561-568.

158. Leichman JG, Aguilar D, King TM, et al. Improvements in systemic metabolism, anthropometrics, and left ventricular geometry 3 months after bariatric surgery. *Surg Obes Relat Dis.* 2006;2:592-599.

159. Ikonomidis I, Mazarakis A, Papadopoulos C, et al. Weight loss after bariatric surgery improves aortic elastic properties and left ventricular function in individuals with morbid obesity: a 3-year follow-up study. *J Hypertens.* 2007;25:439-447.

160. Willens HJ, Chakko SC, Byers P, et al. Effects of weight loss after gastric bypass on right and left ventricular function assessed by tissue Doppler imaging. *Am J Cardiol.* 2005;95:1521-1524.

161. Garza CA, Pellikka PA, Somers VK, et al. Structural and functional changes in left and right ventricles after major weight loss following bariatric surgery for morbid obesity. *Am J Cardiol.* 2010;105:550-556.

162. Shah RV, Murthy VL, Abbasi SA, et al. Weight loss and progressive left ventricular remodelling: the multi-ethnic study of atherosclerosis (MESA). *Eur J Prev Cardiol.* 2015;22:1408-1418.

163. Leichman J, Wilson E, Scarborough T, et al. Dramatic reversal of derangements in muscle metabolism and left ventricular function after bariatric surgery. *Am J Med.* 2008;121:966-973.

164. Kanoupakis E, Michaloudis D, Fraidakis O, Parthenakis F, Vardas P, Melissas J. Left ventricular function and cardiopulmonary performance following surgical treatment of morbid obesity. *Obes Surg.* 2001;11:552-558.

165. Di Bello V, Santini F, Di Cori A, et al. Effects of bariatric surgery on early myocardial alterations in adult severely obese subjects. *Cardiology.* 2008;109:241-248.

166. Koshino Y, Villarraga HR, Somers VK, et al. Changes in myocardial mechanics in patients with obesity following major weight loss after bariatric surgery. *Obesity.* 2013;21:1111-1118.

167. Kaier TE, Morgan D, Grapsa J, et al. Ventricular remodelling post-bariatric surgery: is the type of surgery relevant? A prospective study with 3D speckle tracking. *Eur Heart J Cardiovasc Imaging.* 2014;15:1256-1262.

168. Benotti PN, Wood GC, Carey DJ, et al. Bypass surgery produces a durable reduction in cardiovascular disease risk factors and reduces the long-term risks of congestive heart failure. *J Am Heart Assoc.* 2017;6.

169. Persson CE, Björck L, Lagergren J, Lappas G, Giang KW, Rosengren A. Risk of heart failure in obese patients with and without bariatric surgery in Sweden—a Registry-Based Study. *J Card Fail.* 2017;23:530-537.

170. Sundström J, Bruze G, Ottosson J, Marcus C, Näslund I, Neovius M. Weight loss and heart failure: a nationwide study of gastric bypass surgery versus intensive lifestyle treatment. *Circulation.* 2017;135:1577-1585.

171. Zuber M, Kaeslin T, Studer T, Erne P. Weight loss of 146 kg with diet and reversal of severe congestive heart failure in a young, morbidly obese patient. *Am J Cardiol.* 1999;84:955-956.

172. Iyengar S, Leier C. Rescue bariatric surgery for obesity-induced cardiomyopathy. *Am J Med.* 2006;119:e5-e6.

173. Ristow B, Rabkin J, Haeusslein E. Improvement in dilated cardiomyopathy after bariatric surgery. *J Card Fail.* 2008;14:198-202.

174. Alpert MA, Terry BE, Kelly DL. Effect of weight loss on cardiac chamber size, wall thickness and left ventricular function in morbid obesity. *Am J Cardiol.* 1985;55:783-786.

175. Alpert MA, Terry BE, Mulekar M, Cohen MV, Massey CV, Fan TM. Cardiac morphology and left ventricular function in normotensive morbidly obese patients with and without congestive heart failure, and effect of weight loss. *Am J Cardiol.* 1997;80:736-740.

176. McCloskey CA, Ramani GV, Mathier MA, et al. Bariatric surgery improves cardiac function in morbidly obese patients with severe cardiomyopathy. *Surg Obes Relat Dis.* 2007;3:503-507.

177. Ramani GV, McCloskey C, Ramanathan RC, Mathier MA. Safety and efficacy of bariatric surgery in morbidly obese patients with severe systolic heart failure. *Clin Cardiol.* 2008;31:516-520.

178. Alsabrook GD, Goodman HR, Alexander JW. Gastric bypass for morbidly obese patients with established cardiac disease. *Obes Surg.* 2006;16:1272-1277.

179. Wikiel KJ, McCloskey CA, Ramanathan RC. Bariatric surgery: a safe and effective conduit to cardiac transplantation. *Surg Obes Relat Dis.* 2014;10:479-484.

180. Lim C-P, Fisher OM, Falkenback D, et al. Bariatric surgery provides a "bridge to transplant" for morbidly obese patients with advanced heart failure and may obviate the need for transplantation. *Obes Surg.* 2016;26:486-493.

181. Vest AR, Patel P, Schauer PR, et al. Clinical and echocardiographic outcomes after bariatric surgery in obese patients with left ventricular systolic dysfunction. *Circulation: Heart Failure.* March 2016 [epub ahead of print].

182. Shimada YJ, Tsugawa Y, Brown DFM, Hasegawa K. Bariatric surgery and emergency department visits and hospitalizations for heart failure exacerbation: population-based, self-controlled series. *J Am Coll Cardiol.* 2015;67:895-903.

5 GENETIC TESTING FOR CARDIOMYOPATHY

Amy C. Sturm, MS, LCGC
Ray Hershberger, MD

PATIENT CASE

A 36-year-old Caucasian woman was referred to the Cardiovascular Genetic and Genomic Medicine Clinic for genetic evaluation due to her diagnosis of idiopathic dilated cardiomyopathy (DCM) at 31 years of age. At that time she had presented emergently to cardiology care in advanced heart failure (HF) having had progressive dyspnea on exertion for several weeks. There was no known trigger to her symptom onset. Her echocardiogram revealed a left ventricular end-diastolic dimension (LVEDD) of 7.2 cm and a left ventricular ejection fraction (LVEF) of 10% to 15%. She underwent cardiac magnetic resonance imaging, which showed a dilated left ventricle, severe global hypokinesis, LVEF of 19%, biatrial enlargement, minimal midwall fibrosis with gadolinium enhancement, and no iron overload. She underwent emergent ventricular assist device (VAD) placement, was treated medically, and improved to the point where her VAD was explanted 1 year later. Since her VAD explant, she has continued with full medical therapy and has received close cardiovascular surveillance with her HF cardiologist. An implantable cardioverter defibrillator (ICD), placed after her VAD was removed, has delivered no shocks. A follow-up echocardiogram revealed an LVEDD of 5.8 cm with a LVEF of 30% to 35%.

During the Cardiovascular Genetic and Genomic Medicine Clinic appointment, which included consultation with a HF/heart transplant cardiologist with genetics expertise and a genetic counselor in a multidisciplinary team approach, the genetic counselor constructed a 4-generation pedigree for the proband, the person who serves as the starting point for the genetic evaluation of a family (Figure 5-1). The family history was significant for nonischemic cardiomyopathy (NICM) and heart transplant in a maternal first cousin once removed. A paternal grandfather was reported who died suddenly at 49 years of age. The proband's father and mother were 62 years of age with no reported heart disease. The proband also had 3 siblings, none of whom had undergone cardiovascular screening to date. She also had multiple nieces and nephews. No other relatives were reported with a concerning history.

Genetic testing was discussed with the patient as a useful tool to investigate the underlying etiology of her cardiomyopathy. She had been assigned the diagnosis of idiopathic DCM, acknowledging that no plausible cause had been found. Also informing this discussion was the proband's severe DCM at a young age of onset, and her remote family history of NICM requiring transplant, as well as sudden death in her paternal grandfather. Informed consent was obtained and a blood sample was collected for genetic testing. A comprehensive cardiomyopathy genetic testing panel was ordered that included sequence analysis and deletion/duplication testing of more than 70 genes known to be associated with different types of cardiomyopathy.

The patient tested positive for three variants (Table 5-1). These included a novel, likely pathogenic variant in *TNNC1*, a gene known to be relevant for DCM; a previously reported pathogenic/likely pathogenic variant in *MYBPC3*, a well-established hypertrophic cardiomyopathy (HCM) gene with this specific variant having been identified in HCM patients; and a novel variant of unknown significance (VUS) in *LAMA4*. The genetic testing results were discussed and interpreted by the cardiovascular genetics and genomics team. This thorough assessment included critical review of the available data on each variant, starting with the level of evidence for whether the gene itself has strong, or limited, evidence for association with the patient's phenotype. Specifically, pathogenic variants in *MYBPC3* are a common cause of HCM; however, the role of *MYBPC3* variants in DCM is uncertain and still evolving. At the variant level, the adjudication included whether the variant had previously been reported in the scientific literature, whether it segregated with a cardiomyopathy phenotype, the minor allele frequency of each variant in large databases, as well as whether each variant had a ClinVar entry. The ClinVar entry for the previously reported *MYBPC3* variant stated that it has been reported in 4 individuals with HCM tested across 4 studies, and that it has been identified in 3 probands with HCM and 2 affected relatives tested by 1 large commercial genetic-testing laboratory. It had also been reported in both a proband and an unaffected parent, suggesting incomplete penetrance.[1]

The genetic counselor telephoned the proband to inform her of the results and to present the following plan: (1) Recommend clinical cardiology screening to all first-degree relatives (her parents and siblings). (2) Recommend parental genetic testing for the genetic variants identified in the proband to determine whether they were inherited from 1 parent, both parents, or whether 1 or more were de novo (arose new in the patient).

When the genetic counselor called the proband with her results, remarkably, the proband informed the genetic counselor that her older sister had just been diagnosed with peripartum cardiomyopathy (PPCM). In addition, her father, being prompted by the proband's questioning of possible family history of heart disease for her initial genetics appointment, had recognized that he had been having shortness of breath, fatigue, and pretibial and pedal edema. He informed his primary care physician, who ordered an echocardiogram that showed a reduced LVEF of 25%. Based on this new family history information, the cardiovascular genetics team modified their recommendations to also include full panel cardiomyopathy genetic testing for the sister with PPCM in order to determine whether she had the same variants as the proband, and/or additional variants that may be underlying her PPCM. The

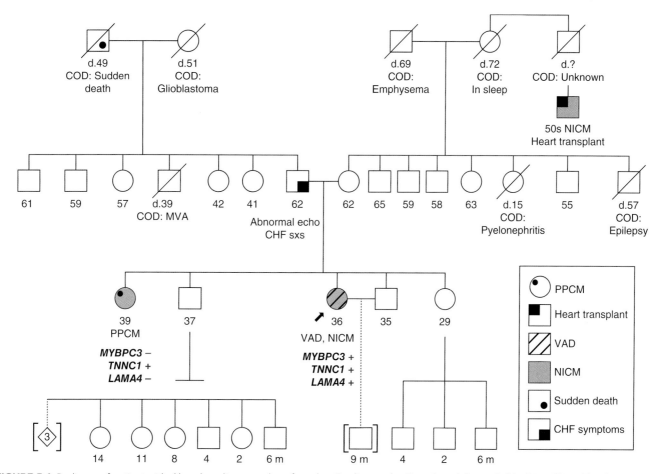

FIGURE 5-1 Pedigree of patient with dilated cardiomyopathy referred to Cardiovascular Genetic and Genomic Medicine Clinic. This 4-generation pedigree utilizes standard pedigree symbols (men are represented by squares; women are represented by circles). The pedigree was constructed by the genetic counselor during the proband's first appointment in the clinic. An arrow points to the proband. A symbol key can be found in the lower right hand corner. The genetic testing results can be found under the proband and her affected sister with PPCM.

Table 5-1 Variants Identified in Proband with Dilated Cardiomyopathy via Cardiomyopathy Panel Clinical Genetic Testing

Gene	cDNA Change	Amino Acid Change/Protein Effect	Minor Allele Frequency[+]	CLIA Lab Interpretation	ClinVar Entry's Clinical Significance
MYBPC3*	c.26-2A>G	IVS1-2A>G	0.005%	Pathogenic	Pathogenic/Likely pathogenic
TNNC1^	c.446A>G	Asp149Gly	Novel (not present in ExAC)	Likely pathogenic	Likely pathogenic
LAMA4~	c.4624A>T	Asn1542Tyr	Novel (not present in ExAC)	Variant of uncertain significance	Variant of uncertain significance

*Reported previously in association with hypertrophic cardiomyopathy; destroys canonical splice acceptor site.

^Novel variant; nonconservative amino acid substitution; conserved position; missense variants in nearby residues have been reported in the Human Gene Mutation Database (HGMD) in association with cardiomyopathy (CMP) (E134D, D145E, I148V).

~Novel variant; semiconservative amino acid substitution; position not well conserved; no nearby variants reported in HGMD in association with CMP.

[+]MAF data from ExAC, the Exome Aggregation Consortium (http://exac.broadinstitute.org/).

sister presented to the clinic, underwent full evaluation, including genetic testing, and was also found to have the novel *TNNC1* variant, not the *MYBPC3* or *LAMA4* variants, and no additional variants. We hypothesize that the *MYBPC3* variant, established as a cause of HCM, may have modified the pathogenicity of the *TNNC1* variant. This may explain the dramatic variability of severity of onset between the 2 sisters, 1 with only the *TNNC1* variant identified, and the other with the *TNNC1* variant in addition to 2 other potentially associated variants.

These additional genetic data allowed us to determine that the proband's *TNNC1* variant was almost certainly inherited from 1 of her parents, because both the proband and her sister with PPCM were found to have this same *TNNC1* variant. Referrals were made for the sister's 6 at-risk children to the local children's hospital's cardiac genetics clinic for both clinical cardiology screening and targeted genetic testing for the *TNNC1* variant. It was also recommended that both of the sisters' parents undergo genetic evaluation, including targeted genetic testing, in order to determine which parent had the *TNNC1* variant, and whether the other 2 variants identified in the proband were inherited from 1 parent, both parents, or were de novo. It is possible that this pedigree represents bilineal inheritance, meaning that the proband inherited cardiomyopathy-predisposing genetic variants from each of her parents that contributed to her phenotype. Parental testing is also indicated to determine whether 1, or both, of her parents may also have underlying genetic predispositions to cardiomyopathy, and in turn, whether the proband's paternal, maternal, or both sides of her family may also be at risk.

CASE COMMENTARY

The heritable cardiomyopathies are relatively common conditions that can lead to HF and sudden cardiac death (SCD). DCM may be the most common heritable cardiomyopathy, estimated to occur in 1 in 250 individuals,[2] and HCM occurs in 1 in 500 individuals.[3] Research discoveries and rapidly dropping costs of DNA sequencing technologies have resulted in the availability of multiple cardiomyopathy genetic testing panels.[4] Genetic testing not only helps in determining the underlying etiology of idiopathic and familial cardiomyopathies, but is also a powerful tool in the determination of which relatives may be at risk, or not, in the preclinical phase. Both pretest and posttest genetic counseling are imperative components of genetic testing, as the many benefits and limitations of genetic testing need to be discussed with each patient undergoing this process.

Position and international consensus statements, as well as practice guidelines, regarding genetic evaluation, including genetic testing and counseling of cardiomyopathy patients, have been published.[5-7] The Heart Failure Society of America practice guideline on genetic evaluation of cardiomyopathy recommends: (1) a careful family history for ≥ 3 generations for all patients with cardiomyopathy; (2) clinical screening for cardiomyopathy in asymptomatic first-degree relatives; (3) genetic and family counseling for all patients and families with cardiomyopathy; and (4) consideration of referral to centers with expertise in the complex processes of genetic evaluation, genetic counseling, genetic testing, and family-based management.[5]

The multidisciplinary clinical cardiovascular genetics evaluation for the proband and her family in the above case presentation resulted in the following:

1. Confirmation of a familial cardiomyopathy with an underlying, identifiable, genetic etiology;

2. Determination that the proband's DCM may be due to bilineal inheritance of multiple variants inherited from both her father and mother;

3. Diagnosis of at-risk relatives with cardiomyopathy;

4. Determination of additional at-risk relatives' risk status through both clinical screening and cascade, family-specific genetic testing;

5. Receipt of information regarding the inheritance pattern of the variants predisposing to familial cardiomyopathy and recurrence risk;

6. Provision of counseling regarding future reproductive options; and

7. Receipt of psychosocial support and resources.

OVERVIEW OF GENETIC CARDIOMYOPATHIES

Genetic forms of cardiomyopathy are often the cause of unexplained, or idiopathic, cardiomyopathy that may lead to HF or SCD. For any cardiomyopathy deemed to be of unknown cause, a genetic basis should always be considered. The types of genetic, or inherited, cardiomyopathies most commonly encountered in the clinical setting include DCM, HCM, and less commonly, arrhythmogenic right ventricular cardiomyopathy (ARVC) and restrictive cardiomyopathy (RCM). Left ventricular noncompaction (LVNC), named as a primary cardiomyopathy by a U.S. consensus panel,[8] was not considered a cardiomyopathy by a European panel as it is a developmental variant observed in all cardiomyopathies and other cardiovascular conditions.[9] Because of improved cardiovascular imaging methods, particularly cardiac magnetic resonance (CMR) imaging, LVNC is now more commonly identified and referred to for genetic evaluation. Whether LVNC drives increased risk for development of cardiomyopathy remains unanswered.

The genetic variants predisposing to the various types of familial cardiomyopathies are usually inherited in an autosomal-dominant Mendelian pattern and display both variable expressivity and age-related penetrance. The term *penetrance* defines whether any evidence of the clinical phenotype is discernable, whereas *variable expressivity* refers to the degree, variability, and/or severity of the clinical phenotype.[2]

The genetic cardiomyopathies have had many genes (termed *locus heterogeneity*) identified in causing disease, and in most genes multiple different pathogenic variants have been implicated (termed *allelic heterogeneity*).[6,10] There is also significant genetic overlap between the different cardiomyopathy phenotypes, both with each other, and with other heritable cardiovascular conditions

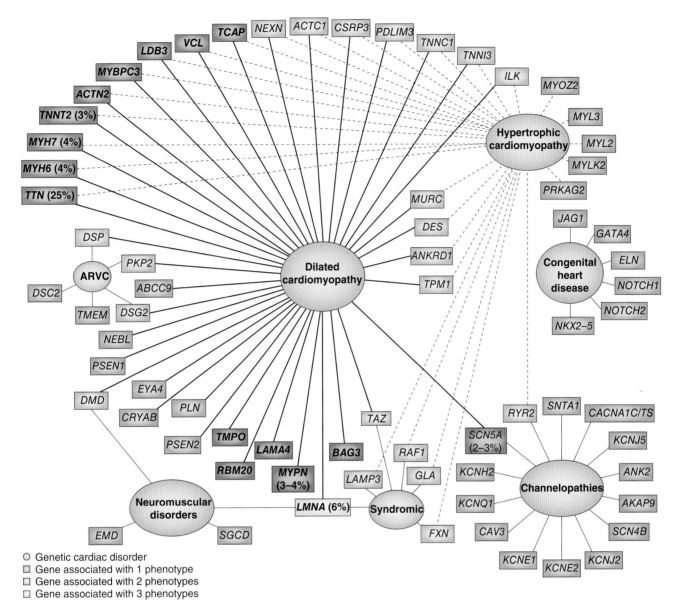

FIGURE 5-2 Relationships between genes associated with cardiomyopathies and related phenotypes. The genetic architecture underlying selected genetic cardiac disorders is shown. Edges (lines) connect each phenotype to the genes that have been implicated in the etiology. Gene nodes associated with familial dilated cardiomyopathy are darker and have bold text if they have been found to cause disease in ≥ 1% of patients, and include frequency information if they have been found to cause disease in ≥ 3% of patients. Abbreviation: ARVC, arrhythmogenic right ventricular cardiomyopathy. (Reproduced, with permission, from Hershberger RE, Jedges DJ, Morales A. Dilated cardiomyopathy: the complexity of a diverse genetic architecture. *Nat Rev Cardiol.* 2013;10(9):531-547.)

including channelopathies, congenital heart disease, and neuromuscular disorders (Figure 5-2).[2] For example, pathogenic variants in genes encoding sarcomere proteins have been shown to be associated with variable presentations of cardiomyopathy, including hypertrophic, dilated, restrictive, and left ventricular noncompaction phenotypes.[11-13] Most families have their own unique, pathogenic variant(s), colloquially labeled "private," meaning that they have never been reported in the publicly available databases or in the research literature, which can lead to difficulty in genetic variant interpretation due to lack of data on multiple probands and families with the same variant.

The heritable cardiomyopathies (DCM, HCM, ARVC, RCM) are in most cases nonsyndromic, that is, they exhibit clinical features that are specific to myocardial structure and function (eg, dilatation, hypertrophy). However, syndromic forms of cardiomyopathy also exist, and it is imperative to diagnose these syndromic conditions because of the important implications for therapeutics (eg, enzyme replacement therapy in Fabry disease, which can masquerade as HCM) as well as differences in inheritance patterns and risk to family members (eg, women with DCM due to mutations in the X-linked *DMD* gene associated with Duchenne and Becker muscular dystrophies). The syndromic forms of cardiomyopathy have been discussed in detail.[14-16] Nonsyndromic DCM, HCM, and ARVC will be discussed below.

DILATED CARDIOMYOPATHY (DCM)

Idiopathic DCM is the most common condition that leads to cardiac transplantation in the United States. Idiopathic DCM is characterized by left ventricular dilatation and systolic dysfunction, with the most common underlying etiologies excluded, including most importantly coronary artery disease, and other causes such as toxin exposure, iron overload, infectious causes such as Chagas disease, and infiltrative disease.[17] Familial DCM can be assigned when 2 or more closely related family members have met stringent criteria for idiopathic DCM diagnoses, or when a first-degree relative of a DCM patient has had unexplained sudden death at 35 years of age or younger.[18] Regarding "apparently sporadic" idiopathic DCM, the true extent of its genetic etiology is uncertain, as family history is often insensitive and affected family members can be asymptomatic and remain undiagnosed unless clinical evaluation commences.[17] Furthermore, prior large clinical series searching for familial DCM by clinically screening large cohorts of family members have not provided comprehensive genetic information. Clinical screening of first-degree relatives of patients with idiopathic DCM revealed familial disease ranging from 20% to 35%.[2,18,19] Family-based DCM studies have implicated genetic etiology with mutations in more than 30 genes of diverse ontology including those encoding the sarcomere, components of the cytoskeleton, ion channels, and others.[2,18,20-22] The current clinical sensitivity of DCM genetic testing reaches approximately 40%,[23] with truncating variants of *TTN* estimated to account for 15% to 25% of familial DCM.[24-26] Variants of uncertain significance are identified in a high percentage of cases.[23]

HYPERTROPHIC CARDIOMYOPATHY (HCM)

HCM is characterized by left ventricular hypertrophy (LVH), myocyte disarray, and fibrosis and has a prevalence of approximately 1 in 500 individuals in the general population.[3] Cardiac sarcomere mutations are identified in approximately 50% of HCM patients with a family history of HCM and in approximately 30% of unselected probands.[27] The majority of cases are due to mutations in the cardiac myosin-binding protein C (*MYBPC3*) and beta-myosin heavy chain (*MYH7*) genes, with more than 15 additional genes identified as rare causes of this condition.[10,27] Similar to DCM, there is a high level of variability of HCM disease expression observed in families; a large cohort study of families with *MYBPC3* mutations[1] found ages at diagnosis ranging from 5 to 80 years, all morphological variants of HCM observed, as well as a significant degree of incomplete penetrance. These findings stress the

importance of the role of additional genetic, epigenetic, and environmental modifiers in the pathogenesis of the HCM phenotype within and between families and also highlight our current inability to provide specific prognostic information to family members who test positive for an HCM-predisposing variant.

ARRHYTHMOGENIC RIGHT VENTRICULAR CARDIOMYOPATHY (ARVC)

The prevalence of ARVC is estimated to be 1 in 1000 to 2000, with >50% of cases being familial.[28] Although ARVC itself is rare, ARVC commonly presents with arrhythmia, presyncope, syncope, or SCD in young adults (≤35 years), although it may also present in later life.[29] The diagnosis of ARVC is made in patients who meet major and minor diagnostic Task Force criteria, revised in 2010.[30] In addition to an arrhythmia presentation, classic manifestations include characteristic electrocardiographic parameters, fibrofatty replacement of the right ventricle, and right ventricular enlargement and dysfunction. Structurally, ARVC is classically described as a disease of the desmosome, the cellular structure for cell-to-cell adhesion and electrophysical communication, which is especially essential in the myocardium. However, both desmosomal and more rarely, nondesmosomal, gene variants have been found in association with ARVC.[29] Left-dominant and biventricular subtypes have also been described and molecularly classified.[31] The yield of genetic testing in probands meeting revised Task Force criteria has been shown to be approximately 50%, with more than 1 desmosomal variant identified in 28% of probands; relatives harboring more than 1 desmosomal variant had a 5-fold increased risk of developing ARVC clinical signs and symptoms.[32]

CARDIOVASCULAR GENETIC AND GENOMIC EVALUATION BEGINS WITH FAMILY HISTORY COLLECTION AND ASSESSMENT

It is recommended that a careful family history for at least 3 generations be taken on all patients with cardiomyopathy.[5,18] Guidelines regarding the collection of family history information in the cardiovascular medicine setting exist.[33] Collection of family history is imperative in aiding diagnosis, identifying at-risk relatives, selecting the most informative family member for genetic testing initiation, and determining inheritance pattern.

While most genetic risk variants predisposing to cardiomyopathies are inherited in an autosomal-dominant pattern, there are important exceptions and this information is necessary for the provision of accurate recurrence risks. Also complicating matters is the fact that many inherited cardiomyopathies display both incomplete and age-related penetrance and variable expressivity of clinical signs and symptoms. Small, or limited, family structures may also mask a genetic pattern of disease (eg, smaller sibships including only children may limit the number of affected individuals in the family, higher number of female relatives in a family can hide an X-linked disease). Because patients' self-reported family history information can have both reduced sensitivity and specificity, it is important to collect medical records, including autopsy reports, whenever possible so that diagnoses can be confirmed. In many cases, it is not until clinical screening commences through a family that a familial, or genetic, condition is able to be diagnosed.[34] Also, family history is not static, but changes over time, and should therefore be updated periodically.

CLINICAL GENETIC TESTING FOR CARDIOMYOPATHY

Technological advances and cardiovascular genetics research discoveries have steadily and rapidly increased the number of clinically available genetic testing options for patients and their families with heritable heart diseases, including the cardiomyopathies.[4] As discussed, due to the dramatic locus and allelic heterogeneities, as well as genetic overlap between phenotypes, clinical genetic testing for cardiomyopathy necessitates both (1) sequencing the entire coding region as well as intron/exon boundaries of large numbers of genes, and (2) the presence of certain genes on more than 1 phenotype-specific genetic testing panel (ie, *MYH7* should be present on HCM, DCM, and comprehensive cardiomyopathy clinical genetic testing panels). Most clinical genetic testing is conducted by ordering multigene DNA sequencing panels developed by commercial genetic testing laboratories. Most genetic testing platforms utilize next-generation sequencing (NGS) technologies, which allow for faster, more comprehensive, and cost-efficient analysis of many genes at the same time from one patient specimen.[35] While many large cardiomyopathy genetic testing panels are now commercially available, expanded gene panels have not substantively increased clinical sensitivity for HCM.[27] While clinical sensitivity has increased for DCM with larger gene panels, so has the number of inconclusive results finding 1 or more variants of uncertain significance.[23] While great strides have been made in this post–Human Genome Project era, not all genetic etiologies have been discovered. This means that a negative genetic test result in a patient with otherwise idiopathic cardiomyopathy does not rule out an underlying genetic etiology. To summarize, current clinical sensitivities of genetic testing panels for HCM reach ~50% in those patients with a positive family history, ~40% in DCM, and ~50% in ARVC. The clinical sensitivities for RCM and LVNC phenotypes are unknown.

When currently available clinical genetic testing panels fail to identify the cause for a patient's likely genetic cardiomyopathy, health care providers (1) can consider large-scale genomic sequencing tests for their patients (ie, whole-exome or whole-genome sequencing), and (2) should inform the patient and the patient's family members of the option to participate in research studies focused on novel gene discovery. Whole-exome sequencing (WES) involves sequencing all of the exons, or coding regions, of a person's genome, whereas whole-genome sequencing (WGS) sequences both the coding and noncoding portions of the genome. WES will have the highest likelihood to identify an underlying genetic etiology by sequencing 3 or more affected individuals in a pedigree, to enhance variant filtering by segregation analysis. WES can also be utilized if the pedigree appears to fit an autosomal recessive pattern, or possibly a de novo mutation in the affected proband, by submitting specimens from the proband and both biological parents.

Up-to-date information on clinical and research genetic testing options can be located in 2 main online genetic testing databases:

- National Institutes of Health Genetic Testing Registry (http://www.ncbi.nlm.nih.gov/gtr) is a resource that provides voluntarily submitted genetic test information including the test's purpose, methodology, validity, usefulness evidence, and contacts and credentials for the laboratory.[36]
- GeneTests (genetests.org) includes an international directory of genetic testing laboratories.[37]

IMPORTANT NUANCES IN ORDERING CARDIOMYOPATHY GENETIC TESTING

Important nuances exist to ordering clinical cardiomyopathy genetic testing, including the value of performing a comprehensive genetic testing panel on the person in the family with the most severe clinical presentation due to the possibility of the presence of more than 1 pathogenic variant. As discussed above, and shown in the clinical case presentation in this chapter, it is possible that patients with genetic cardiomyopathies may have more than 1 underlying pathogenic variant associated with their phenotype (Figure 5-3). For example, 3% to 5% of patients with HCM may be heterozygous for 2 or more pathogenic variants in the same or different genes (ie, compound or double heterozygotes)[38,39] and extreme families with triple sarcomere mutations have also been described.[40] These patients may have a more severe disease presentation, including a younger age of onset. Thus, when disease expression presents more severely in 1 or more relatives within a family (ie, much earlier age of onset compared to other affected family members), the possibility of more than 1 pathogenic variant should be considered and sought. This has major implications for the approach to genetic testing and counseling within such families.

It is also important to understand that for some patients, genetic testing may not be a 1-time test. This is because patients who previously tested negative due to incomplete testing methodologies (ie, the performance of gene sequencing only that did not include the ability to detect large deletions and duplications) or insensitive genetic testing panels (eg, first-generation DCM gene panels that did not include all known DCM-associated genes) may have their pathogenic variant(s) identified when different technology and/or panels with greater clinical sensitivity are applied.

CLINICAL UTILITY AND VALUE OF GENETIC TESTING IN CARDIOMYOPATHY PATIENTS

The clinical utility of genetic testing for multiple inherited cardiac diseases is now well recognized.[41] Clinical utility includes diagnostic confirmation; syndromic cardiomyopathy identification that may reveal specific medical therapies or other management, including guidance on type of device implantation (eg, an implantable cardioverter defibrillator [ICD] versus a pacemaker in patients with an *LMNA* mutation causing conduction system disease and DCM);[5] predictive genetic testing for at-risk relatives when the pathogenic variant(s) is identified; and the ability to provide patients with family planning information and reproductive options, including preimplantation and prenatal genetic diagnosis. Clinical utility can also be derived in some cases with preimplantation genetic diagnosis, which allows couples the option to select mutation-negative embryos for implantation after in vitro fertilization. Also, prenatal genetic testing

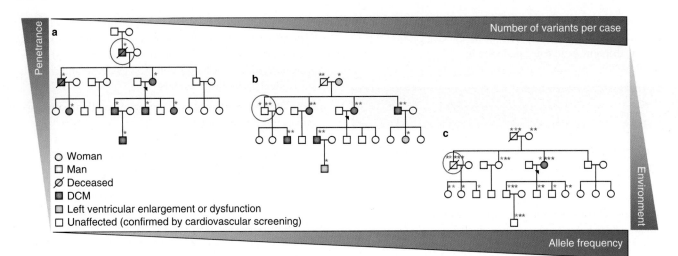

FIGURE 5-3 Variations on the Mendelian disease paradigm relevant to DCM genetics. DCM can be simplex or familial, often with reduced penetrance and variable expressivity. The figure shows the 3 types of pedigree seen in DCM: **(a)** a large family with full penetrance, **(b)** a smaller familial DCM kindred with reduced penetrance and variable expressivity, and **(c)** sporadic DCM where familial disease has been excluded by cardiac clinical screening. The presence of a variant is denoted by an asterisk. Where an asterisk is not shown, the variant is not present. The factors that are thought to influence DCM presentation (penetrance, allele frequency, combinatorial effects of relevant variants, and environmental triggers) are shown on each side of the rectangle surrounding the pedigrees. The position of a pedigree reflects the degree to which each of the 4 factors is thought to contribute to disease. **(a)** Large familial DCM pedigrees are observed when a single, rare, complete-penetrance variant (in this example, one asterisk) is sufficient to cause disease. Little or no environmental influence is required. When this type of mutation occurs de novo, DCM occurs in the absence of family history (sporadic disease), but offspring are at 50% risk of inheriting the mutation (circled individual), leading to an autosomal-dominant pedigree in future generations. **(b)** Smaller families showing reduced penetrance and variable expressivity are observed when the clinical effect of a mutation of low penetrance is influenced by other variants (in this example, two asterisks). Either 1 of the variants leads to partial phenotypes or influence expressivity, for example, isolated left ventricular enlargement without ventricular dysfunction. Individuals harboring a protective variant (purple asterisk) escape overt disease, but their offspring might have DCM or a mild phenotype if they inherit 1 or more mutations in the absence of the protective variant (circled individual). In this type of family, environmental factors can accelerate severe or early-onset disease. **(c)** Sporadic DCM can result from an accumulation of variants that collectively cause disease (in this example, four asterisks). We speculate, on the basis of the rare-variant data, that most or all variants that contribute to sporadic DCM are rare, but can be associated with low degrees of penetrance. One or more protective variants might also have an effect in these pedigrees (circled individual). Abbreviation: DCM, dilated cardiomyopathy. (Reproduced, with permission, from Hershberger RE, Jedges DJ, Morales A. Dilated cardiomyopathy: the complexity of a diverse genetic architecture. *Nat Rev Cardiol.* 2013;10(9):531-547.)

involves testing a sample of fetal DNA to determine whether the fetus carries the disease-associated mutation.

CASCADE GENETIC TESTING

One of the main values in using diagnostic genetic testing in the affected proband is that once his or her causative pathogenic variant(s) has been identified, genetic testing of at-risk family members can commence in order to identify all individuals in the family who are also predisposed to the genetic cardiomyopathy. This type of predictive genetic testing is best performed in a cascade, stepwise fashion, offering family-specific single-site genetic testing to all at-risk first-degree relatives first (parents, siblings, children) and then moving through the pedigree in sequential steps until all at-risk relatives have been identified. This approach can also discern those in the pedigree who did not inherit the genetic predisposition and therefore likely do not require serial clinical screening. Using cascade genetic testing compared to clinical screening alone has been shown to be highly cost-effective in families with HCM.[42]

INTERPRETATION OF GENETIC TESTING RESULTS

The interpretation of genetic testing results, despite progress in the field, remains complex and challenging in many cases. One reason for this is that a significant percentage of variants identified by clinical testing laboratories will be novel missense changes (single nucleotide substitutions) and therefore deemed by the testing laboratory as variants of uncertain clinical significance.[43] Genetic variants identified on clinical genetic testing may be highly penetrant disease-causing variants (pathogenic), lower penetrance modifiers of disease expression (both risk variants and protective variants), or benign variants. Genetic testing laboratories consider multiple factors in determining whether a genetic variant is likely pathogenic or not, and assign classification of a variant's pathogenicity based on published guidelines.[44] These classifications may change over time as new information is learned.[45] The Clinical Genome Resource, also known as ClinGen, includes ClinVar, which is a publicly available database of genetic variation and amasses interpretations of variants from both clinical and research genetic testing laboratories, housed online by the National Center for Biotechnology Information.[46] Accurate, up-to-date interpretations of genetic variants is of the utmost importance, as in order to fully realize the benefit of predictive genetic testing and subsequent risk reduction, clinicians must be sure they are testing at-risk relatives for the pathogenic, disease-associated variant, and not a benign unassociated variant, especially in conditions such as the heritable cardiomyopathies where SCD can be the first presentation of disease. The clinical application of genetic variant information, especially when the variant is novel, can therefore be a challenge that requires additional data, as well as patience in some cases. Determining significance via functional studies can strengthen attributions of pathogenicity; however, this is not always practical or feasible. Further, the range and reliability of functional systems varies greatly, and in the absence of highly relevant, reproducible, and applicable in vivo models, multiple other approaches have been employed to aid in the interpretation of genetic variants. These include cosegregation of the variant with the cardiomyopathy phenotype in large kindreds, amino acid conservation across species, variant frequency in large, ethnically matched control populations, and the use of computational prediction tools. The variants with the highest likelihood of being pathogenic are those that cosegregate with the phenotype, have a high degree of cross-species conservation, are located in a highly significant protein domain, and are absent, or found at a very low frequency, in ethnically matched controls.

With the availability of large, population-based, ethnically variable, genomic sequence datasets, such as the 1000 Genomes Project,[47] the NHLBI Exome Sequencing Project,[48] and the Exome Aggregation Consortium,[49] we have been able to learn more about human genetic variation in cardiomyopathy genes. These datasets have inherent limitations, such as the lack of associated phenotypic information; however, they can be extremely useful in determining the frequency of human genetic variation. One study using this genomic sequence information found that the frequency of predicted pathogenic variants in 3 sarcomere genes (*MYH7*, *MYBPC3*, and *TTN*) exceeded the population estimates for the combined prevalence of HCM and DCM.[50] Relatedly, this study and others have shown that up to 3% of the population has a *TTN* truncating variant,[24,50] significantly exceeding the population-based estimate of 1 in 250 DCM cases. In addition, by comparing ARVC probands to healthy controls of various ethnic backgrounds, it has been shown that the frequency of missense variation in genes associated with ARVC is relatively high.[7]

In sum, the interpretation of the data presented above is that certain genetic variants may serve as risk modifiers for the development of cardiomyopathy, although data to support this contention have not yet been convincingly shown. Further, we and others have suggested that the single-gene Mendelian disease paradigm relevant to genetic cardiomyopathies may be incomplete,[2] although to this point data in support of this hypothesis are limited primarily to case studies such as the 1 presented above. Nevertheless, conceptually it is clear that some single genetic variants may not be sufficient to cause disease on their own, but may require multiple variants, and/or other additive risk factors that contribute to an individual's overall genetic and environmental load to develop cardiomyopathy. Further, some genetic variants interacting with environmental and lifestyle factors may provide risk reduction, or protection, from cardiomyopathy. This important concept has not yet been systematically evaluated.

CLINICAL SCREENING OF AT-RISK RELATIVES

In cases where the pathogenic variant(s) has been identified, but just as importantly, when the underlying genetic etiology has not been identified in a family, clinical screening of at-risk relatives for cardiomyopathy is recommended.[5] Similar to the principles of cascade genetic testing discussed above, clinical screening should commence in a cascade fashion until all at-risk relatives have undergone clinical screening. Also, imperative to the clinical screening process, is the notion of serial screening. A 1-time normal echocardiogram or electrocardiogram is not enough to clear a patient from a possible predisposition to a genetic cardiomyopathy due to reduced and age-dependent penetrance and variable expressivity. For this reason, it must be communicated to the index patient that his or her at-risk relatives should undergo clinical screening, likely in a serial fashion over years, with personalized recommendations for follow-up from their health care providers. Detailed guidelines summarizing recommended clinical testing modalities as well as screening intervals are located in previously referenced guideline statements.[5,6]

CONSENSUS AND POLICY STATEMENTS REGARDING CARDIOMYOPATHY GENETIC TESTING

At the time of writing no guideline-level document has yet provided what we consider to be up-to-date recommendations regarding the availability of very large cardiomyopathy genetic testing panels that include a plethora of genes, some with limited to minimal evidence for association with cardiomyopathy, although we[4] and others[51-53] have provided expert opinion for the field. The 2009 HFSA guideline document[5] remains highly relevant, except for its genetic testing recommendations, which were completed prior to advances in next-generation sequencing (NGS) and the availability of these large gene panels. In 2011, early in the NGS era, an international group of experts published a consensus statement that, in addition to recommendations for genetic testing in the cardiomyopathies,[41] also provided recommendations regarding genetic testing for out-of-hospital cardiac arrest survivors and post-mortem testing in the setting of sudden unexpected death including cardiomyopathies. Specifically, HCM genetic testing was recommended (Class I recommendation) for any patient in whom a cardiologist has established a clinical diagnosis. It was also a Class I recommendation that patients with DCM and significant cardiac conduction disease and/or a family history of premature unexpected sudden death have genetic testing for the genes associated with this phenotype (LMNA, SCN5A, now others). Genetic testing for familial DCM was given the Class IIa (can be useful) designation, as it can be used to confirm a diagnosis, identify those at highest risk of arrhythmia and syndromic features, facilitate cascade testing of at-risk family members, and aid in family planning. It is a Class IIa or IIb (may be considered) recommendation to pursue genetic testing for patients meeting diagnostic criteria for ARVC or with possible ARVC, respectively, according to the 2010 Task Force criteria.[30] Importantly, for all cardiomyopathies reviewed (HCM, ARVC, DCM, LVNC, and RCM), it is a Class I recommendation that following the identification of a causative cardiomyopathy-associated pathogenic variant in the index case, that variant-specific genetic testing be pursued for family members.

A policy statement from the American Heart Association discusses important issues regarding genetic testing from the status of gene patents to the federal regulation of genetic tests and provides multiple recommendations.[54] One section specifically focuses on testing for Mendelian disorders, such as the inherited cardiomyopathies, and advocates for the involvement of physicians and centers with cardiovascular genetics expertise in order to appropriately initiate, interpret, and implement genetic testing. This approach, when feasible, has also been recommended elsewhere.[5] This includes determination of when and how to best pursue clinical genetic testing, pretest and posttest genetic counseling, and evaluation of entire families to aid in the interpretation of testing results (ie, coordination of segregation analysis for pathogenicity evaluation of variants of uncertain clinical significance). Due to the complexity of genetic test technology and result interpretation, it was also recommended that technical validity be regulated and that testing be performed in CLIA-approved laboratories.

GENETIC COUNSELING

Genetic counseling is the process of helping people understand and adapt to the medical, psychological, and familial implications of the genetic contributions to disease[55] and is an imperative component of a cardiovascular genetic medicine clinic.[56] Consensus statements and practice guidelines recommend that genetic counseling be provided to all patients and family members with specific familial heart diseases, including the cardiomyopathies.[5,7,57]

Genetic counselors are health care professionals with specialized graduate degrees and expertise in medical genetics and counseling. Many genetic counselors work as members of a health care team, and provide information and support to families with inherited conditions. Cardiovascular genetic counselors are an important resource and integral health care team members for patients and families with inherited heart disease, including those families that have suffered a sudden death in a young person.[58] It has been suggested that a master's-trained, board-certified genetic counselor, preferably with specialized training in cardiovascular genetics, be part of the multidisciplinary team involved in the care of families with heritable cardiovascular diseases.[59] They can help facilitate the incorporation of genetic medicine into cardiology clinics, by working with subspecialty cardiovascular medicine physicians, such as

HF cardiologists, to provide genetic counseling and testing information to applicable patients.[60]

PRETEST GENETIC COUNSELING

Pretest genetic counseling should include a discussion of all possible results scenarios with the patient undergoing genetic testing, as well as the overall benefits, limitations, and potential risks of testing. This includes the possibility of positive, negative, and uncertain genetic testing results. When possible, pretest probabilities should also be presented (ie, the chance for a pathogenic variant to be identified in familial HCM reaches 50% to 60% with the current testing technology available). Pretest counseling should also include a discussion of the possible psychological ramifications of genetic testing (eg, parental guilt, "survivor guilt"). Baseline levels of anxiety, risk perception, and health beliefs should be assessed.[61] Many patients also have questions regarding genetic discrimination, which should be addressed before genetic testing is ordered. On May 21, 2008, the Genetic Information Nondiscrimination Act (GINA) was signed into law. This federal law prohibits discrimination by health insurers and employers on the basis of genetic information. Life, disability, and long-term care insurance discrimination are not covered under GINA.

POSTTEST GENETIC COUNSELING

Posttest genetic counseling should include a thorough discussion of the genetic testing results and their implications for the proband and family members.[61] Posttest counseling should also include information regarding the proband's "duty to warn" relatives about their own risk. The use of family letters that include information on the diagnosis in the family, risks, genetic and other types of testing and screening, as well as preventive options has been shown to be an effective method to inform relatives of their risk and promote screening for high-risk cardiac diseases.[62] If a pathogenic variant is detected, single-site, family-specific genetic testing should be recommended for all first-degree relatives. If genetic testing is negative, it should be discussed with the proband that his or her diagnosis may still be genetic/familial in nature, that additional genetic testing may be warranted as the sensitivity of genetic testing improves, and that family members should pursue clinical screening. It should be recommended to the proband to inform at-risk relatives of the possibility of family-specific, single-site genetic testing when a pathogenic variant has been identified or if testing was negative, relatives should be informed that while they cannot pursue predictive testing at that time, they should still seek clinical screening evaluations.

During posttest genetic counseling, an assessment of the psychological and emotional response to results should also be performed.[61] A positive result in a clinically affected individual may eliminate doubt and uncertainty, but for those who test positive through predictive testing (ie, they are genotype-positive, phenotype-negative) it may have potential negative impacts including feelings such as increased worry, distress, anxiety, anger, fear of discrimination, alteration of self-esteem, and elimination of autonomy.[61] Genetic testing results can also impact family dynamics and relationships. Parents in particular may have feelings of guilt related to passing a pathogenic variant(s) to their children. In this situation, it may be helpful to emphasize the benefits provided by this type of genetic information (ie, knowledge is power); specifically, clinicians can utilize this information to initiate clinical screening that may lead toward the earliest possible detection of disease and that may provide the opportunity for prophylactic treatment.[63]

A negative family-specific genetic testing result can provide reassurance to at-risk relatives regarding their personal risk level and that of their children and can also eliminate their need for serial cardiac screening. Patients in this category should be counseled that while they may have tested negative for their family's specific variant, they can still develop heart disease, so should not ignore or minimize cardiac symptoms they may have in the future. Patients who test negative may experience feelings of so-called survivor guilt, particularly in families where other siblings are clinically affected or have tested positive and are at risk.[61,63] It has been proposed that follow-up counseling within 3 to 6 months time to assess for persistent or amplified levels of distress over results should be offered to families with inherited cardiovascular diseases.[61]

As part of the genetic counseling process, family planning options should also be discussed, including the option of preimplantation genetic diagnosis (PGD). While deciding to pursue PGD is a personal decision for most couples, a recent article presented the first cumulative experience of PGD for inherited cardiac diseases, including familial cardiomyopathies, which reported that 18 PGD cycles ultimately resulted in the births of 7 disease-free or disease-predisposition-free children.[64]

MULTIDISCIPLINARY APPROACH TO CARE OF FAMILIES WITH GENETIC CARDIOMYOPATHIES

An integrated, structured, multidisciplinary clinical approach to the care of families with inherited cardiac disease and sudden death has been recommended, and should include the expertise of cardiologists, genetic counselors, clinical geneticists, nurses, pathologists, clinical and research molecular genetic testing centers, psychologists, and patient support groups.[58] Such multidisciplinary clinics need not require the actual physical presence of each and every subspecialty during every patient encounter, but instead involve strong, collaborative working relationships and communication between disciplines. Specialized cardiac genetics clinics have been shown to lead to better patient adjustment and less worry.[65] Many academic medical centers have established multidisciplinary cardiovascular genetic medicine clinics; community hospitals and other settings are also beginning to adopt this approach and are including genetic counseling and testing as part of their clinical service offerings.

CARDIOMYOPATHY GENETIC EVALUATION AND TESTING: TOWARD THE FUTURE

The past 20 years have been witness to multitudes of discovery in the field of cardiomyopathy genetics, especially due to the development of novel DNA sequencing technologies. This has led to a vast increase in the number of clinical cardiomyopathy genetic testing options. That being said, much necessary discovery remains, with most cardiomyopathy phenotypes having 50% or less of their underlying genetic etiologies elucidated. Research over the next 20 years should be focused on additional gene discovery as well as the variable expressivity we see in cardiomyopathies by unraveling genetic, epigenetic, and environmental modulators of these phenotypes.

Patients have better access to clinical genetic testing, with many health insurance companies and federally funded insurance plans covering genetic testing for their beneficiaries. In addition, practice guidelines and position statements recommend genetic counseling and genetic testing and provide best practice approaches for the patient and family with genetic cardiomyopathies.

With the costs of DNA sequencing continuing to drop, the $1000 whole genome sequence with concomitant interpretation may very well be close on the horizon for use in even standard clinical care. In the future, cardiologists, cardiovascular genetic and genomic counselors, and patients themselves, may be able to access and utilize their genomic information for true precision medicine (eg, tailored drug therapies) for cardiomyopathy. Affected patients and their at-risk relatives may be able to receive more precise information regarding future cardiovascular health status. The ultimate hope, and goal, is that future research will lead toward additional discoveries that could ameliorate or prevent these conditions altogether.

REFERENCES

1. Page SP, Kounas S, Syrris P, et al. Cardiac myosin binding protein-C mutations in families with hypertrophic cardiomyopathy: disease expression in relation to age, gender, and long term outcome. *Circ Cardiovasc Genet.* 2012;5:156-166.

2. Hershberger RE, Hedges DJ, Morales A. Dilated cardiomyopathy: the complexity of a diverse genetic architecture. *Nat Rev Cardiol.* 2013;10:531-547.

3. Maron BJ, Gardin JM, Flack JM, Gidding SS, Kurosaki TT, Bild DE. Prevalence of hypertrophic cardiomyopathy in a general population of young adults. Echocardiographic analysis of 4111 subjects in the CARDIA Study. Coronary Artery Risk Development in (Young) Adults. *Circulation.* 1995;92:785-789.

4. Sturm AC, Hershberger RE. Genetic testing in cardiovascular medicine: current landscape and future horizons. *Curr Opin Cardiol.* 2013;28:317-325.

5. Hershberger RE, Lindenfeld J, Mestroni L, et al. Genetic evaluation of cardiomyopathy—a Heart Failure Society of America practice guideline. *J Card Fail.* 2009;15:83-97.

6. Charron P, Arad M, Arbustini E, et al. Genetic counselling and testing in cardiomyopathies: a position statement of the European Society of Cardiology Working Group on Myocardial and Pericardial Diseases. *Eur Heart J.* 2010;31:2715-2726.

7. Kapplinger JD, Landstrom AP, Salisbury BA, et al. Distinguishing arrhythmogenic right ventricular cardiomyopathy/dysplasia-associated mutations from background genetic noise. *J Am Coll Cardiol.* 2011;57:2317-2327.

8. Maron BJ, Towbin JA, Thiene G, et al. Contemporary definitions and classification of the cardiomyopathies: an American Heart Association scientific statement from the Council on Clinical Cardiology, Heart Failure and Transplantation Committee; Quality of Care and Outcomes Research and Functional Genomics and Translational Biology Interdisciplinary Working Groups; and Council on Epidemiology and Prevention. *Circulation.* 2006;113:1807-1816.

9. Elliott P, Andersson B, Arbustini E, et al. Classification of the cardiomyopathies: a position statement from the European Society Of Cardiology Working Group on Myocardial and Pericardial Diseases. *Eur Heart J.* 2008;29:270-276.

10. Maron BJ, Maron MS, Semsarian C. Genetics of hypertrophic cardiomyopathy after 20 years: clinical perspectives. *J Am Coll Cardiol.* 2012;60:705-715.

11. Fowler SJ, Napolitano C, Priori SG. The genetics of cardiomyopathy: genotyping and genetic counseling. *Curr Treat Options Cardiovasc Med.* 2009;11:433-446.

12. Klaassen S, Probst S, Oechslin E, et al. Mutations in sarcomere protein genes in left ventricular noncompaction. *Circulation.* 2008;117:2893-2901.

13. Kubo T, Gimeno JR, Bahl A, et al. Prevalence, clinical significance, and genetic basis of hypertrophic cardiomyopathy with restrictive phenotype. *J Am Coll Cardiol.* 2007;49:2419-2426.

14. Hershberger RE, Cowan J, Morales A, Siegfried JD. Progress with genetic cardiomyopathies: screening, counseling, and testing in dilated, hypertrophic, and arrhythmogenic right ventricular dysplasia/cardiomyopathy. *Circ Heart Fail.* 2009;2:253-261.

15. Judge DP. Use of genetics in the clinical evaluation of cardiomyopathy. *JAMA.* 2009;302:2471-2476.

16. Wheeler M, Pavlovic A, DeGoma E, Salisbury H, Brown C, Ashley EA. A new era in clinical genetic testing for hypertrophic cardiomyopathy. *J Cardiovasc Transl Res.* 2009;2:381-391.

17. Hershberger RE, Morales A, Siegfried JD. Clinical and genetic issues in dilated cardiomyopathy: a review for genetics professionals. *Genet Med.* 2010;12:655-667.

18. Hershberger RE, Siegfried JD. Update 2011: clinical and genetic issues in familial dilated cardiomyopathy. *J Am Coll Cardiol.* 2011;57:1641-1649.

19. Baig MK, Goldman JH, Caforio AL, Coonar AS, Keeling PJ, McKenna WJ. Familial dilated cardiomyopathy: cardiac abnormalities are common in asymptomatic relatives and may represent early disease. *J Am Coll Cardiol.* 1998;31:195-201.

20. Grunig E, Tasman JA, Kucherer H, Franz W, Kubler W, Katus HA. Frequency and phenotypes of familial dilated cardiomyopathy. *J Am Coll Cardiol.* 1998;31:186-194.

21. Michels VV, Moll PP, Miller FA, et al. The frequency of familial dilated cardiomyopathy in a series of patients with idiopathic dilated cardiomyopathy. *N Engl J Med.* 1992;326:77-82.

22. Burkett EL, Hershberger RE. Clinical and genetic issues in familial dilated cardiomyopathy. *J Am Coll Cardiol.* 2005;45:969-981.

23. Pugh TJ, Kelly MA, Gowrisankar S, et al. The landscape of genetic variation in dilated cardiomyopathy as surveyed by clinical DNA sequencing. *Genet Med.* 2014;16:601-608.

24. Herman DS, Lam L, Taylor MR, et al. Truncations of titin causing dilated cardiomyopathy. *N Engl J Med.* 2012;366:619-628.

25. Akinrinade O, Alastalo TP, Koskenvuo JW. Relevance of truncating titin mutations in dilated cardiomyopathy. *Clin Genet.* 2016;90:49-54.

26. Roberts AM, Ware JS, Herman DS, et al. Integrated allelic, transcriptional, and phenomic dissection of the cardiac effects of titin truncations in health and disease. *Sci Transl Med.* 2015;7:270ra6.

27. Alfares AA, Kelly MA, McDermott G, et al. Results of clinical genetic testing of 2,912 probands with hypertrophic cardiomyopathy: expanded panels offer limited additional sensitivity. *Genet Med.* 2015;17:880-888.

28. Basso C, Corrado D, Marcus FI, Nava A, Thiene G. Arrhythmogenic right ventricular cardiomyopathy. *Lancet.* 2009;373:1289-1300.

29. Sen-Chowdhry S, Morgan RD, Chambers JC, McKenna WJ. Arrhythmogenic cardiomyopathy: etiology, diagnosis, and treatment. *Annu Rev Med.* 2010;61:233-253.

30. Marcus FI, McKenna WJ, Sherrill D, et al. Diagnosis of arrhythmogenic right ventricular cardiomyopathy/dysplasia: proposed modification of the Task Force Criteria. *Eur Heart J.* 2010;31:806-814.

31. Sen-Chowdhry S, Syrris P, Prasad SK, et al. Left-dominant arrhythmogenic cardiomyopathy: an under-recognized clinical entity. *J Am Coll Cardiol.* 2008;52:2175-2187.

32. Quarta G, Muir A, Pantazis A, et al. Familial evaluation in arrhythmogenic right ventricular cardiomyopathy: impact of genetics and revised task force criteria. *Circulation.* 2011;123:2701-2709.

33. Morales A, Cowan J, Dagua J, Hershberger RE. Family history: an essential tool for cardiovascular genetic medicine. *Congest Heart Fail.* 2008;14:37-45.

34. Baruteau AE, Behaghel A, Fouchard S, et al. Parental electrocardiographic screening identifies a high degree of inheritance for congenital and childhood nonimmune isolated atrioventricular block. *Circulation.* 2012;126:1469-1477.

35. Meder B, Haas J, Keller A, et al. Targeted next-generation sequencing for the molecular genetic diagnostics of cardiomyopathies. *Circ Cardiovasc Genet.* 2011;4:110-122.

36. Genetic Testing Registry. National Center for Biotechnology Information, U.S. National Library of Medicine, 2012. http://www.ncbi.nlm.nih.gov/gtr/. Accessed September 10, 2012.

37. GeneTests. genetests.org. Accessed September 10, 2012.

38. Van Driest SL, Vasile VC, Ommen SR, et al. Myosin binding protein C mutations and compound heterozygosity in hypertrophic cardiomyopathy. *J Am Coll Cardiol.* 2004;44:1903-1910.

39. Richard P, Charron P, Carrier L, et al. Hypertrophic cardiomyopathy: distribution of disease genes, spectrum of mutations, and implications for a molecular diagnosis strategy. *Circulation.* 2003;107:2227-2232.

40. Girolami F, Ho CY, Semsarian C, et al. Clinical features and outcome of hypertrophic cardiomyopathy associated with triple sarcomere protein gene mutations. *J Am Coll Cardiol.* 2010;55:1444-1453.

41. Ackerman MJ, Priori SG, Willems S, et al. HRS/EHRA expert consensus statement on the state of genetic testing for the

channelopathies and cardiomyopathies this document was developed as a partnership between the Heart Rhythm Society (HRS) and the European Heart Rhythm Association (EHRA). *Heart Rhythm.* 2011;8:1308-1339.

42. Ingles J, McGaughran J, Scuffham PA, Atherton J, Semsarian C. A cost-effectiveness model of genetic testing for the evaluation of families with hypertrophic cardiomyopathy. *Heart.* 2012;98:625-630.

43. Lakdawala NK, Funke BH, Baxter S, et al. Genetic testing for dilated cardiomyopathy in clinical practice. *J Card Fail.* 2012;18:296-303.

44. Richards S, Aziz N, Bale S, et al. Standards and guidelines for the interpretation of sequence variants: a joint consensus recommendation of the American College of Medical Genetics and Genomics and the Association for Molecular Pathology. *Genet Med.* 2015;17:405-424.

45. Ho CY. Hypertrophic cardiomyopathy in 2012. *Circulation.* 2012;125:1432-1438.

46. Rehm HL, Berg JS, Brooks LD, et al. ClinGen—the clinical genome resource. *N Engl J Med.* 2015;372:2235-2242.

47. A map of human genome variation from population-scale sequencing. *Nature.* 2010;467:1061-1073.

48. Tennessen JA, Bigham AW, O'Connor TD, et al. Evolution and functional impact of rare coding variation from deep sequencing of human exomes. *Science.* 2012;337:64-69.

49. Lek M, et al. Analysis of protein-coding genetic variation in 60,706 humans. *Nature.* 2016;536:285.

50. Golbus JR, Puckelwartz MJ, Fahrenbach JP, Dellefave-Castillo LM, Wolfgeher D, McNally EM. Population-based variation in cardiomyopathy genes. *Circ Cardiovasc Genet.* 2012;5:391-399.

51. George AL, Jr. Use of contemporary genetics in cardiovascular diagnosis. *Circulation.* 2014;130:1971-80.

52. Mogensen J, van Tintelen JP, Fokstuen S, et al. The current role of next-generation DNA sequencing in routine care of patients with hereditary cardiovascular conditions: a viewpoint paper of the European Society of Cardiology working group on myocardial and pericardial diseases and members of the European Society of Human Genetics. *Eur Heart J.* 2015;36:1367-1370.

53. Teo LY, Moran RT, Tang WH. Evolving approaches to genetic evaluation of specific cardiomyopathies. *Curr Heart Fail Rep.* 2015;12:339-349.

54. Ashley EA, Hershberger RE, Caleshu C, et al. Genetics and cardiovascular disease: a policy statement from the American Heart Association. *Circulation.* 2012;126:142-157.

55. Resta R, Biesecker BB, Bennett RL, et al. A new definition of genetic counseling: National Society of Genetic Counselors' task force report. *J Genet Couns.* 2006;15:77-83.

56. Cowan J, Morales A, Dagua J, Hershberger RE. Genetic testing and genetic counseling in cardiovascular genetic medicine: overview and preliminary recommendations. *Congest Heart Fail.* 2008;14:97-105.

57. Gersh BJ, Maron BJ, Bonow RO, et al. 2011 ACCF/AHA Guideline for the Diagnosis and Treatment of Hypertrophic Cardiomyopathy: a report of the American College of Cardiology Foundation/American Heart Association Task Force on Practice Guidelines. Developed in collaboration with the American Association for Thoracic Surgery, American Society of Echocardiography, American Society of Nuclear Cardiology, Heart Failure Society of America, Heart Rhythm Society, Society for Cardiovascular Angiography and Interventions, and Society of Thoracic Surgeons. *J Am Coll Cardiol.* 2011;58:e212-260.

58. Ingles J, Yeates L, Semsarian C. The emerging role of the cardiac genetic counselor. *Heart Rhythm.* 2011;8:1958-1962.

59. Tester DJ, Ackerman MJ. Genetic testing for potentially lethal, highly treatable inherited cardiomyopathies/channelopathies in clinical practice. *Circulation.* 2011;123:1021-1037.

60. Hershberger RE. Cardiovascular genetic medicine: evolving concepts, rationale, and implementation. *J Cardiovasc Trans Res.* 2008;1:137-143.

61. Aatre RD, Day SM. Psychological issues in genetic testing for inherited cardiovascular diseases. *Circ Cardiovasc Genet.* 2011;4:81-90.

62. van der Roest WP, Pennings JM, Bakker M, van den Berg MP, van Tintelen JP. Family letters are an effective way to inform relatives about inherited cardiac disease. *Am J Med Genet.* Part A 2009;149A:357-363.

63. Ingles J, Zodgekar PR, Yeates L, Macciocca I, Semsarian C, Fatkin D. Guidelines for genetic testing of inherited cardiac disorders. *Heart Lung Circ.* 2011;20:681-687.

64. Kuliev A, Pomerantseva E, Polling D, Verlinsky O, Rechitsky S. PGD for inherited cardiac diseases. *Reprod Biomed Online.* 2012;24:443-453.

65. Ingles J, Lind JM, Phongsavan P, Semsarian C. Psychosocial impact of specialized cardiac genetic clinics for hypertrophic cardiomyopathy. *Genet Med.* 2008;10:117-120.

6 HEART FAILURE WITH PRESERVED EJECTION FRACTION

Shane Nanayakkara, MBBS, FRACP
David Kaye, MBBS, PhD, FRACP, FACC, FESC

PATIENT CASE

A 69-year-old woman was referred to by her local medical practitioner with worsening exertional dyspnea (NYHA III). She found difficulty mobilizing to her mailbox (120 m on a flat surface), as well as doing light housework and dressing. Her background history is relevant for long-standing hypertension (HTN), dyslipidemia, obesity, stage 3 renal impairment, and paroxysmal atrial fibrillation. Her medication profile is listed in Table 6-1. Physical examination revealed a well-looking woman with a blood pressure of 155/80 mm Hg on both arms, a heart rate of 72 in a regular rhythm, and respiratory rate of 20. Anthropomorphic measurements were a height of 162 cm and weight of 84 kg, with a calculated body mass index (BMI) of 32 kg/m^2. Precordial examination revealed the apex beat to be nondisplaced, with no palpable heaves or thrills. No murmurs were auscultated. The jugular venous pressure was estimated at 2 cm, and there was trace pedal edema. The remainder of the physical examination was normal. The electrocardiogram (ECG) confirmed sinus rhythm, with features of left ventricular hypertrophy (LVH) and left axis deviation. Chest radiography demonstrated clear lung fields and borderline cardiomegaly.

Laboratory profile demonstrated a mild anemia, with hemoglobin of 10.5 g/dL and a mean red cell volume of 92. Renal function was impaired with a urea of 22.4 mg/dL and creatinine of 1.02 mg/dL, leading to an estimated glomerular filtration rate (GFR) of 57.2 mL/min/1.73 m^2 via the MDRD equation, or 57.5 mL/min using the Cockcroft-Gault equation adjusted for the overweight patient. A resting N-terminal pro-brain natriuretic peptide (NT-proBNP) was mildly elevated at 385 pg/mL.

A transthoracic echocardiogram demonstrated moderate global concentric hypertrophy with normal systolic function, with an ejection fraction calculated via Simpson's biplane method of 68%. The left atrium was mildly enlarged, with satisfactory valvular function and E/e' ratio of 13. A recently performed stress echocardiogram was negative for inducible ischemia. Respiratory function tests revealed normal ventilatory function with no significant bronchodilator response. Exercise right heart catheterization was performed (Table 6-2), with evidence of a normal pulmonary capillary wedge pressure (PCWP) at rest, and a marked rise with exercise.

Table 6-1 Medication Profile for Introductory Patient Case

Irbesartan 300 mg daily
Amlodipine 10 mg daily

Table 6-2 Invasive Hemodynamics at Rest and with Exercise

	BP	RA	RV	PA	PA mean	PCWP	CO
Rest	144/71	8	28/4	33/15	21	11	4.2
Exercise	188/64			65/30	42	31	8.4

Abbreviations: BP, blood pressure; CO, cardiac output; PA, pulmonary artery; PCWP, pulmonary capillary wedge pressure; RA, right atrium; RV, right ventricle.

In summary, this 69-year-old woman presents with worsening NYHA III exertional dyspnea on a background of long-standing HTN.

DIFFERENTIAL DIAGNOSIS

There are a wide variety of differential diagnoses for exertional dyspnea, as highlighted in Figure 6-1. As the patient ages, the risk of both cardiac and noncardiac comorbidities contributing to dyspnea increases, and it is important to recognize that patients may have more than 1 cause for their dyspnea. Even for patients satisfying the diagnostic criteria of heart failure with preserved ejection fraction (HFpEF), multiple noncardiac contributions are often present.[1,2] In the present case, respiratory function tests and chest radiography were within normal limits, excluding major parenchymal or airway disease; however, computed tomography could be considered if clinical suspicion of respiratory disease was high. The normocytic anemia alone would not be expected to cause such a marked reduction in exercise capacity.

The cardiovascular differential diagnoses in the patient include ischemic heart disease, restrictive cardiomyopathy, hypertrophic cardiomyopathy, and periods of paroxysmal atrial fibrillation with poor rate control or bradycardia.

Ischemic heart disease is common in patients with HFpEF, with over two-thirds of patients having angiographically proven coronary artery disease.[3,4] This patient did not complain of angina with exertion, although dyspnea can be taken as an angina equivalent, and importantly her stress echocardiogram was negative for ischemia. On further questioning, a coronary angiogram had been performed 2 years ago with no significant luminal pathology, making ischemia unlikely.

Restrictive cardiomyopathy can be a difficult diagnosis to make, often a diagnosis of exclusion, in patients with normal systolic function and severe diastolic dysfunction with elevated filling pressures, often with marked biatrial dilatation. The condition can either be familial or acquired, with the latter being caused by conditions such as amyloidosis, endomyocardial fibrosis, radiation, and chemotherapeutic agents. The patient described above had no clinical, laboratory, echocardiographic, or radiographic features consistent with any common etiology, and no relevant family history of heart failure (HF).

Despite the moderate concentric hypertrophy noted on this patient's transthoracic echocardiogram, the pathological loading condition due to the history of long-standing HTN is the most likely etiology rather than a genetic hypertrophic cardiomyopathy. Cardiac magnetic resonance imaging can be useful to assess the scar pattern between these 2 etiologies, along with a relevant family history.

Poor control of the ventricular rate in atrial fibrillation can also lead to marked dyspnea, and underlying structural abnormalities such as atrial dilatation may predispose to its development. In this patient, the baseline ECG revealed sinus rhythm; however, ambulatory monitoring could be considered to exclude a paroxysmal arrhythmia.

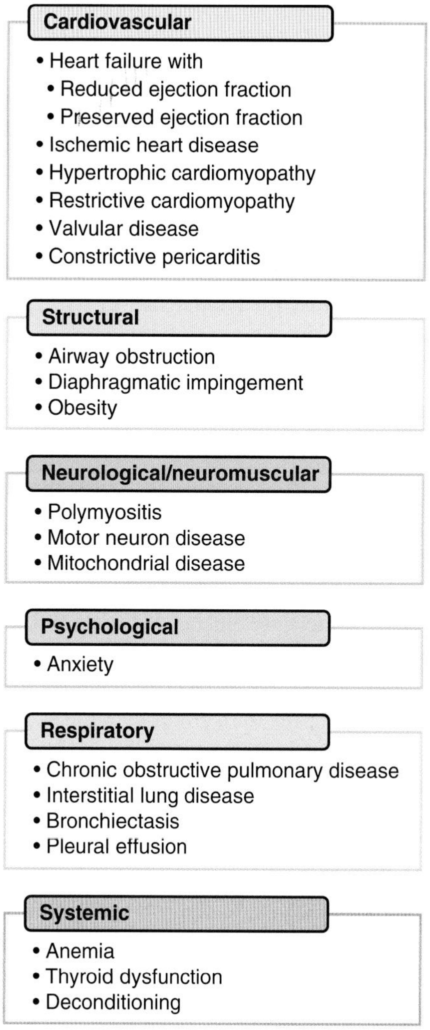

Cardiovascular
- Heart failure with
  - Reduced ejection fraction
  - Preserved ejection fraction
- Ischemic heart disease
- Hypertrophic cardiomyopathy
- Restrictive cardiomyopathy
- Valvular disease
- Constrictive pericarditis

Structural
- Airway obstruction
- Diaphragmatic impingement
- Obesity

Neurological/neuromuscular
- Polymyositis
- Motor neuron disease
- Mitochondrial disease

Psychological
- Anxiety

Respiratory
- Chronic obstructive pulmonary disease
- Interstitial lung disease
- Bronchiectasis
- Pleural effusion

Systemic
- Anemia
- Thyroid dysfunction
- Deconditioning

FIGURE 6-1 Common causes of chronic dyspnea in aging.

In this case, in a hypertensive obese woman with no other significant contributing pathology, with exercise-induced dyspnea and marked pulmonary HTN, HFpEF is the most likely cause.

CLINICAL FEATURES

The cardinal symptom of HFpEF is exercise intolerance, together with classical symptoms and signs of HF as elucidated by history and physical examination. The Framingham criteria for HF, outlined in Figure 6-2, are the most widely used for the clinical diagnosis of HF across studies both for reduced and preserved ejection fraction.

Using phenomapping, a technique involving unsupervised machine learning to understand the intrinsic structure of data, investigators have recently identified 3 primary clinical phenotypes of HFpEF.[5] Each of these groups demonstrates related comorbidities, pathophysiologies, and importantly, different clinical trajectories. The first group were younger patients, with lower levels of natriuretic peptides and better outcomes. The second had more significant comorbidities, including obesity, diabetes, and obstructive sleep apnea. These patients had the worst parameters of left ventricular (LV) relaxation. The third group, with the worst prognosis, were older, had poor renal function, and the most severe electrical and echocardiographic features of myocardial remodelling, including significant right ventricular (RV) dysfunction.

Although there is no single test for the diagnosis of HFpEF, the combination of clinical features of HF together with evidence for elevated filling pressures (in the setting of no other contributory pathology) must be demonstrated. Features of abnormal relaxation and elevated filling pressures can be suggested with abnormal echocardiographic parameters, such as an elevated E/e', or elevated

Major

- Paroxysmal nocturnal dyspnea
- Neck vein distention
- Hepatojugular reflux
- Rales
- Radiographic cardiomegaly
- Acute pulmonary edema
- Third heart sound
- Increased central venous pressure
- Weight loss ≥4.5 kg in 5 days in response to treatment of heart failure
- Autopsy findings including pulmonary edema, visceral congestion, or cardiomegaly

Minor

- Bilateral ankle edema
- Nocturnal cough
- Dyspnea on ordinary exertion
- Hepatomegaly
- Pleural effusion
- Decrease in vital capacity by 33% of maximal value recorded
- Tachycardia >120 beats per minute

FIGURE 6-2 Framingham criteria for the diagnosis of congestive cardiac failure.[41] Either 2 major, or 1 major and 2 minor criteria are required. (Reproduced with permission from McKee PA, Castelli WP, McNamara PM, Kannel WB. The natural history of congestive heart failure: the Framingham study. *N Engl J Med.* 1971;285(26):1441-1446.)

natriuretic peptides; however, invasive hemodynamic measurements are considered definite evidence of HFpEF.[6] Considering the marked contribution of exercise to the developing symptomatology of this patient group, the addition of exercise to the evaluation is critical, particularly when the resting parameters fall within an indeterminate zone (Figure 6-3).[7] The current ESC guidelines recommend a combination of clinical features, exclusion of a normal BNP, and echocardiographic features of functional impairment and structural remodelling.

MECHANISMS OF DISEASE

The reasons for exercise intolerance in HFpEF are multifactorial, and represent an interplay between impaired diastolic function together with peripheral mechanisms and comorbid conditions.

The physiologic parameters involved are highlighted by Houstis and Lewis via the Fick equation (Figure 6-4) demonstrating the variables involved in peak VO_2, a quantitative measure of exercise capacity. Patients with HFpEF demonstrate abnormalities in chronotropic competence and often have smaller stroke volumes; however, the VO_2 may also be limited by variables such as musculoskeletal discomfort or inadequate effort.[8]

Key mechanisms under investigation in HFpEF patients are outlined in Table 6-3.

MANAGEMENT

To date, clinical trials in HFpEF (Table 6-4) have largely been disappointing reflecting variability in trial design,[9–13] heterogeneous population,[5] relatively limited study duration (in comparison to the likely duration required for the development of HFpEF), and that the disease mechanisms are not yet fully understood.

$$VO_2 = CO \times AVO_2$$

$$HR \times SV \quad C_a - C_V$$

FIGURE 6-4 Fick equation. Abbreviations: AVO_2, arteriovenous oxygen difference; Ca, arterial oxygen content; CO, cardiac output; Cv, venous oxygen content; HR, heart rate; SV, stroke volume; VO_2, maximum rate of oxygen consumption.

Table 6-3 Contributing Mechanisms and Potential Therapeutic Targets in HFpEF Patients

Impaired stroke volume augmentation[42]
Elevated filling pressures[8]
Impaired myocardial oxygen utilization[43]
Peripheral oxygen extraction[2]
Myocardial fibrosis[45,46]
Chronotropic incompetence[21,46]
Inspiratory muscle weakness[1]
Microvascular dysfunction[45,47]
Nitrate-nitrite pathway[48–50]
Autonomic dysfunction[21,31]
Left atrial systolic function[51,52]
Functional iron deficiency[53]
Inflammation[54,55]
Right ventricular dysfunction[56,57]
Chronic disease[59,60]
Left ventricular systolic dysfunction[60,61]

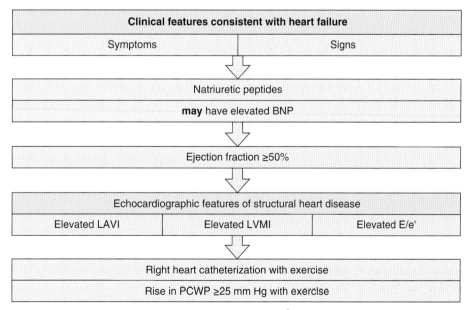

FIGURE 6-3 Diagnostic algorithm for HFpEF incorporating exercise hemodynamics.[7] Abbreviations: BNP, brain natriuretic peptide; HF, heart failure; LAVI, left atrial volume index; LV, left ventricle; LVEF, left ventricular ejection fraction; LVMI, left ventricular mass index; PCWP, pulmonary capillary wedge pressure. (Reproduced with permission from van Empel VPM, Kaye DM. Integration of exercise evaluation into the algorithm for evaluation of patients with suspected heart failure with preserved ejection fraction. *Int J Cardiol*. 2013;168(2):716-722.)

Table 6-4 Major Trials Assessing Therapy in HFpEF

Trial	Year	Therapy	LVEF	Heart Failure	Outcome
TOPCAT[13]	2014	Spironolactone	>45%	Hospitalization or BNP	Modest reduction in hospitalization for HF
					No change to mortality or overall hospitalization
I-PRESERVE[19]	2008	Irbesartan	>45% (median 59%)	Hospitalization or clinical features AND radiographic/ echocardiographic/ electrocardiographic features	No difference in mortality or hospitalization
CHARM-PRESERVED[18]	2003	Candesartan	>40% (median 52%)	Hospitalization for cardiac reason	No change to mortality, modest reduction in hospitalization
RELAX[62]	2013	Sildenafil		Hospitalization OR treatment for heart failure OR loop diuretic + LA enlargement OR PCWP >15 or LVEDP >18 mm Hg (together with VO_2 and BNP criteria)	No change in VO_2 or 6MWT
RELAX-AHF[63]	2014	Serelaxin	>50%	Acutely decompensated HF requiring hospitalization with impaired renal function	
DIG-PEF[64]	2006	Digoxin	>45% (median 53%)		

Abbreviations: 6MWT, 6-minute walk test; BNP, B-type natriuretic peptide; HF, heart failure; LA, left atrium; LVEDP, left ventricular end-diastolic pressure; PCWP, pulmonary capillary wedge pressure; VO_2, maximum rate of oxygen consumption.

The main principles of the management of HFpEF are to maintain strict control of blood pressure, relieve congestion, prevent ischemia, treat comorbid conditions, and maintain atrial function through rate or rhythm control.

NONPHARMACOLOGICAL

Both HFrEF and HFpEF patients are susceptible to volume overload, and strict maintenance of fluid balance through fluid and salt restriction remains important.

Comorbid conditions play a larger role in the HFpEF population, with optimization and management of these conditions leading to improved outcomes.

The vast majority of patients with HFpEF are overweight or obese, which induces structural changes to the left ventricle.[14] A combination of both dietary and exercise therapy has been associated with improvement in peak VO_2, with a minor effect independently and a more substantial additive effect.[15] Exercise training also has been demonstrated to improve quality of life and cardiorespiratory fitness, independent of echocardiographic changes in diastolic function potentially via improved peripheral muscle perfusion and oxygen utilization.[16] Weight loss, either by lifestyle modification or bariatric surgery, has been shown to improve diastolic function; however, this has not been well assessed in the HFpEF population specifically.[17]

PHARMACOLOGICAL

Pharmacological therapies are based around diuretics for the relief of pulmonary venous congestion, strict control of HTN using agents such as angiotensin-converting enzyme (ACE) inhibitors and angiotensin receptor blockers (ARBs), heart rate control, and blockade of the renin-angiotensin-aldosterone system.

Judicious fluid management is particularly well highlighted in the HFpEF patient, due to the reduced stroke volume as well as the sensitivity to a reduction in preload, together with the increased likelihood of underlying renal impairment.

The use of ACE inhibitors and ARBs has been well studied in the HFrEF population, and 3 large-scale trials of these agents in HFpEF[10,18,19] have all failed to show a benefit in regards to mortality. However, a small reduction in hospitalization has been noted.[20]

Aldosterone has also been postulated to play a key role in the pathophysiology of HFpEF and HFrEF. In the TOPCAT trial, the effect of spironolactone on survival and hospitalization was examined. Spironolactone treatment was not associated with improved survival. There was evidence of a modest reduction in HF hospitalization,[13] but importantly blood pressure was also lowered. Importantly, there was significant regional heterogeneity in the performance of the trial limiting interpretability to a degree.

Chronotropic incompetence has been noted as a feature of patients with HFpEF,[21,22] and although beta blockade theoretically would assist by extending diastolic filling time and minimizing the effect of ischemia, trials in this regard have been negative.[24,25] In patients with atrial fibrillation, however, appropriate control of ventricular rate is critical, although the agent of choice has not been well studied.[25] The presence of atrial fibrillation is associated with higher levels of natriuretic peptides, and unlike HFrEF patients, is associated with higher rates of death and hospitalization.[26] Catheter ablation has low first-procedure success rates in this population, rising to 73% after multiple procedures and pharmacotherapy.[27]

DEVICE

Given the limited success of pharmacological interventions, a range of novel devices has been devised to ameliorate physiological targets. Given that an elevation in left atrial pressure is proposed to represent a key mechanism in HFpEF, an iatrogenic interatrial septal shunt device has been developed to allow decompression into the right atrium. This device is positioned percutaneously via the femoral vein using transesophageal or intracardiac echocardiographic guidance. Initial data have shown improvements in functional capacity and a reduction in filling pressures.[28]

Autonomic dysfunction has been implicated in the development and progression of HF, leading to the concept that modulation of sympathetic and parasympathetic activity may lead to improved outcomes. Stimulation of the carotid baroreceptor with baroreflex activation therapy reduces sympathetic outflow and increases parasympathetic activity, and has been shown previously to lower blood pressure significantly.[29] In a multicenter nonblinded trial of 146 patients with HFrEF, there was an improvement in functional status and exercise capacity, and reduction in NT-proBNP.[30] Although it is hypothesized that similar outcomes will occur in HFpEF patients, the outcomes of such trials are still pending.[31,32]

PREVENTION

Control of risk factors is paramount in any chronic disease, and in HFpEF strict blood pressure control and reduction in body fat are likely to provide significant benefit. In the elderly, appropriate blood pressure control has been shown to prevent the onset of clinical symptoms, although echocardiography was not performed in that study.[33] Dietary modification, such as the DASH diet, to lower sodium intake, not only improves blood pressure control but has also been demonstrated to improve echocardiographic parameters of diastolic function.[34]

Exercise training has been shown to improve quality of life measures and cardiorespiratory fitness, likely through a multitude of effects including peripheral muscle perfusion and oxygen utilization.[16,35,36] Similarly, dietary modification to prevent weight gain is likely to have long-lasting effects on LV structure and function, but this has not been assessed.

THE BURDEN OF HEART FAILURE WITH PRESERVED EJECTION FRACTION AND PROGNOSIS

HFpEF affects up to 10% of people over the age of 75 years,[37] and is projected to become the most prevalent form of HF over the next decade,[12] due to the increasing age of the population, epidemics of comorbid conditions such as obesity and diabetes, and the increasing recognition of the condition. Cardiovascular mortality from HFpEF is less than those with HFrEF.[38] However, sudden death and HF are still the most common modes of death in HFpEF. The rate of hospitalization is equivalent, as high as 29% within the first 3 months after hospital discharge.[39] In the case of the patient in this chapter's introductory Patient Case, the MAGGIC score, a predictive score developed using both patients with reduced and preserved ejection fraction, calculated a 12-month mortality of 7.7% and 3-year mortality of 19.1%.

In addition to clinical factors, hemodynamic parameters, particularly PCWP at rest, are significantly associated with mortality, with a 2-fold risk of death in patients with a wedge pressure over 12 mm Hg.[40] Exercise hemodynamics are even more closely linked to mortality, again highlighting the importance of these recordings in patients with normal resting values.

In view of the lack of effective therapeutic options, close follow-up is warranted in these patients. By maintenance and regular optimization of blood pressure, aggressive lifestyle modification, and control of both fluid status as well as maintenance of sinus rhythm, the rate of hospitalization can be reduced.

KEY POINTS

- HFpEF makes up half of all HF, and will become the most prevalent form of HF over the next decade.
- There are currently no treatments that have demonstrated any effect on mortality in HFpEF.
- Diastolic dysfunction is 1 component of a complex interplay of physiological conditions that lead to the syndrome.
- The hallmark of diagnosis is the combination of the clinical features of HF together with evidence of elevated filling pressures.
- Treatment at this stage includes strict control of blood pressure, judicious fluid balance, and optimal management of other comorbidities including atrial fibrillation.

Future Therapies in HFpEF

Therapy	Hypothesized Mechanism	Key Trials	Key Findings in Studies to Date	Future Studies
PHARMACOLOGICAL				
Sildenafil	Reduction in pulmonary pressure Reduction in cardiac fibrosis	RELAX[62]	No effect on clinical or structural measures Potential reduction in left ventricular systolic function	**Sildenafil in HFpEF and PH** (EudraCT 2010-020153-14) **SILICCON** (Eudra CT2011-001674-25) **SIRVEH** (EudraCT 2013-001659-10
Soluble guanylate cyclase agonists	Pulmonary and systemic vasodilation Inhibition of smooth muscle proliferation	DILATE-1[65]	Increased stroke volume No change in PVR or mean PAP	**SOCRATES-PRESERVED**
Endothelin receptor antagonists	Reduction in pulmonary pressure	Effectiveness of sitaxsentan sodium in patients with diastolic HF[66]	Increase in exercise tolerance No change to echocardiographic measures of diastolic function	Nil
Neprilysin inhibition	RAAS and inhibition of breakdown of natriuretic peptides	PARAMOUNT[67]	Reduced natriuretic peptide, left atrial volume, and NYHA class No change in LV volume	**PARAGON-HF** (NCT01920711)

(Continued)

Future Therapies in HFpEF (Continued)

Therapy	Hypothesized Mechanism	Key Trials	Key Findings in Studies to Date	Future Studies
Ivabradine	Increase time for diastolic filling	Effect of If-channel inhibition on hemodynamic status and exercise tolerance in HFpEF[68]	Improvement in exercise capacity	**EDIFY** (EudraCT 2012-002742-20)
Iron supplementation	Antioxidant	Evidence in HFrEF; no human data in HFpEF	No randomized trials	**FAIR-HFPEF**
Ranolazine	Reduce intracellular calcium via reduction in late sodium current	RALI-DHF[69]	Reduced LVEDP and PCWP	**RAZE** (NCT01505179)
Mitochondrial enhancement	Restoration of ATP production and energy deficit	Nil	Recruiting	**MITO-HFPEF**
Serelaxin	Pleiotropic effects	RELAX-AHF[70]	Reduced dyspnea No change to hospitalization Not powered for mortality	**RELAX-AHF-EU** (NCT02064868)
Statins	Endothelial redox balance restoration Effect on collagen turnover	Meta-analysis of the effect of statins on mortality in patients with preserved ejection fraction[71]	Improved survival in observational studies; no randomized controlled trials	Nil
Isosorbide dinitrate and hydralazine	Altered ventricular hemodynamics	No human data	Recruiting	**Vasodilator Therapy for Heart Failure with a Preserved Ejection Fraction** (NCT01516346)
Perhexiline	Correct myocardial energy deficiency	No human data	No randomized trials	**Perhexiline therapy in patients with HFpEF** (EudraCT 2006-001109-28; NCT00839228)

(Continued)

Future Therapies in HFpEF (Continued)

Therapy	Hypothesized Mechanism	Key Trials	Key Findings in Studies to Date	Future Studies
DEVICE				
Interatrial septal device	Reduce left atrial pressure Reduce pulmonary pressures	REDUCE-LAP	Reduced NYHA class Reduced pulmonary pressures	**REDUCE LAP-HF**-2
Atrial pacing	Reduce atrial dyssynchrony Prevent chronotropic incompetence	RESET[46]	Trial terminated prior to completion	**LEAD** (NCT01618981) **RAPID-HF** (NCT02145351)
ICD implantation	Prevention of sudden death	Nil	No randomized trials	**VIP-HF** (NCT01989299)
Renal denervation	Reduce systemic arterial pressure Reduce renal sympathetic activation and consequent sodium retention	Nil	No randomized trials	**RESPECT-HF** (NCT02041130) **DIASTOLE** (NCT01583881) **RDT-PEF** (NCT01840059)
Baroreflex activation	Reduce systemic arterial pressure	Single case report only, with limited data[31,32]	Normalization of echocardiographic parameters and improvement in exercise capacity No randomized trials	**HOPE4HF** (NCT00957073)
Ventricular modification	Enhance diastolic function directly using an elastic spring	Nil	No randomized trials	**CORolla-TAA** (NCT01956526)

REFERENCES

1. Yamada K, Kinugasa Y, Sota T, et al. Inspiratory muscle weakness is associated with exercise intolerance in patients with heart failure with preserved ejection fraction: a preliminary study. *J Card Fail.* 2015;22(1):38-47.

2. Dhakal BP, Malhotra R, Murphy RM, et al. Mechanisms of exercise intolerance in heart failure with preserved ejection fraction: the role of abnormal peripheral oxygen extraction. *Circ Hear Fail.* 2015;8(2):286-294.

3. Nanayakkara S, Haykowsky M, Mariani J, et al. Hemodynamic profile of patients with heart failure and preserved ejection fraction vary by age. *J Am Heart Assoc.* 2017;6:e005434.

4. Hwang S-J, Melenovsky V, Borlaug BA. Implications of coronary artery disease in heart failure with preserved ejection fraction. *J Am Coll Cardiol.* 2014;63(25):2817-2827.

5. Shah SJ, Katz DH, Selvaraj S, et al. Phenomapping for novel classification of heart failure with preserved ejection fraction. *Circulation*. 2014;131(3):269-279.

6. Paulus WJ, Tschöpe C, Sanderson JE, et al. How to diagnose diastolic heart failure: a consensus statement on the diagnosis of heart failure with normal left ventricular ejection fraction by the Heart Failure and Echocardiography Associations of the European Society of Cardiology. *Eur Heart J*. 2007;28(20):2539-2550.

7. van Empel VPM, Kaye DM. Integration of exercise evaluation into the algorithm for evaluation of patients with suspected heart failure with preserved ejection fraction. *Int J Cardiol*. 2013;168(2):716-722.

8. Houstis NE, Lewis GD. Causes of exercise intolerance in heart failure with preserved ejection fraction: searching for consensus. *J Card Fail*. 2014;20(10):762-778.

9. Redfield MM, Borlaug BA, Lewis GD, et al. Phosphdiesterase-5 inhibition to improve clinical status and exercise capacity in diastolic heart failure (RELAX) trial: rationale and design. *Circ Heart Fail*. 2012;5(5):653-659.

10. Cleland JGF, Tendera M, Adamus J, Freemantle N, Polonski L, Taylor J. The perindopril in elderly people with chronic heart failure (PEP-CHF) study. *Eur Heart J*. 2006;27(19):2338-2345.

11. McMurray JJV, Packer M, Desai AS, et al. Angiotensin–neprilysin inhibition versus enalapril in heart failure. *N Engl J Med*. 2014;371(11):993-1004.

12. Shah RV, Desai AS, Givertz MM. The effect of renin-angiotensin system inhibitors on mortality and heart failure hospitalization in patients with heart failure and preserved ejection fraction: a systematic review and meta-analysis. *J Card Fail*. 2010;16(3):260-267.

13. Pitt B, Pfeffer M a., Assmann SF, et al. Spironolactone for heart failure with preserved ejection fraction. *N Engl J Med*. 2014;370(15):1383-1392.

14. Turkbey EB, McClelland RL, Kronmal RA, et al. The impact of obesity on the left ventricle: the Multi-Ethnic Study of Atherosclerosis (MESA). *JACC Cardiovasc Imaging*. 2010;3(3):266-274.

15. Kitzman DW, Brubaker PH, Morgan TM, et al. Effect of caloric restriction or aerobic exercise training on peak oxygen consumption and quality of life in obese older patients with heart failure with preserved ejection fraction: a randomized clinical trial. *JAMA*. 2016;315(1):36-46.

16. Pandey A, Parashar A, Kumbhani DJ, et al. Exercise training in patients with heart failure and preserved ejection fraction: meta-snalysis of randomized control trials. *Circ Hear Fail*. 2014;8(1):33-40.

17. de las Fuentes L, Waggoner AD, Mohammed SF, et al. Effect of moderate diet-induced weight loss and weight regain on cardiovascular structure and function. *J Am Coll Cardiol*. 2009;54(25):2376-2381.

18. Yusuf S, Pfeffer MA, Swedberg K, et al. Effects of candesartan in patients with chronic heart failure and preserved left-ventricular ejection fraction: the CHARM-preserved trial. *Lancet*. 2003;362(9386):777-781.

19. Massie BM, Carson PE, McMurray JJV, et al. Irbesartan in patients with heart failure and preserved ejection fraction. *N Engl J Med*. 2008;359(23):2456-2467.

20. Mujib M, Patel K, Fonarow GC, et al. Angiotensin-converting enzyme inhibitors and outcomes in heart failure and preserved ejection fraction. *Am J Med*. 2013;126(5):401-410.

21. Borlaug BA, Melenovsky V, Russell SD, et al. Impaired chronotropic and vasodilator reserves limit exercise capacity in patients with heart failure and a preserved ejection fraction. *Circulation*. 2006;114(20):2138-2147.

22. Brubaker PH, Joo K-C, Stewart KP, Fray B, Moore B, Kitzman DW. Chronotropic incompetence and its contribution to exercise intolerance in older heart failure patients. *J Cardiopulm Rehabil*. 2006;26(2):86-89.

23. Conraads VM, Metra M, Kamp O, et al. Effects of the long-term administration of nebivolol on the clinical symptoms, exercise capacity, and left ventricular function of patients with diastolic dysfunction: results of the ELANDD study. *Eur J Heart Fail*. 2012;14(2):219-225.

24. Yamamoto K, Origasa H, Hori M. Effects of carvedilol on heart failure with preserved ejection fraction: the Japanese Diastolic Heart Failure Study (J-DHF). *Eur J Heart Fail*. 2013;15(1):110-118.

25. Zakeri R, Borlaug BA, McNulty SE, et al. Impact of atrial fibrillation on exercise capacity in heart failure with preserved ejection fraction: a RELAX trial ancillary study. *Circ Heart Fail*. 2014;7(1):123-130.

26. Linssen GCM, Rienstra M, Jaarsma T, et al. Clinical and prognostic effects of atrial fibrillation in heart failure patients with reduced and preserved left ventricular ejection fraction. *Eur J Heart Fail*. 2011;13(10):1111-1120.

27. Machino-Ohtsuka T, Seo Y, Ishizu T, et al. Efficacy, safety, and outcomes of catheter ablation of atrial fibrillation in patients with heart failure with preserved ejection fractions. *J Am Coll Cardiol*. 2013;62(20):1857-1865.

28. Hasenfuß G, Hayward C, Burkhoff D, et al. A transcatheter intracardiac shunt device for heart failure with preserved ejection fraction (REDUCE LAP-HF): a multicenter, open-label, single-arm, phase 1 trial. *Lancet*. 2016;387:1298-1304.

29. Hoppe UC, Brandt M-C, Wachter R, et al. Minimally invasive system for baroreflex activation therapy chronically lowers blood pressure with pacemaker-like safety profile: results from the Barostim neo trial. *J Am Soc Hypertens*. 2012;6(4):270-276.

30. Abraham WT, Zile MR, Weaver FA, et al. Baroreflex activation therapy for the treatment of heart failure with a reduced ejection fraction. *JACC Heart Fail*. 2015;3(6):487-496.

31. Georgakopoulos D, Little WC, Abraham WT, Weaver FA, Zile MR. Chronic baroreflex activation: a potential therapeutic

approach to heart failure with preserved ejection fraction. *J Card Fail*. 2011;17(2):167-178.

32. Brandt MC, Madershahian N, Velden R, Hoppe UC. Baroreflex activation as a novel therapeutic strategy for diastolic heart failure. *Clin Res Cardiol*. 2011;100(3):249-251.

33. Beckett NS, Peters R, Fletcher AE, et al. Treatment of hypertension in patients 80 years of age or older [Internet]. *N Engl J Med*. 2008;358:1887-1898. http://www.nejm.org/doi/full/10.1056/NEJMoa0801369. Accessed May 29, 2015.

34. Hummel SL, Seymour EM, Brook RD, et al. Low-sodium DASH diet improves diastolic function and ventricular-arterial coupling in hypertensive heart failure with preserved ejection fraction. *Circ Heart Fail*. 2013;6(6):1165-1171.

35. Edelmann F, Gelbrich G, Düngen H-D, et al. Exercise training improves exercise capacity and diastolic function in patients with heart failure with preserved ejection fraction: results of the Ex-DHF (Exercise training in Diastolic Heart Failure) pilot study. *J Am Coll Cardiol*. 2011;58(17):1780-1791.

36. Suchy C, Massen L, Rognmo O, et al. Optimising exercise training in prevention and treatment of diastolic heart failure (OptimEx-CLIN): rationale and design of a prospective, randomised, controlled trial. *Eur J Prev Cardiol*. 2014;21(2 Suppl):18-25.

37. Oktay AA, Rich JD, Shah SJ. The emerging epidemic of heart failure with preserved ejection fraction. *Curr Heart Fail Rep*. 2013;10(4):401-410.

38. MAGGIC Group. The survival of patients with heart failure with preserved or reduced left ventricular ejection fraction: an individual patient data meta-analysis. *Eur Heart J*. 2012;33(14):1750-1757.

39. Fonarow GC, Stough WG, Abraham WT, et al. Characteristics, treatments, and outcomes of patients with preserved systolic function hospitalized for heart failure. a report from the OPTIMIZE-HF registry. *J Am Coll Cardiol*. 2007;50(8):768-777.

40. Dorfs S, Zeh W, Hochholzer W, et al. Pulmonary capillary wedge pressure during exercise and long-term mortality in patients with suspected heart failure with preserved ejection fraction. *Eur Heart J*. 2014;35(44):3103-3112.

41. McKee PA, Castelli WP, McNamara PM, Kannel WB. The natural history of congestive heart failure: the Framingham study. *N Engl J Med*. 1971;285(26):1441-1446.

42. Kitzman DW, Higginbotham MB, Cobb FR, Sheikh KH, Sullıvan MJ. Exercise intolerance in patients with heart failure and preserved left ventricular systolic function: failure of the Frank-Starling mechanism. *J Am Coll Cardiol*. 1991;17(5):1065-1072.

43. van Empel VPM, Mariani J, Borlaug BA, Kaye DM. Impaired myocardial oxygen availability contributes to abnormal exercise hemodynamics in heart failure with preserved ejection fraction. *J Am Heart Assoc*. 2014;3(6):e001293.

44. Su MYM, Lin LY, Tseng YHE, et al. CMR-verified diffuse myocardial fibrosis is associated with diastolic dysfunction in HFpEF. *JACC Cardiovasc Imaging*. 2014;7(10):991–997.

45. Mohammed SF, Hussain S, Mirzoyev SA, Edwards WD, Maleszewski JJ, Redfield MM. Coronary microvascular rarefaction and myocardial fibrosis in heart failure with preserved ejection fraction. *Circulation*. 2015;131(6):550-559.

46. Kass DA, Kitzman DW, Alvarez GE. The restoration of chronotropic competence in heart failure patients with normal ejection fraction (RESET) study: rationale and design. *J Card Fail*. 2010;16(1):17-24.

47. Maréchaux S, Samson R, van Belle E, et al. Vascular and microvascular endothelial function in heart failure with preserved ejection fraction. *J Card Fail*. 2015;22(1):3-11.

48. Chirinos JA, Zamani P. The nitrate-nitrite-NO pathway and its implications for heart failure and preserved ejection fraction. *Curr Heart Fail Rep*. 2016;13(1):47-59.

49. Zakeri R, Levine JA, Koepp GA, et al. Nitrate's effect on activity tolerance in heart failure with preserved ejection fraction trial: rationale and design. *Circ Hear Fail*. 2015;8(1):221-228.

50. Zamani P, Rawat D, Shiva-Kumar P, et al. Effect of inorganic nitrate on exercise capacity in heart failure with preserved ejection fraction. *Circulation*. 2014;131(4):371-380.

51. Fang F, Lee AP-W, Yu C-M. Left atrial function in heart failure with impaired and preserved ejection fraction. *Curr Opin Cardiol*. 2014;29(5):430-436.

52. Sanchis L, Gabrielli L, Andrea R, et al. Left atrial dysfunction relates to symptom onset in patients with heart failure and preserved left ventricular ejection fraction. *Eur Hear J Cardiovasc Imaging*. 2014;16(1):62-67.

53. Kasner M, Aleksandrov AS, Westermann D, et al. Functional iron deficiency and diastolic function in heart failure with preserved ejection fraction. *Int J Cardiol*. 2013;168(5):4652-4657.

54. van Empel V, Brunner-La Rocca HP. Inflammation in HFpEF: key or circumstantial? *Int J Cardiol*. 2015;189:259-263.

55. Westermann D, Lindner D, Kasner M, et al. Cardiac inflammation contributes to changes in the extracellular matrix in patients with heart failure and normal ejection fraction. *Circ Heart Fail*. 2011;4(1):44-52.

56. Mohammed SF, Hussain I, Abou Ezzeddine OF, et al. Right ventricular function in heart failure with preserved ejection fraction: a community-based study. *Circulation*. 2014;130(25):2310-2320.

57. Melenovsky V, Hwang S-J, Lin G, Redfield MM, Borlaug BA. Right heart dysfunction in heart failure with preserved ejection fraction. *Eur Heart J*. 2014;15-17.

58. Kitzman DW, Gardin JM, Gottdiener JS, et al. Importance of heart failure with preserved systolic function in patients > or = 65 years of age. CHS Research Group. Cardiovascular Health Study. *Am J Cardiol*. 2001;87(4):413-419.

59. Dunlay SM, Redfield MM, Weston SA, et al. Hospitalizations after heart failure diagnosis a community perspective. *J Am Coll Cardiol*. 2009;54(18):1695-1702.

60. Kraigher-Krainer E, Shah AM, Gupta DK, et al. Impaired systolic function by strain imaging in heart failure with preserved ejection fraction. *J Am Coll Cardiol*. 2014;63(5):447-456.

61. Aurigemma GP, Zile MR, Gaasch WH. Contractile behavior of the left ventricle in diastolic heart failure: with emphasis on regional systolic function. *Circulation*. 2006;113(2):296-304.

62. Redfield MM, Chen HH, Borlaug BA, et al. Effect of phosphodiesterase-5 inhibition on exercise capacity and clinical status in heart failure with preserved ejection fraction: a randomized clinical trial. *JAMA*. 2013;309(12):1268-1277.

63. Filippatos G, Teerlink JR, Farmakis D, et al. Serelaxin in acute heart failure patients with preserved left ventricular ejection fraction: results from the RELAX-AHF trial. *Eur Heart J*. 2014;35(16):1041-1050.

64. Ahmed A, Rich MW, Fleg JL, et al. Effects of digoxin on morbidity and mortality in diastolic heart failure: the ancillary digitalis investigation group trial. *Circulation*. 2006;114(5):397-403.

65. Bonderman D, Pretsch I, Steringer-Mascherbauer R, et al. Acute hemodynamic effects of riociguat in patients with pulmonary hypertension associated with diastolic heart failure (DILATE-1): a randomized, double-blind, placebo-controlled, single-dose study. *Chest*. 2014;146(5):1274-1285.

66. Zile MR, Bourge RC, Redfield MM, Zhou D, Baicu CF, Little WC. Randomized, double-blind, placebo-controlled study of sitaxsentan to improve impaired exercise tolerance in patients with heart failure and a preserved ejection fraction. *JACC Heart Fail*. 2014;2(2):123-130.

67. Solomon SD, Zile MR, Pieske BM, et al. The angiotensin receptor neprilysin inhibitor LCZ696 in heart failure with preserved ejection fraction: a phase 2 double-blind randomised controlled trial. *Lancet*. 2012;380(9851):1387-1395.

68. Kosmala W, Holland DJ, Rojek A, Wright L, Przewlocka-Kosmala M, Marwick TH. Effect of If-channel inhibition on hemodynamic status and exercise tolerance in heart failure with preserved ejection fraction: A randomized trial. *J Am Coll Cardiol*. 2013;62(15):1330-1338.

69. Maier LS, Layug B, Karwatowska-Prokopczuk E, et al. Ranolazine for the treatment of diastolic heart failure in patients with preserved ejection fraction: the RALI-DHF proof-of-concept study. *JACC Heart Fail*. 2013;1(2):115-122.

70. Teerlink JR, Cotter G, Davison BA, et al. Serelaxin, recombinant human relaxin-2, for treatment of acute heart failure (RELAX-AHF): a randomised, placebo-controlled trial. *Lancet*. 2013;381(9860):29-39.

71. Liu G, Zheng X-X, Xu Y-L, Ru J, Hui R-T, Huang X-H. Meta-analysis of the effect of statins on mortality in patients with preserved ejection fraction. *Am J Cardiol*. 2014;113(7):1198-1204.

7 KIDNEY IN HEART FAILURE

Peter A. McCullough, MD, MPH
Katherine Panettiere-Kennedy, BS, MD

PATIENT CASE

A 75-year-old woman presents with effort intolerance, progressive dyspnea on exertion to minimal activity, and progressive feet, ankle, and lower leg swelling. She has a 3-year history of idiopathic nonischemic cardiomyopathy with a left ventricular ejection fraction (LVEF) of 35% measured within the last year. She also has a history of obesity, type 2 diabetes mellitus for 15 years with diabetic nephropathy, and hypertension (HTN) for 25 years. The medication profile includes: furosemide 40 mg orally twice a day, carvedilol 25 mg orally twice a day, enalapril 10 mg orally twice a day, and glargine insulin 60 units subcutaneously every night at bedtime. Vital signs were blood pressure of 105/70 mm Hg, heart rate 95 beats per minute, respiration rate 20 breaths per minute, weight 82 kg, and body mass index 33 kg/m^2, temperature 98.4°F. Her physical examination reveals jugular venous distention, rales one-half of the way up posteriorly, cardiac enlargement, an S_3, 2/6 murmur consistent with mitral regurgitation, hepatomegaly with hepatojugular reflux, and 4+ pitting edema to the midtibia bilaterally, and no visible rashes. The chest x-ray demonstrated cardiomegaly and pulmonary edema and the electrocardiogram revealed normal sinus rhythm, left axis deviation, left bundle branch block, and QRS duration of 120 ms. Laboratory testing was notable for: Na = 133 mEq/L, K = 5.0 mEq/L, creatinine 1.7 mg/dL (estimated glomerular filtration rate [eGFR] = 29 mL/min/1.73 m^2), BUN = 48 mg/dL, glucose = 235 mg/dL, glycohemoglobin = 7.2% and B-type natriuretic peptide = 2765 pg/mL. The urine albumin to creatinine ratio was 315 mg/g. The patient initially received furosemide 80 mg intravenously twice a day with a good diuresis, but on the third hospital day the creatinine rose to 2.9 mg/dL and the urine output dropped to 4 mL/kg for 12 hours. The patient's pulmonary examination improved somewhat; however, the S_3 and peripheral edema were essentially unchanged. The managing team was confronted with a series of questions regarding the differential diagnosis, prognosis, and next management steps.

DIFFERENTIAL DIAGNOSIS

The differential diagnosis includes type 1 cardiorenal syndrome, interstitial nephritis, subclinical sepsis, and prerenal azotemia. Because the patient has considerable evidence of volume expansion, it is unlikely that there has been enough volume loss to have caused prerenal azotemia. The presence of jugular venous distention suggests she has elevated central venous pressure, which is the strongest hemodynamic determinant of type 1 cardiorenal syndrome. While the kidneys may not be receiving enough forward output and there may transiently be a slowed plasma refill from the extravascular space, the patient is very unlikely to be truly volume depleted.

There was no evidence of fever or focal infection; hence the overlap between infection and heart failure (HF), while common, is probably not the issue in this patient. Interstitial nephritis generally presents with rash, fever, and urinary eosinophils, all of which are absent in this patient. Additionally, she has not taken any medications that commonly induce this syndrome. We are left with a working diagnosis of type 1 cardiorenal syndrome in which the onset of acute heart failure (AHF) has led to an attempt at diuresis and then a marked reduction in glomerular filtration and urine output.[1]

MANAGEMENT

We are in the midst of an HF chronic disease pandemic with the aging of populations in the Western world.[2] Survivorship in the settings of long-standing hypertension, myocardial infarction, valvular disease, and myocardial disease has led to an increased prevalence pool of patients with established HF. Approximately half of patients with HF have reduced LVEF or HFrEF and the other half have HF with preserved LVEF, or HFpEF. HFrEF can be attributed to myocardial ischemia or prior infarction in two-thirds of cases, while approximately one-half of those with HFpEF have a significant contribution to their illness due to ischemia as a result of coronary artery disease (CAD).[3] Because of the considerable overlap between HTN, diabetes, and other risk factors for CAD and myocardial disease with chronic kidney disease (CKD), it is a common occurrence to find HF patients (either HFrEF or HFpEF) who also have evidence of CKD, such as reduced estimated glomerular filtration rate (eGFR <60 mL/min/1.72 m^2), albuminuria (≥30 mg/g albumin to creatinine ratio in spot urine), or structural abnormalities in the kidneys or urological tract (eg, polycystic kidney disease, unilateral kidney).[4] Additionally, it is well known that in the setting of AHF decompensation, that acute kidney injury (AKI) occurs in approximately 25% of hospitalized patients (type 1 cardiorenal syndrome).[5] Finally, evidence suggests that HF itself can set up renal pathophysiology in a way to manifest reduced eGFR or albuminuria. This scenario has been termed type 2 cardiorenal syndrome.[6] Thus there is a considerable interface between cardiac and renal function in both health and disease. This chapter provides a framework to understand the kidney in HF from a graphical and pictorial perspective.

HEMODYNAMICS, RENAL BLOOD FLOW, AND GLOMERULAR FILTRATION

A normal human body has approximately 5 liters of blood volume and a cardiac output of 3 to 5 liters per minute at rest. Cardiac output can increase to ~35 liters per minute with aerobic exercise such as running. There is an important Frank-Starling relationship between end-diastolic volume and forward stroke work, which is analogous to the volume per contraction that would partially perfuse the kidneys as shown in Figure 7-1. At rest the parasympathetic system via acetylcholine release predominates over the sinoatrial node and maintains the heart rate in the 50 to 100 beats per minute range. In athletes, parasympathetic tone can be more pronounced and result in even lower sinus rates. With exercise, the sympathetic nervous system via the release of norepinephrine predominates and the sinus node rate increases. Additionally, contractility of the myocardium becomes more forceful, resulting in greater ventricular systolic pressures. The sympathetic nervous system achieves increased cardiac output by increasing heart rate, end-diastolic volume, and stroke volume (Figure 7-2). In order for these responses to occur there must be increased venous return to the heart.

At rest approximately 60% of blood volume is in the venous system at any given time (Figure 7-3). The veins have much thinner walls than the arteries and thus have a much greater capability to dilate creating potential for pooling of blood volume. The tunica media in veins is innervated by the sympathetic nervous system and stains intensely for norepinephrine from sympathetic neuromuscular terminals. This innervation works to control venous tone, and thus provides minute-to-minute regulation of venous return to the heart, which has an important pressure relationship to the overall cardiovascular system as shown in Figure 7-4. As shown in Figure 7-4, the hemodynamic performance of the right-sided chambers, pulmonary circulation, and left-sided systemic chambers are all highly and dynamically dependent on venous return.

The kidneys receive arterial blood flow through the renal arteries, which arise from the abdominal aorta just inferior to the superior mesenteric artery. Each kidney receives approximately 600 mL/min of flow and together renal blood flow (RBF) represents ~20% of cardiac output. The kidneys receive a disproportionate share of cardiac output positioned distally in the aorta because the renal circulation is a very low resistance circuit. This phenomenon has been termed a "vascular waterfall" and the kidneys allow blood to move in response to a ~100 fall in pressure, which is roughly double that of other organ systems including the heart. The renal artery (Figure 7-5) subdivides into segmental branches, then arcuate branches, and ultimately into afferent arterioles that deliver blood to the glomerular tuft and reconstitute as efferent arterioles that go on to form the peritubular network, vasa recta, and then subsegmental and segmental renal veins, which converge on the main renal veins back to the inferior vena cava. This valveless system carries a large blood volume back to the heart and thus is vulnerable to changes in forward perfusion pressure, back pressure, or changes in organ fluid content. Because the kidneys are in the retroperitoneal space unlike other viscera, there is lesser tolerance for organ expansion in the setting of organ edema. Multiple studies have shown that measures of central venous pressure, inferred renal venous pressure, and reduced outflow are strong determinants of type 1 cardiorenal syndrome in patients with AHF.[7]

Intrarenal autoregulatory mechanisms maintain RBF and glomerular filtration rate (GFR) independent of renal perfusion pressure (RPP) over a broad range of systemic arterial pressure (80-180 mm Hg).[8] Such autoregulation is mediated largely by the myogenic response, in which smooth muscle cells of the afferent arteriole sense changes in arteriolar pressure and adjust their tone

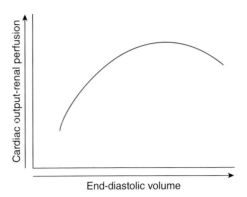

FIGURE 7-1 The Frank-Starling mechanism of the heart as it relates to renal perfusion.

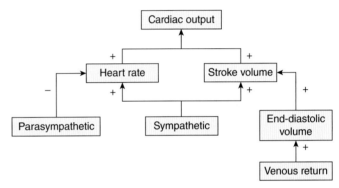

FIGURE 7-2 Determinants of cardiac output.

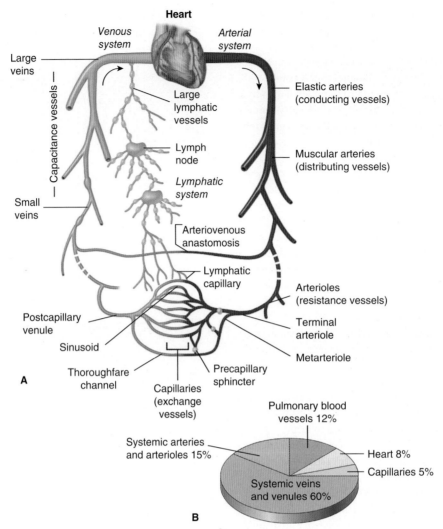

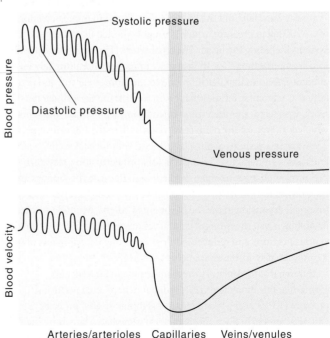

FIGURE 7-3 Proportional distribution of blood in the cardiovascular system.

accordingly to avoid fluctuations in blood flow to the glomerular tuft (Figure 7-6). Additional autoregulation is achieved by the tubuloglomerular feedback mechanism, in which afferent arteriole tone is adjusted in response to changes in NaCl content of tubular fluid. The components of this mechanism will be discussed shortly. The glomerulus is a unique vascular structure with multiple layers that constitute the filtration barrier between plasma and urine, including: (1) glycocalyx, (2) fenestrated endothelium, (3) glomerular basement membrane, formed by fusion of podocyte and endothelial basement membranes, and (4) foot processes of podocytes. The glomerulus also houses the mesangium, juxtaglomerular apparatus, and macula densa cells, which serve a variety of regulatory processes. The mesangial cells have cytosolic contractile proteins that enable them to change shape and regulate blood flow into the glomerulus via the afferent arteriole. Angiotensin II is an important regulator of this function. The juxtaglomerular apparatus refers to the close arrangement of the distal tubule, extraglomerular mesangium, and the afferent arteriole containing specialized juxtaglomerular cells. The juxtaglomerular portion of the distal tubule contains darkly staining, prominently nucleated macula densa cells, which are both the sensing and signaling component of the previously mentioned tubuloglomerular feedback mechanism. In addition to regulating arteriolar tone, the macula

FIGURE 7-4 Blood pressure and velocity throughout the cardiovascular system.

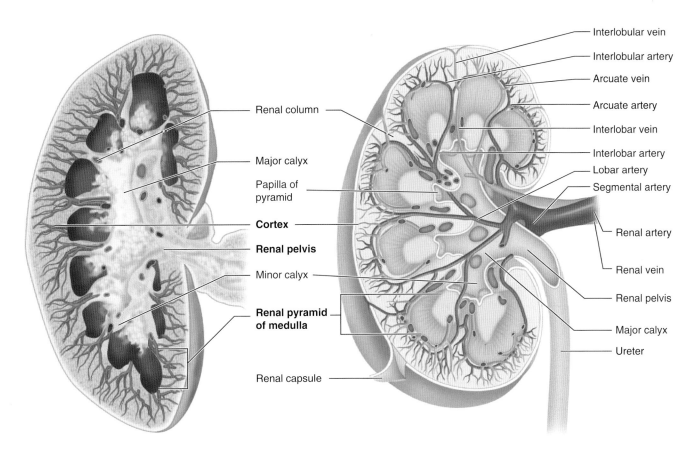

FIGURE 7-5 Vascular anatomy of the kidney.

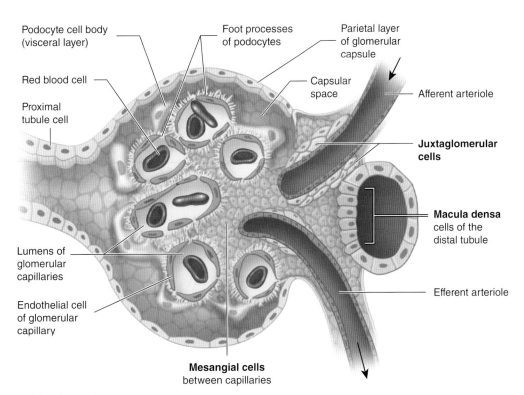

FIGURE 7-6 Structure of the glomerulus.

densa cells respond to changes in distal tubular NaCl by regulating renin release from the nearby juxtaglomerular cells.[9] Thus the anatomy and normal physiology of renal perfusion and glomerular filtration is particularly responsive to changes in both forward flow and venous return. The sodium-glucose transporter-2 channels are located in the proximal tubule and are a major target for a new class of antidiabetic agents, SGLT-2 inhibitors which have been associated with reductions in heart failure hospitalization and cardiovascular death. Additionally, the peritubular network (Figure 7-7) is the site where renal tubules in close proximity to both the tubular lumen and the blood-capillary interface regulate sodium, chloride, ammonium, and bicarbonate in the urine. Each distal convoluted tubule is drained into a collecting duct, and thus, each collecting duct services approximately 4 to 8 nephrons (Figure 7-8). The overall pathway of blood flow through the kidney is depicted in Figure 7-9. The principal cell in the collecting duct has 2 major functions that are relevant in HF: (1) effector response to intranuclear signaling from aldosterone, prompting the cell to reclaim sodium and dump potassium, contingent on distal delivery of sodium, and (2) effector response to cell surface activation of vasopressin 2 receptors to arginine vasopressin, which prompts aquaporin channels to incorporate into the lumen membrane, allowing for reclamation of water.[10] Because of the close proximity of the collecting ducts to the vasa recta, both of these systems work to deliver large amounts of sodium and water to the bloodstream when these hormonal systems are activated.

In summary, the kidneys are positioned to be the most hemodynamically and neurohormonally responsive to changes in blood volume, flow, perfusion, back pressure, sodium, and water in the setting of HF. As a result, both chronic and acute renal filtration function are

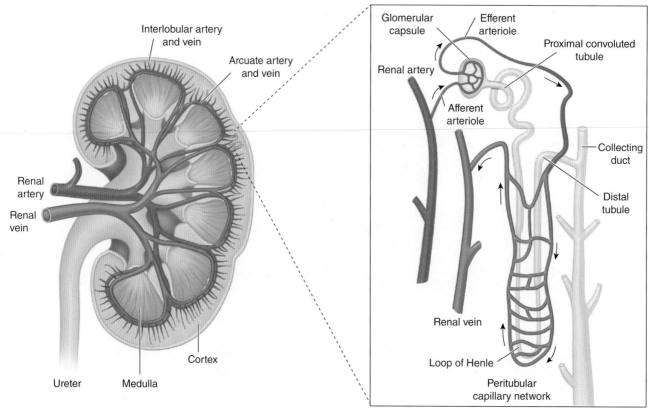

FIGURE 7-7 Blood supply to the nephron.

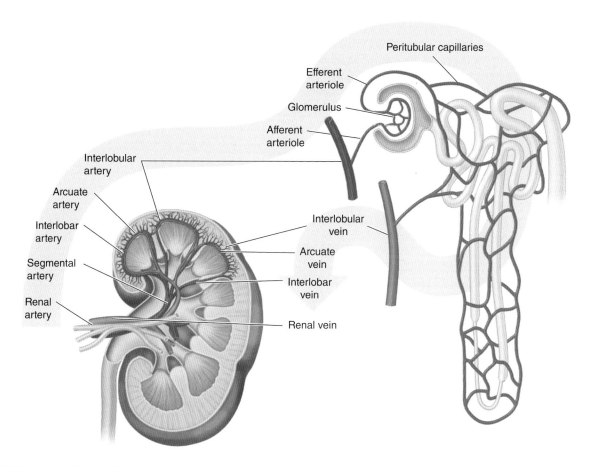

FIGURE 7-8 Schematic of blood flow through the kidney.

2 of the most important parameters in the prognosis and management of patients with all forms of HF.

NEUROHORMONAL REGULATION

It is beyond the scope of this chapter to discuss in detail the role of each neurohormone in detail that is participating in normal physiology, as well as the pathophysiology of HF. In brief, there are multiple important regulatory systems that are activated in HF that work toward preserving perfusion to the brain at the expense of the kidneys, and direct the maximal amount of sodium and water reclamation possible despite the adverse consequences of responses. The sympathetic nervous system releases norepinephrine via peripheral synapses at the neuromuscular junctions within afferent and efferent renal arterioles as well as mesangial cells. This results in stimulation of both alpha- and beta-adrenergic receptors, which in turn decrease RBF, increase intraglomerular pressure, and increase sodium retention. These effects result in a decrease in renal blood flow, an increase in intraglomerular pressure, and increased sodium retention. Norepinephrine is a stimulus for juxtaglomerular cells to release renin, which is the starting point for the renin angiotensin system. In addition to norepinephrine, both epinephrine and dopamine as precursor molecules have effects on the kidneys primarily in the proximal and distal tubule with varying effects depending on the family of receptors. In general, both epinephrine

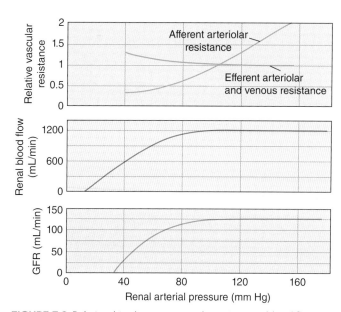

FIGURE 7-9 Relationships between vascular resistance, blood flow, and glomerular filtration.

and norepinephrine stimulate the reabsorption of salt and water. Dopamine, however, acting on a different family of receptors, can stimulate natriuresis and diuresis. In general, the epinephrine and norepinephrine effects are more powerful and the net effect of sympathetic stimulation to the kidneys is release of renin, reduction in RBF, increased salt and water retention, and a slightly reduced GFR.

The renin angiotensin system is integral to renal physiology, not only because the kidneys are the site of renin production and release, but because of the direct effects of angiotensin II on the renal vasculature and renal tubular cells. The results of angiotensin II release include efferent arteriolar vasoconstriction, salt and water retention, and reductions in RBF. Because intraglomerular pressure is elevated, angiotensin II results in maintenance or slight increases in GFR.

Both norepinephrine and angiotensin II stimulate the chromaffin cells in the adrenal glands to synthesize and release aldosterone. Aldosterone has a powerful effect on the principal cells in the collecting ducts, prompting them to reabsorb sodium and release potassium into the urine provided there is adequate delivery of urinary sodium to the distal nephron. In the setting of HF, the result of activation of the sympathetic nervous system and the renin-angiotensin-aldosterone axis is salt and water retention, and over a long period of time, renal fibrosis and drop-out of nephrons with a reduction in GFR.

Arginine vasopressin is secreted by the hypothalamus in response to cardiac afferent signaling to the brain in HF. Vasopressin stimulates V_2 receptors on the principal cell (Figure 7-10) in the collecting

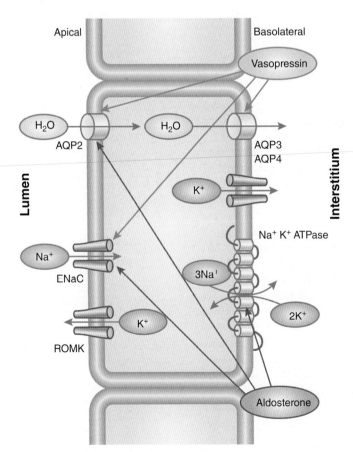

FIGURE 7-10 Collecting duct cell and mechanism of action of aldosterone and arginine vasopressin.

duct, thus stimulating aquaporin channel expression and activation, which work to reclaim free water from the collecting duct. This vasopressin effect raises urine osmolality, lowers plasma osmolality, and represents an inappropriate release of antidiuretic hormone, which can cause hyponatremia in HF patients. When this occurs, this is a poor prognostic sign indicating that systems that work to maintain the plasma concentration of sodium near 140 mEq/L have failed and that short-term cardiac compensation as well as some degree of brain edema are imminent. These changes are common in the setting of multiple forms of hormonal dysregulation including a relative deficiency/resistance to erythropoietin and anemia. Thus there is a vicious cycle of multiple abnormalities that are caused by HF, which beget worsened HF symptoms and are associated with decompensation (Figure 7-11).

Endothelins (ET-1, ET-2, ET-2) are derived from ET precursor (big ET), which is produced by renal tubular cells, and to a lesser extent endothelial and most other cell lines in the kidney, and is a powerful paracrine factor that works on ET-A and ET-B receptors. Endothelin-1 is a potent vasoconstrictor peptide involved in both normal renal physiology and pathology including constriction of cortical and medullary vessels (ET-A), mesangial cell contraction (ET-A), stimulation of extracellular matrix production and fibrosis (ET-B), and inhibition of sodium and water reabsorption along the collecting duct (ET-B).[9] While endothelin receptor antagonists have not proven to be effective in the treatment of HF, they have found a role in the treatment of pulmonary HTN and at very low doses may be effective in reducing the progression of CKD.[10]

Adenosine is another important paracrine substance in the kidney that is produced by multiple cell lines and acts on a family of receptors. Although short-lived in the circulation, adenosine can activate 4 subtypes of G protein-coupled adenosine receptors: A(1), A(2A), A(2B), and A(3). Stimulation of the adenosine A1 receptor on proximal tubular cells results in reabsorption of salt and water and in addition, via tubuloglomerular feedback, increases afferent arterial tone and reduces glomerular blood flow resulting in a reduction in GFR. Recently, adenosine 2B receptors have been implicated in development of fibrosis following renal ischemia in mouse models.[11] Thus adenosine and its effects on receptors, as well as their differential expression probably play roles in hemodynamics, salt and water balance, as well as response to ischemic injury. Dual adenosine A1/A2B inhibition may be a potential therapeutic target for HF in the future.[12]

There are several mediators of vasodilation of the peritubular network in the renal medulla including nitric oxide, bradykinin, and prostaglandins.[13] These substances may be produced by vascular, tubular, or interstitial satellite cells and appear to be important in maintaining the integrity of blood flow and tissue structure in the tubules and peritubular network. Nitric oxide synthase is present in renal tubular cells and appears to be important in maintaining normal salt and water homeostasis as it relates to blood pressure regulation.[14] Bradykinin opposes the effects of aldosterone at the distal nephron epithelial Na channel (ENaC) and results in natriuresis.[15] Prostaglandin E(2) is a major renal cyclooxygenase-derived metabolite of arachidonic acid and interacts with 4 G protein-coupled receptors: EP(1), EP(2), EP(3), and EP(4). EP(1) expression predominates in the collecting duct where it inhibits Na(+) absorption, contributing to natriuresis. The EP(2) receptor regulates vascular reactivity in the peritubular network. The

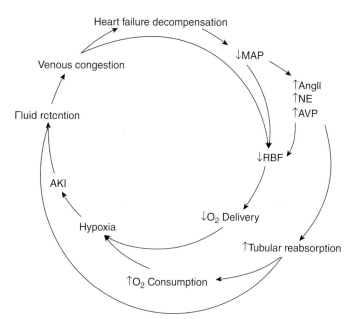

FIGURE 7-11 Multiple processes involved in the pathogenesis of acute heart failure.

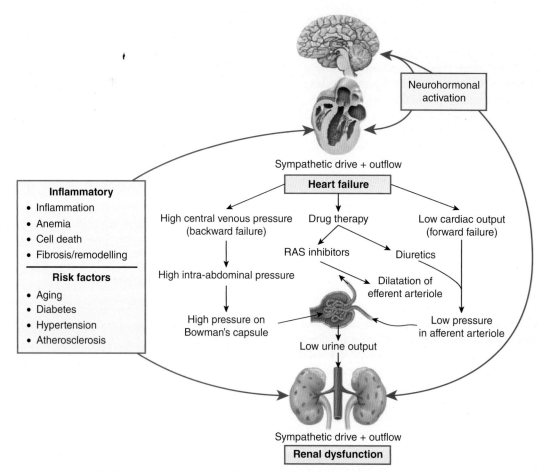

FIGURE 7-12 Factors involved in the development of type 1 and 3 cardiorenal syndromes.

EP(3) receptor is also expressed in vessels as well as in the thick ascending limb and collecting duct, where it partially antagonizes the effect of aquaporin channels in reclaiming water from the collecting duct. EP(4) may regulate glomerular tone and renal renin release. Thus, PGE(2) can be thought of as a buffer, preventing excessive responses to physiological perturbations in the setting of HF. As a result, the use of nonsteroidal anti-inflammatory agents, which impair the production of PGE(2), has been associated with worsened outcomes in patients with HF.[16]

CELL SIGNALING IN CARDIORENAL FAILURE

It has been increasingly appreciated that beyond hemodynamics and neurohormonal derangements (Figure 7-12, Tables 7-1 and 7-2), HF is a condition in which production of cell-signaling peptides (interleukins [ILs], tumor necrosis factor, intracellular transforming growth factor beta) may play a role in directing cell differentiation and proliferation of fibroblasts in the deposition of collagen and tissue fibrosis. Additionally, some cell-signaling molecules may mediate acute tubular dysfunction in the setting of AHF (IL-6, IL-18). The net result may be progressive and simultaneous renal and cardiac fibrosis termed type 4 cardiorenal syndrome. While the production of cell-signaling peptides from adipocytes, endothelial cells, hepatocytes, and immune cells has been termed *inflammation*, this

Table 7-1 Peptide Hormone Actions in the Kidney

Peptide	Localization of Receptors	Intracellular Messenger	Physiological Effects
Atrial natriuretic factor	Mesangium; efferent arteriole	cGMP	↑ GFR
	Inner medullary collecting duct	cGMP	↓ Na reabsorption
Angiotensin II	Mesangium; efferent arteriole	↑ $[Ca^{2+}]_1$	↓ K_f; ↑ glomerular capillary hydrostatic pressure; complex effect on GFR
	Proximal tubule	?↑ $[Ca^{2+}]_1$	
			Stimulates $NaHCO_3$ reabsorption
Vasopressin	V_1—mesangium, renomedullary interstitial cells	↑ $[Ca^{2+}]_1$ cAMP	↓ K_f; stimulates prostaglandin synthesis
	V_2—medullary thick ascending limb;	cAMP	↑ NaCL reabsorption; ↓ HCO_3 reabsorption
	cortical and medullary collecting duct		↑ Water permeability; ↑ K secretion
Y-MSH	(?) Proximal tubule	?	↓ Na reabsorption; natriuresis
Growth hormone	Renal tubule	?	Postulated role in GFR, RBF
Prolactin	Renal tubule	?	Probably no function in mammals
Parathyroid hormone	Mesangium	cAMP	↓ K_f; extracellular fluid volume-related effects on GFR
	Proximal tubule	cAMP; $[Ca^{2+}]_1$	
			↓ $NaHCO_3$ reabsorption; trivial effect on NA excretion
Calcitonin	Thick ascending limb of Henle's loop; distal convolution	cAMP	↑ Ca reabsorption; no major effect on Na reabsorption
Insulin	Proximal convoluted tubule	?	↑ proximal reabsorption;
		?	↑ distal reabsorption; ↓ Na excretion
Glucagon	(?) Mesangium	? cAMP	↑ GFR
	Thick ascending limb of Henle's loop; distal convolution	cAMP	↑ Ca, Mg reabsorption; ↓ HCO_3 reabsorption; no effect on Na excretion other than that related to increases in GFR

GFR = glomerular filtration rate;

$[Ca^{2+}]_1$ = intracellular free cytosolic calcium concentration;

cAMP = cyclic adenosine 3',5'-monophosphate; cGMP, cyclic guanosine 3',5'-monophosphate;

K_f = glomerular ultrafiltration coefficient; RBF, renal blood flow;

Y-MSH = Y-melanocyte stimulating hormone; ↑ = increased; ↓ = decreased.

Table 7-2 Sites of Common Hormonal Action in the Kidney

Hormone	Species	PCT[a]	PR	TDL	TAL	MAL	CAL	DCT$_b$	DCT$_g$	CCT$_g$	CCT$_l$	MCT	Ref.
PTH[b]	Rabbit	III[c]	II	0	—	0	II	0	III	III	0	0	10
	Rat	III	II	0	—	0	III	IIII	II		±[d]	0	45, 46
SCT	Rabbit	0	0	0	0	III	+	IIII	0	0	0	0	11
	Rat	0	0	0	0	II	III	IIII	III		III	0	45, 46
ISO	Rabbit	0	0	0	—	0	0	0	IIII	IIII	II	+	9
	Rat	0	0	0	—	0	II	II	II		II	0	45, 46
AVP	Rabbit	0	0	0	+	II	+	0	0	±	III	IIII	31, 46
	Rat	0	0	0	+	III	II	II	II		III	IIII	45, 46
GLU	Rabbit	0	0	0	0	±	—	0	0	0	0	0	46
	Rat	0	0	0	0	III	III	IIII	—		II	II	2

[a]Abbreviations for nephron segments: CAL, cortical thick ascending limb; CCT$_g$ and CCT$_l$, "granular" and "light" portions, respectively, of the cortical collecting tubule (CNT-connecting tubule, is synonymous with CCT$_g$, initial collecting tubule, or branched collecting tubule); MCT, medullary collecting tubule. In rat nephrons, DCT$_b$ = early DCT; DCT$_g$ = late DCT; DCT$_b$ and DCT$_g$, "bright" and "granular" portions, respectively, of the distal convoluted tubule; MAL, medullary thick ascending limb; PCT, proximal convoluted tubule; PR, pars recta; TAL, thin ascending limb; TDL, thin descending limb.

[b]Abbreviations for hormones: AVP, arginine vasopressin; ISO, isoproterenol; GLU, glucagon PTH, parathyroid hormone; SCT, salmon calcitonin.

[c]Intensity of effect on adenylate cyclase is graded from 0 to IIII; —, data not available.

[d]In rat nephrons, CCT is not further subdivided.

term does not appropriately represent the processes observed in HF. Inflammation classically involves 4 elements: (1) white blood cells, (2) complement, (3) antibodies, and (4) cytokines. Thus inflammation probably does not describe the abnormal cell signaling that is occurring in the heart and kidney, as reflected in the measurement of cytokines or their downstream effects including tubular and myocardial cell dysfunction, apoptosis, and replacement fibrosis. There are a host of hormones that have defined functions along the nephron at specific sites, which are summarized in Table 7-3 and Figure 7-13. As the kidneys fail in the setting of HF, these effector actions can be partially lost causing additional derangements that may become clinically relevant (eg, hyperphosphatemia, hyperparathyroidism).

RENAL RESPONSE TO DIURETICS

Diuretics are a mainstay in the treatment of HF for the relief of systemic congestion and to initiate plasma refill of salt and water from the interstitial space into the venous vasculature. There are a host of diuretics that have different and specific locations of action along the nephron with key issues with respect to their physiological response in HF (Figure 7-14). All available diuretics are tightly bound by albumin and do not undergo glomerular filtration. In order to work, they must get secreted by the S2 segment of the proximal tubule into the urine. Hypoalbuminemia results in an increased volume of distribution of diuretics and lesser delivery to the kidneys and is 1 of many factors related to decreased diuretic

Table 7-3 Binding Site Density of Common Hormones and the Kidney

Hormone	Species	PCT[a]	PR	TDL	TAL	MAL	CAL	DCT$_b$	DCT$_g$	CCT$_g$	CCT$_l$	MCT	Ref.
ALDO[b]	Rabbit	0[c]	0	—	—	0	0	0	—	IIII	II	III	18
CS	Rat	+	±	—	—	±	±	II	—	IIII[d]		II	40
INS	Rabbit	II	II	±	—	IIII	II	IIII	—	II	II	II	52
A$_{II}$	Rat	IIII	II	—	—	+	II	+	—	±		+	49
GLU	Rat	0	—	0	0	IIII	II	II		+		+	7
ANP	Rat	0	0	0	0	0	0	0		0		0	8
	Rabbit	0	0	—	—	0	0	0	0	—	0	0	8
α$_1$-ADR	Rabbit	II	0	—	—	—	—	—	—		0	—	38
	Rat	III	II	—	—	+	+	±	—		0	0	58
DA$_1$	Rat	III	+	—	—	±	±	+	—		+	+	59

[a]Abbreviations for nephron segments are as given in Table 7-2.

[b]Abbreviations for hormones: α$_1$-ADR, α$_1$ adrenergic receptors; A$_{II}$, angiotensin II; ALDO, aldosterone; ANP, atrial natriuretic peptide; CS, corticosterone; DA$_1$, dopamine$_1$; INS, insulin; GLU, glucagon.

[c]Density of specific binding sites is graded 0 to IIII; —, data not available. The table does not include data from microdissected glomeruli, where III binding has been found for A$_{II}$ (49) and ANP (8) and ± for DA$_1$ (58) (see text).

[d]In rat nephrons, CCT is not further subdivided.

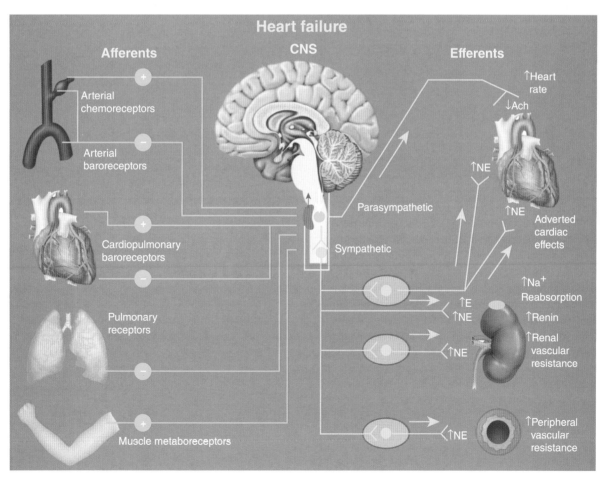

FIGURE 7-13 Neurohormonal activation in heart failure.

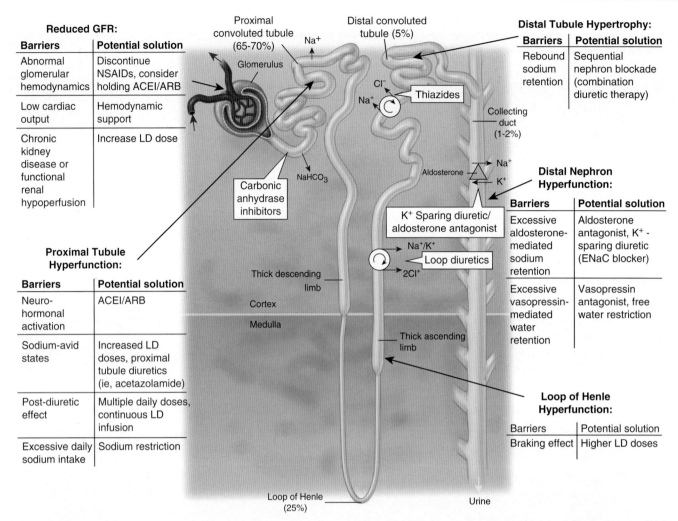

Reduced GFR:

Barriers	Potential solution
Abnormal glomerular hemodynamics	Discontinue NSAIDs, consider holding ACEI/ARB
Low cardiac output	Hemodynamic support
Chronic kidney disease or functional renal hypoperfusion	Increase LD dose

Proximal Tubule Hyperfunction:

Barriers	Potential solution
Neuro-hormonal activation	ACEI/ARB
Sodium-avid states	Increased LD doses, proximal tubule diuretics (ie, acetazolamide)
Post-diuretic effect	Multiple daily doses, continuous LD infusion
Excessive daily sodium intake	Sodium restriction

Distal Tubule Hypertrophy:

Barriers	Potential solution
Rebound sodium retention	Sequential nephron blockade (combination diuretic therapy)

Distal Nephron Hyperfunction:

Barriers	Potential solution
Excessive aldosterone-mediated sodium retention	Aldosterone antagonist, K⁺-sparing diuretic (ENaC blocker)
Excessive vasopressin-mediated water retention	Vasopressin antagonist, free water restriction

Loop of Henle Hyperfunction:

Barriers	Potential solution
Braking effect	Higher LD doses

FIGURE 7-14 Sites of diuretic action and resistance in the nephron. (Jentzer JC, DeWald TA, Hernandez AF. Combination of Loop Diuretics With Thiazide-Type Diuretics in Heart Failure. *J Am Coll Cardiol.* 2010;56(19):1527-1534. doi:https://doi.org/10.1016/j.jacc.2010.06.034.)

responsiveness. Carbonic anhydrase inhibitors (eg, acetazolamide) work in the proximal tubule and cause loss of sodium bicarbonate and thus create a metabolic acidosis. Because of these effects and the relatively large opportunity for upregulation of sodium absorption in the remaining nephron, carbonic anhydrase inhibitors are not a mainstay of therapy for either acute or chronic HF. Loop diuretics (eg, furosemide, bumetanide, torsemide, ethacrynic acid) however, are widely relied upon in most patients with HF at some time or another for the relief of congestion. These agents are the most powerful diuretic class, causing the excretion of 20% to 25% of filtered sodium load.[17] Loop diuretics are secreted by organic anion transporters (OATs), which are expressed in proximal tubule cells and then work in the urinary lumen of the loop of Henle to impair sodium reuptake in the thick ascending limb, which is a major site of sodium reclamation from urine.[18] Furosemide is catabolized by proximal tubular cells and can accumulate in the blood if there is CKD or AKI. Bumetanide and torsemide are broken down by the liver and do not accumulate in renal failure. Use of bolus loop diuretics is equally as effective as continuous infusion for AHF, but with fewer adverse effects such as hyponatremia and hypotension.[19,20] A principal mechanism of loop diuretic upregulation of sodium channel number and function, which undermines channel inhibition by the loop diuretic.[21] Thiazide diuretics exert their mechanism of action in the distal convoluted tubule where they impair reuptake of sodium from the lumen. The thiazide group and metolazone are moderately potent diuretics, resulting in the excretion of 5% to 8% of filtered sodium.[17] Chlorothiazide intravenously and metolazone orally are the most commonly used thiazide diuretics in HF, but usually in conjunction with loop diuretics and as part of "sequential nephron blockade" with pharmacological agents. Diuretics that work proximal to the collecting duct have the potential for causing hypokalemia if distal urinary sodium delivery is increased, because this stimulates the epithelial sodium channel (ENaC) to reabsorb sodium under the control of aldosterone, and causes the renal outer medullary potassium channel (ROMK) channels to excrete potassium in the principal cells. The potassium-sparing drugs are considered mildly potent, causing the excretion of only 2% to 3% of filtered sodium.[17] They spare potassium because they work at the collecting duct and do not influence delivery of sodium to the principal cell as discussed above. Triamterene and amiloride block ENaC on the lumen side of the collecting ducts, whereas mineralocorticoid receptor antagonists work in the principal cells to partially block the effects of endogenous aldosterone and as a result there is less ENaC and ROMK activity with lesser degrees of potassium excretion.

It is common in severe HF to deploy loop diuretics, a thiazide, and an mineralocorticoid receptor antagonist (MRA) agent for control of congestion and for symptom relief in the same patient. As a consequence of sequential nephron blockade with diuretics, volume depletion can occur and electrolyte disturbances, most commonly hyperkalemia, are frequent and must be anticipated with prudent use of the laboratory.[22] Hyperkalemia has multiple causes in the setting of HF as shown in Figure 7-15. There is a clear relationship between the development of hyperkalemia and mortality in patients with critical illness including HF (Figure 7-16). The drug class most commonly implicated is the MRAs; however, many drugs in combination work to sufficiently suppress the release of aldosterone from the adrenal gland and/or antagonize its effects at the collecting ducts to result in insufficient elimination of potassium from the body.[23] Thus, there is a risk-to-benefit equation that must be balanced in patients with HF, CKD, and hyperkalemia as shown in Figure 7-17. Novel strategies employing agents to enable greater gastrointestinal elimination (patiromer calcium, sodium zirconium cyclosilicate) may play a future role in the enablement of drugs that antagonize the renin-angiotensin-aldosterone axis.

PROGNOSIS

Our patient had several clinical features that predict a poor prognosis. Her baseline renal filtration function was moderately impaired, and as a result she was at risk for inpatient and short-term post discharge death or rehospitalization.[24] In multivariate modeling, reduced eGFR or stage of CKD is in general the most important prognostic variable in the setting of HF and is more important than LVEF, type of cardiomyopathy, and treatment received in terms of prognosis for death or hospitalization.[25] The development of type 1 cardiorenal syndrome, which occurs in approximately 25% of patients with AHF is an additional poor prognostic sign and carries a 4- to 7-fold increased risk for death, the need for renal replacement therapy, worsened CKD after discharge, and outpatient mortality.[25]

FOLLOW-UP

Our patient reached a maximum serum creatinine on day 4 of 3.2 mg/dL and then slowly returned to a new baseline of 1.9 mg/dL. The urine was negative for eosinophils. The patient received a 5-day infusion of milrinone and gradually responded with improved diuresis and was discharged on the same baseline medical regimen. While MRA agents were considered, the risk of hyperkalemia was felt to be prohibitive.

PATIENT EDUCATION

It is important for patients to understand their laboratory values that reflect renal function. It is helpful to realize that blood is pumped from the heart to the kidneys and there must be elimination of sodium and water in the urine to stay in good fluid balance. Diuretics help adjust fluid balance, but do not influence the natural history of HF. Long-term dietary, medical, and clinical compliance with office visits and procedures is essential to optimal survival with HF.

PATIENT EDUCATION RESOURCES

American Association of Heart Failure Nurses: https://www.aahfn.org/pdf/awareness2015/AAHFN-15-TipSheet-CardioRenal-Nurse-Web.pdf

SUMMARY

The renal system is integral to the cardiovascular system in health and disease. In the setting of HF, those patients with preserved renal function who do not develop significant reductions in the setting of AHF enjoy good responses to diuretics and optimal outcomes. Those patients with CKD at baseline and who develop acute kidney injury in the setting of hospitalization for HF have increased rates of in-hospital complications, including volume overload, hyperkalemia, and death. Additionally, they face increased risks of readmissions and longer-term mortality, including pump failure and arrhythmic death. Future research into novel diagnostic and therapeutic targets is likely to yield advances in the field of HF given the very close relationships between the cardiovascular and renal organ systems.

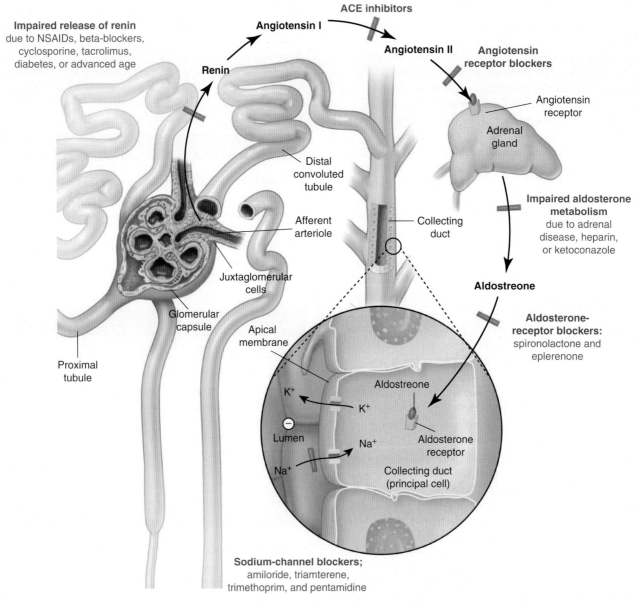

FIGURE 7-15 Renal pharmacological mechanisms in the pathogenesis of hyperkalemia. (Reproduced with permission from Palmer BF. Managing Hyperkalemia Caused by Inhibitors of the Renin-Angiotensin-Aldosterone System. *N Engl J Med*. 2004;351:585-592.)

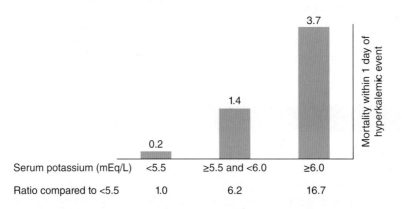

1 day mortality rate for patients with serum potassium >= 5.5 mEq/L was
6 to 17 times higher than for patients with serum potassium <5.5 mEq/L

FIGURE 7-16 Serum potassium and inpatient mortality rate. (Data from Einhorn LM, Zhan M, Hsu VD, et al. The Frequency of Hyperkalemia and Its Significance in Chronic Kidney Disease. *Arch Intern Med*. 2009;169(12):1156 -1162. doi:10.1001/archinternmed.2009.132.)

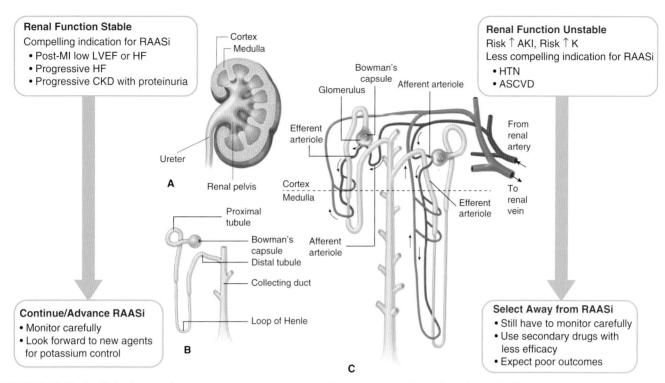

Renal Function Stable
Compelling indication for RAASi
• Post-MI low LVEF or HF
• Progressive HF
• Progressive CKD with proteinuria

Renal Function Unstable
Risk ↑ AKI, Risk ↑ K
Less compelling indication for RAASi
• HTN
• ASCVD

Continue/Advance RAASi
• Monitor carefully
• Look forward to new agents for potassium control

Select Away from RAASi
• Still have to monitor carefully
• Use secondary drugs with less efficacy
• Expect poor outcomes

Cortex
Medulla
Ureter
Renal pelvis
A

Proximal tubule
Bowman's capsule
Distal tubule
Collecting duct
Loop of Henle
Afferent arteriole
B

Bowman's capsule
Glomerulus
Efferent arteriole
Afferent arteriole
From renal artery
To renal vein
Efferent arteriole
Cortex
Medulla
C

FIGURE 7-17 Trade-offs in the use of renin angiotensin system antagonists in patients with very low glomerular filtration rates.

REFERENCES

1. Ronco C, McCullough PA, Anker SD, et al. Cardiorenal syndromes: an executive summary from the consensus conference of the Acute Dialysis Quality Initiative (ADQI). *Contrib Nephrol.* 2010;165:54-67. Epub 2010 Apr 20.

2. McCullough PA, Philbin EF, Spertus JA, Kaatz S, Sandberg KR, Weaver WD. Confirmation of a heart failure epidemic: findings from the Resource Utilization Among Congestive Heart Failure (R.E.A.C.H.) study. *J Am Coll Cardiol.* 2002;39:60-69.

3. Soman P, Lahiri A, Mieres JH, et al. Etiology and pathophysiology of new-onset heart failure: evaluation by myocardial perfusion imaging. *J Nucl Cardiol.* 2009 Jan-Feb;16(1):82-91. Epub 2009 Jan 20.

4. Marinescu V, McCullough PA. Managing comorbidities. Chronic kidney disease. In: Bakris G, Baliga RR, eds. *Hypertension.* New York, NY: Oxford American Cardiology Library, Oxford University Press; 2012:71-81.

5. Ronco C, Cicoira M, McCullough PA. Cardiorenal syndrome type 1: pathophysiological crosstalk leading to combined heart and kidney dysfunction in the setting of acutely decompensated heart failure. *J Am Coll Cardiol.* 2012;60(12):1031-1042.

6. McCullough PA. Cardiorenal syndromes: pathophysiology to prevention. *Int J Nephrol.* 2010;2010:762590.

7. Haase M, Müller C, Damman K, et al. Pathogenesis of cardio-renal syndrome type 1 in acute decompensated heart failure: workgroup statements from the eleventh consensus conference of the Acute Dialysis Quality Initiative (ADQI). *Contrib Nephrol.* 2013;182:99-116. doi:10.1159/000349969. Epub 2013 May 13.

8. Carlström M, Wilcox CS, Arendshorst WJ. Renal autoregulation in health and disease. *Physiol Rev.* 2015;95(2):405-511. doi:10.1152/physrev.00042.2012.

9. Peti-Peterdi J, Harris RC. Macula Densa Sensing and Signaling Mechanisms of Renin Release. *Journal of the American Society of Nephrology : JASN.* 2010;21(7):1093-1096. doi:10.1681/ASN.2009070759.

10. Jameson, J. Larry, DeGroot, L. J., De Kretser, D. M, Giudice, L., Grossman, A., Melmed, S., Potts, J. T., & Weir, G. C. (2016). Chapter 18: Vasopressin, Diabetes Insipidus, and the Syndrome of Inappropriate Antidiuresis, Endocrinology: Adult & Pediatric. 7th edition (pp. 298–311). Philadelphia, PA: Elsevier/Saunders.

11. Speed JS, Fox BM, Johnston JG, Pollock DM. Endothelin and renal ion and water transport. *Semin Nephrol.* 2015;35(2):137-144. doi:10.1016/j.semnephrol.2015.02.003.

12. Kohan DE, Cleland JG, Rubin LJ, Theodorescu D, Barton M. Clinical trials with endothelin receptor antagonists: what went wrong and where can we improve? *Life Sci.* 2012;91(13-14):528-539. doi:10.1016/j.lfs.2012.07.034. Epub 2012 Aug. 6.

13. Roberts V, Lu B, Dwyer KM, Cowan PJ. Adenosine receptor expression in the development of renal fibrosis following ischemic injury. *Transplant Proc.* 2014;46(10):3257-3261. doi:10.1016/j.transproceed.2014.09.151.

14. Tofovic SP, Salah EM, Smits GJ, et al. Dual A1/A2B receptor blockade improves cardiac and renal outcomes in a rat model of heart failure with preserved ejection fraction. *J Pharmacol Exp Ther.* 2015 Nov 19. pii: jpet.115.228841. [Epub ahead of print].

15. Sadowski J, Badzynska B. Intrarenal vasodilator systems: NO, prostaglandins and bradykinin. An integrative approach. *J Physiol Pharmacol.* 2008;59(9):105-119.

16. Hyndman KA, Pollock JS. Nitric oxide and the A and B of endothelin of sodium homeostasis. *Curr Opin Nephrol Hypertens.* 2013;22(1):26-31. doi:10.1097/MNH.0b013e32835b4edc.

17. Mamenko M, Zaika O, Pochynyuk O. Direct regulation of ENaC by bradykinin in the distal nephron. Implications for renal sodium handling. *Curr Opin Nephrol Hypertens.* 2014;23(2):122-129. doi:10.1097/01.mnh.0000441053.81339.61.

18. Ungprasert P, Srivali N, Kittanamongkolchai W. Non-steroidal anti-inflammatory drugs and risk of heart failure exacerbation: a systematic review and meta-analysis. *Eur J Intern Med.* 2015;26(9):685-690. doi:10.1016/j.ejim.2015.09.012. Epub 2015 Oct 1.

19. Puschett JB. Pharmacological classification and renal actions of diuretics. *Cardiology.* 1994;84(2):4-13.

20. Wilcox CS. New insights into diuretic use in patients with chronic renal disease. *J Am Soc Nephrol.* 2002;13(3):798-805.

21. Palazzuoli A, Pellegrini M, Ruocco G, et al. Continuous versus bolus intermittent loop diuretic infusion in acutely decompensated heart failure: a prospective randomized trial. *Crit Care.* 2014;18(3):R134. doi:10.1186/cc13952.

22. Palazzuoli A, Ruocco G, Ronco C, McCullough PA. Loop diuretics in acute heart failure: beyond the decongestive relief for the kidney. *Crit Care.* 2015;19:296. doi:10.1186/s13054-015-1017-3.

23. De Bruyne LK. Mechanisms and management of diuretic resistance in congestive heart failure. *Postgrad Med J.* 2003;79(931):268-271.

24. McCullough PA, Beaver TM, Bennett-Guerrero E, et al. Acute and chronic cardiovascular effects of hyperkalemia: new insights into prevention and clinical management. *Rev Cardiovasc Med.* 2014;15(1):11-23.

25. McCullough PA, Costanzo MR, Silver M, Spinowitz B, Zhang J, Lepor NE. Novel agents for the prevention and management of hyperkalemia. *Rev Cardiovasc Med.* 2015;16(2):140-155.

26. McCullough PA, Soman SS, Shah SS, et al. Risks associated with renal dysfunction in coronary care unit patients. *J Am Coll Cardiol.* 2000;36(3):679-684. PMID: 10987584.

27. Palazzuoli A, Beltrami M, Nodari S, McCullough PA, Ronco C. Clinical impact of renal dysfunction in heart failure. *Rev Cardiovasc Med.* 2011;12(4):186-199. PMID: 22249509.

8 DEPRESSION IN HEART FAILURE

Philip F. Binkley, MD, MPH

PATIENT CASE

A 45-year-old man with a 5-year history of nonischemic cardiomyopathy with an ejection fraction of 30% was seen in routine follow-up in the heart failure (HF) clinic. He had only mild limitation of activity with New York Heart Association (NYHA) Functional Classification I to II symptoms. He had been on a stable regimen of guideline-directed medical therapy for at least 6 months.

In symptom review, he noted that he was having trouble sleeping though he did not have paroxysmal nocturnal dyspnea or orthopnea. He was not noted to snore or have nocturnal apneic episodes according to his wife. It was noted that he had lost 5 pounds and he stated that he had little appetite. He further noted that he had difficulty concentrating on tasks and that, although he had previously engaged in a routine walking regimen, he now had little interest in activity and spent most of his time sitting at home watching television.

He completed the Patient Health Questionnaire 9 (PHQ-9) while waiting for his appointment. The total score on the first part of this depression screening tool was 16, which was consistent with significant depression and suggested the need for treatment. The patient agreed that he was likely depressed and had "felt down" for many days over the past 2 months.

His physician discussed with him the problems of depression in patients with HF and they began discussions of treatment options.

PREVALENCE OF DEPRESSION IN HEART FAILURE

Depression is a comorbidity common to most forms of heart disease.[1] However, it especially affects those with HF. Ferketich and Binkley analyzed a large cohort of respondents to the National Health Interview Survey (NHIS).[1] Of this cohort, 17,541 completed the K6 depression screen, which is a 6-item questionnaire designed for the NHIS. Table 8-1 shows the odds ratios for reporting depression in different cardiovascular disease categories as compared to those who did not report a history of cardiovascular disease. It can be seen that there is a progressive increase in the odds ratio for reporting symptoms of depression with the lowest odds ratio being in those with coronary heart disease and the highest odds ratio in those with HF. Therefore, although all patients with heart disease have an increased risk for having depression, those with HF have a 3.6 to 1 odds ratio compared to those without heart disease. As shown in Table 8-2, smaller studies have further demonstrated the increased prevalence of depression in those with HF.[2] Further, patients with HF and depression have increased mortality and an increase in the risk for hospital admission.

Table 8-1 Odds Ratios and 95% CI for Elevated K6 Scores Associated with the Various Cardiovascular Disease Conditions

Cardiovascular Disease[a]	Odds Ratios (95% CI)[b]
CHD	1.3 (0.9–1.8)
CHD alone	0.7 (0.3–1.5)
CHD and ≥1 other condition	1.5 (0.9–2.2)
Time since last episode	
CHD within past 12 mo	1.3 (0.9–2.0)
CHD >12 mo ago	1.2 (0.6–2.3)
MI	2.0 (1.4–3.0)
MI (± self-reported CHD)	2.0 (1.2–3.4)
MI and ≥1 other condition	2.1 (1.3–3.4)
Time since last episode	
MI within past 12 mo	1.8 (1.0–3.1)
MI >12 mo ago	2.2 (1.4–3.5)
CHF	3.1 (1.8–5.1)
CHF alone	3.6 (1.5–8.6)
CHF and ≥1 other condition	2.9 (1.6–5.1)
Time since last episode	
CHF within past 12 mo	3.4 (2.0–5.9)
CHF >12 mo ago	2.5 (0.9–6.8)

Odds ratios for depression associated with different cardiovascular diseases. Reproduced from Ferketich.[7]

Table 8-2 Prevalence and Prognosis of Depression in Heart Failure

Author (y)	n, Setting	Patient Population	Instrument	Prevalence of Depression	Length of Follow-Up	Relative Risk, Major or Severe Depression vs No Depression	
						Rehospitalization or Functional Decline	Mortality
Koenig (1998)[7]	542, inpatient	Age >60	CES-D, HDRS, interview (DSM-IV)	32% minor, 26% major	12 mo	1.96 (3–6 mo) 2.28 (6–9 mo) $P < 0.05$ for both	1.4 (P = ns)
Jiang et al (2001)[5]	374, inpatient	54% ischemic, 8% NYHA class IV	BDI, interview (DSM-IV) GDS	21.4% mild, 13.9% major	12 mo	2.57 (P = 0.02)*	2.12 (P = 0.07)*
Vaccarino et al (2001)[11]	391, inpatient	Age >50	GDS	35% mild, 33.5% moderate, 9% severe	6 mo	2.51 (P = 0.004)*	2.25 (P = 0.10)*
Faris et al (2002)[8]	396, inpatient	0% ischemic, 10% NYHA class IV	ICD-10 code in patient chart	21%	48 mo	0.25 (P = 0.03)*	3.0 (P = 0.004)*
Freedland et al (2003)[12]	682, inpatient	48% ischemic, 7% NYHA class IV	Interview (DSM-IV)	20% major, 16% minor	None	N/A	N/A
Havranek et al (1999)[10]	45, outpatient	N/A	CED-D	24.4%	None	N/A	N/A
Murberg and Bru (1999)[9]	119, outpatient	65% ischemic, 2.5% NYHA class IV	Zung SDS	27% mild, 13% moderate-severe	24 mo	N/A	1.9
Turvey et al (2002)[13]	199, community	Age >70	CIDI	11%	None	N/A	N/A

Summary of studies investigating the relation of depression to mortality and hospitalization in patients with heart failure. Reproduced from Joynt.[13]

As these data show, clinicians caring for patients with HF will find that depression is a common problem and one that cannot be ignored in their care.

PATHOPHYSIOLOGY

Although patients may feel dysphoric due to the physical limitations imposed by impaired cardiac function, there are clearly physiologic mechanisms that contribute to the concurrence of depression and HF. Figure 8-1 demonstrates 3 of these physiologic pathways. As the figure illustrates, there is a reciprocating cycle of mechanisms that promote both the progression of HF and depression.[3]

Among the mechanisms common to both HF and depression is imbalance of the autonomic nervous system.[4] Increased sympathetic and decreased parasympathetic activity evolve early in the onset of HF and this autonomic imbalance likely contributes to vascular modeling, and promotes myocardial damage and enhanced arrhythmia risk.[5] Similarly, autonomic imbalance is a signature of depression and appears to play a role not only in the progression of depression but also in associated adverse health outcomes.[3,6]

Cytokine mediated inflammation is a second promoter of disease progression common to both depression and HF. Increases in inflammatory cytokines have been consistently demonstrated in

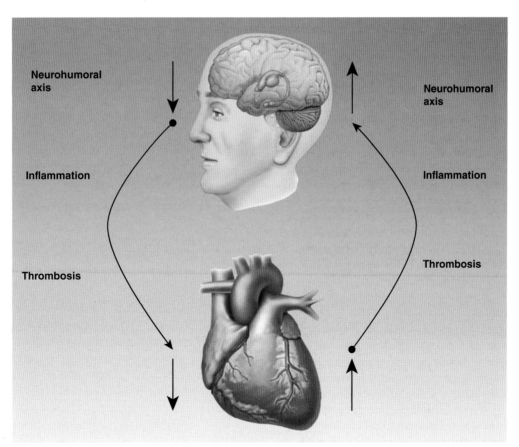

FIGURE 8-1 Heart failure and depression share common pathogenetic mechanisms that may concomitantly advance both disease mechanisms. These include abnormalities of the neurohumoral axis, increases in proinflammatory cytokines, and an increased risk for thrombosis. These pathways emanate from both the brain, top, and the heart bottom, creating a vicious cycle in which both the heart and the brain are affected. Unanswered is whether interruption of any of these pathogenetic pathways in 1 condition will improve the other.

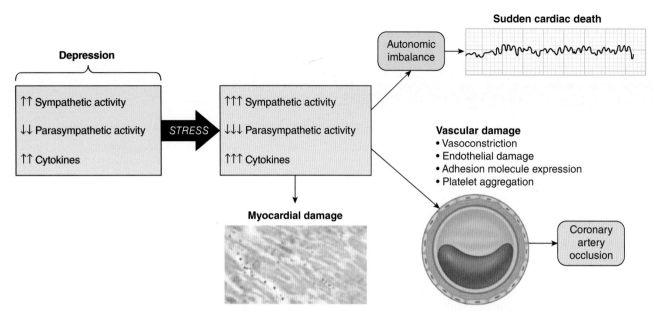

FIGURE 8-2 Abnormal autonomic balance and increases in proinflammatory cytokines that occur in the setting of depression have significant impact on cardiovascular function. These abnormalities can promote further myocardial damage, increase risk for malignant ventricular arrhythmias, and promote vascular damage. (Reproduced from Emani and Binkley; Circulation: Heart Failure.[6])

patients with HF, and likely contribute to progressive myocardial necrosis as well as vascular damage.[3] Cytokines also appear to function as neurotransmitters, and in this capacity have been shown to elicit depressive symptoms in animal models and to be associated with depressed mood in patients.[3]

Finally, both HF and depression are associated with increased risk for platelet aggregation and vascular thrombosis.[2] This hypercoagulability may be due to activation of platelets by both cytokine and sympathetic stimulation as well as increased expression of cell surface activators of platelet aggregation.

As shown in Figure 8-2, these mechanisms can all converge to simultaneously exacerbate depression and HF. Ferketich and Binkley reported that circulating levels of selected circulating cytokines were in fact significantly greater in patients with HF who were depressed as compared to those who were not.[7] This suggests that the coexistence of these mechanisms may have additive detrimental effects in patients with both depression and HF. An intriguing but still unanswered question is whether treatment of either HF or depression will alleviate the symptoms and progression of the other.

SCREENING AND DIAGNOSIS

The high prevalence of depression in coronary artery disease and the associated adverse clinical events motivated an American Heart Association white paper recommending screening of patients for depression.[8] Although this white paper was focused on those with coronary artery disease, the even greater prevalence of depression in patients with HF makes these recommendations even more relevant.

The white paper recommends an initial screen known as the Patient Health Questionnaire 2 (Figure 8-3). If the patient responds yes to either of these questions, a more complete screen provided by the Patient Health Questionnaire 9 (PHQ-9) is recommended (Figure 8-4). This screening instrument asks 9 questions regarding the frequency of symptoms associated with depression experienced over the previous 2 weeks. As shown in Figure 8-4, a range of scores is associated with the possible need for depression treatment.

The PHQ-9 can be administered on paper or electronically on either an inpatient or outpatient basis. Some electronic health records have the PHQ-9 embedded in flow sheets or other components of the system. Figure 8-5 shows a flow diagram for routine computerized inpatient screening of patients with heart disease at the Ross Heart Hospital of The Ohio State University Wexner Medical Center.[9] However, it should be noted that there continues to be controversy regarding whether depression screening in the

---

Patient Health Questionnaire: 2 Items*

Over the past 2 weeks, how often have you been bothered by any of the following problems?

   (1) Little interest or pleasure in doing things.
   (2) Feeling down, depressed, or hopeless.

---

*If the answer is "yes" to either question, then refer for more comprehensive clinical evaluation by a professional qualified in the diagnosis and management of depression or screen with PHQ-9.

FIGURE 8-3 The Patient Health Questionnaire 2. This 2-item depression screen can be used as an initial assessment for symptoms of depression. (Reproduced with permission from Licthman.[5])

PHQ-9 — Nine Symptom Checklist

Patient Name _____ Date _____

1. Over the last 2 weeks, how often have you been bothered by any of the following problems? Read each item carefully, and circle your response.

   a. Little interest or pleasure in doing things
     Not at all   Several days   More than half the days   Nearly every day

   b. Feeling down, depressed, or hopeless
     Not at all   Several days   More than half the days   Nearly every day

   c. Trouble falling asleep, staying asleep, or sleeping too much
     Not at all   Several days   More than half the days   Nearly every day

   d. Feeling tired or having little energy
     Not at all   Several days   More than half the days   Nearly every day

   e. Poor appetite or overeating
     Not at all   Several days   More than half the days   Nearly every day

   f. Feeling bad about yourself, feeling that you are a failure, or feeling that you have let yourself or your family down
     Not at all   Several days   More than half the days   Nearly every day

   g. Trouble concentrating on things such as reading the newspaper or watching television
     Not at all   Several days   More than half the days   Nearly every day

   h. Moving or speaking so slowly that other people could have noticed. Or being so fidgety or restless that you have been moving around a lot more than usual
     Not at all   Several days   More than half the days   Nearly every day

   i. Thinking that you would be better off dead or that you want to hurt yourself in some way
     Not at all   Several days   More than half the days   Nearly every day

2. If you checked off any problem on this questionnaire so far, how difficult have these problems made it for you to do your work, take care of things at home, or get along with other people?

   Not Difficult at All   Somewhat Difficult   Very Difficult   Extremely Difficult

FIGURE 8-4 The Patient Health Questionnaire 9. This 9-question screen for depression may be used as an initial screen for depression or may be triggered by results of PHQ-2. (Reprinted with permission from *Circulation*. 2008;118:1768-1775 ©2008 American Heart Association, Inc.)

PHQ-9 — Scoring Tally Sheet

Patient Name _____ **Date** _____

1. Over the last 2 weeks, how often have you been bothered by any of the following problems? Read each item carefully, and circle your response.

	Not at all	Several days	More than half the days	Nearly every day
	0	1	2	3
a. Little interest or pleasure in doing things				
b. Feeling down, depressed, or hopeless				
c. Trouble falling asleep, staying asleep, or sleeping too much				
d. Feeling tired or having little energy				
e. Poor appetite or overeating				
f. Feeling bad about yourself, feeling that you are a failure, or feeling that you have let yourself or your family down				
g. Trouble concentrating on things such as reading the newspaper or watching television				
h. Moving or speaking so slowly that other people could have noticed. Or being so fidgety or restless that you have been moving around a lot more than usual				
i. Thinking that you would be better off dead or that you want to hurt yourself in some way				
Totals				

2. If you checked off any problem on this questionnaire so far, how difficult have these problems made it for you to do your work, take care of things at home, or get along with other people?

Not Difficult At All	Somewhat Difficult	Very Difficult	Extremely Difficult
0	1	2	3

FIGURE 8-4 (Continued)

inpatient setting accurately reflects the magnitude of depression following hospital discharge.

The American Heart Association white paper provides an algorithm for depression screening, which is shown in Figure 8-6. As indicated in the algorithm, answering yes to Question 9 of the PHQ-9 triggers a further evaluation for possible suicidal ideation. It is important to distinguish suicidal ideation from suicidal behavior.[10] Dube and coauthors published a 4-question follow-up questionnaire that is targeted at stratifying suicide behavior risk. According to this instrument, risk for suicidal action is based on past attempts, having a tangible plan, the patient's assessment of the likelihood that he or she will take action, and whether there are personal factors that would prevent self-harm. It is important that a mental health care professional be consulted to further aid in assessing this risk.

How to Score PHQ-9

Scoring method for diagnosis

Major Depressive Syndrome is suggested if:

- Of the 9 items, 5 or more are circled as at least "More than half the days"
- Either item 1a or 1b is positive, that is, at least "More than the days"

Minor Depressive Syndrome is suggested if:

- Of the 9 items, b, c, or d are circled as at least "More than half the days"
- Either item 1a or 1b is positive, that is, at least "More than half the days"

Scoring method for planning and monitoring treatment

Question One

- To score the first question, tally each response by the number value of each response:

Not at all = 0

Several days = 1

More than half the days = 2

Nearly every day = 3

- Add the numbers together to total the score.
- Interpret the score by using the guide listed below:

Score	Action
≤4	The score suggests the patient may not need depression treatment.
>5-14	Physician uses clinical judgment about treatment, based on patient's duration of symptoms and functional impairment.
≥15	Warrants treatment for depression, using antidepressant, psychotherapy and/or a combination of treatment

Question Two

In question two the patient responses can be one of four: not difficult at all, somewhat difficult, very difficult, extremely difficult. The last two responses suggest that the patient's functionality is impaired. After treatment begins, the functional status is again measured to see if the patient is improving.

FIGURE 8-4 (Continued)

The PHQ-9 and other screening tools are not diagnostic instruments. Diagnosis of depression requires a structured interview with a trained expert to confirm what is suggested by the symptoms detected by screening. However, screening is a critical first step in identifying patients with HF for whom depression is a major comorbidity with significant impact on both quality of life and clinical outcomes.

TREATMENT

There are 2 major approaches to the treatment of mild-to-moderate depression: pharmacologic therapy and psychosocial interventions. There is evidence to suggest that the combination of these 2 modalities may in fact be superior in terms of the breadth and sustainability of symptomatic improvement.[11]

Clinicians vary in their comfort in prescribing antidepressant medications. However, for those who are comfortable, initiating therapy with a selective serotonin reuptake inhibitor (SSRI) can be a simple process as described by a review by Whooley[6] and illustrated in Figure 8-7. The SSRIs sertraline or citalopram may be preferable as initial therapies given their minimal interaction with the P450 cytochrome family that is responsible for the metabolism of many cardiovascular drugs. As shown in Figure 8-7, it is important to assure that the patient does not have a bipolar disorder or suicidal ideation, either of which can be exacerbated by an SSRI. If neither exists, starting doses of either of the above SSRIs can be administered with titration based on symptom control. Whooley noted that failure to respond to the first SSRI does not predict a failure to respond to a second. Therefore, if there is not a beneficial response, the second SSRI can be administered while the dose of the first is reduced.

Psychosocial interventions are the second mainstay of depression treatment. Perhaps the most effective is cognitive behavioral therapy (CBT), which is focused on challenging and eliminating erroneous self-perceptions, event interpretations, and negative

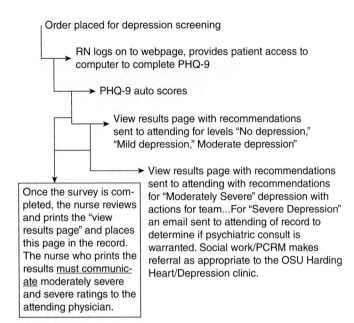

FIGURE 8-5 Schema for an inpatient computer-based screening program implemented at the Ross Heart Hospital of The Ohio State University Wexner Medical Center. (Reproduced with permission Yeager et al. Clinics of Heart Failure.[19])

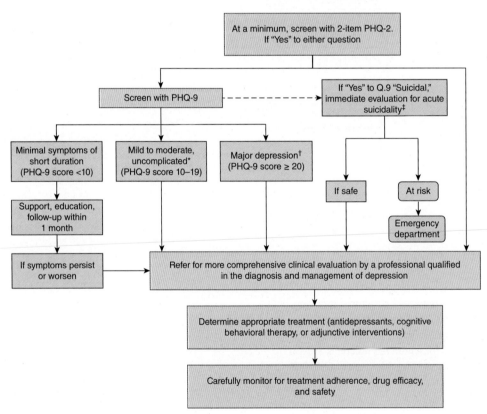

*Meets diagnostic criteria for major depression, has a PHQ-9 score of 10–19, has had no more than 1 or 2 prior episodes of depression, and screens negative for bipolar disorder, suicidality, significant substance abuse, or other major psychiatric problems.

†Meets the diagnostic criteria for major depression and 1) has a PHQ-9 score ≥20; or 2) has had 3 or more prior depressive episodes; or 3) screens positive for bipolar disorder, suicidality, significant substance abuse, or other major psychiatric problem.

‡If "Yes" to Q.9 "suicidal," immediately evaluate for acute suicidality. If safe, refer for more comprehensive clinical evaluation; if at risk for suicide, escort the patient to the emergency department.

FIGURE 8-6 Algorithm for screening and diagnosis of depression as proposed in American Heart Association white paper. (Reprinted with permission from Circulation. 2008;118:1768-1775 ©2008 American Heart Association, Inc.)

thoughts (Figure 8-8).[3,6] As Figure 8-8 shows, interrupting the cycle of inaccurate thoughts and misperceptions, dysphoric mood or anxiety, and associated behaviors has been shown to have a significant impact on depression.[6]

Interventions such as CBT can be limited by access to professionals trained in these methods. However, there are available web-based CBT programs such as Beating the Blues.[12] This program consists of a series of modules teaching cognitive behavioral techniques over an 8-week period. Studies have shown that use of the computerized CBT reduces symptoms of depression and improves social adjustment.[12] In general, this program appears to deliver effective CBT treatment of depression to a wide range of patients and is especially useful for patients for whom direct access to mental health care may be limited.

As discussed above, a combination of pharmacologic and CBT or other interventions may provide optimal results. Collaboration with a mental health care professional is always recommended as the best approach to depression therapy.

TREATMENT OUTCOMES

Table 8-3 summarizes studies identified in the literature that address treatment outcomes in patients with depression and HF. It is apparent that there is mixed evidence for improved HF outcomes with depression treatment. Importantly, the 2 analyses of data from the SADHART-CHF study of sertraline therapy in HF showed improved functional status and reduced adverse events with remission of depression regardless of treatment arm.[13,14] The placebo arm of this study consisted of nurse-facilitated support and is consistent with the known efficacy of psychosocial intervention in depression therapy. The findings are also consistent with the report by Diez-Quevedo et al that showed that depression itself was related to mortality even though antidepressant therapy itself was not independently associated.[15] Of interest is the finding by Veien and coworkers that those patients with HF treated with antidepressants were treated with lower doses of beta blockers.[16] Suboptimal beta blocker treatment may have contributed to the increased mortality rather than depression or depression therapy itself. The MOOD-HF trial of the SSRI escitalopram found no impact on mortality or outcomes in patients with HF and depression.[17] However, there was not a significant improvement in depression in the treatment group.

A substudy of the HF-ACTION trial investigated the impact of aerobic exercise on depression and outcomes in patients with HF.[18] Although aerobic exercise had a modest impact on improvement in depression, improvement in depression symptoms was associated with a reduction in adjusted risk of all-cause mortality or hospitalization. Similar to the SADHART-CHF trial, improvement in depression was associated with improved outcomes regardless of treatment intervention.

As noted in Figure 8-1, the reciprocating cycle of mechanisms that govern both HF and depression suggests that treating 1 disease process can improve the second. It is therefore important that Ploux et al found that depressed patients who responded to biventricular pacing had concomitant improvement in depression.[19] This adds to proof of the concept that treating either depression or HF may lead to improvement in the other.

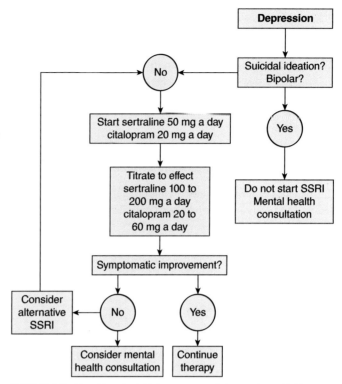

FIGURE 8-7 Algorithm for initial treatment of depression with 2 commonly used SSRIs. (Adapted from Whooley, MA. Depression and cardiovascular disease: healing the broken-hearted. *JAMA.* 2006;295(24):2874-2881.)

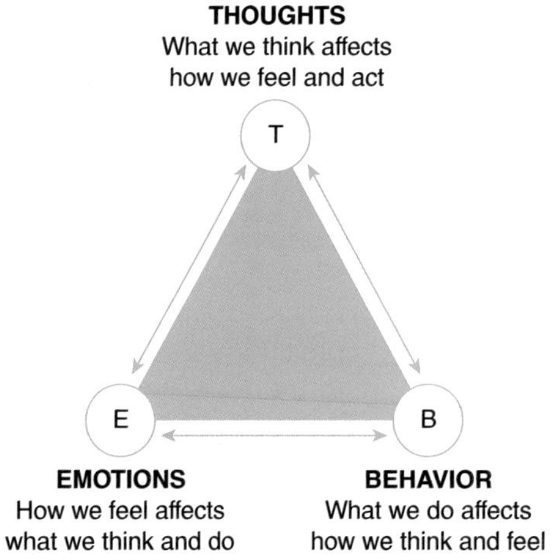

THOUGHTS
What we think affects
how we feel and act

T

E   B

EMOTIONS   **BEHAVIOR**
How we feel affects   What we do affects
what we think and do   how we think and feel

FIGURE 8-8 Triangular model for cognitive behavioral therapy demonstrating the interdependence of thoughts, emotions, and behavior. Challenging inappropriate or erroneous thoughts regarding life challenges or events can trigger emotional responses, including feelings of depression, and subsequent actions and behavior.

There is promising evidence that improvement in depression can reduce adverse outcomes in patients with HF. Studies that have explored this important challenge remain limited and preliminary. There must be continued investigation of the interventions that will optimally treat depression in patients with HF. Regardless of impact on HF outcomes, its treatment is essential to alleviate the painful symptoms of depression and improve quality of life.

PATIENT STORY—CONTINUED

The patient's cardiologist started a low dose of sertraline and referred him to a clinical psychologist specializing in depression. He enrolled in the Beating the Blues online CBT course with the psychologist's supervision. At a visit 3 months later, the patient reported improved energy, better sleep patterns, and had returned to a regimen of exercise. The score on the PHQ-9 had now decreased to 6 consistent with only mild depression.

Table 8-3 Studies Investigating Impact of Depression Treatment on Heart Failure Outcomes

Author/Study	Patient Numbers	Intervention	Outcome	Comments
Diez-Quevedo et al	302	Any antidepressant	Antidepressants not associated with mortality	Depression was related to mortality
Veien et al	3346	Wide range of antidepressants	Increased mortality in those treated with antidepressant	Those receiving antidepressants received lower doses of beta blockers
Xiong et al/ SADHART-CHF	469	SSRI (sertraline) plus nurse-facilitated support vs support only	Improvement in 6-min walk and quality of life in those with remission of depression	Remission of depression did not differ in the 2 treatment groups
Jiang et al/Outcome Analysis SADHART-CHF	469	SSRI (sertraline) plus nurse-facilitated support vs support only	Reduced cardiovascular events in those with remission of depression	Remission of depression did not differ in the 2 treatment groups
Angermann et al/ MOOD-HF	376 randomized to treatment or placebo	SSRI (escitalopram)	No impact on all-cause mortality or outcomes	No improvement in depression symptoms with treatment
Ploux et al	69	Biventricular pacing	Improvement in depression in responders to BiV pacing	Not all subjects who received BiV pacers were depressed
Blumenthal et al/ HF-ACTION	2009	Aerobic exercise	Change in depression associated with reduction in adjusted risk of death or hospitalization	Only modest reduction in depression with exercise; reduction in risk associated with reduction in depression independent of intervention

REFERENCES

1. Binkley PF, Nunziata E, Haas GJ, Nelson SD, Cody RJ. Parasympathetic withdrawal is an integral component of autonomic imbalance in congestive heart failure: demonstration in human subjects and verification in a paced canine model of ventricular failure. *J Am Coll Cardiol.* 1991;18(2):464-472.

2. Blumenthal JA, Babyak MA, O'Connor C, et al. Effects of exercise training on depressive symptoms in patients with chronic heart failure: the HF-ACTION randomized trial. *JAMA.* 2012;308(5):465-474.

3. Christine EA. Effects of selective serotonin re-uptake inhibition on MOrtality, mOrbidity, and mood in depressed heart failure patients: clinical tria–MOOD-HF. 2015.

4. Diez-Quevedo C, Lupon J, Gonzalez B, et al. Depression, antidepressants, and long-term mortality in heart failure. *Int J Cardiol.* 2013;167(4):1217-1225.

5. Dube P, Kroenke K, Bair M, Theobald D, Williams L. The P4 screener: evaluation of a brief measure for assessing potential suicide risk in 2 randomized effectiveness trials of primary care and oncology patients. *Prim Care Companion J Clin Psychiatry.* 2010;12(6):e1-e8.

6. Emani S, Binkley PF. Mind-body medicine in chronic heart failure: a translational science challenge. *Circ Heart Fail.* 2010;3(6):715-725.

7. Ferketich AK, Binkley PF. Psychological distress and cardiovascular disease: results from the 2002 national health interview survey. *Eur Heart J.* 2005;26(18):1923-1929.

8. Ferketich AK, Ferguson JP, Binkley PF. Depressive symptoms and inflammation among heart failure patients. *Am Heart J.* 2005;150(1):132-136.

9. Grippo AJ, Johnson AK. Stress, depression and cardiovascular dysregulation: a review of neurobiological mechanisms and the integration of research from preclinical disease models. *Stress.* 2009;12(1):1-21.

10. Hollon SD, Jarrett RB, Nierenberg AA, Thase ME, Trivedi M, Rush AJ. Psychotherapy and medication in the treatment of adult and geriatric depression: Which monotherapy or combined treatment? *J Clin Psychiatry.* 2005;66(4):455-468.

11. Jiang W, Kuchibhatla M, Clary GL, et al. Relationship between depressive symptoms and long-term mortality in patients with heart failure. *Am Heart J.* 2007;154(1):102-108.

12. Jiang W, O'Connor C, Silva SG, et al. Safety and efficacy of sertraline for depression in patients with CHF (SADHART-CHF): a randomized, double-blind, placebo-controlled trial of sertraline for major depression with congestive heart failure. *Am Heart J.* 2008;156(3):437-444.

13. Joynt KE, Whellan DJ, O'connor CM. Why is depression bad for the failing heart? A review of the mechanistic relationship between depression and heart failure. *J Card Fail.* 2004;10(3):258-271.

14. Lichtman JH, Bigger JT, Jr, Blumenthal JA, et al. Depression and coronary heart disease: recommendations for screening, referral, and treatment: A science advisory from the American heart association prevention committee of the council on cardiovascular nursing, council on clinical cardiology, council on epidemiology and prevention, and interdisciplinary council on quality of care and outcomes research: Endorsed by the american psychiatric association. *Circulation.* 2008;118(17):1768-1775.

15. Ploux S, Verdoux H, Whinnett Z, et al. Depression and severe heart failure: Benefits of cardiac resynchronization therapy. *J Cardiovasc Electrophysiol.* 2012;23(6):631-636.

16. Proudfoot J, Ryden C, Everitt B, et al. Clinical efficacy of computerised cognitive-behavioural therapy for anxiety and depression in primary care: randomised controlled trial. *Br J Psychiatry.* 2004;185:46-54.

17. Veien KT, Videbaek L, Schou M, et al. High mortality among heart failure patients treated with antidepressants. *Int J Cardiol.* 2011;146(1):64-67.

18. Xiong GL, Fiuzat M, Kuchibhatla M, et al. Health status and depression remission in patients with chronic heart failure: patient-reported outcomes from the SADHART-CHF trial. *Circ Heart Fail.* 2012;5(6):688-692.

19. Yeager KR, Binkley PF, Saveanu RV, et al. Screening and identification of depression among patients with coronary heart disease and congestive heart failure. *Heart Fail Clin.* 2011;7(1):69-74.

9 ATHLETIC HEART SYNDROME

Lucy Safi, DO
Asaad Khan, MD
Malissa Wood, MD

PATIENT CASE

A 24-year-old male rower was referred to the cardiologist office for palpitations. He described palpitations that occurred after exercise and denied any lightheadedness or syncope. Echocardiogram was performed, which showed a dilated left ventricle, dilated left atrium, mild concentric left ventricular hypertrophy, and normal left ventricular function. In endurance athletes, cardiac remodeling may occur; distinguishing exercise-induced cardiac adaptations from pathology is important.

PHYSIOLOGIC ADAPTATIONS

Athletic heart syndrome encompasses a variety of significant physiological and morphological changes that occur in a human heart after repetitive strenuous physical exercise. Physical exercise is dependent on the cardiovascular system's ability to provide oxygenated blood to the critical organs, removing deoxygenated blood from tissues, as well as the lungs' ability to clear carbon dioxide (CO_2). With exercise a greater proportion of the oxygen (O_2) is extracted from the blood.

Cardiopulmonary stress testing can be used to assess the athletic performance of an athlete. Gas exchange during rest and exercise can be analyzed. Myocardial oxygen demand is directly related to exercise intensity. The increasing oxygen demands cause an increase in pulmonary oxygen uptake (VO_2). Physiological changes that occur with training include lowered blood pressure and heart rate, enhanced contraction and relaxation of both ventricles, as well as an increase in the VO_2 max. VO_2 max is widely considered to be the gold standard metric for cardiovascular fitness.

Cardiac output is the product of stroke volume and heart rate and may increase 5- to 6-fold during maximal exercise. Heart rate increase accounts for a majority of the augmentation in cardiac output with exercise and may range from 40 bpm at rest to ≥200 bpm in a young maximally exercising athlete.[1] Hemodynamic conditions, specifically changes in cardiac output and peripheral vascular resistance (PVR), vary widely across sporting disciplines.

SPORT-SPECIFIC REMODELING

Structural adaptions of the heart with exercise include increases in heart cavity dimensions, augmentation of cardiac output, and increases in heart muscle mass. Although some overlap exists, exercise activity can be segregated into 2 forms with defining hemodynamic differences.

Isotonic exercise (endurance training) involves sustained elevations in cardiac output with normal or reduced PVR. This hemodynamic effect causes a volume challenge for the heart that affects all 4 chambers. Cardiac adaptations seen with daily sustained exercise include an increase in left ventricular (LV) mass, LV chamber dilation, enhanced LV diastolic function, biatrial enlargement, and right ventricular (RV) dilation with increased systolic and diastolic function. Examples of isotonic sports are long-distance running and swimming.

Isometric exercise (strength training) is characterized by increased PVR and normal or only slightly elevated cardiac output. This increase in PVR causes a pressure load on the ventricle with a transient but potentially marked systolic hypertension and LV afterload. Concentric left ventricular hypertrophy (LVH) and reduction in LV diastolic function occur with repetitive short burst-type power exercises. Football, weightlifting, and discus throwing are some examples of sports involving isometric training. Various sports such as cycling and rowing require both isotonic and isometric forms of training.

Routine athletic training causes alterations in chamber sizes with associated normal systolic and diastolic function in approximately 50% of athletes.[2] The Morganroth hypothesis is based on a study that compared M-mode echocardiographic LV measurements in wrestlers (strength training), swimmers (endurance training), and sedentary control subjects and found significant LV differences across the groups. Athletes exposed to strength training demonstrated concentric LVH whereas individuals exposed to endurance training demonstrated eccentric LV enlargement. This study led to the concept of sport-specific cardiac remodeling.[3] LV ejection fraction is generally normal among athletes.[4,5]

The pattern of LVH may help to distinguish between pathology and an athletic heart. The heart of an athlete is almost always symmetrical; whereas, pathology such as hypertrophic cardiomyopathy (HCM) results in asymmetric hypertrophy of the left ventricle. In an athletic heart, LVH and concomitant left ventricular cavity dilatation results in preservation of the LV relative wall thickness or the ratio between the posterior LV wall thickness and the LV end-diastolic diameter. Patients with hypertrophic cardiomyopathy have pathological hypertrophy, which results in a reduced LV cavity size in athletes.

Left atrial remodeling is a physiological adaptation present in highly trained endurance athletes and usually seen accompanying LV cavity enlargement.[6] Increased transverse left atrial dimensions (≥40 mm) occur in 20% of athletes where larger dimensions (≥45 mm) occur in approximately 2% of athletes.[2] Although increased in size, the overall left atrium should remain proportional to the left ventricular cavity size. There is an increased risk of atrial fibrillation in endurance athletes.[7,8]

Physiological adaptations occur in both male and female athletes; however, the degree of physiological remodeling varies among genders. Women exhibit less physiological remodeling compared to men.[9,10] Race is also a variable in physiological remodeling and black athletes have more LVH than their white counterparts.[11,12]

COMMONLY CONFUSED PATHOLOGIES

Echocardiography is a useful modality when working to evaluate athletic adaptations from the differential diagnosis of diseases that can cause sudden cardiac death (SCD). This portable and noninvasive modality can analyze the left ventricle for pathologies such as hypertrophy cardiomyopathy, dilated cardiomyopathy, and left ventricle noncompaction, and analyze the right ventricle for arrhythmogenic right ventricular cardiomyopathy.

A commonly encountered ECG-based diagnostic dilemma is that of increased QRS voltage, which occurs in both healthy athletes and pathologic cardiac hypertrophy. A number of echocardiographic studies have documented increases in LV chamber dimensions, wall thickness, and mass among healthy, highly trained individuals.[13-15] The increase in LV wall thickness that can result from exercise training has received particular attention because it can share similarities with that caused by HCM.

Hypertrophic cardiomyopathy (HCM) is a well-recognized cause of exercise-related SCD among athletes. This condition is the most common cardiovascular cause of sudden death among athletes in the United States and has the propensity to affect individuals at all levels of competition.[16] Affected individuals have characteristic myofibrillar disarray on histologic inspection of the myocardium while gross analysis demonstrates LVH with increased wall thickness of either symmetric or asymmetric distribution. Roughly 80% of individuals with HCM have electrocardiographic (ECG) abnormalities including interventricular conduction delay, voltage criteria for LVH, ST-segment depression, T-wave inversion, and anterior/inferior Q waves producing a pseudo-infarct pattern.[17,18] While such findings are typical of HCM, they are encountered commonly among trained athletes with no underlying structural heart disease.

Echocardiography is the preferred method of diagnosis for HCM. Findings seen on echocardiography that are suggestive of HCM include increased LV wall thickness, small or normal LV chamber size (LV end-diastolic diameter <45 mm), altered diastolic filling pattern, and systolic anterior motion (SAM) of the mitral valve with associated mitral regurgitation. When reporting HCM it is important to describe area of maximum hypertrophy along with left ventricular outflow tract gradient at rest and with valsalva.

Research has been done to evaluate the magnitude of LVH in athletes without HCM. Pelliccia et al performed echocardiographic assessment of LV wall thicknesses among 947 elite athletes and found that 1.7% of athletes have LV wall thickness >13 mm and all those patients had concomitant LV cavity dilation, a combination not typically found among individuals with HCM.[19] This has been shown again in other studies suggesting that adaptive remodeling can be differentiated from structural heart disease by consideration of LV cavity dimensions.[20] LV wall thickness ≥16 mm is very rare among healthy athletes and this finding must be considered as highly suggestive of HCM. Atrial dilation is less likely to occur in HCM patients compared to patients with exercise-induced LV remodeling. Caselli et al found that LA transverse diameter

measurement >40 mm was highly reliable (sensitivity 92% and specificity 71%) in excluding HCM.[21]

Other echocardiographic data can be used to differentiate between HCM and cardiac adaptations of an athlete. Several studies have shown that diastolic tissue velocities are reduced among individuals with HCM.[22-24] In contrast, a number of authors have independently shown that diastolic tissue velocities are normal or elevated among athletic individuals even in the context of LV enlargement.[21,22]

Other echocardiographic techniques such as strain can be helpful in differentiating an athletic heart from HCM. Strain measurements define changes in muscle fiber length as they contract and relax during the cardiac cycle while strain rate measures these length changes as a function of time. A study by Serri et al found that those with HCM have lower LV systolic strain values than normal controls.[25] In contrast, individuals with adaptive remodeling have strain values that are normal or higher than those found in sedentary healthy controls.[26,27]

SCD in an athlete is tragic and often occurs as a first manifestation of disease. Although HCM is the most common etiology of SCD, other LV pathologies, such as left ventricular noncompaction (LVNC), need to be excluded in athletes.

LVNC cardiomyopathy is a rare condition characterized by increased LV trabeculations and intertrabecular recesses (crypts). LVNC cardiomyopathy is thought to occur due to failure of myocardial compaction during embryological development. Coronary circulation is usually normal and is not associated with the intratrabecular recesses. Clinical presentation of LVNC is variable and can present with HF, thromboembolic events, arrhythmia, or SCD; or it can be asymptomatic. Bhatia et al reported a yearly cardiovascular event rate of 4% in 241 adults with lone LVNC diagnosed by echocardiography with a familial inheritance in first-degree family members of 30%.[28]

Towbin et al described variables of LVNC and classified as LVNC with or without arrhythmias, dilated LVNC, hypertrophic LVNC, right ventricular or biventricular LVNC, and LVNC with congenital heart disease.[29] These variable forms of LVNC have multiple overlapping features with athletic heart syndrome. LVNC diagnosis is usually performed via echocardiography or cardiac magnetic resonance (CMR). Echocardiographic findings of LVNC include a ratio of end systolic noncompacted to compacted layers of >2, color Doppler evidence of intertrabecular recesses, and hypokinesis of the left ventricle.[30]

In athletes regular exercise increases cardiac preload leading to physiological adaptations of LV dilation. This dilation creates a pronounced appearance of LV trabeculations, which may be confused with the pronounced trabeculations seen with LVNC. Gati et al compared 1146 athletes, 75 patients with LVNC, and 415 sedentary patients.[31] They found that 20% of the athletes had a higher amount of trabeculations compared to controls and 10% of the athlete cohort fulfilled their LVNC criteria. Prominent trabeculations were more commonly found in African/Afro-Caribbean compared to Caucasian subjects suggesting a possible genetic component. Also seen were ECG changes, specifically T-wave inversions in the inferior and lateral leads in patients with LVNC.

It is important to consider LVNC when evaluating an athlete with a dilated left ventricle. Occasionally this diagnosis is missed and the patient is thought to have athletic heart syndrome or dilated cardiomyopathy. Marked dilation of the LV cavity may raise suspicion for a dilated cardiomyopathy, especially in the setting of a depressed ejection fraction. Pelliccia et al found that despite the LV dilation in athletes, none of their athletes had LV dysfunction, wall motion abnormalities, or an abnormal diastolic filling pattern. No absolute cutoff value for LV cavity size was provided in that study as cavity enlargement varies between gender, body surface area, as well as the type of exercise performed.[32] Continued surveillance of ejection fraction with continued follow-up with cessation of exercise is recommended.

Arrhythmogenic right ventricular cardiomyopathy (ARVC), also known as arrhythmogenic right ventricular dysplasia (ARVD), is an inherited cardiomyopathy that predominately affects the right ventricle with progressive replacement of the right ventricular myocardium with fibrofatty tissue, RV dilation with or without the presence of RV sacculations, or aneurysms. Of those diagnosed with ARVC, 80% are younger than 40 years of age. ARVC is the most common and potentially serious cause of paroxysmal ventricular tachycardia originating from the right heart in otherwise healthy athletes and should be suspected in all young patients presenting with syncope, ventricular tachycardia, or cardiac arrest. Typically the ventricular tachycardia has a left bundle branch block morphology with origins from the right ventricle. ECG may show a QRS >110 ms in lead V1 and a terminal deflection within or at the end of the QRS complex called an epsilon wave.

The genetic defect is due to altered desmosomes that provide mechanical coupling between myocardial cells binding them together, so called defective glue. The natural history of ARVC includes progressive right ventricle (RV) dysfunction and cardiac electrical instability. Fontaine et al looked at the natural history of the disease and found that of 130 ARVC patients, there were 21 cardiac deaths—14 of which were due to progressive HF and 7 to SCD. This gave an annual mortality rate of 2.3%. In most patients, the mechanism of sudden death was ventricular tachycardia (VT) that ultimately degenerated into ventricular fibrillation. RV failure and LV dysfunction were independently associated with cardiovascular mortality.[33]

Transthoracic echocardiography is a low-cost and easily available diagnostic modality and is a useful tool for establishing the diagnosis of ARVC. The most conspicuous findings on echocardiography are RV and right atrial dilation, increased reflectivity of the moderator band, decreased RV fractional area change, and akinesis/dyskinesis of the RV. The gold standard for diagnosis of ARVC is endomyocardial biopsy. The most striking morphologic feature of the disease is the diffuse or segmental loss of RV myocytes with replacement by fibrofatty tissue and thinning of RV wall. Extensive fibrofatty tissue replacement with myocardial atrophy is seen. The usual site of involvement is found in the so-called triangle of dysplasia located between the RV outflow tract, apex, and infundibulum. The affected areas may form an electrophysiologic hole, potentially constituting a substrate for re-entrant arrhythmias.

Exercise-induced cardiac remodeling is not confined to the LV. Endurance exercise requires both the LV and RV to accept and eject relatively large quantities of blood. In the absence of significant shunting, both chambers must augment function to accomplish this task.

RV structure in collegiate endurance-trained (rowers) and strength-trained (football players) athletes was recently assessed before and after 90 days of team-based exercise training. There was a statistically significant RV dilation in the endurance-trained athletes but no changes in RV architecture were seen in the strength-trained athletes.[34] In an effort to differentiate between athletic remodeling, athletic adaptations, and control subjects, comparisons were made using clinical, ECG, and echocardiographic findings by Bauce et al.[35] They found that RV enlargement as well as a thickened moderator band was present in both athletes and patients with ARVC. The patients with ARVC exhibited RV outflow tract enlargement and reduced RV fractional shortening compared with athletes.

Ventricular tachyarrhythmias can be seen on cardiac rhythm monitors in athletes without cardiovascular abnormalities.[36] In athletes other etiologies for ventricular ectopy such as myocarditis should be excluded. Forced deconditioning will reduce ventricular ectopy in those with athletic adaptations as well as in pathologic heart disease and may not be helpful in determining the etiology.[37]

SCREENING AND IMAGING RECOMMENDATIONS

The term *athlete* suggests someone of excellent health and the unexpected sudden death of an athlete is a great catastrophe. SCD in athletes is rare. Identifying those athletes at risk remains a great challenge because of the adaptive changes seen in response to regular physical exercise that can mimic pathology.

Careful thought needs to be placed in the balance between testing those patients at highest risk and also avoiding unnecessary testing in athletes. There is debate on the amount of screening needed prior to athletic participation in sports. Based on the large number of athletes, the low rate of SCD, and cost-efficiency considerations, routine large-scale cardiac imaging in athletes is not recommended. The widespread use of echocardiography and electrocardiography in athletic populations could result in many false-positive test results creating unnecessary anxiety for the athletes and their families, as well as unjustified exclusion from competitive sports or future insurance coverage.

Multiple screening modalities have been suggested including ECG and limited echocardiogram coupled with a detailed history and physical examination. Harmon et al assessed more than 47,000 athletes and found the most effective screening strategy of athletes to be ECG, with a false-positive rate of 6%.[38] The ECG false-positive rate was less than the lone use of a history (8%) or a physical examination (10%). If there is concern for pathology, more advanced screening modalities and referral to a cardiologist may be warranted.

Newer functional myocardial imaging techniques such as tissue Doppler echocardiography and strain echocardiography indicate that exercise training may lead to changes in LV systolic function that are not detected by assessment of a global index such as LV ejection fraction.[39,40] Mitral valve inflow patterns seen with Doppler and tissue Doppler imaging of the LV walls can reveal impairment of relaxation and global longitudinal function that usually precedes the development of pathological LVH. On the contrary, early diastolic relaxation velocities are usually normal or increased in athletes with exercise-induced LVH.[41] Studies by Afonso et al have shown that global longitudinal strain (GLS) is normal in athletes and abnormal in HCM.[42]

EXERCISE AND CARDIOVASCULAR RISK FACTORS

Regular physical exercise results in improvements in physiologic, psychological, and biochemical parameters, which all lead to a reduction in overall cardiovascular risk. Routine physical exercise is of great value in reducing established cardiovascular risk factors including obesity, diabetes mellitus, serum cholesterol, and hypertension. Furthermore, exercise improves function with less stiffening of the large and small blood vessels and reduction in the risk of pathologic blood clots. In contrast, physical inactivity and poor physical fitness are associated with coronary heart disease.

LONG-TERM CONSEQUENCES OF EXERCISE

Concern exists regarding long-term sequelae of significant LV remodeling evident in some highly trained athletes. Approximately 15% of highly trained athletes show striking LV cavity enlargement, with end-diastolic dimensions ≥60 mm, similar in magnitude to that evident in pathological forms of dilated cardiomyopathy.[43]

One longitudinal echocardiographic study reported incomplete reversal of extreme LV cavity dilatation with deconditioning. In that study, significant chamber enlargement persisted in 20% of retired and deconditioned former elite athletes after 5 years.[44]

Left atrial remodeling is an important physiological adaptation present in highly trained athletes, most commonly those in combined static and dynamic sports (ie, cycling and rowing), and is largely explained by associated LV cavity enlargement and volume overload. In an athletic heart, the overall left atrium may measure large but should remain proportional to the LV cavity size.[45]

CONCLUSIONS

Athletic heart syndrome encompasses a variety of cardiac morphological changes. Sport-specific remodeling occurs and it is pertinent that a complete detailed history of the amount of exercise and the quality of exercise be obtained when evaluating an athlete. The variation from normal cardiac physiology found within the athletic population is similar to some pathologic conditions discussed above. Familiarity of the differentiating characteristics is paramount in discriminating between pathology and normal physiologic changes seen in an athlete's heart.

REFERENCES

1. Baggish AL, Wood MJ. Athlete's heart and cardiovascular care of the athlete scientific and clinical update. *Circulation.* 2011;123:2723-2735.

2. Maron BJ, Pelliccia A. The heart of trained athletes. *Circulation.* 2006;114:1633-1644.

3. Morganroth J, Maron BJ, Henry WL, Epstein SE. Comparative left ventricular dimensions in trained athletes. *Ann Intern Med.* 1975;82:521-524.

4. Maron BJ. Structural features of the athlete heart as defined by echocardiography. *J Am Coll Cardiol.* 1986;7:190-203.

5. Gilbert CA, Nutter DO, Felner JM, Perkins JV, Heymsfield SB, Schlant RC. Echocardiographic study of cardiac dimensions and function in the endurance-trained athlete. *Am J Cardiol.* 1977;40:528-533.

6. Pelliccia A, Maron BJ, Di Paolo FM, et al. Prevalence and clinical significance of left atrial remodeling in competitive athletes. *J Am Coll Cardiol.* 2005;46:690-696.

7. Mont L, Elosua R, Brugada J. Endurance sport practice as a risk factor for atrial fibrillation and atrial flutter. *Europace.* 2009;11(1):11-17.

8. Furlanello F, Bertoldi A, Dallago M, et al. Atrial fibrillation in elite athletes. *J Cardiovasc Electrophysiol.* 1998;9:S63-68.

9. D'Andrea A, Riegler L, Cocchia R, et al. Left atrial volume index in highly trained athletes. *Am Heart J.* 2010;159:1155-1161.

10. Pelliccia A, Maron BJ, Culasso F, Spataro A, Caselli G. Athlete's heart in women: echocardiographic characterization of highly trained elite female athletes. *JAMA.* 1996;276:211-215.

11. Basavarajaiah S, Boraita A, Whyte G, et al. Ethnic differences in left ventricular remodeling in highly trained athletes: relevance to differentiating physiologic left ventricular hypertrophy from hypertrophic cardiomyopathy. *J Am Coll Cardiol.* 2008;51:2256-2262.

12. Rawlins J, Carre F, Kervio G, et al. Ethnic differences in physiological cardiac adaptation to intense physical exercise in highly trained female athletes. *Circulation.* 2010;121:1078-1085.

13. Morganroth J, Maron BJ, Henry WL, Epstein SE. Comparative left ventricular dimensions in trained athletes. *Ann Intern Med.* 1975;82:521-524.

14. Pelliccia A, Culasso F, Di Paolo FM, Maron BJ. Physiologic left ventricular cavity dilatation in elite athletes. *Ann Intern Med.* 1999;130:23-31.

15. Abernethy WB, Choo JK, Hutter AM Jr. Echocardiographic characteristics of professional football players. *J Am Coll Cardiol.* 2003;41:280-284.

16. Baggish A, Yared K, Wood M, Hutter A. Echocardiography and advanced cardiac imaging in athletes. In: Lawless C, ed. *Sports Cardiology Essentials.* New York, NY: Springer; 2011.

17. Savage DD, Seides SF, Clark CE, et al. Electrocardiographic findings in patients with obstructive and nonobstructive hypertrophic cardiomyopathy. *Circulation.* 1978;58:402-408.

18. Maron BJ, Mathenge R, Casey SA, Poliac LC, Longe TF. Clinical profile of hypertrophic cardiomyopathy identified de novo in rural communities. *J Am Coll Cardiol.* 1999;33:1590-1595.

19. Pelliccia A, Maron BJ, Spataro A, Proschan MA, Spirito P. The upper limit of physiologic cardiac hypertrophy in highly trained elite athletes. *N Engl J Med.* 1991;324:295-301.

20. Sharma S, Maron BJ, Whyte G, et al. Physiologic limits of left ventricular hypertrophy in elite junior athletes: relevance to

differential diagnosis of athlete's heart and hypertrophic cardiomyopathy. *J Am Coll Cardiol*. 2002;40:1431-1436.

21. Caselli S, Maron MS, Urbano-Moral JA, et al. Differentiating left ventricular hypertrophy in athletes from that in patients with hypertrophic cardiomyopathy. *Am J Cardiol*. 2014 Nov 1;114(9):1383-1389.

22. McMahon CJ, Nagueh SF, Pignatelli RH, et al. Characterization of left ventricular diastolic function by tissue Doppler imaging and clinical status in children with hypertrophic cardiomyopathy. *Circulation*. 2004;109:1756-1762.

23. Cardim N, Oliveira AG, Longo S, et al. Doppler tissue imaging: regional myocardial function in hypertrophic cardiomyopathy and in athlete's heart. *J Am Soc Echocardiogr*. 2003;16:223-232.

24. Matsumura Y, Elliott PM, Virdee MS, et al. Left ventricular diastolic function assessed using Doppler tissue imaging in patients with hypertrophic cardiomyopathy: relation to symptoms and exercise capacity. *Heart*. 2002;87:247-251.

25. Serri K, Reant P, Lafitte M, et al. Global and regional myocardial function quantification by two-dimensional strain: application in hypertrophic cardiomyopathy. *J Am Coll Cardiol*. 2006;47:1175-1181.

26. Neilan TG, Ton-Nu TT, Jassal DS, et al. Myocardial adaptation to short-term high-intensity exercise in highly trained athletes. *J Am Soc Echocardiogr*. 2006;19:1280-1285.

27. Saghir M, Areces M, Makan M. Strain rate imaging differentiates hypertensive cardiac hypertrophy from physiologic cardiac hypertrophy (athlete's heart). *J Am Soc Echocardiogr*. 2007;20:151-157.

28. Bhatia NL, Tajik AJ, Wilansky S, Steidley DE, Mookadam F. Isolated noncompaction of the left ventricular myocardium in adults: a systematic overview. *J Card Fail*. 2011;17:771-778.

29. Towbin J, Lorts A, Jefferies JL. Left ventricular noncompaction cardiomyopathy. *Lancet*. 2015;386:813-825.

30. Jenni R, Oechslin E, Schneider J, Attenhofer Jost C, Kaufmann PA. Echocardiographic and pathoanatomical characteristics of isolated left ventricular non-compaction: a step towards classification as a distinct cardiomyopathy. *Heart*. 2001;86:666-671.

31. Gati S, Chandra N, Bennet RL, et al. Increased left ventricular trabeculation in highly trained athletes: do we need more stringent criteria for the diagnosis of left ventricular non-compaction in athletes? *Heart*. 2013;99:401-408.

32. Pelliccia A, Culasso F, Di Paolo FM, Maron BJ. Physiologic left ventricular cavity dilatation in elite athletes. *Ann Intern Med*. 1999;130:23-31.

33. Hubot JS, Jouven X, Fontaine G, et al. Natural history and risk stratification of arrhythmogenic right ventricular dysplasia/cardiomyopathy. *Circulation*. 2004;110:1879-1884.

34. Baggish AL, Wang F, Weiner RB, et al. Training-specific changes in cardiac structure and function: a prospective and longitudinal assessment of competitive athletes. *J Appl Physiol*. 2008;104:1121-1128.

35. Bauce B, Frigo G, Benini G, et al. Differences and similarities between arrhythmogenic right ventricular cardiomyopathy and athlete's heart adaptations. *Br J Sports Med*. 2010;44:148-154.

36. Biffi A, Pelliccia A, Verdile L, et al. Long-term clinical significance of frequent and complex ventricular tachyarrhythmias in trained athletes. *J Am Coll Cardiol*. 2002;40:446-452.

37. Biffi A, Maron BJ, Verdile L, et al. Impact of physical deconditioning on ventricular tachyarrhythmias in trained athletes. *J Am Coll Cardiol*. 2004;44:1053-1058.

38. Harmon KG, Zigman M, Drezner JA. The effectiveness of screening history, physical exam, and ECG to detect potentially lethal cardiac disorders in athletes: a systemic review/meta-analysis. *J Electrocardiol*. 2015;48:329-338.

39. Baggish AL, Yared KL, Wang F, et al. The impact of endurance exercise training on left ventricular systolic mechanics. *Am J Physiol Heart Circ Physiol*. 2008;295:H1109-H1116.

40. Cardim N, Oliveira AG, Longo S, et al. Doppler tissue imaging: regional myocardial function in hypertrophic cardiomyopathy and in athlete's heart. *J Am Soc Echocardiogr*. 2003;16:223-232.

41. Pela G, Bruschi G, Montagna L, Manara M, Manca C. Left and right ventricular adaptation assessed by Doppler tissue echocardiography in athletes. *J Am Soc Echocardiogr*. 2004;17:205-211.

42. Afonso L, Kondur A, Simegn M, et al. Two-dimensional strain profiles in patients with physiological and pathological hypertrophy and preserved left ventricular systolic function: a comparative analyses. *BMJ Open*. 2012 Aug 17;2(4).

43. Pelliccia A, Culasso F, Di Paolo F, Maron BJ. Physiologic left ventricular cavity dilatation in elite athletes. *Ann Intern Med*. 1999;130:23-31.

44. Pelliccia A, Maron BJ, de Luca R, et al. Remodeling of left ventricular hypertrophy in elite athletes after long-term deconditioning. *Circulation*. 2002;105:944-949.

45. Pelliccia A, Maron BJ, Di Paolo FM, et al. Prevalence and clinical significance of left atrial remodeling in competitive athletes. *J Am Coll Cardiol*. 2005;46:690-696.

10 HYPERTROPHIC CARDIOMYOPATHY

Darshan H. Brahmbhatt, MB BChir, MA, MPhil, MRCP
Katharine Tweed, MB BS, BMedSci, FRCR
Lynne K. Williams, MBBCh, FRCP, PhD

PATIENT CASE

A 17-year-old adolescent boy presented to the general cardiology clinic for family screening after a maternal aunt had been diagnosed with hypertrophic cardiomyopathy (HCM). He had no history of chest pain, breathlessness, or syncope. He reported mild symptoms of postural hypotension. Examination revealed normal first and second heart sounds with an audible and palpable fourth heart sound, but no murmurs. His electrocardiogram (ECG) demonstrated left ventricular hypertrophy (LVH) with repolarization abnormalities, and echocardiographic and cardiac magnetic resonance imaging (MRI) features of severe asymmetric LVH are noted in this patient (Figure 10-1). He had no evidence of arrhythmia on ambulatory Holter monitoring, but exercise testing demonstrated an abnormal blood pressure response on exercise. Familial genetic testing was performed and identified a pathogenic mutation in the sarcomere gene *MYL3*. Given his risk factor profile for sudden cardiac death (SCD), an automatic implantable cardioverter defibrillator (AICD) was implanted for primary prevention.

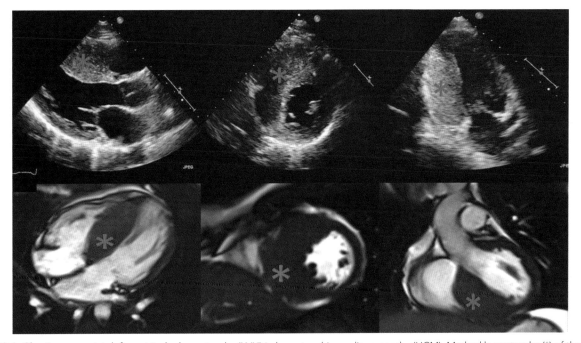

FIGURE 10-1 Classic asymmetric left ventricular hypertrophy (LVH) in hypertrophic cardiomyopathy (HCM). Marked hypertrophy (*) of the interventricular septum is noted on both echocardiography (upper panel) and cardiac magnetic resonance imaging (MRI) (lower panel).

EPIDEMIOLOGY

- HCM represents the most common inherited cardiac disorder and is a global disease with no racial or ethnic preponderance.[1] A reported prevalence of approximately 0.2% (1:500) has been reported consistently in epidemiological studies.[1]
- Age-related penetrance is a key feature of the disease, with onset and progression of hypertrophy occurring at virtually any age.
- Importantly, it is the most common cause of SCD in young people (<35 years of age) and athletes.[2]

CLINICAL DEFINITION

- HCM represents a primary disease of the myocardium. The hallmark of the disease is the presence of increased left ventricular (LV) wall thickness in the absence of another cardiac or systemic disease that could result in a similar degree of myocardial hypertrophy.
- On a microscopic level there is extensive disarray of myocytes and myofibrils, as well as thickening of the intramural microvessels and interstitial fibrosis.

ETIOLOGY

- In adults and adolescents, the disease typically exhibits an autosomal dominant pattern of inheritance. In around 40% to 60% of cases, a mutation in 1 of the genes encoding sarcomeric proteins is identified.
- In up to 10% of cases in adults another underlying genetic disorder may be the cause of the HCM phenotype. In addition, nongenetic causes also account for some cases of unexplained LVH.[3,4]

DIFFERENTIAL DIAGNOSIS

- LVH can represent either a physiologic (athlete's heart) or pathologic cardiac response that can occur in a variety of cardiac, genetic, and systemic diseases (Figure 10-2), or in response to hemodynamic loading of the ventricle (arterial hypertension and aortic stenosis).
- Accurate identification of the underlying etiology is critical given that HCM is a common cause of premature SCD and can lead to considerable morbidity. Specific therapeutic strategies are available for certain mimics of HCM, such as the inborn errors of metabolism, Anderson-Fabry disease, and amyloidosis; early and accurate diagnosis allows timely institution of appropriate therapy.

PATHOPHYSIOLOGY

The symptoms and clinical presentation in patients with HCM result from a complex interplay between several structural and hemodynamic underlying abnormalities.

DIASTOLIC DYSFUNCTION

- Hypertrophy and fibrosis of the myocardium result in an increase in myocardial stiffness, ultimately causing an impairment in LV relaxation. Delayed LV relaxation results both in an inability to increase stroke volume during exercise and an increase in left ventricular end-diastolic pressure (LVEDP).
- Impaired passive filling of the left ventricle due to stiffness leads to an increased reliance on active filling during atrial systole, which is why atrial fibrillation is often poorly tolerated.
- The chronic increase in LVEDP and atrial pressures results in left atrial dilatation over time.

LEFT VENTRICULAR OUTFLOW TRACT OBSTRUCTION

- Left ventricular outflow tract (LVOT) obstruction is an important and frequent manifestation of HCM. While in most cases the level of obstruction is subvalvular in the outflow tract, in a subset of patients the obstruction is primarily at the midventricular level (resulting from a combination of septal hypertrophy and hypertrophy of the papillary muscles).[5]
- Obstruction is a major cause of symptoms such as dyspnea, chest pain, presyncope, and syncope, and is associated with a higher risk of progressive heart failure (HF) and death.[6]
- LVOT obstruction is classically dynamic and variable, affected by the hemodynamic changes that occur in day-to-day life (heart rate, inotropic or contractile state of the heart, systemic vascular resistance, and loading conditions).
- The cause is multifactorial and includes both vigorous ejection of the left ventricle as well as the alterations in chamber geometry and morphology caused by hypertrophy. Hypertrophy of the interventricular septum and systolic anterior motion of the mitral valve contribute to obstruction. Abnormalities of the mitral valve and subvalvular apparatus/papillary muscles frequently coexist and further aggravate obstruction.

MYOCARDIAL ISCHEMIA

- Unlike common forms of ischemia related to epicardial coronary artery disease, ischemia in HCM is multifactorial. It arises not only from a supply/demand mismatch (as a result of increased myocardial mass), but also due to abnormalities of the myocardial microvasculature.
- A reduction in arteriolar density, small intracoronary arteriole dysplasia (SICAD), vessel intimal and/or medial thickening, and proliferation and disorganization of smooth muscle cells have all been described (Figure 10-3). The reduction in luminal cross-sectional area of the small vessels is further aggravated by dense perivascular collagen and increased collagen content in the media of the vessels.
- Raised intracavitary left ventricular end-diastolic pressure (LVEDP) also serve to cause a reduction in transcoronary perfusion gradient, which further compromises coronary blood flow.

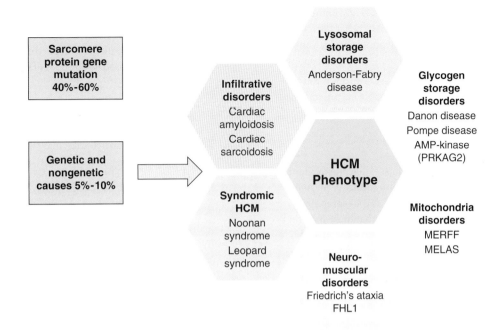

FIGURE 10-2 Etiology and differential diagnosis of hypertrophic cardiomyopathy (HCM). Causes of HCM include both genetic and nongenetic disorders.

AUTONOMIC DYSFUNCTION

- Disturbances of reflex control of the vasculature and systemic vascular resistance have been demonstrated in HCM. Inappropriate firing of LV mechanoreceptors can occur, particularly during exercise. The resulting sudden and inappropriate vasodilatation can precipitate a fall in blood pressure.[7] These episodes of hypotension may lead to recurrent presyncope, syncope, or even act as a trigger for SCD.

- Approximately 30% of patients demonstrate an abnormal blood pressure response to exercise (failure to increase systolic pressure by >20 mm Hg, or even a fall in blood pressure).[8,9]

ARRHYTHMIA

- Supraventricular arrhythmias are common, with up to 20% to 25% of patients experiencing episodes of atrial fibrillation. Risk factors for atrial fibrillation include the presence of LVOT obstruction, significant mitral regurgitation, and diastolic dysfunction. The risk of atrial fibrillation is related to the degree of left atrial dilatation and to abnormalities of left atrial function.[10-12]

- Bradycardias secondary to sinus node dysfunction or atrioventricular block are relatively uncommon. In younger patients, they may suggest the presence of certain genotypes (desmin, FHL1, PRKAG2). In older patients, they should raise the suspicion of a mimic of HCM such as cardiac amyloidosis or Anderson-Fabry disease.

- Nonsustained ventricular tachycardia (NSVT; defined as ≥3 ventricular extrasystoles at a rate of ≥120 bpm, of <30 seconds duration) is a relatively common finding on ambulatory Holter monitoring. NSVT increases in frequency with age, occurring in around 25% of patients over the age of 40 years. NSVT is a risk factor for SCD (particularly in adults and young children),[13] and is related to the degree of LVH and myocardial fibrosis.

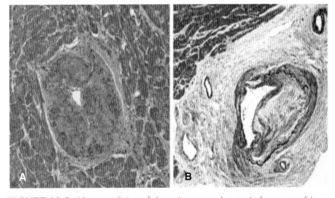

FIGURE 10-3 Abnormalities of the microvasculature in hypertrophic cardiomyopathy (HCM). Histopathologic section of myocardium removed from the basal interventricular septum during surgical myectomy. Panel A demonstrates hyperplasia of the smooth muscle cells of the media, and panel B demonstrates hyperplasia of the intima with increased mucopolysaccharide and collagen deposition. A reduction in the luminal cross-sectional area is noted. (Reprinted from Kwon DH, Smedira NG, Rodriguez ER, et al. Cardiac magnetic resonance detection of myocardial scarring in hypertrophic cardiomyopathy: correlation with histopathology and prevalence of ventricular tachycardia. *J Amer Coll of Cardiol.* 2009;54(3):242-249, with permission from Elsevier.)

- Sustained ventricular tachycardia, in contrast, is uncommon. However, in high-risk patients in whom an AICD has been fitted for primary prevention of SCD, sustained monomorphic ventricular tachycardia is seen more frequently on device interrogation.

- Exercise-induced ventricular arrhythmias are rare, but when present have been associated with a significantly increased risk of sudden death or AICD discharge.[14]

SYSTOLIC DYSFUNCTION

- A small proportion of patients can develop systolic impairment, with a reported prevalence of between 2.4% and 15%.[15,16] A left ventricular ejection fraction (LVEF) of <50% represents significant impairment of LV function, given that these patients typically have a supranormal LVEF. Similar to other causes of LV dysfunction, there is progressive wall thinning and chamber dilatation (end-stage or burnt-out HCM).

CLINICAL FEATURES

AGE

- Age is important and may give a clue to the underlying cause of HCM. Inherited metabolic disorders and congenital syndromes (eg, Noonan syndrome) are much more common in neonates and infants. Similarly, transthyretin cardiac amyloidosis is more common with advancing age.

FAMILY HISTORY

- A thorough family history spanning 3 to 4 generations is crucial in order to establish and confirm the genetic nature of the disease (Figure 10-4). Most genetic forms of HCM are autosomal dominant and an affected individual will be present in every generation. When transmission occurs only from the mother, a mitochondrial DNA mutation should be suspected.

- Family history should include a history of premature SCD, unexplained HF, pacemaker or defibrillator implantation, or heart transplantation.

SYMPTOMS

Many patients are either asymptomatic or minimally symptomatic, with severe medically refractory symptoms occurring in only a small proportion. Asymptomatic patients may come to attention due to the incidental finding of a heart murmur or an abnormal ECG. An increasing number of cases come to attention through family screening of an affected individual.

DYSPNEA

- Breathlessness is common in patients with HCM, and is typically the result of diastolic dysfunction and LVOT obstruction.

- An increase in breathlessness and NYHA class may be precipitated by the acute onset of atrial fibrillation, or more insidiously by the development of LV systolic dysfunction.

CHEST PAIN

- Chest pain may present as typical angina (often with postprandial exacerbation, typically in patients with obstructive physiology) or as atypical pain, and is caused by episodes of myocardial ischemia.

PALPITATIONS

- Palpitations are most commonly associated with the development of atrial fibrillation, particularly if paroxysmal. In addition, NSVT and sustained ventricular arrhythmias may be the underlying cause.

PRESYNCOPE AND SYNCOPE

- Episodes can occur at rest or with exertion.

- The underlying causes are myriad, including arrhythmia, outflow tract obstruction, and autonomic dysfunction resulting in episodic hypotension.

- Syncope, particularly if recent (within the preceding 6 months) or recurrent, is associated with an increased risk of SCD.[17]

STROKE

- Occasionally the first presentation of HCM may be a stroke in the setting of atrial fibrillation or thrombus associated with an LV apical aneurysm.

CLINICAL EXAMINATION AND PHYSICAL FINDINGS

- In many patients the clinical examination may be entirely normal, particularly in patients without obstruction.

- The apex beat is typically sustained and forceful, and a palpable fourth heart sound (S_4) may be present.

- In patients with obstruction, an ejection systolic murmur, which is heard best at the left sternal edge, is present. The murmur will increase in intensity in the standing position and with performance of a Valsalva maneuver (reduction in preload), and will decrease in intensity with squatting and handgrip maneuvers (increase in afterload/systemic vascular resistance).

- If significant mitral regurgitation is present, a pansystolic murmur will be heard best at the apex, with radiation to the axilla.

- A thorough clinical examination may give clues to the underlying etiology of hypertrophy, with certain clinical signs associated with specific underlying conditions (angiokeratoma in Anderson-Fabry disease, multiple lentigines in LEOPARD syndrome, neuropathic pain and parasthesia in Anderson-Fabry disease and amyloidosis).

DIAGNOSTIC INVESTIGATIONS

ELECTROCARDIOGRAPHY

- The resting ECG may be normal in a minority of patients, but typically demonstrates a combination of LVH, ST segment and T-wave changes (typically T-wave inversion), and pathological Q waves (Figure 10-5). In apical HCM there is giant negative T-wave inversion (>10 mm).

- Left atrial enlargement may be surmised by the presence of a P-mitrale pattern.

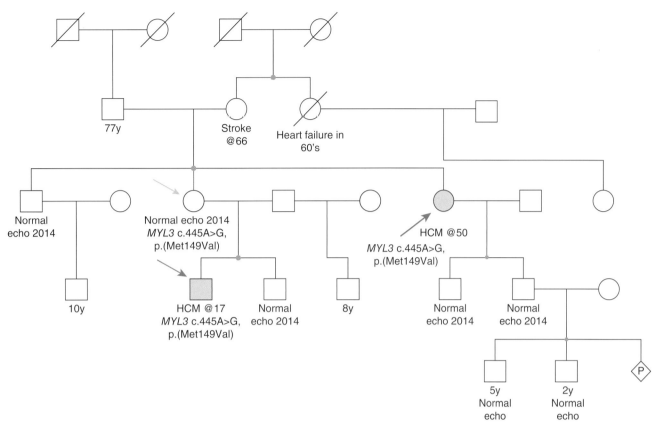

FIGURE 10-4 Family pedigree in a patient with hypertrophic cardiomyopathy (HCM). The patient described in the clinical scenario (blue arrow) was diagnosed during routine family screening after a diagnosis of HCM in his maternal aunt (red arrow). His mother (gold arrow) is an obligate carrier, and despite a positive genetic test for the *MYL3* mutation, she has no evidence of disease expression on either ECG or echocardiography at this stage (genotype positive, phenotype negative carrier).

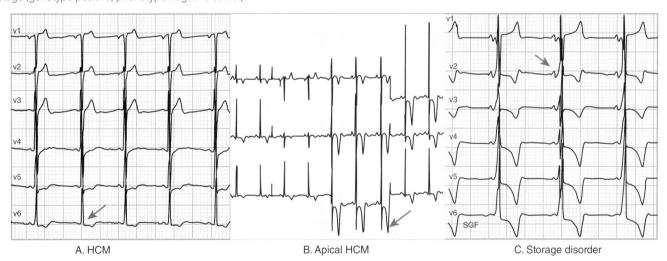

FIGURE 10-5 Electrocardiographic (ECG) findings in hypertrophic cardiomyopathy (HCM). Classically there is evidence of left ventricular hypertrophy (LVH) by voltage criteria, with repolarization abnormalities and changes in the ST segment (A). In apical HCM, giant T-wave inversion is noted across the precordial leads (B). A short PR interval and pre-excitation (slurring of the upstroke of the QRS complex) may provide clues to an underlying storage or mitochondrial disorder (C).

- The presence of a short PR interval and pre-excitation may give a clue to the underlying etiology (storage disorders, mitochondrial disorders, and Anderson-Fabry disease).

- Ambulatory Holter monitoring is recommended in all patients at first clinical assessment and subsequently at periodic intervals for both risk stratifications for SCD (NSVT) and stroke (paroxysmal or sustained atrial fibrillation).

ECHOCARDIOGRAPHY

Transthoracic echocardiography (TTE) is the primary imaging modality for diagnosis and monitoring of patients with HCM. Given that the pattern of hypertrophy can be variable in HCM, all imaging windows should be used to assess myocardial thickness.

Ventricular Hypertrophy

- The diagnosis of HCM is based on the demonstration of a maximal wall thickness of >15 mm in any myocardial segment. In the pediatric population, a wall thickness ≥2 standard deviations above the mean (z score) after correction for age and body surface area should be demonstrated. In family members undergoing screening, a wall thickness of >13 mm may signify the presence of underlying disease, and should be interpreted in conjunction with the ECG and clinical symptoms. However, any wall thickness is compatible with the presence of an HCM genetic mutation.[3,4]

- The most common pattern of hypertrophy is asymmetric hypertrophy of the ventricular septum, resulting in a septal to posterior wall thickness ratio of >1.3:1 in normotensive patients, and >1.5:1 in hypertensive patients.[18] However, hypertrophy may be concentric, or primarily involve the apex of the left ventricle (Figure 10-6).

- The LV cavity is small and the systolic function hyperdynamic with a normal or supranormal LVEF.

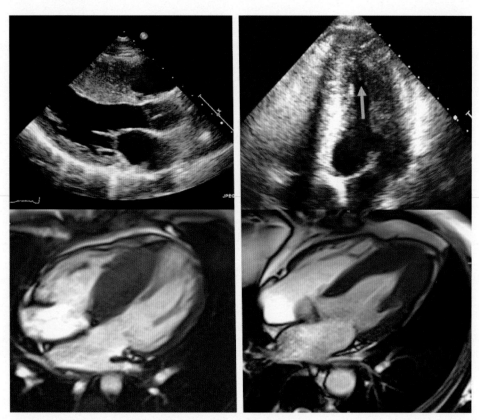

FIGURE 10-6 Patterns of hypertrophy in hypertrophic cardiomyopathy (HCM). The classic pattern of asymmetric left ventricular hypertrophy (LVH) involving predominantly the interventricular septum is shown on the left. In some patients the hypertrophy is localized to the apex of the left ventricle (gold arrow), resulting in an ace-of-spades shape to the left ventricular (LV) cavity.

Obstruction

- Outflow tract obstruction is present in 30% of patients at rest, and in a further 40% of patients a gradient can be demonstrated with provocation (standing, Valsalva maneuver, exercise).[19]

- Turbulent blood flow can be seen in the LVOT, along with systolic anterior motion (SAM) of the mitral valve. This can be visualized on both echocardiography and cardiac MRI (Figures 10-7 and 10-8). A posteriorly directed jet of mitral regurgitation is typically seen in association with SAM.

- Gradients can be measured using either pulse-wave or continuous-wave Doppler and the gradient across the midcavity or outflow tract calculated. The Doppler profile is typically late-peaking and dagger-shaped, in contrast to the Doppler profile of either aortic stenosis or mitral regurgitation, which both have a more rounded envelope. Typically, the Doppler profile of mitral regurgitation will commence at onset of systole, and will be of high velocity (>5.5 m/sec).

- If the resting gradient is <30 mm Hg, provocation maneuvers should be performed to unmask dynamic obstruction.

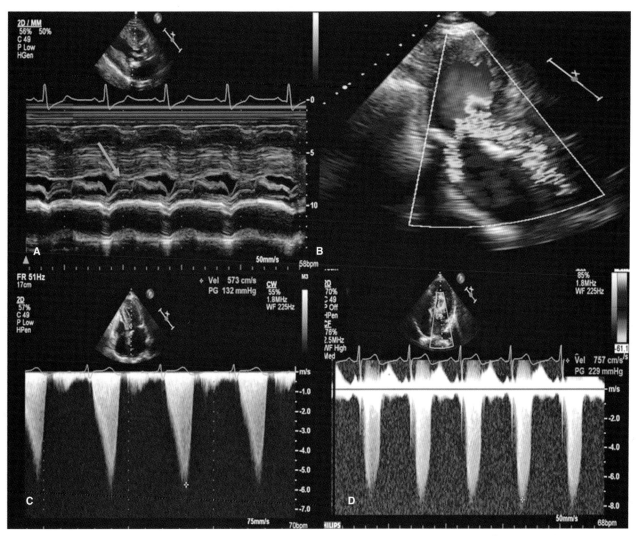

FIGURE 10-7 Obstructive hypertrophic cardiomyopathy on echocardiography. Systolic anterior motion (SAM) of the mitral valve is seen in panel A, with contact between the anterior mitral valve leaflet and the basal interventricular septum (arrow). Obstruction can occur at the level of the outflow tract (B) or in the midventricle. The Doppler profile is typically late-peaking and dagger-shaped (C) with a resting gradient of 132 mm Hg. The Doppler profile of mitral regurgitation (D) has a rounded envelope and a high velocity (7.6 m/sec).

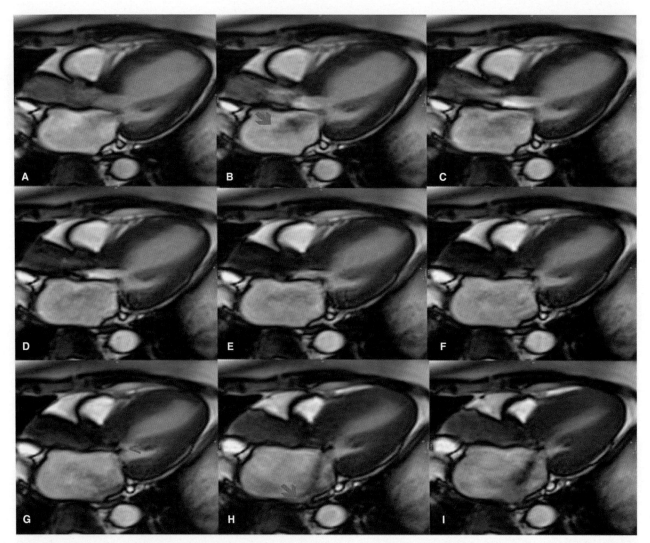

FIGURE 10-8 Obstruction in hypertrophic cardiomyopathy on magnetic resonance imaging (MRI). The 3-chamber view SSFP images (A-I) are demonstrated throughout the cardiac cycle. Initially in early systole there is a central jet of mitral regurgitation (B, blue arrow). There is increased turbulence in the LVOT with flow acceleration (D, blue asterisk). Systolic anterior motion of the mitral valve then develops (G, blue arrowhead), resulting in moderate to severe posteriorly directed mitral regurgitation (H, blue arrow).

Mitral Valve Abnormalities

- Abnormalities include elongated and redundant leaflets, mitral annular calcification, thickened mitral valve leaflets and chordae, as well as abnormalities of the subvalvular apparatus (bifid papillary muscles and papillary muscle malposition).

- In any patients in whom significant mitral regurgitation is noted which is not posteriorly directed (related to SAM of the mitral valve), a search for intrinsic mitral valve disease should be made.

Left Ventricular Diastolic Dysfunction and Left Atrial Dilatation

- LV diastolic dysfunction is almost universal, and is typically reflected as elevated filling pressures.

- Left atrial dilatation occurs secondary to this chronic elevation in LV filling pressures, and is further aggravated by the concomitant presence of LVOT obstruction and mitral regurgitation. Left atrial size and volume have been correlated with the risk of development of atrial fibrillation and progression to HF.[10,20,21]

CARDIAC MAGNETIC RESONANCE IMAGING

- Cardiac magnetic resonance (CMR) imaging, via complete imaging of the entire LV myocardium, allows for detailed assessment of the distribution and extent of LV hypertrophy, with a higher spatial resolution and contrast between the myocardium and blood pool than transthoracic echocardiography. This is particularly helpful in patients with suboptimal echocardiographic windows, or in patients with suspected apical hypertrophy.

- CMR imaging is also helpful in identifying apical infarction and aneurysm formation, a complication that can occur in patients with midcavity obstruction or apical HCM. This complication can be associated both with thrombus formation and embolism, or with monomorphic ventricular tachycardia arising from the site of the scar and aneurysm.[5,22,23]

- The use of gadolinium contrast agents allows for the visualization of myocardial scar and fibrosis (Figure 10-9). There is a growing body of evidence demonstrating the association between scar burden and risk of HF, arrhythmia, and SCD.[24,25]

- Occasionally the pattern and degree of scarring will alert the clinician to the possibility of an alternate diagnosis, most importantly cardiac amyloidosis or Anderson-Fabry disease.

- In cardiac amyloidosis there is typically concentric LVH and right ventricular involvement. Diffuse LV subendocardial enhancement and enhancement of the atrial wall are shown in Figure 10-10.[26]

- In Anderson-Fabry disease the pattern of involvement involves particularly the basal inferior and inferolateral walls, where late gadolinium enhancement can be demonstrated (Figure 10-11).[27]

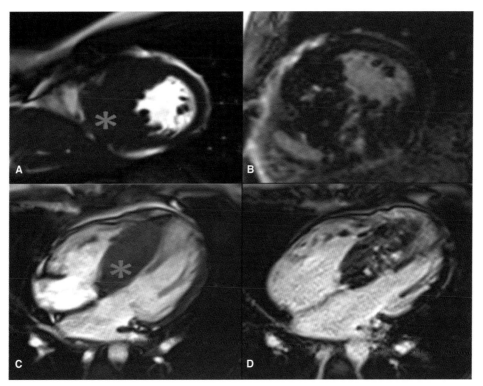

FIGURE 10-9 Late gadolinium enhancement on cardiac magnetic resonance (CMR) imaging. Short-axis (A) SSFP image with matched late gadolinium enhancement images demonstrating severe myocardial fibrosis (B), also seen in the horizontal long-axis 4-chamber view (C) SSFP and (D) post-gadolinium imaging. Blue asterisks denote the area of gross asymmetric left ventricular hypertrophy.

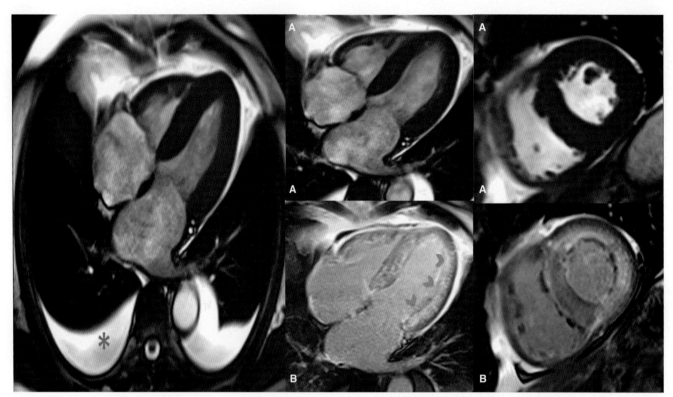

FIGURE 10-10 Cardiac amyloidosis on cardiac magnetic resonance (CMR) imaging. The axial images of the chest demonstrate the constellation of biatrial enlargement, concentric left ventricular and right ventricular hypertrophy, a small pericardial, and bilateral pleural effusions (green asterisk) (A). There is extensive global subendocardial late gadolinium enhancement (B), a pattern that is rarely seen in hypertrophic cardiomyopathy (HCM).

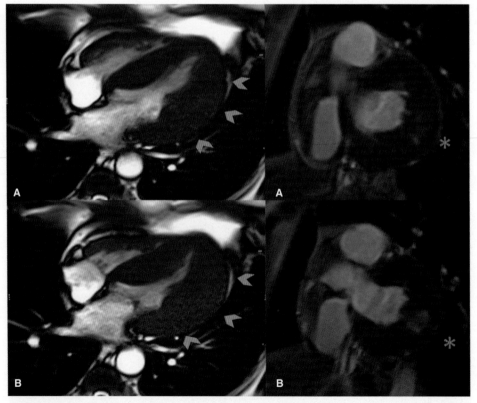

FIGURE 10-11 Anderson-Fabry disease on cardiac magnetic resonance (CMR) imaging. Marked hypertrophy of the basal inferior and inferolateral wall is noted (orange arrowheads) involving the papillary muscles. Midmyocardial late gadolinium enhancement is noted in the basal inferolateral wall (orange asterisk).

EXERCISE TESTING

- Exercise testing plays a useful role in determining exercise capacity, assessing blood pressure response to exercise, and documenting exercise-induced arrhythmias. ECG changes and ST depression may occur in the absence of epicardial coronary disease as a result of supply-demand mismatch and microvascular ischemia.

- Echocardiography can be combined with exercise testing in order to assess for dynamic LVOT obstruction. This is indicated in all patients with symptoms who have an LVOT gradient of <50 mm Hg at rest or with Valsalva maneuver.[3]

- Cardiopulmonary exercise testing with calculation of peak oxygen consumption will demonstrate a reduction in peak VO_2 max in nearly all patients with HCM. However, a profound impairment with early lactic acidosis may raise the possibility of an underlying mitochondrial disorder.

CARDIAC COMPUTED TOMOGRAPHY

- In patients with poor echocardiographic imaging windows who cannot undergo CMR imaging procedures, due to the presence of implanted devices or claustrophobia, computed tomography (CT) can provide an alternative means to measure ventricular wall thickness, confirm the presence of hypertrophy, and demonstrate evidence of complications such as apical aneurysm formation (Figure 10-12).

- Coronary CT angiography (CTA) is a noninvasive method of imaging the epicardial coronary arteries to exclude atherosclerotic disease. CTA is useful for the assessment of underlying coronary artery disease in patients with chest pain with a low likelihood of coronary disease.[4]

CORONARY ANGIOGRAPHY

- In patients with symptoms suggestive of angina, particularly in the presence of other cardiac risk factors, angiography is helpful in excluding epicardial coronary artery disease as a cause of

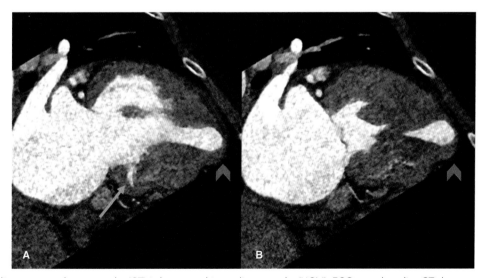

FIGURE 10-12 Cardiac computed tomography (CT) in hypertrophic cardiomyopathy (HCM). ECG-gated cardiac CT demonstrating a 2-chamber view in end diastole (A) and end systole (B). The hypertrophy is causing dynamic obstruction at midventricular level. A noncontractile apical aneurysm (red arrowhead) is noted, without evidence of apical thrombus. In addition, there is a basal inferior wall myocardial crypt with typical appearances (gold arrow).

symptoms. In patients with an intermediate to high likelihood of coronary disease, angiography should be performed particularly when the identification of concomitant disease may impact management decisions.[4]

ETIOLOGICAL TESTING

- Given the wide differential diagnosis, a panel of biochemistry testing can be helpful to identify nonsarcomeric disease. A routine full blood count, renal and liver function, thyroid function, plasma BNP, and serum Troponin should ideally be performed in all patients at initial evaluation.

- A reduction in renal function and proteinuria may be seen in cases of systemic amyloidosis, Anderson-Fabry disease, and a mitochondrial disorder.

- Similarly, abnormal liver function and an elevation in serum creatine phosphokinase may be seen in mitochondrial disorders and storage disorders such as Danon disease.

- Testing of plasma/leukocyte alpha galactosidase A should be performed in all men aged >30 years, and in any other patient in whom a diagnosis of Anderson-Fabry disease is clinically suspected. Low (<10% normal) or undetectable plasma and leukocyte alpha galactosidase A activity confirms the diagnosis in male patients. Enzyme levels are often within the normal range in affected women and so genetic testing should be considered.

- In cases of suspected cardiac amyloidosis, serum immunoglobulins and serum and urine protein electrophoresis should be performed.

MANAGEMENT

- In patients with symptoms, management is determined principally by the presence or absence of LVOT obstruction, and can be broadly divided into pharmacologic and interventional.

- Risk stratification for SCD should be performed in all patients regardless of the presence or absence of symptoms.

- Risk factors for coronary artery disease should be managed as per medical guidelines.

PHARMACOLOGIC

- A significant proportion of HCM patients are asymptomatic, and despite the presence or absence of obstruction there is no clear demonstration of benefit for the use of beta blockers and calcium channel antagonists in the absence of symptoms.

- Beta blockers are first-line therapy for the treatment of symptoms in adult patients with both obstructive or nonobstructive HCM, and should be titrated up to a maximum tolerated dose (aiming for a resting heart rate of 60-65 bpm).

- Calcium channel antagonists such as verapamil should be used in patients in whom beta-blockade is contra-indicated or ineffective. Diltiazem can be used in patients in whom verapamil is ineffective or contra-indicated.

- In patients with obstruction who remain symptomatic, a second-line agent such as disopyramide can be used in combination with a beta blocker or verapamil. It should not be used alone as disopyramide may enhance atrioventricular conduction and increase the ventricular rate during episodes of atrial fibrillation. The initiation of disopyramide should be undertaken under close cardiac monitoring for potential arrhythmias and lengthening of the QT interval on surface ECG.[4]

- Vasodilators such as angiotensin-converting emzyme inhibitors (ACE-i) and alpha blockers should be used with caution as they may aggravate outflow tract obstruction. In addition, high-dose diuretics are potentially harmful and should be avoided or used with caution.

- Oral diuretics can be added in patients with nonobstructive HCM when symptoms of dyspnea persist despite first-line therapy with either a beta blocker or verapamil.

INTERVENTIONAL

- Approximately two-thirds of patients can be managed with medical therapy with relief or amelioration of symptoms and >50% reduction in the LVOT gradient. However, a significant proportion of patients require an interventional strategy for relief of LVOT obstruction. Given the potential complications of invasive therapies, it is important that patients fulfill clinical, anatomic and hemodynamic criteria when determining suitability for a particular procedure.

- The ACCF/AHA 2011 guidelines recommend that septal reduction therapies only be performed by experienced operators in centers with a multidisciplinary HCM program.[4]

- Eligible patients should have severe medically refractory symptoms and evidence of a resting or provocable LVOT gradient ≥50 mm Hg. In addition, the degree of septal hypertrophy should be sufficient to perform the procedure safely and effectively.

Surgical Septal Myectomy

- Septal myectomy is considered the most appropriate treatment for the majority of patients, and allows for concomitant coronary artery bypass grafting and mitral valve surgery (required in up to one-third of patients undergoing surgery).

- Results for myectomy are unmatched for both early efficacy and low procedural mortality and morbidity when performed in high-volume specialized centers (<1%).

- Surgical approaches typically involve an "extended myectomy" with resection of muscle from the interventricular septum, allowing physical enlargement of the LVOT and abolition of systolic anterior motion of the mitral valve. Resection is often extended down to the midventricular level. In some cases, papillary muscle repositioning or shaving of hypertrophied papillary muscles may be required.

- In selected cases a concomitant mitral valve repair or replacement may be required, particularly if the anterior leaflet of the mitral valve is elongated, or if intrinsic mitral valve disease (prolapse, ruptured chordae, annular dilatation) is present.

- Transesophageal echocardiography is crucial in the identification of mitral valve disease preoperatively, and in guiding the depth and extent of resection perioperatively. In addition, postoperative

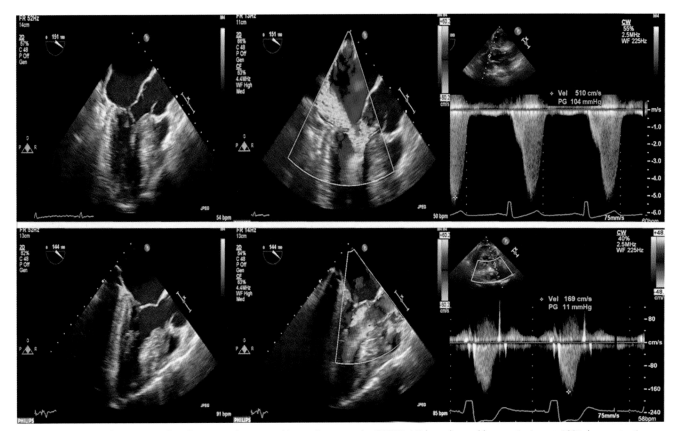

FIGURE 10-13 Surgical myectomy for obstructive hypertrophic cardiomyopathy (HCM). Midesophageal long-axis view at 120° demonstrating systolic anterior motion of the mitral valve and posteriorly directed mitral regurgitation prior to surgery, with an LVOT gradient of 104 mm Hg (upper panel). Immediately after coming off of bypass there is now laminar flow in the LVOT with resolution of mitral regurgitation. A residual gradient of only 11 mm Hg is measured after myectomy.

imaging allows confirmation not only of abolition of the LVOT gradient, but also of mitral valve competency. Immediate exclusion of complications such as iatrogenic ventricular septal defects, aortic valve injury, and residual mitral regurgitation is essential so that they can be addressed immediately (Figure 10-13).

Alcohol Septal Ablation

- Alcohol septal ablation (ASA) is performed through a percutaneous approach, and provides a suitable alternative for patients of advanced age or with significant comorbidities that would lead to an increased or unacceptably high surgical risk.

- ASA, via injection of ethanol into a septal perforator vessel identified as supplying the myocardium of the hypertrophied basal interventricular septum adjacent to the point of anterior mitral valve leaflet-basal septum contact, creates infarction and subsequent regression of hypertrophy of the targeted area with scar formation over a 6- to 12-month period.

- ASA should be discouraged in cases of severe septal hypertrophy (>30 mm). It should not be performed in patients <21 years of age, and should be discouraged in those <40 years of age if surgical myectomy is a viable alternative.[4]

- Contrast echocardiography is essential during the procedure to ensure that the selected septal perforator supplies only the targeted area of myocardium, and to ensure that no enhancement of

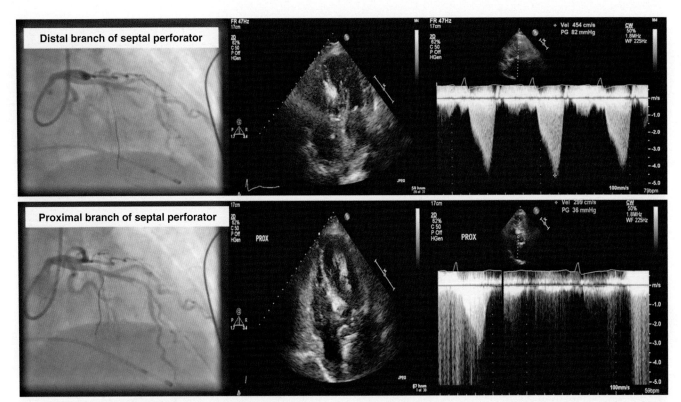

FIGURE 10-14 Alcohol septal ablation for obstructive hypertrophic cardiomyopathy (HCM). Contrast echocardiography helps to identify the septal perforator vessel supplying the basal interventricular septum. Note the distal vessel results in opacification of the midseptum with no effect on LVOT obstruction after balloon occlusion of the selected vessel (82 mm Hg), but when the proximal vessel is selected there is opacification of the target basal myocardium, associated with a significant decrease in LVOT gradient (36 mm Hg).

other regions of remote myocardium occurs (papillary muscles, free wall of the left or right ventricle) (Figure 10-14).

- A decrease in both resting and provocable LVOT gradients is seen immediately as a result of myocardial stunning, with progressive declines in LVOT gradients over 3 to 6 months due to myocardial thinning.

- Transient complete atrioventricular block can occur during the procedure, with persistent complete heart block necessitating permanent pacemaker occurring in 10% to 20% of patients.

- Because of the potential for creating a ventricular septal defect, septal ablation should not be performed if the septal thickness of the myocardium is <15 mm.[4]

Dual-Chamber Pacing

- Dual-chamber pacing is a potential therapy for those patients who have an unacceptably high risk for either surgical myectomy or ASA, or in patients without appropriate septal perforator anatomy for ASA.[4]

- Randomized controlled trials have demonstrated only a modest benefit. In patients who already have a dual-chamber pacemaker implanted, it is reasonable to consider a trial of short AV delay dual-chamber pacing from the RV apex for the relief of symptoms attributable to LVOT obstruction.

TREATMENT OF SYSTOLIC DYSFUNCTION

- Development of systolic dysfunction can occur in the setting of HCM in a small proportion of patients. A reduction in LVEF should prompt investigations and exclusion of other potential contributing causes such as coronary artery disease, valvular heart disease, and metabolic disorders.

- Patients with nonobstructive HCM who develop systolic dysfunction should be treated according to clinical guidelines for other forms of HF (ie, angiotensin-converting enzyme inhibitors, angiotensin receptor blockers, beta blockers, and other indicated drugs).[3,4]

- Referral for assessment for heart transplantation should be considered early in patients with advanced heart failure symptoms (NYHA class III or IV symptoms refractory to pharmacologic and nonpharmacologic interventions), particularly in the presence of a decline in LVEF to <50%.[4]

RISK STRATIFICATION FOR SUDDEN CARDIAC DEATH

- SCD may be the first presentation of the disease, and remains the most feared complication. Identification of the minority of patients at high risk for SCD remains a major challenge. An AICD can offer protection to those patients deemed to be at high risk for SCD.

- All patients should undergo a comprehensive risk stratification at initial evaluation, with periodic reassessment every 12 to 24 months during follow-up.[3,4]

- Established risk factors for SCD individually have a low positive predictive value, and as such overall risk is best assessed in terms of total burden of risk as opposed to the presence or absence of any single risk factor alone.

SECONDARY PREVENTION AICD IMPLANTATION

- A patient who has previously experienced a high-grade potentially fatal arrhythmia should undergo implantation of an AICD, as this group is at highest risk of recurrence of arrhythmic events (in the order of 10% annual event rate). However, even in this high-risk group, arrhythmia-free intervals may be long and individuals may never suffer a further arrhythmia.[3,4]

PRIMARY PREVENTION AICD IMPLANTATION

- Established risk factors and potential risk modifiers for SCD are shown in Table 10-1. While the presence of multiple risk markers in an individual patient would intuitively suggest greater risk for SCD, the majority of patients with ≥1 risk marker will not experience SCD. In the international HCM-ICD registry the cumulative number of risk factors did not correlate with the rate of subsequent appropriate defibrillator discharges among presumably high-risk patients selected for AICD placement.

- Decisions need to be individualized with regard to patient age, the strength of the risk factor, and the risk versus benefit of life-long AICD therapy.

- The current ACCF/AHA guidelines consider it reasonable to recommend an AICD in patients with 1 of the following risk factors:

Table 10-1 Sudden Cardiac Death: Established Risk Factors and Potential Risk Modifiers

Risk Factor	2014 ESC Guidelines[3]	2011 ACCF/ AHA Guidelines[4]
Maximal wall thickness (MWT)	Included	Included MWT >30 mm Major risk factor
Family history of sudden cardiac death	Included	Included Major risk factor
Unexplained syncope	Included	Included Major risk factor
Nonsustained ventricular tachycardia	Included	Included Minor risk factor
Left ventricular outflow tract obstruction	Included	Not included
Abnormal blood pressure response to exercise	Not included	Included Minor risk factor
Age	Included	Not included
Left atrial size	Included	Not included
Late gadolinium enhancement on cardiac MRI	Not included	Included Risk modifier
Apical aneurysm	Not included	Included Risk modifier

Established risk factors for sudden cardiac death and potential modifiers of risk are listed above. Two risk stratification algorithms are currently advocated in clinical practice, and the various risk factors incorporated into these algorithms is illustrated.

a family history of sudden death, a maximum wall thickness ≥30 mm, or 1 or more recent unexplained syncopal episodes. The presence of NSVT (especially in patients younger than 30 years of age) and abnormal blood pressure response to exercise should justify AICD implantation only in the presence of other SCD risk factors or modifiers.[4]

- The 2014 ESC guidelines endorse a novel clinical risk-prediction model, which gives a prognostic score and is accessible as an interactive online calculator. The formula includes 7 clinical variables, 4 of which are conventional risk factors (family history of SCD, maximum wall thickness, NSVT, and unexplained syncope). Three novel risk factors are included, notably left atrial diameter, LVOT gradient at rest or with Valsalva provocation, and age at evaluation.[3]

- The online calculator produces a 5-year risk for SCD, based upon which patients are stratified into 3 groups: >6% (AICD should be considered), <4% (AICD generally not indicated), and 4% to 6% (AICD may be considered).

- AICD decision-making in these complex cases cannot be solely done by a risk calculator or a checklist of risk factors, both of which can overestimate or underestimate the risk in an individual patient. These risk assessment models should be integrated with, rather than substitute for, the clinical assessment of the physician.

PROGNOSIS

Historically, HCM was felt to be a rare disease with a high risk of adverse events, but current evidence suggests that with contemporary management strategies the natural history of the HCM population as a whole is relatively benign. This is clearly contingent of the identification of patients at an elevated risk of SCD and other complications, and appropriate and timely intervention.

- SCD occurs over a wide age range, but tends to be more frequent in younger patients. It may be the first presentation of disease, with up to two-thirds of patients having no or very little in the way of symptoms prior to death. Exercise-related sudden death appears to occur more commonly in younger patients compared to exercise-unrelated deaths.

- Over the past decades, the annual risk of SCD has fallen from around 3% to 1%, with a concomitant decrease in all-cause mortality from 5% to 3%.[28-30]

- Three distinct modes of death occur: (1) sudden and unexpected (accounting for up to half of all cases), (2) progressive HF (approximately one-third of cases), and (3) HCM-related ischemic stroke associated with atrial fibrillation (more commonly seen in elderly patients).[31]

FOLLOW-UP

Patients require lifelong follow-up, with monitoring of symptoms, LV function, and development of arrhythmias. In addition, risk stratification is a dynamic and ongoing process throughout the follow-up process. The frequency of monitoring should be individualized based on the age of the patient, presence of symptoms, and severity of disease expression. In stable patients the follow-up interval should be every

1 to 2 years, with a 12-lead ECG, transthoracic echocardiogram, ambulatory 48-hour ECG monitoring, and clinical examination. In patients with significant left atrial dilatation, in whom the risk of atrial arrhythmia is higher, ambulatory monitoring should be performed more frequently (every 6-12 months).[3]

PATIENT EDUCATION

EXERCISE RESTRICTIONS

- Patients with HCM should avoid all competitive sports, but should maintain a healthy lifestyle. These restrictions apply regardless of the presence or absence of outflow tract obstruction or implantation of an AICD.[4]

- Aerobic exercise is preferable to isometric exercise. Any activities involving sudden bursts of exertion (associated with sudden and rapid changes in heart rate) should be avoided. Patients should maintain good levels of hydration when exercising, as periods of dehydration can aggravate intracavitary and outflow tract obstruction.

PREGNANCY AND CONTRACEPTION

- Most women with HCM tolerate the physiologic and hemodynamic changes of pregnancy without complication. However, the increase in circulating blood volume can be tolerated poorly in the presence of significant diastolic dysfunction or LVOT obstruction, and these patients require closer monitoring during pregnancy. Maternal mortality rates are extremely low, other than in women with advanced HF symptoms, in whom pregnancy is associated with higher rates of morbidity and mortality.

- Oral contraception can safely be used in all patients with HCM (unless otherwise contraindicated) other than those with HF or atrial fibrillation (unless fully anticoagulated).

- The risk of transmission of a pathogenic mutation to the fetus should be discussed with all women of childbearing age.

PATIENT EDUCATION RESOURCES

Hypertrophic Cardiomyopathy Association: www.4hcm.org

Cardiomyopathy UK—The Heart Muscle Charity: www.cardiomyopathy.org

PROVIDER RESOURCES (PRACTICE GUIDELINES)

- 2011 ACCF/AHA guideline for the diagnosis and treatment of hypertrophic cardiomyopathy: executive summary: a report of the American College of Cardiology Foundation/American Heart Association Task Force on Practice Guidelines.[4]

- 2014 ESC guidelines on diagnosis and management of hypertrophic cardiomyopathy: The Task Force for the Diagnosis and Management of Hypertrophic Cardiomyopathy of the European Society of Cardiology (ESC).[3]

- 2011 American Society of Echocardiography clinical recommendations for multimodality cardiovascular imaging of patients with hypertrophic cardiomyopathy: Endorsed by the American Society of Nuclear Cardiology, Society for Cardiovascular Magnetic Resonance, and Society of Cardiovascular Computed Tomography.[32]

REFERENCES

1. Maron BJ, Ommen SR, Semsarian C, Spirito P, Olivotto I, Maron MS. Hypertrophic cardiomyopathy: present and future, with translation into contemporary cardiovascular medicine. *J Am Coll Cardiol.* 2014;64:83-99.

2. Maron BJ, Doerer JJ, Haas TS, Tierney DM, Mueller FO. Sudden deaths in young competitive athletes: analysis of 1866 deaths in the United States, 1980-2006. *Circulation.* 2009;119:1085-1092.

3. Elliott PM, Anastasakis A, Borger MA, et al. 2014 ESC Guidelines on diagnosis and management of hypertrophic cardiomyopathy: the Task Force for the Diagnosis and Management of Hypertrophic Cardiomyopathy of the European Society of Cardiology (ESC). *Eur Heart J.* 2014;35:2733-2779.

4. Gersh BJ, Maron BJ, Bonow RO, et al. 2011 ACCF/AHA guideline for the diagnosis and treatment of hypertrophic cardiomyopathy: a report of the American College of Cardiology Foundation/American Heart Association Task Force on Practice Guidelines. *Circulation,* 2011;124:e783-e831.

5. Minami Y, Kajimoto K, Terajima Y, et al. Clinical implications of midventricular obstruction in patients with hypertrophic cardiomyopathy. *J Am Coll Cardiol.* 2011;57:2346-2355.

6. Maron MS, Olivotto I, Betocchi S, et al. Effect of left ventricular outflow tract obstruction on clinical outcome in hypertrophic cardiomyopathy. *N Engl J Med.* 2003;348:295-303.

7. Prasad K, Williams L, Campbell R, Elliott PM, McKenna WJ, Frenneaux M. Episodic syncope in hypertrophic cardiomyopathy: evidence for inappropriate vasodilation. *Heart.* 2008;94:1312-1317.

8. Frenneaux MP, Counihan PJ, Caforio AL, Chikamori T, McKenna WJ. Abnormal blood pressure response during exercise in hypertrophic cardiomyopathy. *Circulation.* 1990;82:1995-2002.

9. Sadoul N, Prasad K, Elliott PM, Bannerjee S, Frenneaux MP, McKenna WJ. Prospective prognostic assessment of blood pressure response during exercise in patients with hypertrophic cardiomyopathy. *Circulation.* 1997;96:2987-2991.

10. Maron BJ, Haas TS, Maron MS, et al. Left atrial remodeling in hypertrophic cardiomyopathy and susceptibility markers for atrial fibrillation identified by cardiovascular magnetic resonance. *Am J Cardiol.* 2014;113:1394-1400.

11. Olivotto I, DiDonna P, Baldi M, Sgalambro A, Maron BJ, Cecchi F. [Atrial fibrillation in hypertrophic cardiomyopathy: determinants, clinical course and management]. *Zhonghua Xin Xue Guan Bing Za Zhi.* 2009;37:303-307.

12. Siontis KC, Geske JB, Ong K, Nishimura RA, Ommen SR, Gersh BJ. Atrial fibrillation in hypertrophic cardiomyopathy: prevalence, clinical correlations, and mortality in a large high-risk population. *J Am Heart Assoc.* 2014;3:e001002.

13. Monserrat L, Elliott PM, Gimeno JR, Sharma S, Penas-Lado M, McKenna WJ. Non-sustained ventricular tachycardia in hypertrophic cardiomyopathy: an independent marker of sudden death risk in young patients. *J Am Coll Cardiol.* 2003;42:873-879.

14. Gimeno JR, Tome-Esteban M, Lofiego C, et al. Exercise-induced ventricular arrhythmias and risk of sudden cardiac death in patients with hypertrophic cardiomyopathy. *Eur Heart J.* 2009;30:2599-2605.

15. Harris KM, Spirito P, Maron MS, et al. Prevalence, clinical profile, and significance of left ventricular remodelling in the end-stage phase of hypertrophic cardiomyopathy. *Circulation.* 2006;114:216-225.

16. Melacini P, Basso C, Angelini A, et al. Clinicopathological profiles of progressive heart failure in hypertrophic cardiomyopathy. *Eur Heart J.* 2010;31:2111-2123.

17. Spirito P, Autore C, Rapezzi C, et al. Syncope and risk of sudden death in hypertrophic cardiomyopathy. *Circulation.* 2009;119:1703-1710.

18. Cardim N, Galderisi M, Edvardsen T, et al. Role of multimodality cardiac imaging in the management of patients with hypertrophic cardiomyopathy: an expert consensus of the European Association of Cardiovascular Imaging Endorsed by the Saudi Heart Association. *Eur Heart J Cardiovasc Imaging.* 2015;16:280.

19. Maron MS, Olivotto I, Zenovich AG, et al. Hypertrophic cardiomyopathy is predominantly a disease of left ventricular outflow tract obstruction. *Circulation.* 2006;114:2232-2239.

20. Tani T, Yagi T, Kitai T, et al. Left atrial volume predicts adverse cardiac and cerebrovascular events in patients with hypertrophic cardiomyopathy [abstract]. *Cardiovascular Ultrasound.* 2011;9.

21. Yang W, Shim CY, Kim YJ, et al. Left atrial volume index: a predictor of adverse outcome in patients with hypertrophic cardiomyopathy [abstract]. *J Am Soc Echocardiogr.* 2009;22:1338-1343.

22. Efthimiadis GK, Pagourelias ED, Parcharidou D, et al. Clinical characteristics and natural history of hypertrophic cardiomyopathy with midventricular obstruction. *Circ J.* 2013; Epub May 31.

23. Hanneman K, Crean AM, Williams L, et al. Cardiac magnetic resonance imaging findings predict major adverse events in apical hypertrophic cardiomyopathy. *J Thorac Imaging.* 2014;29:331-339.

24. Briasoulis A, Mallikethi-Reddy S, Palla M, Alesh I, Afonso L. Myocardial fibrosis on cardiac magnetic resonance and cardiac outcomes in hypertrophic cardiomyopathy: a meta-analysis. *Heart.* 2015;101:1406-1411.

25. Chan RH, Maron BJ, Olivotto I, et al. Prognostic value of quantitative contrast-enhanced cardiovascular magnetic resonance for the evaluation of sudden death risk in patients with hypertrophic cardiomyopathy. *Circulation.* 2014;130:484-495.

26. Maceira AM, Joshi J, Prasad SK, et al. Cardiovascular magnetic resonance in cardiac amyloidosis. *Circulation.* 2005;111:186-193.

27. Moon JC, Sachdev B, Elkington AG, et al. Gadolinium enhanced cardiovascular magnetic resonance in Anderson-Fabry disease. Evidence for a disease specific abnormality of the myocardial interstitium. *Eur Heart J.* 2003;24:2151-2155.

28. Maron BJ, Rowin EJ, Casey SA, et al. Hypertrophic cardiomyopathy in adulthood associated with low cardiovascular mortality with contemporary management strategies. *J Am Coll Cardiol.* 2015;65:1915-1928.

29. Maron BJ, Rowin EJ, Casey SA, et al. Hypertrophic cardiomyopathy in children, adolescents, and young adults associated with low cardiovascular mortality with contemporary management strategies. *Circulation.* 2016;133:62-73.

30. Maron MS, Rowin EJ, Olivotto I, et al. Contemporary natural history and management of nonobstructive hypertrophic cardiomyopathy. *J Am Coll Cardiol.* 2016;67:1399-1409.

31. Maron BJ, Olivotto I, Spirito P, et al. Epidemiology of hypertrophic cardiomyopathy-related death: revisited in a large nonreferral based patient population. *Circulation.* 2000;102:858-864.

32. Nagueh SF, Bierig SM, Budoff MJ, et al. American Society of Echocardiography clinical recommendations for multimodality cardiovascular imaging of patients with hypertrophic cardiomyopathy: endorsed by the American Society of Nuclear Cardiology, Society for Cardiovascular Magnetic Resonance, and Society of Cardiovascular Computed Tomography. *J Am Soc Echocardiogr.* 2011;24:473-498.

11 AMYLOID HEART DISEASE

Taimur Sher, MD
Morie A. Gertz, MD

PATIENT CASE

JS, a 45-year-old Caucasian man, was referred to the Mayo Clinic in consultation for progressive congestive heart failure (CHF) of unclear etiology. A year prior to his symptoms, he had been a healthy and active person playing tennis 4 times a week and leading a very busy life as a farmer in the Midwest and as a father of 3 young children with no medical problems except for well-controlled essential hypertension (HTN). Six to eight months prior to presentation he experienced a decline in exercise capacity and gradually gave up tennis. Three months prior to presentation he developed dyspnea on moderate exertion and intermittent swelling of his legs. Medical evaluation included normal renal function, blood counts, and pulmonary computed tomography (CT) angiogram. Nuclear medicine cardiac stress test was normal; pulmonary function tests indicated a mild reversible obstructive defect and 2D echocardiogram revealed mildly thickened left ventricle with an ejection fraction of 60% and borderline diastolic dysfunction. Treatment with bronchodilators was empirically started for a provisional diagnosis of atypical asthma. His symptoms progressed rather rapidly over the course of 2 to 3 weeks and he underwent a coronary angiogram, which demonstrated normal coronary arteries. At his evaluation at Mayo Clinic he was found to be in New York Heart Association (NYHA) class III CHF. Based on the review of his electrocardiograph (ECG) and echocardiogram a diagnosis of infiltrative cardiomyopathy was suspected and further work demonstrated an immunoglobulin lambda light chain gammopathy in the serum with 8% lambda restricted plasma cells in the bone marrow. Congo red staining of the bone marrow and abdominal fat aspirate was positive for extracellular amorphous material that demonstrated apple green birefringence under polarized microscope. He was diagnosed with immunoglobulin lambda light chain amyloidosis (AL) with stage IV cardiac disease.

AMYLOIDOSIS

HISTORY AND INTRODUCTION

Matthias Schleiden, a German botanist, first used the term *amyloid* in 1838 to describe a normal constituent of plants.[1] In 1858, Rudolph Virchow described amyloid deposits in spleen that stained blue with iodine and sulfuric acid, similar to the chemical reaction markers of starch. Virchow concluded that the substance was composed of starch and used the word *amyloid* to describe it.[2] In 1859, Friedreich, Nikolau, and Kekule recognized that the waxy spleen described by Virchow did not contain any starchlike substances and that the deposits probably were derived from modified proteins.[3]

Amyloidosis, as understood today, is a unique, yet remarkably heterogeneous group of diseases characterized by the deposition of misfolded protein precursors in a beta-pleated sheet configuration in the extracellular space in various tissues. This characteristically conserved structure renders the amyloid fibrils of different origins resistant to proteolytic cleavage under physiological condition and forms the basis of characteristic staining of amyloid fibrils by Congo red, thioflavin T, and Alcian blue, a feature essential for establishing the diagnosis on histopathologic examination (Figure 11-1).[4] Widely divergent precursor proteins (more than 30 currently known) can cause amyloidosis and can lead to diseases belonging to infectious (prion disease), neoplastic (immunoglobulin light chain systemic amyloidosis), neurodegenerative (Alzheimer disease), and hereditary (familial amyloidosis) groups of disorders (Figure 11-2).[5] Clinically, amyloidosis manifests as localized or systemic disease with disease manifestations resulting from type and extent of organ involvement. The heart is a frequently involved organ in systemic amyloidosis and amyloid cardiomyopathy is the most common cause of death in these patients.

AMYLOID CARDIOMYOPATHY

The heart is one of the most common organs involved in amyloidosis. With the exception of localized atrial amyloidosis derived from natriuretic peptide, cardiac amyloidosis almost always indicates systemic disease.

Amyloidogenic proteins can involve any anatomical region of the heart, including the myocardium (atrial, ventricular, and interventricular septum), valvular tissue, the perivascular space around and within small blood vessels, and the conduction system. Gross pathologic examination of the heart infiltrated with amyloidosis reveals characteristic thickening of all 4 cardiac chambers and interventricular septum (Figure 11-3). Microscopically, amyloid deposition is seen in the extracellular space, which results in separation and distortion of myocardial cells and electromechanical dissociation. Myocardial damage results from physical deposition of the amyloid material and from direct cellular cytotoxicity of the circulating amyloidogenic protein. No histologic pattern is specific for a particular form of amyloid cardiomyopathy and different amyloid proteins can result in similar pathological findings. Cardiac involvement can occur at any stage of the disease and may be the initial presentation, incidentally discovered during evaluation of other symptoms, or discovered on postmortem examination.[6]

COMMON TYPES OF AMYLOID CARDIOMYOPATHIES

All forms of cardiac amyloidosis can result in similar cardiac presentations; however, they progress at different rates and important clinical clues can help to differentiate them (Table 11-1).

Immunoglobulin Light Chain Amyloid Cardiomyopathy

Immunoglobulin light chain amyloidosis (primary systemic amyloidosis or AL), the most common systemic amyloidosis in the United States and western Europe, is a plasma cell dyscrasia, where transformed plasma cells in the bone marrow produce amyloidogenic light chains. With 2500 new cases each year, AL is an orphan disease.[7] Most commonly, AL occurs de novo, but in a minority of patients it can evolve from preexisting multiple myeloma (the most common plasma cell malignancy) and non-Hodgkin lymphomas such as Waldenström macroglobulinemia. Cardiac involvement is often very advanced and is seen in half of the cases.[8] AL cardiomyopathy presents with restrictive physiology and patients frequently present with CHF with a nondilated, thickened left ventricle on echocardiogram. Peripheral edema from right heart dysfunction is a very common feature. In advanced stage, ascites, hepatomegaly, and jugular venous distension are common. Atrial dysrhythmias are common and can be complicated by mural atrial thrombus; embolic stroke may be the first presentation of the disease.[9] Ventricular arrhythmias also occur, but are not a common presenting feature, possibly because patients succumb to sudden cardiac arrest before the diagnosis is established. Angina pectoris from myocardial ischemia from amyloid infiltration of small vessel walls can, at times, be very frustrating as cardiac catheterization reveals normal epicardial coronaries.[10] Multiorgan involvement is very commonly seen in AL patients and kidney, peripheral nerves, autonomic nerves, and the liver and GI tract are frequent extracardiac sites of disease (Table 11-2).[8] Soft tissue infiltration can give rise to rare but classic clinical exam findings such as shoulder pad sign, muscle infiltration, macroglossia, and raccoon eyes (Figure 11-4 through Figure 11-6). Small- and medium-sized blood vessel ischemia from involvement by amyloid can cause symptoms of jaw claudication and patients can be misdiagnosed as having giant cell arteritis. Mucocutaneous bleeding due to failure of hemostasis resulting

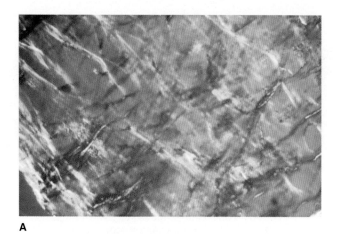

A

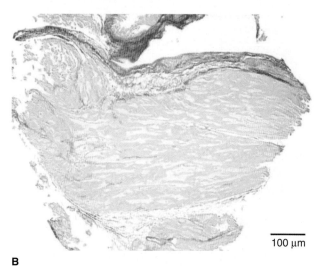

B

FIGURE 11-1 Diagnosis of amyloidosis must be established on histologic examination. (A) Apple green birefringence of a Congo red stained fat aspirate as seen through polarized microscope. (B) Extracellular amyloid deposits in a section of endomyocardial biopsy stained with Alcian blue.

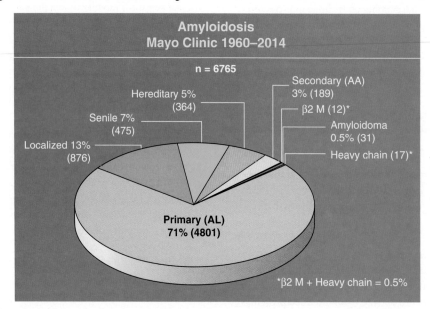

FIGURE 11-2 Number of cases of various types of amyloidosis seen at the Mayo Clinic. Beta-2-microglobulin-related amyloidosis is seen in patients undergoing chronic renal replacement therapy. Localized amyloidosis almost always remains limited and commonly involves the head and neck region, tracheobronchial tree, and urinary bladder and may cause clinically significant local symptoms requiring local intervention such as surgical, laser guided, or radiation therapy.

from altered blood vessel wall integrity and acquired deficiency of circulating coagulation factors, in particular factor X, can be a prominent presenting feature.[11] AL cardiomyopathy is the most aggressive form of amyloid heart disease and is the sole reason for the poor prognosis associated with amyloidosis.

Senile Systemic Amyloid (Wild-Type ATTR) Cardiomyopathy

Senile systemic amyloidosis (SSA) is caused by systemic deposition of amyloid fibrils derived from a native (wild-type) circulating plasma protein transthyretin (TTR).[12] With the increasing availability and more common use of echocardiography, the incidence of SSA is expected to increase significantly in coming years. Interestingly, for unclear reasons, SSA is almost exclusively seen in men. Autopsy series have commonly identified wild-type TTR amyloid deposits in the hearts of older men with some series reporting an incidence as high as 25% in subjects 80 years of age or older. Many patients with SSA may not develop clinically significant end-organ damage, despite histological or radiological evidence of amyloidosis. When clinically apparent, SSA typically presents with progressive decline in energy and symptoms of CHF, often with normal systolic function.[13] The diagnosis is often delayed in these patients until they have multiple hospitalizations for CHF. Increased myocardial thickness is often blamed on systemic HTN, a very prevalent condition in this age group. Almost half of SSA patients may have symptomatic median neuropathy presenting as carpal tunnel syndrome. This is in contrast to familial TTR amyloidosis, where manifestations of peripheral neuropathy and gastrointestinal (GI) involvement are frequently seen in addition to cardiomyopathy.

Familial Amyloid Cardiomyopathy

Familial/hereditary amyloidosis results from mutant misfolded forms of several proteins such as TTR, apolipoprotein, fibrinogen, and leukocyte chemotactic factor 2, among others.[14] With more than 100 pathogenic mutations described in the *TTR* gene on chromosome 18, amyloidosis of TTR type (familial-ATTR) is the most common familial amyloid cardiomyopathy.[15] In familial ATTR, the specific TTR mutant determines the clinical presentation, but peripheral nerves and the heart are the most common sites of involvement. Autonomic dysfunction and GI tract involvement can be severe and can cause significant malabsorption and protein-losing enteropathy.[16,17] One particular variant allele, Val122Ile, is found in 1 out of every 25 African Americans (carrier rate of 4%) and is a frequently overlooked cause of cardiomyopathy in African American men.[18] Despite the high prevalence of this variant, the overall prevalence and incidence of familial amyloid cardiomyopathy in African Americans remains low, possibly owing to failure to recognize the etiology of the CHF. In Caucasians, the Val30Met mutant is the most commonly reported variant with high penetrance presenting as early onset (30-40 years of age) peripheral neuropathy and relatively late onset (50-60 years of age) cardiomyopathy.[19]

In addition to TTR, mutant fibrinogen A-α and apoA-I and A-II can involve the heart; however, renal involvement predominates in these very rare forms of non-TTR familial amyloidoses.[20,21]

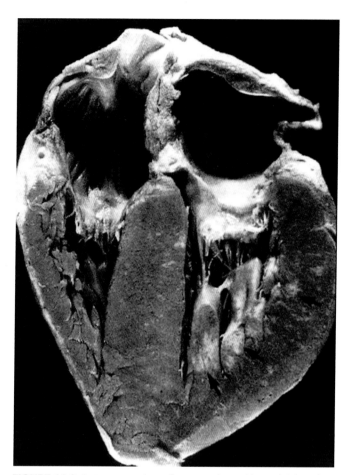

FIGURE 11-3 Autopsy specimen from a patient with amyloid cardiomyopathy. Thickened interventricular septum and left ventricular posterior wall is obvious. Interestingly this thickness is more pronounced in ATTR than in AL indicating that poor prognosis of AL is not related to the mechanical phenomenon of myocardial infiltration. Preclinical studies have shown that amyloidogenic light chain from patients with AL can cause rapid reduction in myocardial function when infused in mice.

Table 11-1 Common Types of Cardiac Amyloidosis

Characteristics	AL	ATTR Mutant	ATTR Wild	AA	AANF
Common name	Primary (immuno-globulin light chain) systemic amyloidosis	Familial tran-sthyretin amyloidosis	Senile systemic amyloidosis	Secondary amyloidosis	Isolated atrial amyloidosis
Incidence / prevalence	2000-3000 cases/yr	Variable in differ-ent races: Val-122Ile variant in 4% of African Americans. Val30Met variant in Caucasians.	Males older than 70 y Incidence increases with age.	Uncommon	Common
Precursor protein	Immunoglobulin light chain	Mutant TTR	Wild-type TTR	SAA protein	Atrial natriuretic peptide
Clinical organ involvement	Heart, kidney, liver, peripheral nerves, autonomic nerves, GI tract, soft tissue	Heart, nerves, GI tract, auto-nomic nerves	Heart, rarely nerves	Kidney, liver, GI tract. Very rarely heart.	Cardiac atria
Salient features	Low QRS voltage. Pseudoinfarct pat-tern on ECG. IVS thickness sel-dom more than 1.9 cm. Rapid progression.	IVS thickness fre-quently severe	IVS thickness frequently severe. Relatively indolent disease.		
Treatment	Chemotherapy (standard or stem cell transplant)	Liver transplant	Supportive care	Treat inflammation	No specific treatment
Prognosis/ survival	Poor. 3-5 mo if present with CHF.	8-10 y from presentation	5-8 y from diagnosis	Generally good	Good

Abbreviations: CHF, congestive heart failure; ECG, electrocardiogram; GI, gastrointestinal; IVS, interventricular septum; TTR, transthyretin.

Secondary Systemic Amyloid Cardiomyopathy

Secondary systemic (AA) amyloidosis results from excessive pro-duction and misfolding of the acute-phase reactant serum amyloid A protein. AA is a very common form of systemic amyloidosis in developing countries and in the Mediterranean basin due to a high prevalence of chronic infections (chronic osteomyelitis and mycobacterial infections) and auto-inflammatory disorders, such as familial periodic fever syndromes.[22] In the United States and Western Europe, it is rare and usually results from unrec-ognized or untreated chronic autoimmune disorders such as rheumatoid arthritis and inflammatory bowel disease. Nephrotic syndrome is the most common presentation but involvement of GI and hepatobiliary systems leading to malabsorption syndrome

Table 11-2 Syndromes in AL Amyloidosis (Mayo Clinic Experience)

Syndrome	Patients, %
Nephrotic or nephrotic and renal failure	30
Hepatomegaly	24
Congestive heart failure	22
Carpal tunnel syndrome	21
Neuropathy	17
Orthostatic hypotension	12

and/or hepatosplenomegaly can be a presenting feature. Involvement of endocrine organs, such as the thyroid and adrenal gland, can be seen and may result in adrenal insufficiency.[23] Cardiac involvement in AA is rare and even if severe by echocardiogram, seldom results in clinically significant cardiomyopathy.

Isolated Atrial Amyloidosis

Isolated atrial amyloidosis (IAA) is a relatively recently recognized entity and results from atrial deposits of atrial natriuretic peptide.[24] Unlike other cardiac amyloidoses, this is almost always localized to the atria and can be diagnosed only on histologic examination of atrial tissue. The incidence of IAA increases with age and appears to be more common in patients with atrial diseases such as rheumatic heart disease. Intriguingly, recent studies have reported a very high incidence of IAA on the histopathologic examination of the explanted hearts from patients with dilated and hypertrophic cardiomyopathies and raise important questions about the possible role of IAA in the pathogenesis of these conditions.[25]

DIAGNOSIS OF AMYLOID CARDIOMYOPATHY

Like many rare diseases, amyloid cardiomyopathy is very often diagnosed at late stages. This is especially true in AL where the rapid disease course coupled with a lack of specificity in the patient's symptoms results in delayed diagnosis and poor outcomes. Amyloidosis should be included in the differential diagnosis of all patients presenting with proteinuria; unexplained CHF (especially diastolic heart failure); new-onset peripheral neuropathy, especially with bilateral carpal tunnel syndrome; new-onset autonomic dysfunction; otherwise unexplained weight loss; and hepatomegaly in the absence of known liver disease (Table 11-2).

Patients suspected of amyloidosis should undergo a thorough physical examination with particular attention to signs of volume overload, orthostatic hypotension, macroglossia, amyloid purpura, hepatosplenomegaly, peripheral edema, and sensory neuropathy. Initial laboratory studies should include complete blood counts, renal and liver function profiles, serum electrolytes, coagulation profile, serum protein electrophoresis with immunofixation,

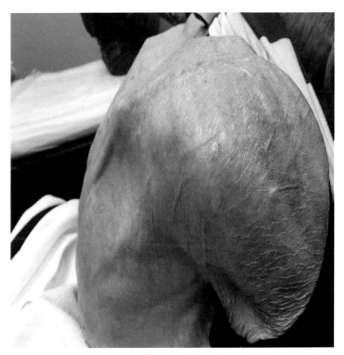

FIGURE 11-4 Periarticular infiltration of joints by amyloid can result in pseudohypertrophy. This particular patient has lambda light chain AL amyloidosis that presented with progressive and painful enlargement of shoulders and weakness of arm muscles over the course of 6 weeks. Note generalized cachexia as indicated by the loss of muscle and subcutaneous fat in the infraspinatus region of scapula.

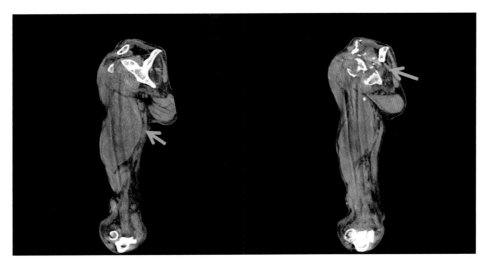

FIGURE 11-5 CT scan from the same patient reveals pseudohypertrophy of the biceps muscle leading to "Popeye" sign as noted on the left. Severe destructive arthropathy of shoulder and free-floating bony tissue in the periarticular effusion is noted on the right.

24-hour urine protein electrophoresis, immunofixation and nephelometric measurement of serum immunoglobulin-free light chains (Table 11-3).[26] The common abnormalities noted in these initial studies in amyloidosis, particularly in AL patients, are summarized in (Table 11-4). The diagnosis of amyloidosis must be confirmed by histological examination of an optimal biopsy. Sites for the biopsy include abdominal wall subcutaneous fatty tissue (fat pad aspirate, fat pad biopsy), vascular submucosa of the GI tract (minor salivary glands in mouth, labial soft tissue, rectal biopsy), or bone marrow biopsy. In our experience, at the Mayo Clinic, a combination of bone marrow biopsy and abdominal subcutaneous fat pad aspirate yields the diagnosis of AL amyloidosis in 85% of patients.[8]

Endomyocardial biopsy (EMB) is the gold standard for the diagnosis of cardiac amyloidosis. While it can be safely performed through right heart catheterization at experienced centers (incidence of major procedure-related complications is <5%), EMB is not needed in patients with less invasive biopsy sufficing to establish a diagnosis of amyloidosis with strong evidence of cardiac involvement by noninvasive investigations.[27] EMB is needed if the heart is the only site of amyloidosis (ie, negative peripheral biopsies), an unequivocal diagnosis is needed before heart transplantation, or if post-transplant cardiac rejection is suspected. The biopsy tissue should be stained with amyloid-binding stains such as Congo red or sulfated Alcian blue. Once a histological diagnosis is established, the next step should be determination of the amyloid type. Immunohistochemistry has been most commonly used for amyloid typing; however, its sensitivity is relatively low, unless performed in experienced centers with appropriate tissue processing and staining. The gold standard for determining the type of amyloidosis is detection of amyloidogenic protein in microdissected specimens of involved tissue by immunogold electron microscopy or proteomic analysis by mass spectrometry. At the Mayo Clinic, we use laser capture microdissection and mass spectrometry to determine the subtype in all patients with amyloidosis.[28,29] The accurate determination of amyloid type is especially important to exclude familial ATTR as it can clinically mimic light chain amyloidosis and up to 10% of patients with non-AL cardiomyopathy can have coexisting monoclonal gammopathy of undetermined significance (MGUS), which can lead to the misdiagnosis of AL in these patients.[30] If TTR is identified as the precursor protein, DNA testing should be performed on peripheral blood to identify a possible gene mutation to differentiate between SSA and familial ATTR.

Once the diagnosis and type of amyloidosis are confirmed, the next step in the management of patients is to determine the extent of organ involvement. The heart is the most important organ involved in amyloidosis; therefore determination of the presence and degree of cardiac amyloidosis is imperative. Various diagnostic procedures providing critical clues to the diagnosis and severity of cardiac amyloidosis are briefly reviewed below.

Electrocardiography

ECG abnormalities are frequent in amyloidosis and often overlooked. Low QRS voltage is a fairly common abnormality and can be seen in up to two-thirds of patients with AL.[31] It is less common in non-AL amyloid heart disease; in fact, recent evidence indicates that, with the increasing availability of advanced cardiac imaging,

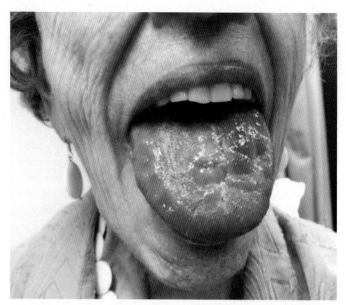

FIGURE 11-6 Macroglossia is fairly specific for AL and is seen in 15% to 20% of cases. Usually the lingual involvement is uniform but at times nodular deposits or amyloidomas can be seen. It can be a particularly difficult problem to manage and patients can experience significant weight loss from dysfunction of deglutition and suffer from severe sleep apnea and choking.

Table 11-3 Recommended Diagnostic Testing for a Histologic Diagnosis of Amyloidosis

- Complete blood cell count, creatinine level, alkaline phosphatase level
- Serum and 24-h urine total protein, electrophoresis, and immunofixation
- Serum immunoglobulin free light chain assay
- Marrow biopsy
- Quantitative immunoglobulins
- N-terminal pro-B natriuretic peptide level, serum troponin levels, uric acid level
- Echocardiography with Doppler
- Confirmation that amyloid deposits are of immunoglobulin origin (ie, laser capture microdissection followed by mass spectroscopy)

patients with ATTR amyloidosis are seen earlier in their disease course, with ECG demonstrating voltage criteria for left ventricular (LV) hypertrophy in up to 29% of patients.[32] Low ECG voltage in the presence of the ECG findings of increased myocardial thickness is highly suggestive of advanced amyloid heart disease. Bundle branch abnormalities are uncommon in AL, but can be seen in up to 40% of patients with ATTR. Additional ECG abnormalities include loss of the R wave in leads V1 to V3, resulting in a pseudo-infarction pattern. Patients with a pseudoinfarction pattern on ECG frequently undergo an unrevealing coronary angiogram. Rarely, patients can present with true myocardial ischemia due to amyloid infiltration of small intramyocardial arteries.

Cardiac Biomarkers

Myocardial damage from amyloidosis results in leakage of intracellular proteins and enzymes into the systemic circulation. Availability of serum cardiac biomarkers such as cardiac troponin T (cTnT) and N-terminus of the prohormone-brain natriuretic peptide (NT-proBNP) has made a significant impact in the care of patients with AL cardiomyopathy. A 4-stage prognostic scoring system has been developed from 801 previously untreated AL patients seen at the Mayo Clinic. Median survival of patients with stage I, II, III, and IV disease was 94, 40.3, 14, and 5.8 months, respectively. In patients with non-AL amyloid cardiomyopathy, BNP or NT-proBNP is useful for following CHF and its treatment (Figure 11-7).[33]

Cardiac Imaging

Cardiac imaging remains the cornerstone of evaluation of patients suspected of having amyloid heart disease.

Echocardiograhy

A 2D echocardiogram is widely available and can be an invaluable tool for evaluating patients with amyloid cardiomyopathy. While echocardiography can provide critical information that aids in the management of these patients, cardiologists may frequently overlook echocardiographic findings of amyloid heart disease.[10,34] Increased LV thickness from amyloid infiltration may be attributed to hypertensive heart disease—the most common cause of increased LV thickness. Normal ejection fraction and absence of LV dilatation in patients presenting with HF should strongly lead cardiologists to suspect cardiac amyloidosis. Thickening of the right ventricular free wall and biatrial enlargement, along with diffuse valvular thickening, are all features suggestive of amyloid cardiomyopathy.[34] In advanced stages, atrial standstill and intramural thrombus can be seen (Figure 11-8).

Doppler studies also provide important clues to the presence of amyloid heart disease. Measurement of myocardial flow velocities with Doppler almost always reveals longitudinal systolic dysfunction, despite preserved LV ejection fraction calculated from myocardial contraction along its short axis.[35] The impairment of long-axis LV contraction is especially visible in strain and strain rate imaging.[36]

Echocardiography with standard Doppler also provides important prognostic information. In a Mayo Clinic series of 132 AL patients, an interventricular septal (IVS) thickness of more than

Table 11-4 Common Abnormalities in AL Cardiomyopathy and Their Prognostic Impact

Prognostic Factor	Comment
Clinical findings:	
• Congestive heart failure and exertional syncope	• Patients presenting with exertional syncope have a median survival of 2 mo
• Jaundice	• Jaundice and hyperbilirubinemia is usually a pre-terminal finding
Laboratory findings:	
• Thrombocytosis	• Indicator of splenic involvement
• Howell-Jolly bodies	
• Elevated bilirubin	• Indicator of advanced disease
• Elevated creatinine	
• Elevated free light chain levels	• Often a preterminal finding
• Elevated troponin T	• Important factors that have been incorporated into 4-stage prognostic model
• Elevated BNP (NTpro-BNP)	
Echocardiogram findings:	
• Interventricular septum thickness	• Median survival 1 y (if thickness >1.5 cm) vs 4 y (if thickness <1.5 cm)
• Short mitral deceleration time	• Poor outcome for patients with deceleration <150 ms
• Decreased fractional shortening	• Poor outcomes for patients with fractional shortening <20%

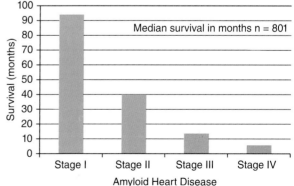

FIGURE 11-7 Revised prognostic score derived from 801 previously untreated AL patients seen at the Mayo Clinic. Patients were assigned a score of 1 for each of dFLC (difference between involved and uninvolved free light chain) ≥ 18 mg/dL, cTnT ≥ 0.025 ng/mL, and NT-proBNP ≥ 1800 pg/mL, creating stages I to IV with scores of 0 to 3 points, respectively. The proportions of patients with stages I, II, III, and IV disease were 189 (25%), 206 (27%), 186 (25%), and 177 (23%).

(Modified and reproduced with permission from Kumar et al. Revised prognostic staging system for light chain amyloidosis incorporating cardiac biomarkers and serum free light chain measurements. *J Clin Oncol.* 2012 Mar 20;30(9):989-995.)

1.5 cm was associated with a median survival of less than 1 year as compared to that of 4 years in patients with an IVS thickness of less than 1.5 cm.[37] Transmitral Doppler studies serve as a good index of restrictive physiology seen in amyloid cardiomyopathy and a short mitral deceleration time (<150 ms) has been associated with shorter survival in AL patients. Basal systolic strain measured on regional strain and strain rate assessments is superior to Doppler flow measurements in predicting clinical outcomes. A large observational study identified longitudinal strain and 2D global longitudinal strain as important prognostic factors in patients with amyloid cardiomyopathy. Importantly, the 2D global longitudinal strain remained an independent predictor of prognosis even in patients with preserved LV ejection fraction.[36] Novel echocardiographic techniques, such as feature- and speckle-tracking imaging, allow dynamic frame-by-frame myocardial motion analysis during the cardiac cycle, and can help to distinguish between amyloid cardiomyopathy, hypertensive heart disease, and hypertrophic cardiomyopathy.[34] Evolving echocardiographic techniques are expected to help differentiate between various forms of diastolic dysfunction and represent an opportunity for early diagnosis of amyloid heart disease that can have a profound impact on outcome in amyloid cardiomyopathy.

Magnetic Resonance Imaging

Contrast-enhanced cardiac MRI is a promising diagnostic modality and is being increasingly utilized in the assessment of myocardial diseases. Besides accurate measurements of myocardial thickness, the kinetics of gadolinium enhancement can provide very specific clues about cardiac amyloidosis. The finding of ventricular wall and IVS thickening associated with diffuse, delayed gadolinium enhancement of the subendocardium is very suggestive of cardiac amyloidosis (Figure 11-9).[38] Phase-contrast MRI, such as Doppler echocardiography, can provide useful information about the flow dynamic parameters such as mitral deceleration times, early to late ratio of LV diastolic filling, and mitral peak inflow velocity.[39] Novel techniques, such as magnetic resonance (MR) relaxometry, can characterize the physical composition of the tissues and assess their dynamic properties.[40] By providing functional assessment of the heart, these newer MR techniques can not only help establish early diagnosis, but also serve as a useful tool for assessment of organ response to treatment. Despite these important advancements, the use of cardiac MR in amyloidosis may be limited due to the presence of pacemakers and defibrillators. Renal impairment increases the risk of gadolinium-induced nephrogenic systemic sclerosis.

Nuclear-Medicine Based Imaging

Advances in radiotracer nuclear-based imaging appear promising in systemic amyloidosis. ^{123}I-labeled SAP component scanning (SAP scan) is the prototype of nuclear medicine tests used for imaging tissue amyloid burden.[41] This test can measure systemic amyloid burden, but does not accurately assess myocardial involvement and is not used in the United States. Technetium (^{99m}Tc)-based isotopes can identify cardiac involvement with TTR amyloidosis, but have variable sensitivity and specificity for different types; for example, ^{99m}Tc-3,3-diphos-phono-1,2-propanol carboxylic

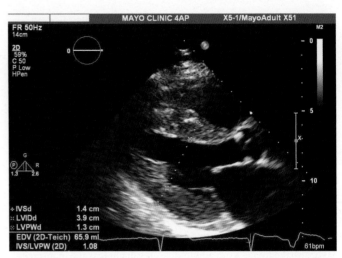

FIGURE 11-8 Transthoracic echocardiogram from a patient with AL cardiomyopathy demonstrating thickened interventricular septum and posterior wall of left ventricle.

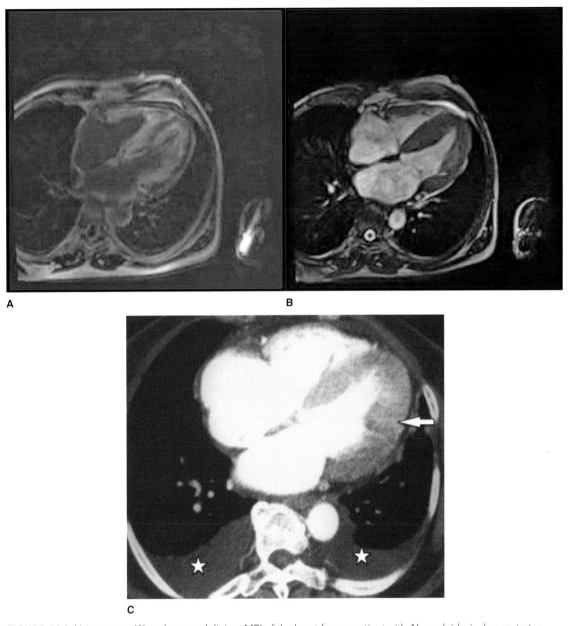

FIGURE 11-9 Noncontrast (A) and postgadolinium MRI of the heart from a patient with AL amyloidosis demonstrates thickened myocardium and delayed sub-endocardial enhancement—a feature highly suggestive of infiltrative cardiomyopathy. (C) CT scan in the same patient also shows myocardial thickening and bilateral pleural effusions.

acid, an agent not available in the United States, has a preference for cardiac uptake in ATTR versus AL.[42] Similarly, technetium pyrophosphate is a sensitive marker of cardiac amyloidosis with preferential myocardial uptake in ATTR compared with AL (Figure 11-10). Recently, in a small study, N-[methyl-^{11}C]2(4'-methylaminophenyl)-6-hydroxybenzothiazole ([11]CPIB) based positron-emission tomography (PET) imaging appeared promising as it identified cardiac amyloid deposits in all patients with AL or ATTR amyloid heart disease, while it was negative in healthy controls.[43,44] The role of nuclear-based techniques in assessing systemic and, more importantly, cardiac amyloid burden, is evolving. Additional studies are needed to help identify the appropriate isotope-scanning technique that can not only assess the disease burden, but also reliably differentiate between various types of amyloidosis.

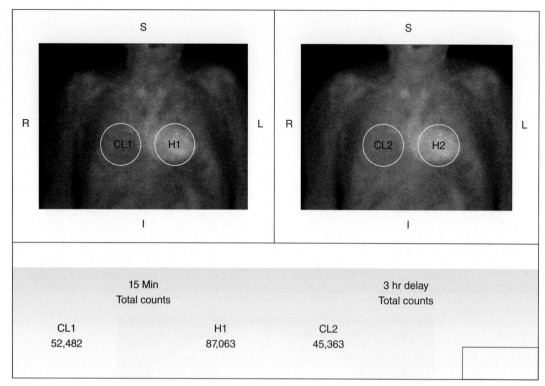

FIGURE 11-10 Technetium 99 pyrophosphate scan in a patient with senile ATTR presenting with congestive heart failure and bilateral carpal tunnel syndrome. Congo red staining of the fat aspirate confirmed presence of amyloid. Mass spectrometric analysis confirmed wild-type TTR sequence of the amyloid. Tc99PYP scintigraphy is strongly positive for myocardial uptake both immediately and 3-hour postinjection as indicated by relatively clear CL 1 and 2 circles compared to "hot" H1 and H2 circles. CL refers to contralateral blood pool that serves as control.

MANAGEMENT OF AMYLOID CARDIOMYOPATHY

Management of amyloid heart disease depends upon the type of amyloid.

MANAGING AL CARDIOMYOPATHY

Primary treatment of AL involves the use of systemic chemotherapy to treat the underlying plasma cell dyscrasia to eliminate the production of amyloidogenic light chains. Systemic therapy improves organ function, quality of life, and survival of patients. Serum-free light-chain assay and cardiac biomarkers (cTnT and NT-proBNP) are invaluable in monitoring response to treatment.[45] The ultimate goal of therapy in AL is improvement in organ function, which can take a median of 6 to 12 months and does not happen in all patients. Hematological response precedes the organ response and has been shown to be a strong predictor of not only organ improvement, but also overall survival.[46] Patients who achieve a complete hematologic remission (CR; ie, normal serum-free light chain levels and a normal K to L ratio and no evidence of clonal plasma cells) have a 66% to 86% chance of organ improvement and 5-year survival approaches 70%.[47] Improvement in organ function and survival is also noted in patients who achieve partial hematological remission (ie, at least 50% reduction from baseline in involved free light chain levels).

Oral melphalan and dexamethasone (Mel-Dex) has been the most common regimen used for the treatment of AL and has demonstrated hematological response rates of over 60%, with 30% to

40% of patients achieving CR. Organ improvement is noted in one-third of patients with median survival as long as 5 years in some series.[48,49] Newer antiplasma cell agents, such as proteasome inhibitors and immunomodulatory drugs, have demonstrated significant activity in patients with relapsed AL. Bortezomib has demonstrated hematological response rates of 80% or more in combination with steroids and alkylating agents, and these combinations are rapidly moving to the front-line treatment of AL.[50] Lenalidomide and pomalidomide are thalidomide analogs and have demonstrated response rates of over 50% in patients with relapsed disease.[51] While these newer agents are highly effective in AL, their use can be challenging because of potential cardiotoxicity, and their safety and superiority over Mel-Dex has not been prospectively demonstrated. Myeloablative chemotherapy followed by autologous peripheral blood stem cell rescue (stem cell transplant [SCT]) has demonstrated very high efficacy in amyloidosis. In a large series of patients, SCT has demonstrated overall hematological response rates of 75% and CR rates of 38% (Figure 11-11).[52] Median overall survival of patients who achieved CR was not reached, while it was 107 months for those with partial hematological remission. Patients who achieved CR after SCT have been reported to have a 10-year survival approaching 60%.[53] While SCT is very effective, it is associated with a high risk of complications including a high treatment-related mortality. Early experience reported mortality in excess of 20% in the United States and more than 40% in a small European series. A randomized study of 100 patients comparing Mel-Dex to SCT in amyloidosis patients did not report any significant difference in outcomes.[54] In fact, patients with advanced cardiac disease did particularly poorly with SCT. High transplant-related mortality has largely been attributed to inclusion of patients with advanced cardiac disease. The availability of cardiac biomarkers and the use of stringent selection criteria have significantly improved the transplant-related mortality to less than 5% in experienced centers.[55,56] At the Mayo Clinic, active New York Heart Association class III or IV heart failure, an LV ejection fraction <45%, advanced cardiac stage by biomarkers, and more than 2 organ involvement is considered a contraindication for SCT. In patients with less severe involvement, a risk-adapted approach is used to select an appropriate dose of melphalan as conditioning for SCT. Using these stringent criteria, only 25% of amyloidosis patients qualify for SCT at diagnosis.

Emerging evidence suggests that using bortezomib and alkylating agents in combination with steroids can result in significant improvements in organ function in patients with contraindications to SCT who can subsequently become eligible for SCT.[57] Generally, if an AL patient is a suitable candidate, we recommend proceeding with SCT as soon as the diagnosis is made. In all other patients, combination therapy with Mel-Dex or with newer agents is recommended.

In a recent phase I/II study, NEOD 001—a monoclonal antibody against epitopes expressed by amyloidogenic light chains—has been found to be well tolerated by AL patients who achieved control of their plasma cell dyscrasia with systemic therapy. Intriguingly, improvement in biomarkers of organ dysfunction was seen in several patients and this is undergoing active investigation in combination with systemic therapy in newly diagnosed patients in a phase III study.[58]

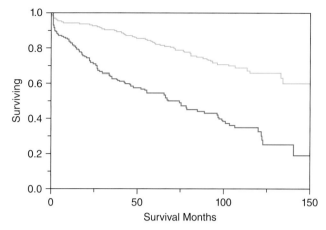

FIGURE 11-11 Survival stratified by NT-proBNP ≥1000 ng/mL in 600 patients that underwent stem cell transplant at the Mayo Clinic.

Supportive care remains the cornerstone of management of AL cardiomyopathy and includes managing the cardiac manifestations of the disease and complications of systemic chemotherapy. Management of HF is a particular challenge in AL, as these patients cannot tolerate several medications used for routine therapy of HF from other causes. Use of angiotensin-converting enzyme (ACE) inhibitors is particularly difficult due to significant hypotension. We have seen patients develop significant hypotension after low doses of ACE inhibitors. The negative inotropic effect of beta blockers can precipitate acute CHF in a patient with stable HF. Digitalis derivatives and atrioventricular nodal-blocking calcium channel blockers can cause significant dysrhythmias as their intracardiac concentration may increase due to increased binding to amyloid fibrils. Patients with atrial hypokinesis and standstill are at risk of developing mural thrombus and subsequent embolization and stroke. These patients should be treated with anticoagulation with close attention to the risk of bleeding as it is significantly increased in AL patients. Orthostatic hypotension can become particularly problematic and patients benefit from compression stockings and use of the alpha-adrenergic agonist midodrine. Volume overload can be a recurrent and difficult-to-treat problem; salt restriction and judicious use of loop diuretics and metolazone along with strict monitoring of blood pressure and orthostatic responses can be helpful in difficult cases. Patients with dysrhythmias pose a particular challenge. The role of cardiac pacemakers in AL cardiomyopathy is highly controversial, as no clear survival advantage has been demonstrated with their use as primary prevention or as treatment of common cardiac dysrhythmia in this setting. Pacemaker placement should be considered on an individual basis especially in patients who present with high-grade atrioventricular block. Unlike non-AL cardiomyopathies, even an automatic implantable cardioverter-defibrillator (AICD) may not help the failing heart in AL as electromechanical dissociation is common.

Heart transplantation is an option in AL; however, the vast majority of patients with AL cardio-myopathy will not qualify for a heart transplant due to significant extracardiac involvement and rapid disease progression.[59,60] Moreover, the outcomes of heart transplantation in AL cardiomyopathy have been inferior compared with outcomes for other cardiomyopathies. These poor outcomes are primarily due to progression of AL, as a heart transplant does not address the production of amyloidogenic light chains. Use of SCT after heart transplant has been reported in a small series with 1- and 5-year heart transplant survival rates of 82% and 65%, respectively.[61] Median survival from heart and stem cell transplantation was 76 and 57 months, respectively; again these numbers do not compare favorably to the outcomes achieved by heart transplant for other conditions. In summary, a heart transplant is feasible in highly selected patients with AL cardiomyopathy; the ideal candidate will be a younger patient with isolated or predominant heart involvement who is also a candidate for SCT within 6 to 12 months after cardiac transplant.

Outcomes of relapsed AL are generally poor. The best option for these patients is enrollment in clinical trials whenever possible or the use of the same or non-cross-resistant chemotherapy regimens, depending upon the length of initial response to the first regimen prior to disease relapse.

MANAGING FAMILIAL/HEREDITARY AMYLOID CARDIOMYOPATHY

Like other amyloidoses, the management of familial amyloid cardiomyopathy consists of supportive care and addressing the source of amyloidogenic protein. The liver is the most common source of production of amyloidogenic protein precursors and, as such, orthotopic liver transplantation (OLT) is the only definitive treatment for ATTR, fibrinogen related, and apolipoprotein-related amyloidosis.[62] Mutant ATTR is the most common indication for liver transplantation for familial amyloidosis worldwide. OLT is most effective in Val30Met mutant and 5-year survivals of 82% have been reported with this variant compared with 59% in non-Val30Met patients. Interestingly, progression of amyloid heart disease may occur in patients with ATTR after liver transplantation.[63] This is caused by deposition of wild-type TTR produced from the transplanted liver on already established amyloid deposits in the heart. This phenomenon is particularly noticeable in cases involving the Ala60 mutation where progression of amyloid cardiomyopathy is common after liver transplantation. Combined liver and heart transplantation should be considered in this situation if no other significant systemic involvement is noted. Unlike ATTR, fibrinogen and apolipoprotein A-related amyloid cardiomyopathy does not appear to progress significantly after liver transplantation.

Recent advancements in our understanding of the pathogenesis of amyloidosis have resulted in the emergence of novel therapies in ATTR. Tafamidis meglumine, a small molecule that stabilizes the native TTR and thus inhibits its aggregation to an amyloid fibril, is 1 such example.[64] It has been approved in Europe and Japan for the treatment of familial amyloid polyneuropathy (caused by ATTR) by demonstrating improved symptom control in these patients and is under active clinical testing in FAC patients. Diflunisal, an NSAID, has also been shown to stabilize native TTR and is under active clinical investigations.[65] Recently, messenger RNA-based silencing of the TTR mRNA with short interfering RNA (siRNA) has been shown to significantly decrease the levels of circulating transthyretin.[66] Early clinical trials have confirmed the feasibility of this therapy and an ongoing large phase III study will help assess the effectiveness of this modality compared to current standard of supportive care. This may obviate the need for liver transplantation.

HF in ATTR is generally milder and medications such as ACEIs and beta blockers are better tolerated in ATTR compared with AL, if advanced autonomic neuropathy is not present. Salt restriction and diuretics are the mainstay of symptomatic treatment. Outcomes of cardiac transplant in non-AL amyloid cardiomyopathies are significantly better compared with those in AL cardiomyopathy; therefore, a diagnosis of cardiac amyloidosis early in the disease course will result in better organ transplantation outcomes. All patients with familial amyloid cardiomyopathy must be offered genetic counseling and testing for early diagnosis in relatives.

MANAGING SENILE SYSTEMIC AMYLOIDOSIS

Treatment of SSA is predominantly supportive. The usual principles of management of CHF apply in SSA. As a majority of these patients are older, cardiac transplantation is not routinely used in

SSA, except in the occasional younger patient with good organ system function and absence of advanced systemic amyloidosis. Trials of tafamidis and siRNA are being planned in SSA.

PROGNOSIS OF AMYLOID CARDIOMYOPATHY

The prognosis of cardiac amyloidosis is highly dependent upon the underlying amyloid protein. AL patients with symptomatic CHF and advanced cardiac stage, as determined by biomarkers, have a median survival of 3 to 5 months. Despite significant advancements made in antiplasma therapy in the last 2 decades, the early mortality (~40% in 1 year) has not significantly changed in AL, with death usually resulting from progressive cardiac failure and/or fatal arrhythmias. In patients with less severe cardiac involvement, systemic chemotherapy improves survival. The staging system based on cardiac biomarkers and serum-free light chains provides critical information about prognosis as patients with stage I cardiac disease have a median survival of 94 months compared with 5.8 months for stage IV disease (see Figure 11-7).[33] The prognosis is significantly better in familial and SSA cardiac amyloidosis despite advanced cardiac infiltration as assessed by imaging studies compared with AL. In familial ATTR, the type of mutation in the *TTR* gene influences prognosis; for example, in a large series of patients with the Ala60 variant, median survival from the time of diagnosis was 3.4 years. Generally, median survival in SSA and familial ATTR ranges between 5 and 8 years.

REFERENCES

1. Franke WW. Matthias Jacob Schleiden and the definition of the cell nucleus. *Eur J Cell Biol*. 1988;47(2):145-156.

2. Sipe JD, Cohen AS. Review: history of the amyloid fibril. *J Struct Biol*. 2000;130(2-3):88-98.

3. Cohen AS. History of amyloidosis. *J Intern Med*. 1992;232(6):509-510.

4. Picken MM. Amyloidosis—where are we now and where are we heading? *Arch Pathol Lab Med*. 2010;134(4):545-551.

5. Sipe JD, Benson MD, Buxbaum JN, et al. Amyloid fibril protein nomenclature: 2012 recommendations from the Nomenclature Committee of the International Society of Amyloidosis. *Amyloid*. 2012;19(4):167-170.

6. Falk RH. Diagnosis and management of the cardiac amyloidoses. *Circulation*. 2005;112(13):2047-2060.

7. Kyle RA, Linos A, Beard CM, et al. Incidence and natural history of primary systemic amyloidosis in Olmsted County, Minnesota, 1950 through 1989. *Blood*. 1992;79(7):1817-1822.

8. Gertz MA, Lacy MQ, Dispenzieri A. Amyloidosis: recognition, confirmation, prognosis, and therapy. *Mayo Clin Proc*. 1999;74(5):490-494.

9. Seldin DC, Berk JL, Sam F, Sanchorawala V. Amyloidotic cardiomyopathy: multidisciplinary approach to diagnosis and treatment. *Heart Fail Clin*. 2011;7(3):385-393.

10. Falk RH, Dubrey SW. Amyloid heart disease. *Prog Cardiovasc Dis*. 2010;52(4):347-361.

11. Choufani EB, Sanchorawala V, Ernst T, et al. Acquired factor X deficiency in patients with amyloid light-chain amyloidosis: incidence, bleeding manifestations, and response to high-dose chemotherapy. *Blood*. 2001;97(6):1885-1887.

12. Westermark P, Sletten K, Johansson B, Cornwell GG 3rd. Fibril in senile systemic amyloidosis is derived from normal transthyretin. *Proc Natl Acad Sci U S A*. 1990;87(7):2843-2845.

13. Ng B, Connors LH, Davidoff R, Skinner M, Falk RH. Senile systemic amyloidosis presenting with heart failure: a comparison with light chain-associated amyloidosis. *Arch Intern Med*. 2005;165(12):1425-1429.

14. Gertz MA, Kyle RA, Thibodeau SN. Familial amyloidosis: a study of 52 North American-born patients examined during a 30-year period. *Mayo Clin Proc*. 1992;67(5):428-440.

15. Connors LH, Richardson AM, Theberge R, Costello CE. Tabulation of transthyretin (TTR) variants as of 1/1/2000. *Amyloid*. 2000;7(1):54-69.

16. Plante-Bordeneuve V, Said G. Transthyretin related familial amyloid polyneuropathy. *Curr Opin Neurol*. 2000;13(5):569-573.

17. Benson MD. Ostertag revisited: the inherited systemic amyloidoses without neuropathy. *Amyloid*. 2005;12(2):75-87.

18. Jacobson DR, Pastore RD, Yaghoubian R, et al. Variant-sequence transthyretin (isoleucine 122) in late-onset cardiac amyloidosis in black Americans. *N Engl J Med*. 1997;336(7):466-473.

19. Tojo K, Sekijima Y, Machida K, Tsuchiya A, Yazaki M, Ikeda S-I. Amyloidogenic transthyretin Val30Met homozygote showing unusually early-onset familial amyloid polyneuropathy. *Muscle Nerve*. 2008;37(6):796-803.

20. Benson MD, Liepnieks JJ, Yazaki M, et al. A new human hereditary amyloidosis: the result of a stop-codon mutation in the apolipoprotein AII gene. *Genomics*. 2001;72(3):272-277.

21. Hamidi Asl L, Fournier V, Billerey C, et al. Fibrinogen A alpha chain mutation (Arg554 Leu) associated with hereditary renal amyloidosis in a French family. *Amyloid*. 1998;5(4):279-284.

22. van der Hilst JC, Simon A, Drenth JP. Hereditary periodic fever and reactive amyloidosis. *Clin Exp Med*. 2005;5(3):87-98.

23. Hazenberg BP, van Rijswijk MH. Where has secondary amyloid gone? *Ann Rheum Dis*. 2000;59(8):577-579.

24. Millucci L, Ghezzi L, Bernardini G, Braconi D, Tanganelli P, Santucci A. Prevalence of isolated atrial amyloidosis in young patients affected by congestive heart failure. *ScientificWorldJournal*. 2012;2012:293863.

25. Millucci L, Paccagnini E, Ghezzi L, et al. Different factors affecting human ANP amyloid aggregation and their implications in congestive heart failure. *PLoS One*. 2011;6(7):e21870.

26. Gertz MA. I don't know how to treat amyloidosis. *Blood*. 2010;116(4):507-508.

27. Pellikka PA, Holmes DR Jr, Edwards WD, Nishimura RA, Tajik AJ, Kyle RA. Endomyocardial biopsy in 30 patients with

primary amyloidosis and suspected cardiac involvement. *Arch Intern Med.* 1988;148(3):662-666.

28. Klein CJ, Vrana JA, Theis JD, et al. Mass spectrometric-based proteomic analysis of amyloid neuropathy type in nerve tissue. *Arch Neurol.* 2011;68(2):195-199.

29. Brambilla F, Lavatelli F, Di Silvestre D, et al. Reliable typing of systemic amyloidoses through proteomic analysis of subcutaneous adipose tissue. *Blood.* 2012;119(8):1844-1847.

30. Comenzo RL, Zhou P, Fleisher M, Clark B, Teruya-Feldstein J. Seeking confidence in the diagnosis of systemic AL (Ig light-chain) amyloidosis: patients can have both monoclonal gammopathies and hereditary amyloid proteins. *Blood.* 2006;107(9):3489-3491.

31. Hongo M, Yamamoto H, Kohda T, et al. Comparison of electrocardiographic findings in patients with AL (primary) amyloidosis and in familial amyloid polyneuropathy and anginal pain and their relation to histopathologic findings. *Am J Cardiol.* 2000;85(7):849-853.

32. Rapezzi C, Merlini G, Quarta CC, et al. Systemic cardiac amyloidoses: disease profiles and clinical courses of the 3 main types. *Circulation.* 2009;120(13):1203-1212.

33. Kumar S, Dispenzieri A, Lacy MQ, et al. Revised prognostic staging system for light chain amyloidosis incorporating cardiac biomarkers and serum free light chain measurements. *J Clin Oncol.* 2012;30(9):989-995.

34. Tsang W, Lang RM. Echocardiographic evaluation of cardiac amyloid. *Curr Cardiol Rep.* 2010;12(3):272-276.

35. Elliott PM, Mahon NG, Matsumura Y, Mckenna WJ, Hawkins PN, Gillmore JD. Tissue Doppler features of cardiac amyloidosis. *Clin Cardiol.* 2000;23(9):701.

36. Koyama J, Falk RH. Prognostic significance of strain Doppler imaging in light-chain amyloidosis. *JACC Cardiovasc Imaging.* 2010;3(4):333-342.

37. Klein AL, Hatle LK, Taliercio CP, et al. Prognostic significance of Doppler measures of diastolic function in cardiac amyloidosis. A Doppler echocardiography study. *Circulation.* 1991;83(3):808-816.

38. vanden Driesen RI, Slaughter RE, Strugnell WE. MR findings in cardiac amyloidosis. *AJR Am J Roentgenol.* 2006;186(6):1682-1685.

39. Maceira AM, Joshi J, Prasad SK, et al. Cardiovascular magnetic resonance in cardiac amyloidosis. *Circulation.* 2005;111(2):186-193.

40. Rubinshtein R, Glockner JF, Feng D, et al. Comparison of magnetic resonance imaging versus Doppler echocardiography for the evaluation of left ventricular diastolic function in patients with cardiac amyloidosis. *Am J Cardiol.* 2009;103(5):718-723.

41. Hawkins PN, Aprile C, Capri G, et al. Scintigraphic imaging and turnover studies with iodine-131 labelled serum amyloid P component in systemic amyloidosis. *Eur J Nucl Med.* 1998;25(7):701-708.

42. Koizumi K, Monzawa S, Shindo C, Hosaka M. Primary hepatic amyloidosis well delineated by Tc-99m DTPA galactosyl HSA liver SPECT. *Clin Nucl Med.* 1999;24(4):271-273.

43. Glaudemans AW, Slart RH, Zeebregts CJ, et al. Nuclear imaging in cardiac amyloidosis. *Eur J Nucl Med Mol Imaging.* 2009;36(4):702-714.

44. Antoni G, Lubberink M, Estrada S, et al. In vivo visualization of amyloid deposits in the heart with 11C-PIB and PET. *J Nucl Med.* 2013;54(2):213-220.

45. Gertz MA, Comenzo R, Falk RH, et al. Definition of organ involvement and treatement response in immunoglobulin light chain amyloidosis (AL): a consensus opinion from the 10th International Symposium on Amyloid and Amyloidosis. *Am J Hematol.* 2005;79:319-328.

46. Gertz MA, Lacy MQ, Dispenzieri A, et al. Effect of hematologic response on outcome of patients undergoing transplantation for primary amyloidosis: importance of achieving a complete response. *Haematologica.* 2007;92(10):1415-1418.

47. Dispenzieri A, Lacy MQ, Katzmann JA, et al. Absolute values of immunoglobulin free light chains are prognostic in patients with primary systemic amyloidosis undergoing peripheral blood stem cell transplantation. *Blood.* 2006;107(8):3378-3383.

48. Palladini G, Perfetti V, Obici L, et al. Association of melphalan and high-dose dexamethasone is effective and well tolerated in patients with AL (primary) amyloidosis who are ineligible for stem cell transplantation. *Blood.* 2004;103(8):2936-2938.

49. Sanchorawala V, Seldin DC, Berk JL, Sloan JM, Doros G, Skinner M. Oral cyclic melphalan and dexamethasone for patients with AL amyloidosis. *Clin Lymphoma Myeloma Leuk.* 2010;10(6):469-472.

50. Kastritis E, Wechalekar AD, Dimopoulos MA, et al. Bortezomib with or without dexamethasone in primary systemic (light chain) amyloidosis. *J Clin Oncol.* 2010;28(6):1031-1037.

51. Palladini G, Russo P, Foli A, et al. Salvage therapy with lenalidomide and dexamethasone in patients with advanced AL amyloidosis refractory to melphalan, bortezomib, and thalidomide. *Ann Hematol.* 2012;91(1):89-92.

52. Gertz MA, Lacy MQ, Dispenzieri, et al. Autologous stem cell transplant for immunoglobulin light chain amyloidosis: a status report. *Leuk Lymphoma.* 2010;51(12):2181-2187.

53. Sanchorawala V, Skinner M, Quillen K, Finn KT, Doros G, Seldin DC. Long-term outcome of patients with AL amyloidosis treated with high-dose melphalan and stem-cell transplantation. *Blood.* 2007;110(10):3561-3563.

54. Jaccard A, Moreau P, Leblond V, et al. High-dose melphalan versus melphalan plus dexamethasone for AL amyloidosis. *N Engl J Med.* 2007;357(11):1083-1093.

55. Gertz MA, Lacy MQ, Dispenzieri A, et al. Trend toward improved day 100 and two-year survival following stem cell transplantation for AL: a comparison before and after 2006. *Amyloid.* 2011;18 (Suppl 1):132-133.

56. Comenzo RL, Gertz MA. Autologous stem cell transplantation for primary systemic amyloidosis. *Blood.* 2002;99(12):4276-4282.

57. Cornell RF, Zhong X, Arce-Lara C, et al. Bortezomib-based induction for transplant ineligible AL amyloidosis and feasibility of later transplantation. *Bone Marrow Transplant.* 2015;50(7):914-917.

58. Gertz MA, Landau H, Comenzo RL, et al. First-in-Human Phase I/II Study of NEOD001 in Patients With Light Chain Amyloidosis and Persistent Organ Dysfunction. *J Clin Oncol.* 2016;34(10):1097-1103.

59. Kpodonu J, Massad MG, Caines A, Geha AS. Outcome of heart transplantation in patients with amyloid cardiomyopathy. *J Heart Lung Transplant.* 2005;24(11):1763-1765.

60. Hosenpud JD, DeMarco T, Frazier OH, et al. Progression of systemic disease and reduced long-term survival in patients with cardiac amyloidosis undergoing heart transplantation. Follow-up results of a multicenter survey. *Circulation.* 1991;84(5 Suppl):III338-111343.

61. Lacy MQ, Dispenzieri A, Hayman SR, et al. Autologous stem cell transplant after heart transplant for light chain (Al) amyloid cardiomyopathy. *J Heart Lung Transplant.* 2008;27(8):823-829.

62. Suhr OB, Friman S, Ericzon BG. Early liver transplantation improves familial amyloidotic polyneuropathy patients' survival. *Amyloid.* 2005;12(4):233-238.

63. Herlenius G, Wilczek HE, Larsson M, Ericzon BG; Familial Amyloidotic Polyneuropathy World Transplant Registry. Ten years of international experience with liver transplantation for familial amyloidotic polyneuropathy: results from the Familial Amyloidotic Polyneuropathy World Transplant Registry. *Transplantation.* 2004;77(1):64-71.

64. Lozeron P, Theaudin M, Mincheva Z, et al. Effect on disability and safety of Tafamidis in late onset of Met30 transthyretin familial amyloid polyneuropathy. *Eur J Neurol.* 2013;20(12):1539-1545.

65. Castano A, Helmke S, Alvarez J, Delisle S, Maurer MS. Diflunisal for ATTR cardiac amyloidosis. *Congest Heart Fail.* 2012;18(6):315-319.

66. Suhr OB, Coelho T, Buades J, et al. Efficacy and safety of patisiran for familial amyloidotic polyneuropathy: a phase II multi-dose study. *Orphanet J Rare Dis.* 2015;10:109.

12 HEART FAILURE IN MINORITIES

Shannon Willis, MD
Quinn Capers IV, MD, FACC, FSCAI
R. R. Baliga, MD, MBA, FACP, FRCP (Edin), FACC
Khadijah Breathett, MD, MS, FACC

PATIENT CASE

Ms. Jones is a 64-year-old African American woman with a history of hypertension (HTN), type 2 diabetes mellitus, and remote tobacco usage who works as a teller at a bank. She presents with complaints of increased dyspnea on exertion after walking 25 feet. She has noticed bilateral lower extremity edema and has been sleeping in a recliner on the first floor of her home rather than in her bed on the second floor for the past month because of shortness of breath when climbing stairs. Should the diagnosis of heart failure (HF) and management be based upon the patient's race and ethnicity?

OVERVIEW

The prevalence of HF in the United States is on the rise, and it disproportionately affects racial/ethnic minorities.[1-5] Currently 5.1 million individuals in the United States have HF.[6] While the risk of developing HF is 1 in 5 after age 40 years, the prevalence is expected to approach 46% in 2030.[6,7] African Americans have the highest risk of developing HF (4.6 per 1000 person-years), followed by Hispanic/Latinos (3.5 per 1000 person-years), Caucasians (2.4 per 1000 person-years), and Chinese Americans (1.0 per 1000 person-years).[6,7] With the growing populations of racial/ethnic minorities in the United States, including Hispanics and Asians, these minorities will represent an emerging number of HF patients.[8,9] This chapter reviews the burden of HF on different racial and ethnic groups in the United States and appropriate management.

ETIOLOGY AND PATHOPHYSIOLOGY

The etiology of HF differs based on racial and ethnic backgrounds.[10] Ischemic disease and HTN are the most common causes of HF in the general population and should be assessed for independent of race and ethnicity upon diagnosis.[1,5,10] In the Multi-Ethnic Study of Atherosclerosis, the development of HF was linked to coronary calcification with Caucasians having the highest prevalence followed by African Americans, Hispanics, and then Chinese Americans.[7] African Americans who developed HF more commonly had left ventricular (LV) hypertrophy, HTN, diabetes, and obesity, whereas Chinese Americans had rare incidence of LV hypertrophy.[6,7,11] These differences may also be attributed to physiologic (salt sensitivity, vascular reactivity, nocturnal dipping in blood pressure, renin angiotensin-aldosterone activation system), genetic, and environmental factors, which will be discussed later in this review.[10,12,13] Unfortunately many of the large HF clinical trials have failed to include sufficient numbers of racial and ethnic minorities, which limits precision-based care (Table 12-1).[14]

HEART FAILURE IN AFRICAN AMERICANS IN THE UNITED STATES

The greatest risk factor for HF in African Americans is HTN.[13] African Americans may have an increased risk factor profile at the time of diagnosis of HF, including HTN, diabetes, and obesity although they present with similar signs of volume overload as other races and ethnicities.[13,15] In the Losartan Intervention for Endpoint Reduction in Hypertension Study, patients with HTN were followed for 2 years post antihypertensive therapy.[16] At the end of the study, LV mass and relative wall thickness were significantly greater in African American than in non-African American patients.[16] The unfavorable remodeling and HTN were hypothesized to be mediated by polymorphisms of the corin I555 allele, which is found commonly in African Americans and rarely in Caucasians.[16] In addition to increased LV mass, studies have shown that African Americans have higher levels of pro-brain natriuretic peptide, which confer increased risk of development of HF.[12]

Genetic predispositions for HF exist in the African American population. African Americans possessing the α2CDel322–325 and β1Arg389 adrenergic receptors have higher risk of developing HF.[17] A dual receptor polymorphism in the beta 1 and alpha adrenergic receptors is seen more commonly in African Americans with HF and is associated with worse outcomes.[13] A mutation of the beta 3 subunit of the G1 type protein is also overexpressed in some African Americans, and it correlates with HTN, renal disease, and salt sensitivity.[13] The Genetic Risk Assessment Sub-Study of the African American HF Trial (A-HeFT) has shown that a specific polymorphism of aldosterone synthase exists in a higher frequency in self-identified African Americans.[18] This polymorphism is associated with greater responsiveness to the combination of isosorbide dinitrate and hydralazine.[18]

Cardiopulmonary exercise testing is a form of clinical assessment in the HF population, but interpretation should be influenced by race/ethnicity. Peak oxygen consumption and ventilator efficiency are important independent prognostic indicators in HF.[19] However in multivariable analyses, a minute ventilation (VE)/carbon dioxide

Table 12-1 Ethnicty of Participants in Heart Failure Treatment/Prevention Trials

Trial	Entry Criteria	Intervention	Main Outcome—%(95%CI)	White	Black	Asian	Other
SOLVD Prevention	EF < 35%, asymptomatic	Enalapril (2.5-20 mg/d) vs. placebo	29% (21-36) reduction in combined endpoint of death/development of HF, 20% (9-30) reduction in hospitalization	86.5%	9.6%	3.9%	
SOLVD Treatment	EF < 35%, with HF	Enalapril (2.5-20 mg/d) vs. placebo	16% (5-26) reduction in mortality	80.3%	15.4%	4.3%	
SAVE	Post MI, EF < 40%, no overt HF	Captopril (6.25-50 mg three times/d) vs. placebo	19% (3-32) reduction in mortality	Not reported			
CONSENSUS-I	NYHA IV	Enalapril (2.5-40 mg/d)	40% reduction in mortality (P = 0.002)	Not reported			
MERIT-HF	NYHA II-IV, EF < 40%	Metoprolol (12.5-25 mg/d)	Hazard ratio for death 0.66 (0.53-0.81)	94%	5%	1%	
CIBIS-II	NYHA III/IV, EV < 35%	Bisoprolol (up to 10 mg/d) vs. placebo	Hazard ratio for death 0.66 (0.54-0.81)	Not reported			
RALES	NYHA III/IV, EF < 35%	Spironolactone (25 mg/d) vs. placebo	30% (18-40) reduction in mortality	86%	14%	Non-White	
V-HeFT-I	History of HF, or EF < 45% or increased CTR, and decreased VO$_2$ max	Prazosin (5 mg four times/d) or Hydralazine and ISDN (75 mg/40 mg four times/d) vs. placebo	Decreased mortality with Hydralazine/ISDN vs. placebo (26% vs. 34%)	71%	29%	0%	0%
V-HeFT-II		Enalapril (10 mg twice/d) or Hydralazine and ISDN (75 mg/40 mg four times/d)	28% reduction in mortality with Enalapril vs. Hydralazine/ISDN (P = 0.016)	73%	27%	0%	0%

CTR, x-ray cardiothoracic ratio; VO$_2$ max, peak oxygen consumption; SAVE, Survival And Ventricular Enlargement; MERIT-HF, MEtoprolol Randomized Intervention Trial in congestive Heart Failure; CIBIS, cardiac insufficiency bisoprolol study; RALES, randomized aldactone evaluation study; "CONSENSUS, Cooperative North Scandinavian Enalapril Survival Study; SOLVD, Studies of Left Ventricular Dysfunction; V-HeFT, Vasodilator Heart Failure Trial." This table was reproduced with permission from Sosin, MD, et al, Heart failure—the importance of ethnicity. *Eur J Heart Fail.* 2004;6(7):p. 831-843.

output (VCO_2) slope provided the most prognostic information independent of race/ethnicity and sex.[19] Furthermore the combination of VE/VCO$_2$ and oxygen consumption (VO_2) provided additive prognostic information only in Caucasians, and the combination of VE/VCO$_2$ and LV ejection fraction provided additive prognostic information in African Americans.[19]

Key considerations in management of HF in the African American population pertaining to the HF stages set by the guidelines and recommended therapies are reviewed below.[13,20] For complete management and treatment recommendations, providers should look toward the HF guidelines.[13,20]

Stage A represents a critically important group because many of the risk factors can be effectively controlled and may prevent the development of cardiac disease and ultimately HF especially in African Americans.[1] Lifestyle modifications for the prevention of HTN include weight reduction, adoption of Dietary Approaches to Stop Hypertension, restriction of dietary sodium, inclusion of daily physical activity, and moderation of alcohol consumption.[13] Thiazide diuretics represent the cornerstone of HTN therapy in all patients especially African Americans.[13]

Asymptomatic LV dysfunction, stage B, progresses to symptomatic HF much more aggressively in African Americans.[1,13,21] At this stage, specific cardiac structural changes (LV remodeling, LV dilation) may occur including those caused by myocardial infarction, HTN, cardiomyopathies, and valvular heart disease.[13,20] Therapeutic recommendations from HF guidelines for stage B include lifestyle modifications as described for stage A, and patients should be on evidence-based therapy including beta blockers, angiotensin-converting enzyme (ACE) inhibitors, and angiotensin II receptor blockers (ARBs) irrespective of race/ethnicity.[20]

In stage C HF, there is evidence of structural heart disease and symptoms of HF.[1] At this stage, the guidelines recommend continuing medication therapy, as in stage B patients, and adding an aldosterone antagonist.[1] There are some key differences in response to HF medications in the African American population. In the Beta-Blocker Evaluation in Survival Trial (BEST) study, the use of bucindolol was associated with a nonsignificant increase in the risk of serious clinical events in African American patients, but reduced death or hospitalization in non-African American patients.[22] However in the United States Carvedilol Heart Failure Trial with symptomatic HF and ejection fraction <35%, the benefit was of similar magnitude in both African American and non-African American patients.[23,24] The authors proposed that, as compared with other beta blockers, carvedilol might be more effective in African American patients because of its additional alpha adrenergic receptor blocking activity.[24] Subanalysis of the Studies of Left Ventricular Dysfunction (SOLVD) study data showed that the response to treatment with the ACE inhibitor, enalapril, was decreased in African Americans.[13,24] Current HF guidelines stress that although African Americans may not achieve the same level of benefit from ACE inhibitors, this class of drugs has been shown to significantly reduce risks of renal disease and cardiovascular mortality and is indicated in the long-term management of HF.[13,20,25] Studies have demonstrated that African Americans receive additional mortality benefit not seen in other races/ethnicities with the addition of hydralazine and long-acting nitrates (Figure 12-1).[13] The African American

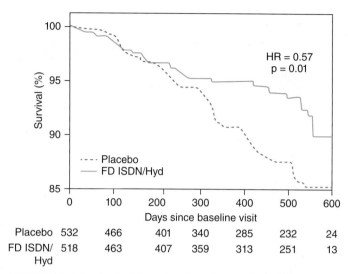

Placebo	532	466	401	340	285	232	24
FD ISDN/Hyd	518	463	407	359	313	251	13

FIGURE 12-1 Survival in African American Heart Failure Trial. (Reproduced with permission from Taylor AL, Ziesche S, Yancy C, et al. Combination of isosorbide dinitrate and hydralazine in blacks with heart failure. *N Engl J Med.* 2004;351(20):2049-2057.)

Heart Failure Trial and its substudies demonstrated improvements in echocardiographic parameters, rehospitalization, and mortality.[26] A possible explanation for the greater efficacy of the isosorbide dinitrate and hydralazine combination in African Americans may be that nitric oxide levels are reduced more and angiotensin II levels are increased less in African Americans with HF compared to Caucasians.[26] Genetic studies support this hypothesis, showing that African Americans are more likely to have polymorphisms in certain endothelial nitric oxide synthase genes compared with other ethnic groups.[13,18,25-28] Although there is strong evidence for the benefits of isosorbide dinitrate and hydralazine in self-described African American patients, this therapy remains underused.[26] Trials evaluating the aldosterone antagonists spironolactone and eplerenone in chronic severe HF and post myocardial infarction LV dysfunction have demonstrated clinical efficacy, but the numbers of African American participants in those studies have been too few to allow meaningful subset analysis by race.[28] However, there is no reason to assume a lack of efficacy, and these agents should be used per published guideline statements in patients irrespective of race/ethnicity.[13]

Patients with stage D HF are defined as those with refractory HF, end-stage HF, requiring specialized interventions. Despite having higher rates of HF, African Americans are the least likely to receive a heart transplant or LV assist device.[29,30] This is secondary to a myriad of etiologies including: underinsurance, education, social support, patient-centered decision, referral, and adherence.[30-33] Race/ethnicity should not impact the decision to offer advanced therapies for HF.

Arrhythmias in HF have a variable presence based upon race/ethnicity.[13] Atrial fibrillation is a common occurrence and can aggravate HF.[13] For reasons not yet clear, atrial fibrillation occurs less commonly in African Americans with HF.[13] Ventricular arrhythmias are potentially life threatening and often less prominent across race/ethnicity in the setting of effective evidence-based treatment and overall improvement in LV ejection fraction. However the disparate receipt of implantable cardiac defibrillators for sudden cardiac death (SCD) in African Americans compared to Caucasians is of greater concern.[13]

HEART FAILURE IN HISPANICS IN THE UNITED STATES

Hispanic Americans lead all ethnic groups in number and rate of population growth and have high rates of new HF.[6,34] Hispanics in the United Sates are comprised of the following populations: Mexican (63%), Puerto Rican (9.2%), Cuban (3.5%), and Dominican (2.8%).[34] The potential HF burden of the population remains challenging as Hispanics have a disproportionate cardiometabolic risk burden, underrepresentation in HF trials, and additional cultural and health disparity barriers (Table 12-1).[8] Hispanics have a relatively higher prevalence of abnormal ejection fraction (Figure 12-2).[8] The predominate etiology of HF in the Hispanic population has yet to be elucidated.[8,35] In contrast to non-Hispanic Caucasians, some data have shown Hispanics have a lower atherosclerotic burden demonstrated by lower prevalence

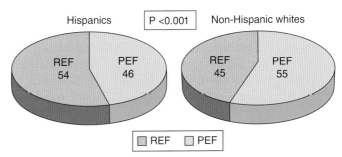

FIGURE 12-2 Percentage of Hispanic and non-Hipanic Caucasians with heart failure. PEF, Preserved Ejection Fraction; REF, Reduced Ejection Fraction (Reproduced with permission from Vivo RP, Krim SR, Krim NR, et al. Care and outcomes of Hispanic patients admitted with heart failure with preserved or reduced ejection fraction: findings from get with the guidelines-heart failure. *Circ Heart Fail.* 2012;5(2):167-175.)

of obstructive coronary artery disease (CAD), abnormal coronary artery calcium score, and common carotid artery intima-media thickening.[36,37] Further evidence demonstrated an unexpectedly lower cardiovascular mortality among Hispanics despite their high cardiometabolic risk indicating a Hispanic paradox.[37] The answers to this paradox may lie in environmental or genetic factors that have yet to be identified.[38]

Retrospective and observational studies have revealed that Hispanic patients have more risk factors for HF than non-Hispanic Caucasians.[38-40] Hispanics compared to non-Hispanic Caucasians are more likely to be younger, underinsured, and have higher rates of metabolic syndrome, diabetes, dyslipidemia, and kidney disease.[38-40] Data from the Multi-Ethnic Study of Atherosclerosis (MESA) indicated than Hispanics had greater LV abnormalities associated with diabetes when compared to non-Hispanic populations.[41] A genetic linkage of increased susceptibility to insulin resistance in the Hispanic population has been reported.[35] Given the cardiovascular risk burden in this population, Hispanics may be at increased risk for non ischemic cardiomyopathy from diabetic cardiomyopathy.[35] Metabolic syndrome is a significant predictor of LV dysfunction and incident HF independent of blood pressure or myocardial infarction; there is high likelihood for increasing incidence of HF in Hispanics.[8] Additional risk factors in Hispanics, especially in the immigrant Hispanic population, include rheumatic heart disease and Chagas disease.[8] The changing demographics of the U.S. population warrant health care professionals to consider and embrace the diverse patient population that is encountered while providing evidence-based care per HF guidelines.[42]

The electrocardiograph (ECG) of Hispanics often differ from other races/ethnicities with HF.[40] A study of HF with reduced Ejection fraction management revealed that African American patients had less evidence of myocardial infarction than Caucasians and Hispanics.[39] African American patients had more evidence of LV hypertrophy than Hispanics and Caucasians.[39] Hispanics had more evidence of ischemic changes than African Americans and Caucasians.[39] These variations may have implications for further diagnostic testing and potential treatment regimens.[39]

Further studies on the efficacy of standard HF medications should aim to include a substantial percentage of racial/ethnic minorities including Hispanics. In one study, investigators determined that Hispanics demonstrated less of a response to the effects of β-adrenergic blockade and less-than-expected improvement in LV function when compared to Caucasian participants.[43] Problems also exist in adherence to and prescription of therapy. One study demonstrated that Hispanic patients with HF and systolic dysfunction had an 82% use of ACE inhibitors and 89% use of beta blockers.[44] Additional studies have revealed that Hispanic patients are least likely to have an assessment of LV ejection fraction or be discharged on an ACE inhibitor compared with non-Hispanic Caucasian patients and African Americans.[44] Despite the lack of adequate Hispanic participants in clinical trials, the recommendations are to treat Hispanic patients in the various stages of HF according to existing guidelines.[1]

HEART FAILURE IN ASIANS IN THE UNITED STATES

Asian Americans represent a diverse heterogeneous population and little is known about their epidemiology of HF particularly in the United States. In China, 4.2 million individuals have HF, and cardiovascular disease is the leading cause of death.[45] In Japan, 1.0 million individuals were estimated to have HF in 2005, and this figure is expected to rise to 1.3 million by 2035.[45] Among North Asian Canadian patients, fewer Chinese patients had a history of myocardial infarction, 3-vessel CAD, or LV ejection fraction <39%, and more North Asian patients had a lower prescription rate of ACE inhibitors compared with non-Chinese/non-South Asian patients.[46] In contrast, South Asian patients more frequently had a past history of myocardial infarction, 3-vessel disease on angiogram, and treatment with coronary revascularization compared with non-Chinese/non-South Asian patients.[46] Previous studies have shown that South Asians are at an increased risk of developing HF due to premature CAD.[14] A recent longitudinal study of Asian Americans with HF revealed that Asian Americans were more likely to be younger, male, uninsured, and have higher risk of diabetes, HTN, and kidney disease than non-Hispanic Caucasians.[47]

In East Asia, the most common comorbidities were coronary artery disease, HTN, and diabetes mellitus.[45] Dilated cardiomyopathy, valvular heart disease, and atrial fibrillation were common comorbidities in Chinese populations with HF.[45] Chinese patients diagnosed with HF generally exhibited higher LV ejection fraction than Caucasian patients.[9] Among Chinese patients, HF was less commonly associated with ischemic disease and more commonly due to HTN and valvular etiologies.[45] Chinese patients were less frequently prescribed ACE inhibitors and more frequently prescribed ARBs.[9] In a study of 1-year mortality among patients hospitalized with HF, after a baseline adjustment, Chinese patients had a significantly higher hazard ratio of 1-year mortality compared with Caucasian patients (Figure 12-3).[48] However, a small American study suggested that mortality in Asians was no different from Caucasians with HF.[47] In the same study, multivariable analysis showed no disparities in receipt of evidence-based therapies in Asian Americans compared to Caucasians with the exception of reduced receipt of aldosterone antagonist and anticoagulation for atrial fibrillation.[47] While there are differences in the prevalence of comorbidities across these Asian ethnic groups, they do not entirely explain the high risk of mortality among Chinese patients.[9] There may be an HF gene predilection in Asians, as the angiotensinogen polymorphisms in Asians may be associated with HF.[49] Additional research is required to identify the reasons for the higher mortality among Chinese patients.

No HF beta blocker trials have involved sufficient Asian patients to provide comparative data.[10] Nitrates, diuretics, digitalis, ACE inhibitors, and beta blockers were the most commonly used agents in Chinese patients with chronic HF.[45] Nearly half of the patients with NYHA class III-IV HF were treated with a combination of ACE

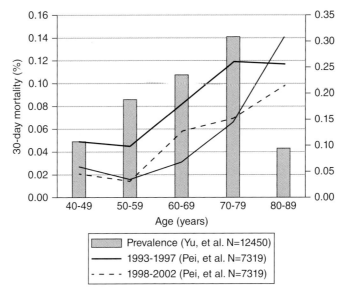

FIGURE 12-3 Prevalence and mortality of heart failure in Chinese population. (Reproduced with permission from Guo Y, Lip GYH, Banerjee A. Heart failure in East Asia. *Curr Cardiol Rev.* 2013;9:112-122.)

inhibitor and beta blocker or diuretic, digitalis, ACE inhibitor, and beta blocker.[45] To date, the use of aldosterone antagonist in South Asian patients has received little research attention (Table 12-1).[10]

CONCLUSION

HF affects all races and ethnicities with a variable prevalence and presentation. However, the diagnosis of HF and staging is the same. Unfortunately, response to known evidence-based therapies is not consistent across races and ethnicities. More inclusive research is needed with diverse patients to judge the efficacy of HF management across populations. Until that time regardless of the patient's race and ethnicity, equitable access to evidence-based therapy (ACE inhibitors, ARBs, beta blockers, aldosterone antagonists, and device therapy) should be provided per ACCF/AHA Guidelines.

REFERENCES

1. Yancy CW, Jessup M, Bozkurt B, et al. 2013 ACCF/AHA guideline for the management of heart failure: a report of the American College of Cardiology Foundation/American Heart Association Task Force on Practice Guidelines. *J Am Coll Cardiol.* 2013.

2. Kociol RD, Liang L, Hernandez AF, et al. Are we targeting the right metric for heart failure? Comparison of hospital 30-day readmission rates and total episode of care inpatient days. *Am Heart J.* 2013;165:987-994.e1.

3. Trends in Healthcare Costs and the Concentration of Medical Expenditures. http://www.ahrq.gov/news/events/nac/2012-07-nac/cohenmeyers/cohenmeyers.html. Accessed November 17, 2015.

4. Desai AS, Stevenson LW. Rehospitalization for heart failure predict or prevent? *Circulation.* 2012;126:501-506.

5. Heart Failure Fact Sheet|Data & Statistics|DHDSP|CDC. http://www.cdc.gov/dhdsp/data_statistics/fact_sheets/fs_heart_failure.htm. Accessed October 10, 2013.

6. Mozaffarian D, Benjamin EJ, Go AS, et al. Heart disease and stroke statistics—2015 update a report from the American Heart Association. *Circulation*. 2015;131(4):e29-322.

7. Bahrami H, Kronmal R, Bluemke DA, et al. Differences in the incidence of congestive heart failure by ethnicity. *Arch Intern Med*. 2008;168:2138-2145.

8. Vivo RP, Krim SR, Cevik C, Witteles RM. Heart failure in Hispanics. *J Am Coll Cardiol*. 2009;53:1167-1175.

9. Yeung DF, Van Dyke NK, Maclagan LC, et al. A comparison of Chinese and non-Chinese Canadian patients hospitalized with heart failure. *BMC Cardiovasc Disord*. 2013;13:114.

10. Sosin MD, Bhatia GS, Davis RC, Lip GYH. Heart failure—the importance of ethnicity. *Eur J Heart Fail*. 2004;6:831-843.

11. Domanski MJ, Krause-Steinrauf H, Massie BM, et al. A comparative analysis of the results from 4 trials of beta-blocker therapy for heart failure: BEST, CIBIS-II, MERIT-HF, and COPERNICUS. *J Card Fail*. 2003;9:354-363.

12. Choi E-Y, Bahrami H, Wu CO, et al. N-terminal pro-B-type natriuretic peptide, left ventricular mass, and incident heart failure: multiethnic study of atherosclerosis. *Circ Heart Fail*. 2012;5:727-734.

13. Franciosa JA, Ferdinand KC, Yancy CW; Group O behalf of the CS on HF in AAW. Treatment of heart failure in African Americans: a consensus statement. *Congest Heart Fail*. 2010;16:27-38.

14. Pina IL, Ventura HO. Heart failure in ethnic minorities: slow and steady progress. *JACC Heart Fail*. 2014;2:400-402.

15. Sharma A, Colvin-Adams M, Yancy CW. Heart failure in African Americans: disparities can be overcome. *Cleve Clin J Med*. 2014;81:301-311.

16. Okin PM, Kjeldsen SE, Dahlöf B, Devereux RB. Racial Differences in Incident Heart Failure During Antihypertensive Therapy. *Circ Cardiovasc Qual Outcomes*. 2011;4:157-164.

17. Small KM, Wagoner LE, Levin AM, Kardia SLR, Liggett SB. Synergistic polymorphisms of beta1- and alpha2C-adrenergic receptors and the risk of congestive heart failure. *N Engl J Med*. 2002;347:1135-1142.

18. McNamara DM, Tam SW, Sabolinski ML, et al. Aldosterone synthase promoter polymorphism predicts outcome in African Americans with heart failure results from the A-HeFT trial. *J Am Coll Cardiol*. 2006;48:1277-1282.

19. Arena R, Myers J, Abella J, et al. Prognostic characteristics of cardiopulmonary exercise testing in Caucasian and African American patients with heart failure. *Congest Heart Fail*. 2008;14:310-315.

20. Lindenfeld J, Albert NM, Boehmer JP, et al. HFSA 2010 comprehensive heart failure practice guideline. *J Card Fail*. 2010;16:e1-194.

21. Dries DL, Strong MH, Cooper RS, Drazner MH. Efficacy of angiotensin-converting enzyme inhibition in reducing progression from asymptomatic left ventricular dysfunction to symptomatic heart failure in black and white patients. *J Am Coll Cardiol*. 2002;40:1019.

22. A trial of the beta-blocker bucindolol in patients with advanced chronic heart failure. *N Engl J Med*. 2001;344:1659-1667.

23. Packer M, Bristow MR, Cohn JN, et al. The effect of carvedilol on morbidity and mortality in patients with chronic heart failure. *N Engl J Med*. 1996;334:1349-1355.

24. Yancy CW, Fowler MB, Colucci WS, et al. Race and the response to adrenergic blockade with carvedilol in patients with chronic heart failure. *N Engl J Med*. 2001;344:1358-1365.

25. Cuyjet AB, Akinboboye O. Acute heart failure in the African American patient. *J Card Fail*. 2014;20:533-540.

26. Ferdinand KC, Elkayam U, Mancini D, et al. Use of isosorbide dinitrate and hydralazine in African-Americans with heart failure 9 years after the African-American Heart Failure Trial. *Am J Cardiol*. 2014;114:151-159.

27. Li R, Lyn D, Lapu-Bula R, et al. Relation of endothelial nitric oxide synthase gene to plasma nitric oxide level, endothelial function, and blood pressure in African Americans. *Am J Hypertens*. 2004;17:560-567.

28. Ishizawar D, Yancy C. Racial differences in heart failure therapeutics. *Heart Fail Clin*. 2010;6:65-74.

29. Johnson MR, Meyer KH, Haft J, Kinder D, Webber SA, Dyke DB. Heart transplantation in the United States, 1999-2008. *Am J Transplant Off J Am Soc Transplant Am Soc Transpl Surg*. 2010;10:1035-1046.

30. Aggarwal A, Gupta A, Pappas PS, Tatooles A, Bhat G. Racial differences in patients with left ventricular assist devices. *ASAIO J*. 2012;58:499-502.

31. Coughlin SS, Halabi S, Metayer C. Barriers to cardiac transplantation in idiopathic dilated cardiomyopathy: the Washington, DC, Dilated Cardiomyopathy Study. *J Natl Med Assoc*. 1998;90:342-348.

32. Disparities in Solid Organ Transplantation for Ethnic Minorities. Medscape. http://www.medscape.com/viewarticle/547386. Accessed August 17, 2015.

33. Singh TP, Givertz MM, Semigran M, DeNofrio D, Costantino F, Gauvreau K. Socioeconomic position, ethnicity, and outcomes in heart transplant recipients. *Am J Cardiol*. 2010;105:1024-1029.

34. Blair JEA, Huffman M, Shah SJ. Heart failure in North America. *Curr Cardiol Rev*. 2013;9:128-146.

35. Hayat SA, Patel B, Khattar RS, Malik RA. Diabetic cardiomyopathy: mechanisms, diagnosis and treatment. *Clin Sci (Lond)*. 2004;107:539-557.

36. Budoff MJ, Yang TP, Shavelle RM, Lamont DH, Brundage BH. Ethnic differences in coronary atherosclerosis. *J Am Coll Cardiol*. 2002;39:408-412.

37. Agostino RB D', Burke G, O'Leary D, et al. Ethnic differences in carotid wall thickness. The Insulin Resistance Atherosclerosis Study. *Stroke J Cereb Circ*. 1996;27:1744-1749.

38. Perez MV, Yaw TS, Myers J, Froelicher VF. Prognostic value of the computerized ECG in Hispanics. *Clin Cardiol.* 2007;30:189-194.

39. Hebert K, Lopez B, Dias A, et al. Prevalence of electrocardiographic abnormalities in a systolic heart failure disease management population by race, ethnicity, and sex. *Congest Heart Fail.* 2010;16:21-26.

40. Hebert K, Quevedo HC, Tamariz L, et al. Prevalence of conduction abnormalities in a systolic heart failure population by race, ethnicity, and gender. *Ann Noninvasive Electrocardiol.* 2012;17:113-122.

41. Bertoni AG, Goff DC, Agostino RB DRB Dt Soc Holter Noninvasive Electrocardiol Inc S, Arce M, Tracy RP, Siscovick DS. Diabetic cardiomyopathy and subclinical cardiovascular disease: the Multi-Ethnic Study of Atherosclerosis (MESA). *Diabetes Care.* 2006;29:588-594.

42. McLean RC, Jessup M. The challenge of treating heart failure: a diverse disease affecting diverse populations. *JAMA.* 2013;310:2033-2034.

43. Kelesidis I, Varughese CJ, Hourani P, Zolty R. Effects of B-adrenergic blockade on left ventricular remodeling among Hispanics and African Americans with chronic heart failure. *Clin Cardiol.* 2013;36:595-602.

44. Ventura HO, Piña I. Heart failure in Hispanic patients: coming together? *Congest Heart Fail Greenwich Conn.* 2010;16:187-188.

45. Guo Y, Lip GYH, Banerjee A. Heart failure in East Asia. *Curr Cardiol Rev.* 2013;9:112-122.

46. Choi D, Nemi E, Fernando C, Gupta M, Moe GW. Differences in the clinical characteristics of ethnic minority groups with heart failure managed in specialized heart failure clinics. *JACC Heart Fail.* 2014;2:392-399.

47. Qian F, Fonarow GC, Krim SR, et al. Characteristics, quality of care, and in-hospital outcomes of Asian-American heart failure patients: findings from the American Heart Association Get With The Guidelines-Heart Failure Program. *Int J Cardiol.* 2015;189:141-147.

48. Kaul P, McAlister FA, Ezekowitz JA, Grover VK, Quan H. Ethnic differences in 1-year mortality among patients hospitalised with heart failure. *Heart Br Card Soc.* 2011;97:1048-1053.

49. Jiang W, He H, Yang Z. The angiotensinogen gene polymorphism is associated with heart failure among Asians. *Sci Rep.* 2014;4:4207.

13 PERIPARTUM CARDIOMYOPATHY

Rahul Chaudhary, MD
Jalaj Garg, MD, FESC
Gregg M. Lanier, MD, FACC

PATIENT CASE

A 29-year-old Caucasian woman presents to the emergency department 5 days post delivery with complaints of dyspnea and fatigue for 2 days. She reports it to be her first pregnancy, the course of which was complicated with gestational hypertension (HTN) (without other features of preeclampsia), and dependent bilateral pedal edema. She was treated with labetalol 200 mg by mouth twice a day for gestational HTN during her antepartum period. On physical examination, she was found to be dyspneic with respiratory rate of 25 breaths per minute and hypoxic with 80% saturation on room air. She was afebrile and had a blood pressure of 156/88 mm Hg and a pulse rate of 98 beats per minute. Her neck examination demonstrated a jugular venous distention of 17 cm water and grade 2+ pedal edema on both lower extremities. On systemic examination, lungs had diffuse bilateral inspiratory crackles; cardiac examination demonstrated regular heart rate with an S_3 summation gallop. No calf tenderness was observed and the rest of her physical examination was unremarkable.

Her laboratory investigation demonstrated urinalysis negative for protein. Cardiac enzymes, D-dimer, and thyroid function were within normal range and antinuclear antibodies were absent. The circulating levels of B-type natriuretic peptide (BNP) were 864 pg/mL. An electrocardiogram (ECG) showed a normal sinus rhythm with no conduction delays and no ectopy. Chest radiograph showed cardiomegaly with increased vascular congestion bilaterally (Figure 13-1). A computed tomography (CT) chest scan with contrast was negative for pulmonary embolism, but did show small bilateral pleural effusions and cardiomegaly. Subsequently an echocardiogram was obtained, which showed an ejection fraction (EF) of 35%.

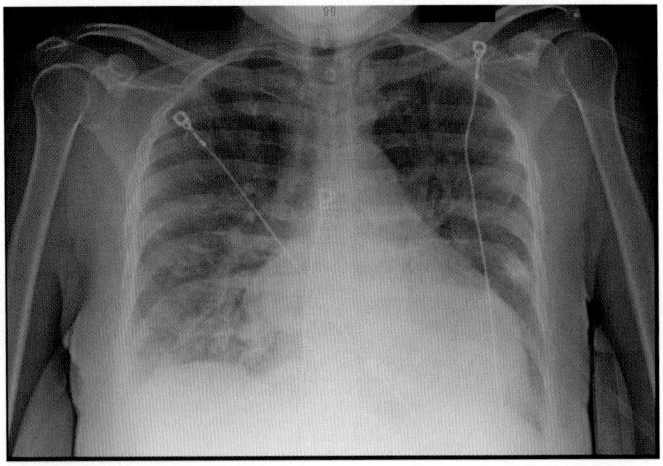

FIGURE 13-1 Chest x-ray showing pulmonary edema, pleural effusion with cardiomegaly.

DIFFERENTIAL DIAGNOSIS

At this point, the patient appears to have a new onset congestive heart failure (HF). The differential diagnosis to consider includes:

1. Peripartum cardiomyopathy (PPCM)

2. Cardiomyopathy including dilated, hypertrophic, or restrictive

3. Myocardial infarction

4. Pulmonary embolism (less likely given a negative CT scan)

5. Other cardiomyopathies: Drug-induced (alcoholic or cocaine-induced, although our patient denies usage of both)

6. Valvular heart disease (rheumatic mitral stenosis, aortic stenosis)

7. Noncardiogenic pulmonary edema

8. Primary pulmonary disease (asthma, chronic obstructive pulmonary disease, pulmonary fibrosis)

9. Others, including: Arrhythmogenic right ventricular dysplasia; infiltrative cardiac disease; toxic or metabolic disorders.

The diagnosis of PPCM is often missed as the signs and symptoms of a normal pregnancy coincide with findings of HF. These findings include dyspnea, dizziness, orthopnea, and decreased exercise capacity. Patients often do not show any indication of the syndrome until after delivery. Elkayam et al[1] and Sliwa et al[2] showed that patients could manifest similar symptoms even before the last gestational month and hence represent a continuum in the spectrum of this disease. The diagnostic criteria for peripartum cardiomyopathy are as follows: development of cardiac failure in the last month of pregnancy or within 5 months of delivery; absence of an identifiable cause for the cardiac failure other than pregnancy; absence of recognizable heart disease before the last month of pregnancy; and left ventricular (LV) systolic dysfunction with left ventricular ejection fraction (LVEF) <45%, fractional shortening below 30%, or both.

The risk factors of PPCM include age >30 years;[1,3,4] African descent;[1] multiple pregnancy;[1] history of preeclampsia, eclampsia, or postpartum HTN;[5,6] maternal cocaine abuse;[7] or long-term (>4 weeks) oral tocolytic therapy with beta adrenergic agonists such as terbutaline.[8] The presenting history of patients with PPCM includes symptoms consistent with systolic dysfunction in nonpregnant patients.[9] Dyspnea and tachycardia are the most common initial complaints in these patients.[10] However, a new or rapid onset of the following symptoms requires prompt evaluation: cough, orthopnea, paroxysmal nocturnal dyspnea, chest pain, and nonspecific symptoms of fatigue, palpitations, hemoptysis, and abdominal pain. The physical examination findings may include hypoxia, tachypnea, tachycardia with a normal blood pressure, elevated jugular venous pressure, worsening bilateral peripheral pedal edema, cardiomegaly, pulmonary crackles, ascites, hepatomegaly, and thromboembolism. Cardiac examination is consistent with loud pulmonic component of the second heart sound, mitral or tricuspid regurgitation,[11] and often S_3 and/or S_4 summation gallop.

For aiding in an early diagnosis of PPCM, Fett[12] suggested a screening tool consisting of 6 clinical categories that were scored based on their symptom severity from 0 to 2 and comprised of orthopnea, dyspnea, unexplained cough, lower extremity swelling, excessive weight gain, and palpitations (Table 13-1).

Table 13-1 Screening Tool for Peripartum Cardiomyopathy[12]

Symptom	0 points	1 point	2 points
Orthopnea	None	Need to elevate head	Elevation ≥45 degrees
Dyspnea	None	Climbing ≥8 steps	Walking on level ground
Unexplained cough	None	At night	Day and night
Pedal edema (pitting)	None	Below knee	Above and below knee
Excessive weight gain during last month of pregnancy	<2 lbs/wk	2-4 lbs/wk	≥4 lbs/wk
Palpitations	None	When lying down at night	Day and night, any position

MANAGEMENT

DIAGNOSTIC WORKUP

The diagnostic workup of these individuals includes blood tests such as complete blood count, serum electrolytes, lipid profile, liver function chemistries, thyroid profile, cardiac enzymes, antineutrophil antibody, and viral serology as a baseline (although none of these are specific for diagnosing PPCM). Additional diagnostic tools include 12-lead ECG, chest x-ray, and echocardiogram for assessment of HF.

Cardiac Protein Assays

Cardiac biomarkers such as cardiac troponins, BNP, and N-terminal proBNP (NT-proBNP), although nonspecific, are useful for initial assessment in patients with HF. In the postpartum period, Forster et al[13] demonstrated a significant elevation of NT-proBNP in patients with PPCM compared with healthy postpartum controls. Elevation of cardiac troponin T (≥0.04 ng/mL) within 2 weeks of PPCM onset has been shown to be a predictor of LV systolic dysfunction (sensitivity 55% and specificity 91%).[14]

Electrocardiogram

No specific ECG findings have been associated with PPCM. However, an ECG is useful in ruling out myocardial ischemia as an etiology of systolic dysfunction. The most common abnormalities noted on ECG are LV hypertrophy and ST-T wave changes. Although less frequently, other ECG findings notable with PPCM include arrhythmias such as atrial fibrillation, atrial flutter, and ventricular tachycardia; prolonged PR interval; and bundle branch block,[15] but these changes are highly nonspecific. There has also been a case report on unmasking of inherited long QT interval via dyselectrolytemia and structural changes due to PPCM.[16]

Echocardiogram

Echocardiography is an essential tool in these patients as it not only aids in making the diagnosis of PPCM but also helps assess the degree of cardiac dysfunction. Some common findings seen include dilatation of LV cavity with moderate to severely reduced EF mitral and/or tricuspid regurgitation, right ventricle (RV) and/or biatrial dilatation, increased pulmonary artery pressures, and, in severe cases, LV thrombus (Figures 13-2 and 13-3).[2,9-11]

A majority of women have a full recovery of their cardiac function over a time period ranging from 6 months to 48 months. However, it has been suggested that even after normalization of LV function after pregnancy, patients might continue to have decreased contractile reserves as demonstrated by a reduced rate-corrected velocity of fiber shortening on dobutamine stress echocardiogram.[17] A study by Fett et al[18] identified markers of persistent LV dysfunction and poor prognosis[19] on echocardiogram as LV end-diastolic diameter of 6 cm or more and M mode fractional shortening of 20% or less. In another study by Karaye,[20] a higher prevalence of RV dysfunction was noted in patients with PPCM, as measured by a reduction in tricuspid annular plane systolic excursion

Apical 4-chamber view

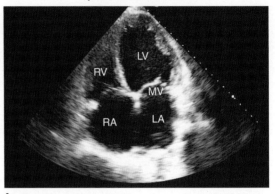

A

Parasternal long-axis view

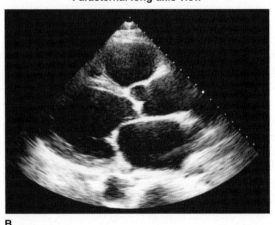

B

FIGURE 13-2 Echocardiographic appearance of dilated left ventricle on (a) apical 4-chamber view. (b) Parasternal long-axis view.

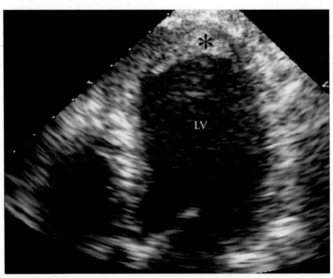

FIGURE 13-3 Echocardiographic appearance of left ventricular thrombus of apical 4 chamber view. (Reproduced with permission from Kim TS, Youn HJ. Role of echocardiography in the emergency department. *J Cardiovasc Ultrasound.* 2009 Jun;17(2):40-53.)

(TAPSE) ≤14 mm (54.6% vs 37.1%, respectively, p = 0.05). Novel echocardiographic techniques such as strain, strain rate, and speckle tracking have not yet been adequately explored in PPCM patients.

The follow-up and monitoring of disease progression has been suggested to be done by serial echocardiograms at regular intervals including at the time of discharge, 6 weeks, 6 months, and annually subsequently until normalization of LV function.[2]

Cardiac Magnetic Resonance Imaging

The modality of choice for assessment of myocardial fibrosis is cardiac magnetic resonance imaging (MRI).[21] Cardiac MRI has been shown to be helpful in prognostication of patients with HF based on presence or absence of late gadolinium enhancement.[22] In patients with PPCM, cardiac MRI has been demonstrated to have a more accurate assessment of chamber volume and ventricular function, LV thrombus, and myocardial fibrosis compared with echocardiography (Figure 13-4).[23] Additionally, cardiac MRI is able to distinguish between inflammatory and noninflammatory cardiomyopathy on the basis of late gadolinium enhancement in these patients and also helps to delineate PPCM from other cardiomyopathies such as ischemic heart disease or Takotsubo cardiomyopathy or infiltrative diseases such as hemochromatosis or amyloidosis. The identification of myocarditis-like PPCM from the gadolinium enhancement patterns may help direct therapy with intravenous immunoglobulins (IVIGs) and other immunosuppressive therapies.[24]

However, gadolinium contrast has been shown to have teratogenic effects in pregnancy and according to the American College of Radiology, gadolinium should be avoided during pregnancy.[25] Given the limited data for use of MRI with gadolinium contrast in the diagnosis and further management of PPCM and its teratogenic effects in pregnancy, it is not yet an approved diagnostic modality of choice in this patient population.

Endomyocardial Biopsy

There is no clear role of endomyocardial biopsy in establishing the diagnosis of PPCM. For diagnosis of dilated cardiomyopathy, its role is controversial[26-28] except in patients with a strong clinical suspicion of myocarditis (Figure 13-5) or no improvement after 2 weeks of optimal medical therapy for HF, especially if malignant ventricular arrhythmias are present and the diagnosis of giant cell myocarditis is being considered. The disadvantages of the procedure include its invasive nature, availability, complication rates, and nonspecific pathologic findings (edema, inflammation, hypertrophy, and fibrosis).[28]

TREATMENT OF PERIPARTUM CARDIOMYOPATHY

Treatment of PPCM in pregnant women is analogous to the management of HF with a few exceptions, which are described below in the relevant subsections (Figure 13-6). The overall management comprises nonpharmacological, medical, complementary/alternative therapy, and experimental therapies.

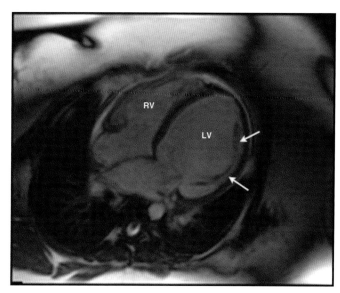

FIGURE 13-4 Cardiac MRI showing a large area of full-thickness delayed enhancement in the lateral wall of the left ventricle with some involvement of the anterolateral and inferolateral walls. (Source: Altuwaijri WA, Kirkpatrick IDC, Jassal DS, et al. Vanishing left ventricular thrombus in a woman with peripartum cardiomyopathy: a case report. *BMC Research Notes.* 2012;5:554.)

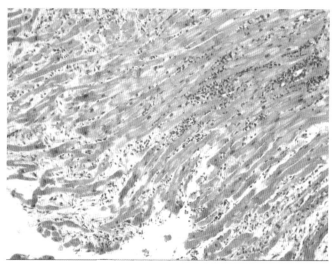

FIGURE 13-5 Histological appearance of myocarditis showing a dense infiltrate of lymphocytes and myocyte necrosis. (Reproduced from Gonzalez J, Salgado F, Azzato F, Ambrosio G, Milei J. Endomyocardial biopsy: a clinical research tool and a useful diagnostic method. In: Milei J, Ambrosio G. *Diagnosis and Treatment of Myocarditis.* InTechOpen, 2013. http://www.intechopen.com/books/diagnosis-and-treatment-of-myocarditis. Accessed June 20, 2017. Figure 2.)

NONPHARMACOLOGICAL

The nonpharmacological therapy involves lifestyle modification. This entails low-salt diet to <1.5 g/day, fluid restriction in patients with volume overload, daily monitoring of weight, and optimum blood pressure control. These measures form the main pillars in the management of PPCM presenting as HF.[3] Physical activity should not be restricted unless limited by disease severity.[29]

MEDICAL MANAGEMENT

The medical therapy should always be tailored to choose drugs safe in pregnancy and lactation for avoiding maternal and fetal morbidity.

Diuretics

The most commonly used diuretics in patients with HF are loop diuretics, for example, furosemide, which reduces preload and improves pulmonary vascular congestion and peripheral edema. Furosemide has been shown to be a category C drug during pregnancy (animal reproduction studies show an adverse effect on the fetus with absence of well-controlled studies in human beings, but the potential benefits may warrant use of the drug in pregnant women despite risks). While administering in pregnancy, it is essential to closely monitor the patient's volume status, as diuretic-induced dehydration can cause adverse fetal outcomes with oligohydroamnios, decreased uterine perfusion, and subsequent worsening of maternal metabolic acidosis.[30] During lactation, although furosemide has been shown to be excreted in breast milk, no case of furosemide toxicity in infants has been reported to date.[31] Other diuretic agents that can be used are thiazide diuretics and potassium-sparing diuretics. Thiazide diuretics have been labeled category B (animal reproduction studies failed to show a risk to the fetus, and insufficient data on usage in pregnant women; or animal studies have shown an adverse effect, but current data in pregnant women failed to demonstrate a risk to the fetus in any trimester) and potassium-sparing diuretics have been labeled category D (positive evidence of human fetal risk from studies in human beings). Thiazide diuretics have been deemed safe to administer during pregnancy and lactation. However, due to the teratogenic effects of potassium-sparing diuretics (such as spironolactone), their role and use in PPCM is controversial.[31] During lactation, canrenone, an active metabolite of spironolactone, is minimally secreted in breast milk and is of likely no clinical significance. Hence, spironolactone has currently been approved by the American Academy of Pediatrics for management of HF in the postpartum period.[32]

Angiotensin-Converting Enzyme Inhibitors and Angiotensin II Receptor Blockers

Angiotensin-converting enzyme (ACE) inhibitors and Angiotensin II receptor blockers (ARBs) form the cornerstone of therapy in patients with HF in the general population. However, they have been shown to be highly teratogenic both during pregnancy and lactation periods. Their teratogenic effects range from oligohydroamnios, intrauterine growth retardation, limb contractures, patent ductus arteriosus, hypocalvaria, fetal renal failure, and fetal death.[33] Due to these severe effects, these agents have been

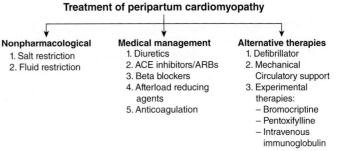

FIGURE 13-6 Overview of management strategies in peripartum cardiomyopathy.

contraindicated during pregnancy in patients with PPCM.[34-36] However, enalapril and captopril have been deemed to be safe to administer during the lactation period by the American Academy of Pediatrics.

Other Afterload Reducing Agents

Other agents include digoxin, nitrates, and hydralazine. Digoxin has been shown to be relatively safe in both pregnancy and lactation when its levels are within therapeutic range between 0.5 and 0.8 ng/mL.[37,38] Digoxin levels between 1.1 and 1.5 ng/mL have been shown to be associated with increased mortality as demonstrated in the Digitalis Investigation Group Trial.[39] Both nitrates and hydralazine are classified as category C drugs, but they are considered relatively safe during pregnancy and serve as an effective combination for afterload reduction.[2,11]

Beta Blockers

The most commonly used beta-blocking agents are metoprolol, carvedilol, and bisoprolol. These agents have been shown to reduce the risk of ventricular arrhythmias, sudden cardiac death, and mortality in patients with HF. These agents are classified as category C during pregnancy. Also, it is imperative to use beta-1 selective blockers during pregnancy to avoid antitocolytic activity (mediated via beta-2 blockage).[40] The most commonly used beta blocker in pregnancy is metoprolol tartrate. These agents have been shown to have beneficial effects on cardiomyopathy from reduction in myocardial expression of tumor necrosis factor (TNF)-α and decrease in its circulating levels.[41] The American Academy of Pediatrics has classified metoprolol tartrate as compatible during the lactation period. However, it recommends monitoring the growth curve in neonates (due to the medication's secretion in breast milk compared to carvedilol and bisoprolol)[32] and fetuses during the second and third trimesters of pregnancy.[31]

Anticoagulation

Patients suffering from LV dysfunction have been shown to have a 1 to 2.5 per 100 patient-years risk of developing thromboembolic events.[42,43] Pregnancy further adds to the risk as both pregnancy and puerperium are hypercoagulable states.[44,45] Multiple case reports of thromboembolic phenomena have been reported associated with PPCM complicated by pulmonary emboli,[46] coronary emboli,[47] biventricular emboli,[48,49] and peripheral embolization.[50] However, the current data are inconclusive on the utility of anticoagulation therapy (either antiplatelet or anticoagulation) in reduction of thromboembolic events or mortality in patients with PPCM who are in sinus rhythm and without an LV thrombus. In pregnant women who do require anticoagulation due to presence of an intracardiac thrombus or an arrhythmia such as atrial fibrillation, the decision to choose the agent and regimen is challenging because of varying risks during different stages of pregnancy. According to the American College of Cardiology/American Heart Association, "warfarin is probably safe during the first 6 weeks of gestation, but there is a risk of embryopathy if warfarin is taken between 6 and 12 weeks of gestation."[51] Warfarin is considered relatively safe during the second and third trimester of gestation; however, it needs to be changed to unfractionated heparin before delivery.

In the postpartum period, both warfarin and heparin are equally efficacious, as both these drugs are not secreted in breast milk.

Duration of Medical Therapy

Although recovery of LV function typically occurs over a period of 6 months to 48 months, recurrence of HF has been documented after initial normalization. Continuation of an ACE inhibitor and a beta blocker may be required indefinitely. However, if it is decided to stop these agents after normalization of the EF, serial echocardiograms may be necessary for monitoring cardiac function.

COMPLEMENTARY/ALTERNATIVE THERAPY

Defibrillators

Due to scant evidence on use of defibrillators in patients with PPCM, specific indications on their use have not been established. Because approximately 20% to 60% of patients undergo a complete recovery of LV function by 6 months to 5 years, patients with reduced EF of <35% with New York Heart Association class II, or class III for longer than 3 months on optimal medical therapy, should be considered for implantation of primary prevention implantable cardioverter defibrillators. In the first 3 months before implantation of a defibrillator, the utility of a wearable cardiac defibrillator is untested.[52]

There is no clear role for cardiac resynchronization therapy (CRT) in these patients unless they have electrical dyssynchrony manifested by a wide QRS duration (>150 ms with left bundle branch morphology). In an observational case series of 8 patients, 2 patients with persistently reduced EF, CRT led to a remarkable improvement in EF from 28% to 55% in 1 patient and 25% to 45% in the second patient.[53] Currently, no randomized trials support CRT in patients with PPCM and a narrow QRS complex.

Mechanical Assist Device and Heart Transplantation

Mechanical circulatory support with a left ventricular assist device (LVAD) or heart transplantation is a treatment option in patients with symptomatic HF refractory to optimal medical management. In patients with PPCM, baseline LVEF <30% has been shown to be associated with the likelihood of recovery of LVEF with medical management.[54] However, it is a poor predictor of recovery in individual patients. LVADs can be used as either a destination therapy or, more commonly, as a bridge-to-transplant while the patient awaits the arrival of a new heart, especially in patients dependent on inotropes. Studies evaluating outcomes with LVAD support showed a better 2-year survival in women with PPCM (83%) compared to women without PPCM receiving circulatory support.[54]

Cardiac transplantation is another treatment option for patients with HF refractory to optimal medical therapy. The rate of heart transplantation in women suffering from PPCM ranges from 4% to 23%.[1,55-58] Hence, it is important to note that women with PPCM should be managed in a center with transplant capabilities. Studies have shown a higher rate of graft failure and death in patients with PPCM undergoing cardiac transplantation.[55] The factors contributing to poorer outcomes in these patients included a younger age of the patient, higher allosensitization, higher pretransplant acuity, and increased rate of rejection.

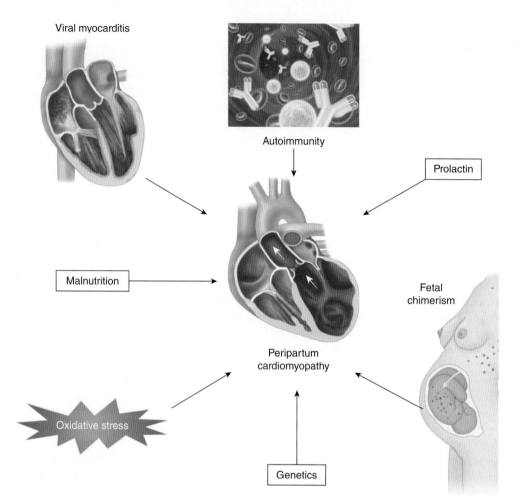

Viral myocarditis

Autoimmunity

Prolactin

Malnutrition

Fetal chimerism

Peripartum cardiomyopathy

Oxidative stress

Genetics

FIGURE 13-7 Proposed pathophysiological mechanisms contributing to development of peripartum cardiomyopathy.

EXPERIMENTAL THERAPIES

Bromocriptine

Treatment with dopamine-receptor agonists such as bromocriptine and cabergoline, which reduce secretion of prolactin from the anterior pituitary (Figure 13-7), may facilitate ventricular recovery in PPCM. Several observational studies and a small randomized study have shown beneficial effects of bromocriptine in these patients given at the dosage of 2.5 mg twice daily for 2 weeks followed by 2.5 mg daily for 6 weeks.[59-63] Safety of this drug remains a concern in both the peripartum and postpartum periods. A survey of 1400 pregnant women found no increased evidence of spontaneous abortion or congenital malformations in patients who used bromocriptine.[64] However, many cases of increased thrombotic events including myocardial infarction, strokes, seizures, and retinal vein occlusion have been reported presumed secondary to bromocriptine usage.[65-69] Although the results of studies have been promising so far, owing to its role in inhibiting breast milk production, thereby depriving the mothers and newborns from the emotional and physical benefits of breastfeeding and the potential to cause maternal complications, the current literature does not support use of this agent and it remains an unlabeled treatment option.

Pentoxifylline

The overexpression of inflammatory cytokines TNF-α, interferon-γ, interleukin-6, and C-reactive protein (CRP) has been implicated in LV dysfunction, pulmonary edema, ventricular remodeling, and cardiomyopathy (Figure 13-7).[70] Pentoxifylline is a xanthine derivative, which inhibits TNF-α production and also impedes apoptosis in vitro as well as in vivo.[31] A prospective trial evaluated this agent in 59 black women with new diagnoses of PPCM and found a significant improvement of LV end-diastolic (p = 0.0005) and end-systolic dimensions (p < 0.00001) and subsequently improved EF (p < 0.00001) with use of pentoxifylline given at 400 mg 3 times a day (for 6 months) in addition to standard medical therapy (n = 30) compared to standard therapy alone (n = 29).[71] However, this study was not randomized and small scale. Large double-blind randomized controlled trials are needed to confirm the efficacy of this agent in PPCM.

Immunoglobulins

IVIGs have been tried in patients with recent-onset dilated cardiomyopathy or myocarditis with no clear clinical benefits. In a few patients with PPCM, myocarditis has been shown to be the underlying pathology on endomyocardial biopsy (Figures 13-5 and 13-7). The IMAC trial (Controlled Trial of Intravenous Immune Globulin in Recent-Onset Dilated Cardiomyopathy) evaluated 111 patients with histological diagnoses of myocarditis and reduced LVEF (<45%). These patients were randomized to receive either conventional medical therapy or conventional medical therapy with a 24-week regimen of immunosuppressive therapy. The study demonstrated an improvement in LV function regardless of the immunosuppressive regimen.[72] This was challenged in a study by Bozkurt et al[73] in patients with PPCM, where they showed a significant improvement of LVEF with IVIG (2 g/kg over 2 days) compared to optimal medical therapy (26% vs 13%, respectively, p = 0.04). Due to the lack of sufficient clinical data from randomized controlled studies, the efficacy of this agent remains largely unknown.

HOSPITALIZATION AND DELIVERY

The timing and mode of delivery in women suffering from PPCM has not been well studied. Prompt delivery should be undertaken in women with PPCM and advanced HF for maternal cardiovascular indications. Urgent delivery is indicated in women with PPCM and advanced HF who develop hemodynamic instability.[2] In patients requiring inotropic or mechanical circulatory support, a planned cesarean delivery is preferred.[2,74] An early delivery is not indicated if the maternal and fetal conditions are stable.[2]

PROGNOSIS

The prognosis of PPCM varies globally and broadly encompasses maternal, obstetric, and neonatal outcomes in addition to the effects of subsequent pregnancy. There is a global variation in the maternal mortality rates of these patients, with the 1-year mortality rate ranging from 6% to 10% in the United States;[57] 6-month and 2-year mortality rates in South Africa between 10% and 28%, respectively; 6-month rates of 14% to 16% in Brazil and Haiti;

and up to 30% over 4 years in Turkey. The major causes of death in PPCM include sudden cardiac death, pump failure, or thromboembolic events. Multiple studies have identified predictors of poor prognosis in these patients including worse New York Heart Association class,[75] LVEF ≤25%,[60] multiparity,[76] black race,[76,77] Asian race,[78] age >35 years,[79] and low socioeconomic status.[80]

The usual recovery period of LV dysfunction is within 6 months after diagnosis of PPCM.[1,3,77] However, some studies have also shown a late recovery in LVEF in these patients beyond 1 year after diagnosis.[18,80-82] Interestingly, some studies have also shown patients to develop late deterioration of ventricular function after an initial recovery.[81] At follow-up, LVEF ≤30%,[1] fractional shortening of less than 20%,[10] LV end-diastolic diameter (LVEDD) ≥6 cm,[10] elevated cardiac troponin-T,[14] black race,[82,83] a diagnosis during pregnancy,[82] and presence of LV thrombus[58] have been shown to be predictors of persistent LV dysfunction. In a prospective cohort study of 100 patients by McNamara et al, no women with both an EF <30% and LVEDD ≥6 cm had recovery of cardiac function at 1 year.[54] Favorable prognostic indicators in patients with PPCM include smaller LV end-systolic and end-diastolic diameter,[58,85] higher baseline EF,[80,86,87] older age,[88] and white race.[78] Studies evaluating inotropic contractile reserve (demonstrated by dobutamine stress echocardiography) have yielded mixed results for assessing recovery of LV function.[89,90] There is a recent shift in focus to identify biomarkers for predicting prognosis in patients suffering from PPCM. Two such biomarkers evaluated by Damp et al were observed to be associated with the prognosis in patients with PPCM.[91] Relaxin-2 is a hormone produced in the corpus luteum of the ovary and in the heart.[92,93] The levels of relaxin-2 increase during pregnancy and have been shown to have anti-inflammatory, angiogenic, and antifibrotic properties.[92] Another biomarker, soluble fms-like tyrosine kinase 1 (sFlt1), is an anti-angiogenic factor released from the placenta during the peripartum phase. In translational research, it has been shown that sFlt1 and other vascular endothelial growth factor (VEGF) inhibitors combine to create an anti-angiogenic environment that impairs both systolic and diastolic function of heart.[94] In a recent study by Damp et al, these biomarkers were seen to be associated with recovery period and major adverse clinical events in 98 patients with PPCM enrolled in the Investigation in Pregnancy Associated Cardiomyopathy study.[91] Higher relaxin-2 levels soon after delivery were observed to be associated with myocardial recovery at a follow-up of 2 months. However, higher sFlt1 levels correlated with more severe symptoms and major adverse clinical events.

PROGNOSIS IN SUBSEQUENT PREGNANCIES

There is a higher recurrence risk of PPCM in patients with history of or persistent PPCM on subsequent pregnancies; these patients should undergo prenatal counseling.[2] In patients with persistent LV dysfunction (LVEF ≤50% or LVEF ≤25% at the time of diagnosis), a higher risk of progressively worsening HF and mortality (17%-19%) has been observed.[95,96] In women with complete recovery of LV function, the risk of developing PPCM with subsequent pregnancy has been seen to be lower than patients with persistent LV dysfunction but higher than the general population.[95,97] This persistent risk in these patients could be from subclinical residual dysfunction not detected on resting echocardiogram (which can also be assessed by measuring contractile reserve using dobutamine stress echocardiogram).[17] Although exercise or dobutamine stress echocardiography may be useful in the risk stratification of patients with a history of PPCM,[96] the current guidelines recommend against any future pregnancies.[2] However, if pregnancy recurs, women who are on ACE inhibitors or ARBs should be changed to an isosorbide dinitrate-hydralazine combination and metoprolol tartrate instead of carvedilol.

FOLLOW-UP

BREASTFEEDING

Although the 2010 European Society of Cardiology working group suggest that breastfeeding should be avoided postpartum due to potential effects of prolactin subfragments,[98] there is paucity of clinical data to support this recommendation. Elkayam et al examined the predictors of ventricular recovery in 37 of 55 patients with PPCM who decided to breastfeed and none had any adverse maternal effects. In fact, the observed rate of recovery of LV function was significantly higher in lactating women. Given the benefits of breastfeeding and lack of clinical data to show adverse outcomes, clinically stable women with PPCM should not be discouraged from breastfeeding as long as it is compatible with their HF regimen.[99]

CONTRACEPTION

Women with a history of PPCM should undergo counseling regarding risk of recurrence with family planning and contraception options. With absence of guideline recommendations, in women with high risk of recurrence of PPCM (persistently reduced LVEF <50% or ≤25% at diagnosis) it is safer to avoid future pregnancies.[2] The safety of various forms of contraception has not been studied in this patient population. Due to the adverse outcomes and poorer prognoses with recurrent PPCM, use of highly effective forms of contraception is suggested including a sterilization procedure or non-estrogen method of contraception (eg, intrauterine device implants). Due to the risk of exacerbating symptoms of HF (due to fluid retention), and the prothrombotic effect with estrogen-progestin contraceptives, these agents should be avoided.[100,101]

MEDICAL MANAGEMENT AFTER RECOVERY OF LV FUNCTION

Patients with persistent LV dysfunction should be continued on standard HF treatment indefinitely. It is important to note that in the subset of patients with full recovery of LV function (LVEF >50%), there is still a chance of recurrence of LV dysfunction even in the absence of subsequent pregnancies. However, there is limited data in such patient populations and no societal guidelines to assess the effects of therapy withdrawal and clinical outcomes. It is suggested that patients who demonstrate **persistently normal LV function** (LVEF >50%) **for a period of at least 6 months**, a stepwise weaning of the HF regimen can be undertaken. If utilizing this approach, it is imperative to have close clinical follow-up (every 3-4 months) and echocardiographic monitoring (every 6 months) to ensure stability of LVEF for the first 1 to 2 years after weaning medications. A decline in LVEF as documented by echocardiographic assessment or recurrence in symptoms of HF should lead to reinstitution of standard HF therapy.

PATIENT EDUCATION

Children's Cardiology Associates: http://www.cca-austin.com/blank.cfm?id=58&action=detail&AEArticleID=000188&AEProductID=Adam2004_1&AEProjectTypeIDURL=APT_1

PATIENT RESOURCES (ADVOCACY ORGANIZATIONS, WEBSITES)

American Heart Association: http://www.heart.org/HEARTORG/Conditions/More/Cardiomyopathy/Peripartum-Cardiomyopathy-PPCM_UCM_476261_Article.jsp#.VvtyKuIrJD8

MedlinePlus: https://www.nlm.nih.gov/medlineplus/ency/article/000188.htm

https://en.wikipedia.org/wiki/Peripartum_cardiomyopathy

PROVIDER RESOURCES (PRACTICE GUIDELINES, WEBSITES)

1. Current state of knowledge on etiology, diagnosis, management, and therapy of peripartum cardiomyopathy: a position statement from the Heart Failure Association of the European Society of Cardiology working group on peripartum cardiomyopathy. *Eur J Heart Fail.* 2010;12(8):767-778.

2. Peripartum cardiomyopathy: review and practice guidelines. *Am J Crit Care.* 2012;21(2):89-98.

REFERENCES

1. Elkayam U, Akhter MW, Singh H, et al. Pregnancy-associated cardiomyopathy: clinical characteristics and a comparison between early and late presentation. *Circulation.* 2005;111:2050-2055.

2. Sliwa K, Hilfiker-Kleiner D, Petrie MC, et al. Current state of knowledge on aetiology, diagnosis, management, and therapy of peripartum cardiomyopathy: a position statement from the Heart Failure Association of the European Society of Cardiology working group on peripartum cardiomyopathy. *Eur J Heart Fail.* 2010;12:767-778.

3. Demakis JG, Rahimtoola SH, Sutton GC, et al. Natural course of peripartum cardiomyopathy. *Circulation.* 1971;44:1053-1061.

4. Seftel H, Susser M. Maternity and myocardial failure in african women. *Br Heart J*. 1961;23:43-52.

5. Bello N, Rendon IS, Arany Z. The relationship between pre-eclampsia and peripartum cardiomyopathy: a systematic review and meta-analysis. *J Am Coll Cardiol*. 2013;62:1715-1723.

6. Lanier GM. New insights and clarity for peripartum heart failure and recovery in the modern era. *J Am Coll Cardiol*. 2015;66:915-916.

7. Mendelson MA, Chandler J. Postpartum cardiomyopathy associated with maternal cocaine abuse. *Am J Cardiol*. 1992;70:1092-1094.

8. Lampert MB, Hibbard J, Weinert L, Briller J, Lindheimer M, Lang RM. Peripartum heart failure associated with prolonged tocolytic therapy. *Am J Obstet Gynecol*. 1993;168:493-495.

9. Hibbard JU, Lindheimer M, Lang RM. A modified definition for peripartum cardiomyopathy and prognosis based on echocardiography. *Obstet Gynecol*. 1999;94:311-316.

10. Chapa JB, Heiberger HB, Weinert L, Decara J, Lang RM, Hibbard JU. Prognostic value of echocardiography in peripartum cardiomyopathy. *Obstet Gynecol*. 2005;105:1303-1308.

11. Ro A, Frishman WH. Peripartum cardiomyopathy. *Cardiol Rev*. 2006;14:35-42.

12. Fett JD. Validation of a self-test for early diagnosis of heart failure in peripartum cardiomyopathy. *Crit Pathw Cardiol*. 2011;10:44-45.

13. Forster O, Hilfiker-Kleiner D, Ansari AA, et al. Reversal of IFN-gamma, oxLDL and prolactin serum levels correlate with clinical improvement in patients with peripartum cardiomyopathy. *Eur J Heart Fail*. 2008;10:861-868.

14. Hu CL, Li YB, Zou YG, et al. Troponin t measurement can predict persistent left ventricular dysfunction in peripartum cardiomyopathy. *Heart*. 2007;93:488-490.

15. Adesanya CO, Anjorin FI, Adeoshun IO, Davidson NM, Parry EH. Peripartum cardiac failure. A ten year follow-up study. *Trop Geogr Med*. 1989;41:190-196.

16. Nishimoto O, Matsuda M, Nakamoto K, et al. Peripartum cardiomyopathy presenting with syncope due to torsades de pointes: a case of long qt syndrome with a novel kcnh2 mutation. *Intern Med*. 2012;51:461-464.

17. Lampert MB, Weinert L, Hibbard J, Korcarz C, Lindheimer M, Lang RM. Contractile reserve in patients with peripartum cardiomyopathy and recovered left ventricular function. *Am J Obstet Gynecol*. 1997;176:189-195.

18. Fett JD, Sannon H, Thelisma E, Sprunger T, Suresh V. Recovery from severe heart failure following peripartum cardiomyopathy. *Int J Gynaecol Obstet*. 2009;104:125-127.

19. Witlin AG, Mabie WC, Sibai BM. Peripartum cardiomyopathy: an ominous diagnosis. *Am J Obstet Gynecol*. 1997;176:182-188.

20. Karaye KM. Right ventricular systolic function in peripartum and dilated cardiomyopathies. *Eur J Echocardiogr*. 2011;12:372-374.

21. Mahrholdt H, Wagner A, Judd RM, Sechtem U, Kim RJ. Delayed enhancement cardiovascular magnetic resonance assessment of non-ischaemic cardiomyopathies. *Eur Heart J*. 2005;26:1461-1474.

22. Assomull RG, Prasad SK, Lyne J, et al. Cardiovascular magnetic resonance, fibrosis, and prognosis in dilated cardiomyopathy. *J Am Coll Cardiol*. 2006;48:1977-1985.

23. Mouquet F, Lions C, de Groote P, et al. Characterisation of peripartum cardiomyopathy by cardiac magnetic resonance imaging. *Eur Radiol*. 2008;18:2765-2769.

24. Ntusi NB, Mayosi BM. Aetiology and risk factors of peripartum cardiomyopathy: a systematic review. *Int J Cardiol*. 2009;131:168-179.

25. Kanal E, Barkovich AJ, Bell C, et al. ACR guidance document for safe MR practices: 2007. *AJR Am J Roentgenol*. 2007;188:1447-1474.

26. Zimmermann O, Kochs M, Zwaka TP, et al. Myocardial biopsy based classification and treatment in patients with dilated cardiomyopathy. *Int J Cardiol*. 2005;104:92-100.

27. Rizeq MN, Rickenbacher PR, Fowler MB, Billingham ME. Incidence of myocarditis in peripartum cardiomyopathy. *Am J Cardiol*. 1994;74:474-477.

28. Fett JD. Inflammation and virus in dilated cardiomyopathy as indicated by endomyocardial biopsy. *Int J Cardiol*. 2006;112:125-126.

29. Burch GE, McDonald CD, Walsh JJ. The effect of prolonged bed rest on postpartal cardiomyopathy. *Am Heart J*. 1971;81:186-201.

30. Lindheimer MD, Katz AI. Sodium and diuretics in pregnancy. *N Engl J Med*. 1973;288:891-894.

31. Garg J, Palaniswamy C, Lanier GM. Peripartum cardiomyopathy: definition, incidence, etiopathogenesis, diagnosis, and management. *Cardiol Rev*. 2015;23:69-78.

32. American Academy of Pediatrics Committee on Drugs. Transfer of drugs and other chemicals into human milk. *Pediatrics*. 2001;108:776-789.

33. Shotan A, Widerhorn J, Hurst A, Elkayam U. Risks of angiotensin-converting enzyme inhibition during pregnancy: experimental and clinical evidence, potential mechanisms, and recommendations for use. *Am J Med*. 1994;96:451-456.

34. Hunt SA, Abraham WT, Chin MH, et al. 2009 focused update incorporated into the ACC/AHA 2005 guidelines for the diagnosis and management of heart failure in adults: a report of the American College of Cardiology Foundation/American Heart Association task force on practice guidelines: developed in collaboration with the international society for heart and lung transplantation. *Circulation*. 2009;119:e391-e479.

35. Lavoratti G, Seracini D, Fiorini P, et al. Neonatal anuria by ace inhibitors during pregnancy. *Nephron*. 1997;76:235-236.

36. Alwan S, Polifka JE, Friedman JM. Angiotensin ii receptor antagonist treatment during pregnancy. *Birth Defects Res A Clin Mol Teratol*. 2005;73:123-130.

37. Rathore SS, Wang Y, Krumholz HM. Sex-based differences in the effect of digoxin for the treatment of heart failure. *N Engl J Med*. 2002;347:1403-1411.

38. Adams KF Jr, Patterson JH, Gattis WA, et al. Relationship of serum digoxin concentration to mortality and morbidity in women in the digitalis investigation group trial: a retrospective analysis. *J Am Coll Cardiol*. 2005;46:497-504.

39. The effect of digoxin on mortality and morbidity in patients with heart failure. *N Engl J Med*. 1997;336:525-533.

40. Easterling TR, Carr DB, Brateng D, Diederichs C, Schmucker B. Treatment of hypertension in pregnancy: effect of atenolol on maternal disease, preterm delivery, and fetal growth. *Obstet Gynecol*. 2001;98:427-433.

41. Ohtsuka T, Hamada M, Hiasa G, et al. Effect of beta-blockers on circulating levels of inflammatory and anti-inflammatory cytokines in patients with dilated cardiomyopathy. *J Am Coll Cardiol*. 2001;37:412-417.

42. Dunkman WB, Johnson GR, Carson PE, Bhat G, Farrell L, Cohn JN. Incidence of thromboembolic events in congestive heart failure. The V-HeFT VA cooperative studies group. *Circulation*. 1993;87:VI94-VI101.

43. Freudenberger RS, Hellkamp AS, Halperin JL, et al. Risk of thromboembolism in heart failure: an analysis from the sudden cardiac death in heart failure trial (scd-heft). *Circulation*. 2007;115:2637-2641.

44. Kane A, Mbaye M, Ndiaye MB, et al. [Evolution and thromboembolic complications of the idiopathic peripartal cardiomyopathy at Dakar University hospital: forward-looking study about 33 cases]. *J Gynecol Obstet Biol Reprod*. 2010;39:484-489.

45. Simeon IA. Echocardiographic profile of peripartum cardiomyopathy in a tertiary care hospital in Sokoto, Nigeria. *Indian Heart J*. 2006;58:234-238.

46. Jha P, Jha S, Millane TA. Peripartum cardiomyopathy complicated by pulmonary embolism and pulmonary hypertension. *Eur J Obstet Gynecol Reprod Biol*. 2005;123:121-123.

47. Box LC, Hanak V, Arciniegas JG. Dual coronary emboli in peripartum cardiomyopathy. *Tex Heart Inst J*. 2004;31:442-444.

48. Koc M, Sahin DY, Tekin K, Cayli M. [Development of biventricular large apical thrombi and cerebral embolism in a young woman with peripartum cardiomyopathy]. *Turk Kardiyol Dern Ars*. 2011;39:591-594.

49. Nishi I, Ishimitsu T, Ishizu T, et al. Peripartum cardiomyopathy and biventricular thrombi. *Circ J*. 2002;66:863-865.

50. Bennani SL, Loubaris M, Lahlou I, et al. [Postpartum cardiomyopathy revealed by acute lower limb ischemia]. *Ann Cardiol Angeiol*. 2003;52:382-385.

51. Bonow RO, Carabello BA, Chatterjee K, et al. 2008 focused update incorporated into the ACC/AHA 2006 guidelines for the management of patients with valvular heart disease: a report of the American College of Cardiology/American Heart Association task force on practice guidelines (writing committee to revise the 1998 guidelines for the management of patients with valvular heart disease): endorsed by the society of cardiovascular anesthesiologists, society for cardiovascular angiography and interventions, and society of thoracic surgeons. *Circulation*. 2008;118:e523-e661.

52. Saltzberg MT, Szymkiewicz S, Bianco NR. Characteristics and outcomes of peripartum versus nonperipartum cardiomyopathy in women using a wearable cardiac defibrillator. *J Card Fail*. 2012;18:21-27.

53. Mouquet F, Mostefa Kara M, Lamblin N, et al. Unexpected and rapid recovery of left ventricular function in patients with peripartum cardiomyopathy: impact of cardiac resynchronization therapy. *Eur J Heart Fail*. 2012;14:526-529.

54. Loyaga-Rendon RY, Pamboukian SV, Tallaj JA, et al. Outcomes of patients with peripartum cardiomyopathy who received mechanical circulatory support. Data from the interagency registry for mechanically assisted circulatory support. *Circ Heart Fail*. 2014;7:300-309.

55. Rasmusson K, Brunisholz K, Budge D, et al. Peripartum cardiomyopathy: post-transplant outcomes from the united network for organ sharing database. *J Heart Lung Transplant*. 2012;31:180-186.

56. Habli M, O'Brien T, Nowack E, Khoury S, Barton JR, Sibai B. Peripartum cardiomyopathy: prognostic factors for long-term maternal outcome. *Am J Obstet Gynecol*. 2008;199:415 e411-e415.

57. Felker GM, Jaeger CJ, Klodas E, et al. Myocarditis and long-term survival in peripartum cardiomyopathy. *Am Heart J*. 2000;140:785-791.

58. Amos AM, Jaber WA, Russell SD. Improved outcomes in peripartum cardiomyopathy with contemporary. *Am Heart J*. 2006;152:509-513.

59. Carlin AJ, Alfirevic Z, Gyte GM. Interventions for treating peripartum cardiomyopathy to improve outcomes for women and babies. *Cochrane Database Syst Rev*. 2010:CD008589.

60. Haghikia A, Podewski E, Libhaber E, et al. Phenotyping and outcome on contemporary management in a german cohort of patients with peripartum cardiomyopathy. *Basic Res Cardiol*. 2013;108:366.

61. Hilfiker-Kleiner D, Meyer GP, Schieffer E, et al. Recovery from postpartum cardiomyopathy in 2 patients by blocking prolactin release with bromocriptine. *J Am Coll Cardiol*. 2007;50:2354-2355.

62. Habedank D, Kuhnle Y, Elgeti T, Dudenhausen JW, Haverkamp W, Dietz R. Recovery from peripartum cardiomyopathy after treatment with bromocriptine. *Eur J Heart Fail*. 2008;10:1149-1151.

63. Sliwa K, Blauwet L, Tibazarwa K, et al. Evaluation of bromocriptine in the treatment of acute severe peripartum cardiomyopathy: a proof-of-concept pilot study. *Circulation.* 2010;121:1465-1473.

64. Turkalj I, Braun P, Krupp P. Surveillance of bromocriptine in pregnancy. *JAMA.* 1982;247:1589-1591.

65. Hopp L, Haider B, Iffy L. Myocardial infarction postpartum in patients taking bromocriptine for the prevention of breast engorgement. *Int J Cardiol.* 1996;57:227-232.

66. Loewe C, Dragovic LJ. Acute coronary artery thrombosis in a postpartum woman receiving bromocriptine. *Am J Forensic Med Pathol.* 1998;19:258-260.

67. Katz M, Kroll D, Pak I, Osimoni A, Hirsch M. Puerperal hypertension, stroke, and seizures after suppression of lactation with bromocriptine. *Obstet Gynecol.* 1985;66:822-824.

68. Nagaki Y, Hayasaka S, Hiraki S, Yamada Y. Central retinal vein occlusion in a woman receiving bromocriptine. *Ophthalmologica.* 1997;211:397-398.

69. Dutt S, Wong F, Spurway JH. Fatal myocardial infarction associated with bromocriptine for postpartum lactation suppression. *Aust N Z Obstet Gynaecol.* 1998;38:116-117.

70. Paulus WJ. How are cytokines activated in heart failure? *Eur J Heart Fail.* 1999;1:309-312.

71. Sliwa K, Skudicky D, Candy G, Bergemann A, Hopley M, Sareli P. The addition of pentoxifylline to conventional therapy improves outcome in patients with peripartum cardiomyopathy. *Eur J Heart Fail.* 2002;4:305-309.

72. Mason JW, O'Connell JB, Herskowitz A, et al. A clinical trial of immunosuppressive therapy for myocarditis. The myocarditis treatment trial investigators. *N Engl J Med.* 1995;333:269-275.

73. Bozkurt B, Villaneuva FS, Holubkov R, et al. Intravenous immune globulin in the therapy of peripartum cardiomyopathy. *J Am Coll Cardiol.* 1999;34:177-180.

74. van Schaik SM. Do pediatric patients with septic shock benefit from steroid therapy? A critical appraisal of "low-dose hydrocortisone improves shock reversal and reduces cytokine levels in early hyperdynamic septic shock" by Oppert et al. (Crit Care Med 2005; 33:2457-2464). *Pediatr Crit Care Med.* 2007;8:174-176.

75. Sliwa K, Forster O, Libhaber E, et al. Peripartum cardiomyopathy: inflammatory markers as predictors of outcome in 100 prospectively studied patients. *Eur Heart J.* 2006;27:441-446.

76. Murali S, Baldisseri MR. Peripartum cardiomyopathy. *Crit Care Med.* 2005;33:S340-S346.

77. Sliwa K, Skudicky D, Bergemann A, Candy G, Puren A, Sareli P. Peripartum cardiomyopathy: analysis of clinical outcome, left ventricular function, plasma levels of cytokines and fas/apo-1. *J Am Coll Cardiol.* 2000;35:701-705.

78. Krishnamoorthy P, Garg J, Palaniswamy C, et al. Epidemiology and outcomes of peripartum cardiomyopathy in the United States: findings from the Nationwide Inpatient Sample. *J Cardiovasc Med (Hagerstown).* 2016;17:756-761.

79. Harper MA, Meyer RE, Berg CJ. Peripartum cardiomyopathy: population-based birth prevalence and 7-year mortality. *Obstet Gynecol.* 2012;120:1013-1019.

80. Modi KA, Illum S, Jariatul K, Caldito G, Reddy PC. Poor outcome of indigent patients with peripartum cardiomyopathy in the United States. *Am J Obstet Gynecol.* 2009;201:e171-e175.

81. Biteker M, Ilhan E, Biteker G, Duman D, Bozkurt B. Delayed recovery in peripartum cardiomyopathy: an indication for long-term follow-up and sustained therapy. *Eur J Heart Fail.* 2012;14:895-901.

82. Pillarisetti J, Kondur A, Alani A, et al. Peripartum cardiomyopathy: predictors of recovery and current state of implantable cardioverter-defibrillator use. *J Am Coll Cardiol.* 2014;63:2831-2839.

83. Cooper LT, Mather PJ, Alexis JD, et al. Myocardial recovery in peripartum cardiomyopathy: prospective comparison with recent onset cardiomyopathy in men and nonperipartum women. *J Card Fail.* 2012;18:28-33.

84. McNamara DM, Elkayam U, Alharethi R, et al. Clinical outcomes for peripartum cardiomyopathy in North America: results of the IPAC study (Investigations of Pregnancy-Associated Cardiomyopathy). *J Am Coll Cardiol.* 2015;66:905-914.

85. Witlin AG, Mabie WC, Sibai BM. Peripartum cardiomyopathy: a longitudinal echocardiographic study. *Am J Obstet Gynecol.* 1997;177:1129-1132.

86. Duran N, Gunes H, Duran I, Biteker M, Ozkan M. Predictors of prognosis in patients with peripartum cardiomyopathy. *Int J Gynaecol Obstet.* 2008;101:137-140.

87. Goland S, Bitar F, Modi K, et al. Evaluation of the clinical relevance of baseline left ventricular ejection fraction as a predictor of recovery or persistence of severe dysfunction in women in the United States with peripartum cardiomyopathy. *J Card Fail.* 2011;17:426-430.

88. Blauwet LA, Libhaber E, Forster O, et al. Predictors of outcome in 176 South African patients with peripartum cardiomyopathy. *Heart.* 2013;99:308-313.

89. Dorbala S, Brozena S, Zeb S, et al. Risk stratification of women with peripartum cardiomyopathy at initial presentation: a dobutamine stress echocardiography study. *J Am Soc Echocardiogr.* 2005;18:45-48.

90. Barbosa MM, Freire CM, Nascimento BR, et al. Rest left ventricular function and contractile reserve by dobutamine stress echocardiography in peripartum cardiomyopathy. *Rev Port Cardiol.* 2012;31:287-293.

91. Damp J, Givertz MM, Semigran M, et al. Relaxin-2 and soluble Flt1 levels in peripartum cardiomyopathy: results of the multicenter IPAC study. *JACC Heart Fail.* 2016;4:380-388.

92. Wilson SS, Ayaz SI, Levy PD. Relaxin: a novel agent for the treatment of acute heart failure. *Pharmacotherapy.* 2015;35:315-327.

93. Conrad KP. Maternal vasodilation in pregnancy: the emerging role of relaxin. *Am J Physiol Regul Integr Comp Physiol.* 2011;301:R267-R275.

94. Patten IS, Rana S, Shahul S, et al. Cardiac angiogenic imbalance leads to peripartum cardiomyopathy. *Nature*. 2012;485:333-338.

95. Elkayam U, Tummala PP, Rao K, et al. Maternal and fetal outcomes of subsequent pregnancies in women with peripartum cardiomyopathy. *N Engl J Med*. 2001;344:1567-1571.

96. Fett JD, Fristoe KL, Welsh SN. Risk of heart failure relapse in subsequent pregnancy among peripartum cardiomyopathy mothers. *Int J Gynaecol Obstet*. 2010;109:34-36.

97. Sutton MS, Cole P, Plappert M, Saltzman D, Goldhaber S. Effects of subsequent pregnancy on left ventricular function in peripartum cardiomyopathy. *Am Heart J*. 1991;121:1776-1778.

98. Safirstein JG, Ro AS, Grandhi S, Wang L, Fett JD, Staniloae C. Predictors of left ventricular recovery in a cohort of peripartum cardiomyopathy patients recruited via the internet. *Int J Cardiol*. 2012;154:27-31.

99. Elkayam U. Clinical characteristics of peripartum cardiomyopathy in the United States: diagnosis, prognosis, and management. *J Am Coll Cardiol*. 2011;58:659-670.

100. Tepper NK, Paulen ME, Marchbanks PA, Curtis KM. Safety of contraceptive use among women with peripartum cardiomyopathy: a systematic review. *Contraception*. 2010;82:95-101.

101. Update to CDC's U.S. Medical eligibility criteria for contraceptive use, 2010: Revised recommendations for the use of hormonal contraception among women at high risk for HIV infection or infected with HIV. *MMWR Morb Mortal Wkly Rep*. 2012;61:449-452.

14 HEART FAILURE IN THE ELDERLY

Kumar Dharmarajan, MD, MBA
Michael W. Rich, MD

PATIENT CASE

An 86-year-old woman with a history of heart failure with preserved ejection fraction (HFpEF) is admitted to the hospital for worsening shortness of breath and fatigue. She has multiple coexisting conditions including hypertension (HTN), chronic kidney disease, chronic obstructive pulmonary disease (COPD), anemia, mild cognitive impairment, gait instability, and urinary incontinence. She lives in an assisted living facility and requires help with her medications, grocery shopping, and housework. She uses a walker and had a mechanical fall 4 months prior to admission. She has been hospitalized 3 times in the past year and will require subacute rehabilitation after hospital discharge to regain the ability to perform self-care activities including toileting, bathing, and dressing. She wants to discuss her long-term prognosis.

EPIDEMIOLOGY

- The prevalence of heart failure (HF) increases with age and exceeds 1 in 10 persons over the age of 80 years in the United States (Figure 14-1).[1]

- The risk of hospitalization for HF increases markedly with age for men and women (Figure 14-2).

- Persons 85 years of age and older make up an increasing proportion of all hospitalizations for HF in the United States (Figure 14-3).

- Although the majority of older persons hospitalized with HF in the United States have HFpEF,[2] most persons with heart failure with reduced ejection fraction (HFrEF) are also over 65 years of age.

- More than 80% of deaths attributable to HF in the United States occur in persons over 65 years of age, and approximately 60% occur in persons over 75 years of age.

AGE-RELATED PHYSIOLOGIC CHANGES

- Cardiovascular changes with aging contribute to the development of HF, in particular HFpEF. These changes include the following:[3]
  - Increased arterial stiffness as manifested by rising arterial pulse wave velocity (Figure 14-4), systolic blood pressure, and pulse pressure.
  - Impaired endothelium-mediated vasodilatation with reduced peak coronary blood flow.

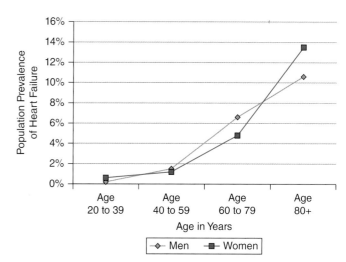

FIGURE 14-1 Prevalence of heart failure in the United States by age and gender: National Health and Nutrition Examinations Survey, 2009-2012. (Data from Mozaffarian D, Benjamin EJ, Go AS, et al. Heart disease and stroke statistics—2015 update. A report from the American Heart Association. *Circulation.* 2015;131(4):e275.)

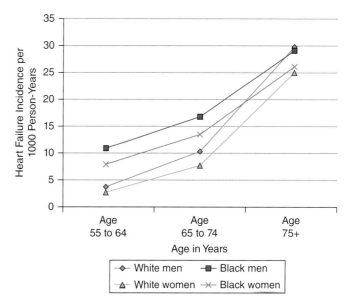

FIGURE 14-2 Incidence of heart failure hospitalization in the United States by age, gender, and race, 2005-2011: The Atherosclerosis Risk in Communities study. (Data from Mozaffarian D, Benjamin EJ, Go AS, et al. Heart disease and stroke statistics—2015 update. A report from the American Heart Association. *Circulation.* 2015;131(4):e276.)

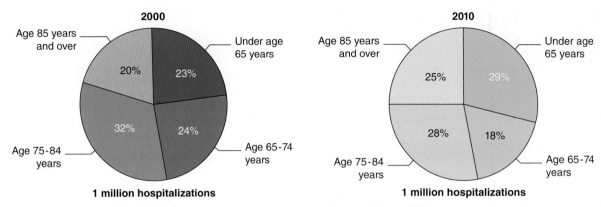

FIGURE 14-3 Age distribution of hospitalizations for heart failure in the United States, 2000 and 2010. (Reproduced from National Center for Health Statistics, Data brief no. 108, October 2012.)

- ○ Impaired active relaxation of the myocardium in diastole coupled with increased passive myocardial stiffness.
- ○ Reduced myocardial response to beta-adrenergic stimulation.
- ○ Impaired sinus node function.
- Older persons are therefore less able to augment cardiac output in response to stress due to the following:
  - ○ Insufficient preload or sufficient preload at the expense of elevated left ventricular (LV) diastolic pressure.
  - ○ Reduced stroke volume from impaired contractile reserve and increased vascular stiffness.
  - ○ Reduced peak heart rate (ie, 220 – age).
- Concomitant age-related changes to other organ systems include the following:
  - ○ Lungs: Reduced elastic recoil, reduced vital capacity, increased ventilation/perfusion mismatching.
  - ○ Kidneys: Declining glomerular filtration rate, impaired water and electrolyte homeostasis.
  - ○ Musculoskeletal system: Sarcopenia, osteopenia.
  - ○ Central nervous system: Impaired baroreceptor responsiveness, impaired thirst mechanism.

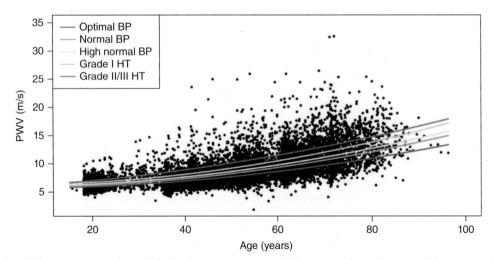

FIGURE 14-4 Relationship between age and carotid-femoral pulse wave velocity. Pulse wave velocity increases with age regardless of baseline blood pressure. Abbreviations: BP, blood pressure; HT, hypertension. (Reproduced with permission from the Reference Values for Arterial Stiffness' Collaboration. Determinants of pulse wave velocity in healthy people and in the presence of cardiovascular risk factors: 'establishing normal and reference values'. *Eur Heart J.* 2010 Oct;31(9):2338-2350.)

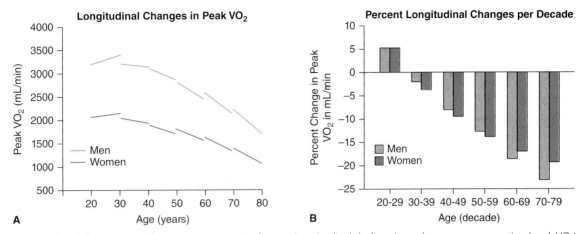

FIGURE 14-5 Age-related changes in peak oxygen consumption by sex. Longitudinal declines in peak oxygen consumption (peak VO_2) accelerate with age for both sexes. Abbreviation: VO_2: oxygen consumption. (Reproduced with permission from Strait JB, Lakatta EG. Aging-associated cardiovascular changes and their relationship to heart failure. *Heart Fail Clin.* 2012;8:143-164.)

- ○ Hemostatic system: Shift in balance between thrombosis and fibrinolysis toward thrombosis, increased risk for both thrombosis and hemorrhage.
- Physiologic changes with aging contribute to the decline in peak oxygen consumption (peak VO_2) (Figure 14-5) and to the increase in treatment-related side effects with age.[3]

GERIATRIC SYNDROMES COMMON IN HEART FAILURE

- Multimorbidity
  - ○ The majority of older persons with HF have 5 or more chronic conditions.
  - ○ The average number of chronic conditions increases with age.
  - ○ The average number of chronic conditions is increasing over time (Figure 14-6).
  - ○ The most common chronic conditions among Medicare beneficiaries 65 years of age or older with HF are HTN (86%), ischemic heart disease (72%), hyperlipidemia (63%), anemia

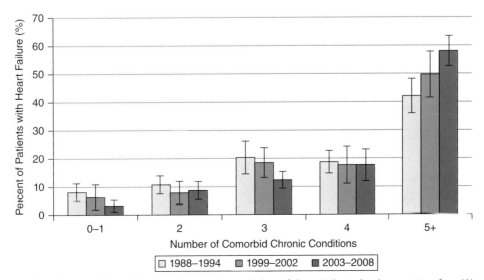

FIGURE 14-6 Trend in number of comorbid conditions among persons with heart failure. (Adapted with permission from Wong CY, Chaudhry SI, Desai MM, Krumholz HM. Trends in comorbidity, disability, and polypharmacy in heart failure. *Am J Med.* 2011;124:136-143.)

(51%), diabetes (47%), arthritis (46%), chronic kidney disease (45%), COPD (31%), atrial fibrillation (29%), and cognitive impairment (29%).[4]

- Polypharmacy
  - The median number of unique medications taken each day by persons with HF is 11 (Figure 14-7).
  - The number of medications taken daily is increasing over time.[5]
  - Medication adherence declines as complexity of the medical regimen increases.
  - Risk of drug-drug interactions exceeds 90% with 10 or more concomitant medications.

- Cognitive impairment
  - More than 1 in 4 older persons with HF have cognitive impairment.[4]
  - Among older persons hospitalized with HF, almost 1 in 2 have cognitive impairment. More than 1 in 5 has moderate to severe cognitive impairment.[6]

- Functional impairment
  - Almost 3 in 5 persons newly diagnosed with HF have difficulty in performing at least 1 of the following tasks: Feeding themselves, dressing, using the toilet, housekeeping, climbing stairs, bathing, walking, using transportation, and managing medications.[7]
  - Almost 2 in 5 older persons hospitalized with HF require assistance with walking.[8]

- Frailty
  - The phenotype of frailty may result from varied pathways, including the age-associated activation of inflammatory cells and decline in androgen hormones that result in loss of muscle quality and quantity, as well as increasing impairments across multiple organ systems (Figure 14-8).
  - One in four older persons with HF has at least 3 of the following hallmarks of frailty: Weak grip strength, physical exhaustion, slow gait speed, low activity level, and unintentional weight loss of 10 or more pounds in the past year.[9]

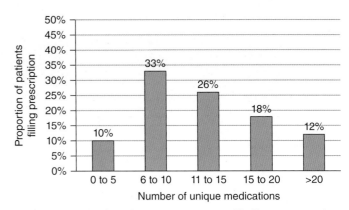

FIGURE 14-7 Number of unique prescriptions filled by patients with heart failure. (Adapted with permission from Dunlay SM, Eveleth JM, Shah ND, McNallan SM, Roger VL. Medication adherence among community-dwelling patients with heart failure. *Mayo Clin Proc.* 2011;86:273-281.)

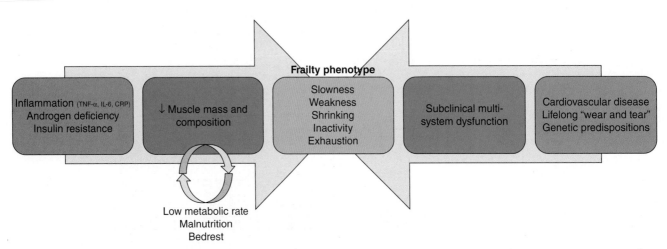

FIGURE 14-8 Two pathways leading to the phenotype of frailty. Abbreviations: CRP, C-reactive protein; IL, interleukin; TNF, tumor necrosis factor. (Reproduced with permission from Afilalo J, Alexander KP, Mack MJ, et al. Frailty assessment in the cardiovascular care of older adults. *J Am Coll Cardiol.* 2014;63:747-762.)

- Impact on outcomes
  - Increased comorbidities are associated with a higher risk of hospitalization.
  - Geriatric syndromes, especially frailty, mobility disability, and cognitive impairment, are associated with a higher risk of short- and long-term mortality after hospitalization for HF.[8]
  - Comorbid conditions contribute to the majority of hospitalizations[10] and rehospitalizations[11] among older persons with HF.

DIAGNOSTIC CHALLENGES

- Diagnosis of HF is more challenging in older persons.
- Many alternative sources of dyspnea and exercise intolerance may exist including coronary artery disease, atrial fibrillation and flutter, chronic lung disease, pneumonia, pulmonary HTN, pulmonary embolism, obesity, anemia, thyroid disorders, deconditioning, etc.
- Many alternative sources of fatigue and weakness may also exist including depression, infections, obstructive sleep apnea, frailty, sarcopenia, etc.
- Diagnostic test results are less specific in the elderly:
  - Natriuretic peptide levels increase with age (Figure 14-9).
  - Echocardiographic diastolic relaxation abnormalities increase with age.[12]

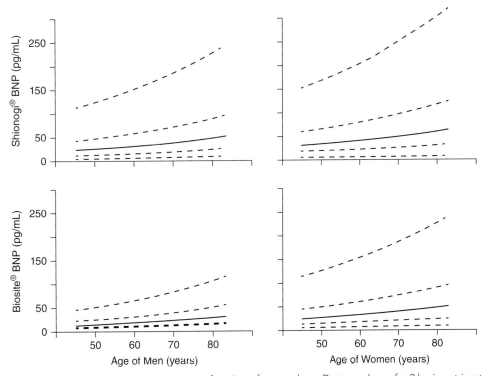

FIGURE 14-9 Plasma brain natriuretic peptide concentration as a function of age and sex. Data are shown for 2 brain natriuretic peptide assay systems. The nomogram demonstrates the 5th, 25th, 50th, 75th, and 95th percentiles for brain natriuretic peptide according to age. Abbreviation: BNP: brain natriuretic peptide. (Reproduced with permission from Redfield MM, Rodeheffer RJ, Jacobsen SJ, Mahoney DW, Bailey KR, Burnett JC Jr. Plasma brain natriuretic peptide concentration: impact of age and gender. *J Am Coll Cardiol.* 2002;40:976-982.)

TREATMENT PRINCIPLES

- Focus on universal health outcomes such as symptoms, functional status, health-related quality of life, all-cause hospitalization, and death rather than disease-specific outcomes such as cardiovascular hospitalization.[13]
- Emphasize nonpharmacologic modalities wherever possible to minimize likelihood of drug-drug and drug-disease interactions.
- Engage patients and their caregivers to make shared decisions that are consistent with their values and preferences.

GENERAL MANAGEMENT APPROACHES

- Encourage regular physical activity and exercise.
  - Exercise may improve health-related quality of life (Figure 14-10).
  - Exercise may improve functional status as measured by peak oxygen consumption.[14]
  - Exercise may improve noncardiac symptoms and outcomes related to mood, breathing difficulties, and lower extremity claudication.
  - See Table 14-1 for sample exercise prescription.
  - Contraindications to exercise in older patients are few and include ongoing myocardial ischemia, persistently decompensated HF, life-threatening arrhythmias that are not adequately treated, severe aortic stenosis or hypertrophic cardiomyopathy, any serious acute illness (eg, pneumonia), or any condition precluding safe participation in an exercise program (eg, severe disequilibrium or gait instability).
- Provide coordinated multidisciplinary care.
  - Medicare demonstration projects that have reduced preventable hospitalizations through care coordination have had common features (Table 14-2).[15]
  - Hospitals with the lowest 30-day readmission rates after HF hospitalization have implemented the greatest number of transitional care interventions (Table 14-3).[16]
  - Multidisciplinary HF clinics and high-intensity home visit programs have lowered readmissions after HF hospitalization.[17]
- Actively monitor patients for adverse drug effects, which are more common in the elderly:
  - Beta blockers can increase fatigue and worsen exercise intolerance.

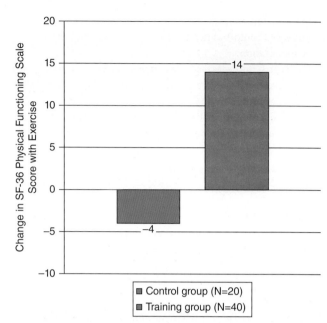

FIGURE 14-10 Changes in quality of life with exercise training among persons with heart failure with preserved ejection fraction. Abbreviations: SF-36, Short Form (36) Health Survey; MLWHFQ, Minnesota Living with Heart Failure Questionnaire. (Reproduced with permission from Edelmann F, Gelbrich G, Dungen HD, et al. Exercise training improves exercise capacity and diastolic function in patients with heart failure with preserved ejection fraction: results of the Ex-DHF (Exercise training in Diastolic Heart Failure) pilot study. *J Am Coll Cardiol.* 2011;58:1780-1791.)

Table 14-1 Exercise Prescription for Older Patients with Heart Failure

Components of conditioning program:

Aerobic conditioning exercises

Strengthening exercises

Flexibility and balance exercises

Frequency of exercise: Daily, if possible

Duration of exercise: Individualized within comfort range of patient

Intensity of exercise: Start at low intensity from patient perspective

Rate of progression in duration and intensity: Gradual over weeks to months

Monitoring: Perceived exertion most practical; start with very light or light exertion on perceived exertion scale

Table 14-2 Common Features of Medicare Demonstration Projects that Have Reduced Preventable Hospitalizations

Frequent in-person meetings between care coordinators and patients

In-person meetings between care coordinators and health providers

Supplemental educational sessions for patients and caregivers

Medication management services

Timely and comprehensive transitional care after hospitalization

- Angiotensin-converting enzyme (ACE) inhibitors, angiotensin II receptor blockers (ARBs), and potassium-sparing diuretics (including mineralocorticoid receptor antagonists) can cause severe hyperkalemia, especially in the setting of chronic kidney disease.
  - Loop diuretics can cause dehydration, orthostasis, and severe electrolyte abnormalities.
  - Nitrates can worsen dizziness and reduce activity level.[18]
- Carefully consider the use of pharmacologic and device-based interventions in the context of weak or negative trial data and higher competing risks of death in the elderly.
  - No pharmacologic intervention has been shown to improve mortality in older persons with HFpEF (Table 14-4).
  - Most trials in HFpEF and HFrEF have excluded very elderly persons and persons with complex or poorly controlled comorbid conditions, so benefits and risks are uncertain in these populations.
  - The benefit of implantable cardioverter defibrillators (ICDs) appears to be less among older persons when used in both primary[19] and secondary prevention[20] (Figure 14-11).
  - Shared decision-making is therefore particularly important for guiding treatment strategies in the elderly.

PROGNOSIS

- Overall mortality within 5 years of a diagnosis of HF is approximately 50% and increases with age.[1]
- Among older persons hospitalized for HF, more than 1 in 3 die and more than 2 in 3 are rehospitalized in the year after hospital discharge.[21]
- Mortality at 1 year is >1 in 2 for older patients discharged to a skilled nursing facility.[22]
- Approximately 1 in 2 deaths are due to noncardiovascular conditions, which may account for the reduced benefit of ICDs among older persons.[23]
- Predictors of mortality at the time of hospitalization include older age, lower systolic blood pressure, higher respiratory rate, serum sodium concentration <136 mEq/L, hemoglobin <10 g/dL, higher blood urea nitrogen, worse functional status, and history of cerebrovascular disease, chronic obstructive pulmonary disease, dementia, hepatic cirrhosis, or cancer.[24]

PALLIATIVE AND END-OF-LIFE CARE

- Palliative care and supportive care to address symptoms and psychosocial distress should be provided concurrently with evidence-based and disease-modifying interventions (Figure 14-12).
  - Early in HF care, supportive efforts should focus on education around self-management.
  - As the patient progresses to end of life (anticipated survival less than 6 to 12 months), the major focus should be on palliation.
- Benefits of palliative care for patients and caregivers include management of physical symptoms; strategies to address anxiety, depression, spiritual, and existential needs; clarification of goals

Table 14-3 Transitional Care Interventions Associated with Lower 30-day Readmissions After Heart Failure Hospitalization

Partner with community physicians or physician groups to reduce readmission

Partner with local hospitals to reduce readmissions

Systematized medication reconciliation

Arrange follow-up appointments before discharge

Send all discharge summaries directly to the patient's primary physician

Assign staff to follow-up on test results that return after the patient is discharged

Table 14-4 Negative Clinical Trials for Mortality Endpoint in Heart Failure with Preserved Ejection Fraction

Trial Acronym	Agent
SENIORS	Nebivolol
PEP-CHF	Perindopril
CHARM-Preserved	Candesartan
I-PRESERVE	Irbesartan
TOPCAT	Spironolactone
Aldo-DHF	Spironolactone
DIG-Ancillary	Digoxin
RELAX	Sildenafil

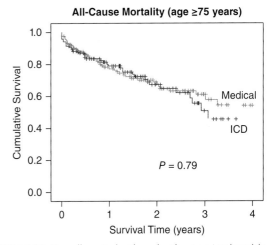

FIGURE 14-11 Overall survival with and without an implantable cardioverter defibrillator in persons with heart failure greater than 75 years of age. Abbreviation: ICD: implantable cardioverter defibrillator. (Reproduced with permission from Healey JS, Hallstrom AP, Kuck KH, et al. Role of the implantable defibrillator among elderly patients with a history of life-threatening ventricular arrhythmias. *Eur Heart J.* 2007;28:1746-1749.)

of care; development of strategies to manage the dying process; and decisions on plans after death.

- Palliative care can also provide caregivers with bereavement services after the patient's death.

- Frequently reassess goals of care as disease progress. Patients' willingness to trade survival time for freedom from symptoms (ie, quantity vs quality of life) and desire to avoid resuscitation often change as disease severity worsens.[25]

- All patients with an ICD should have the opportunity to deactivate their device.

SUMMARY FRAMEWORK

- Care of HF in elderly patients requires melding of cardiovascular perspectives with knowledge of multimorbidity, polypharmacy, cognitive decline, functional decline, frailty, and other clinical, social, financial, and psychological dimensions of aging.

- To accomplish these goals, clinicians caring for older patients with HF need to develop additional skills related to diagnosis, risk assessment, prognostication, treatment de-escalation, care coordination, collaborative care, communication, and end-of-life care (Figure 14-13).

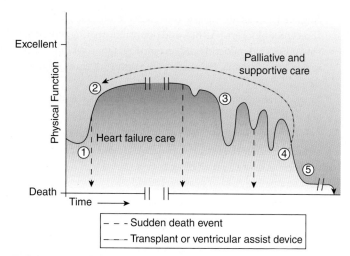

FIGURE 14-12 Schematic description of comprehensive heart failure care. (Reproduced with permission from Goodlin SJ. Palliative care in congestive heart failure. *J Am Coll Cardiol.* 2009;54:386-396.)

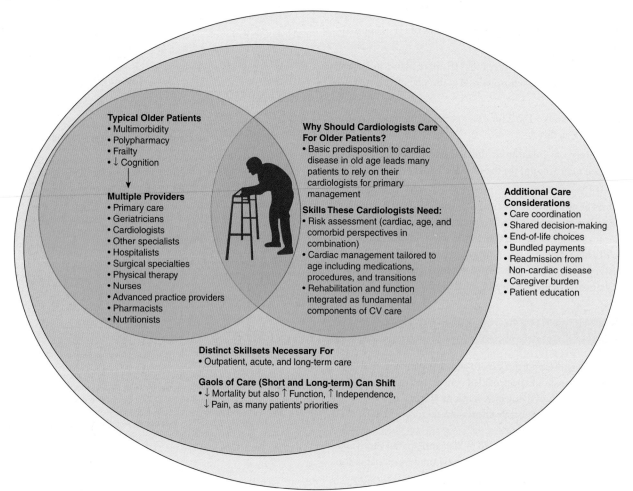

FIGURE 14-13 Summary framework for caring for older adults with heart failure. (Reproduced with permission from Bell SP, Orr NM, Dodson JA, et al. What to expect from the evolving field of geriatric cardiology. *J Am Coll Cardiol.* 2015;66:1286-1299.)

REFERENCES

1. Yancy CW, Jessup M, Bozkurt B, et al. 2013 ACCF/AHA guideline for the management of heart failure: a report of the American College of Cardiology Foundation/American Heart Association Task Force on practice guidelines. *Circulation.* 2013;128(16):e240-e327.

2. Owan TE, Hodge DO, Herges RM, Jacobsen SJ, Roger VL, Redfield MM. Trends in prevalence and outcome of heart failure with preserved ejection fraction. *N Engl J Med.* 2006;355(3):251-259.

3. Strait JB, Lakatta EG. Aging-associated cardiovascular changes and their relationship to heart failure. *Heart Fail Clin.* 2012;8(1):143-164.

4. Arnett DK, Goodman RA, Halperin JL, Anderson JL, Parekh AK, Zoghbi WA. AHA/ACC/HHS strategies to enhance application of clinical practice guidelines in patients with cardiovascular disease and comorbid conditions: from the American Heart Association, American College of Cardiology, and US Department of Health and Human Services. *Circulation.* 2014;130(18):1662-1667.

5. Wong CY, Chaudhry SI, Desai MM, Krumholz HM. Trends in comorbidity, disability, and polypharmacy in heart failure. *Am J Med.* 2011;124(2):136-143.

6. Dodson JA, Truong TT, Towle VR, Kerins G, Chaudhry SI. Cognitive impairment in older adults with heart failure: prevalence, documentation, and impact on outcomes. *Am J Med.* 2013;126(2):120-126.

7. Dunlay SM, Manemann SM, Chamberlain AM, et al. Activities of daily living and outcomes in heart failure. *Circ Heart Fail.* 2015;8(2):261-267.

8. Chaudhry SI, Wang Y, Gill TM, Krumholz HM. Geriatric conditions and subsequent mortality in older patients with heart failure. *J Am Coll Cardiol.* 2010;55(4):309-316.

9. McNallan SM, Chamberlain AM, Gerber Y, et al. Measuring frailty in heart failure: a community perspective. *Am Heart J.* 2013;166(4):768-774.

10. Dunlay SM, Redfield MM, Weston SA, et al. Hospitalizations after heart failure diagnosis a community perspective. *J Am Coll Cardiol.* 2009;54(18):1695-1702.

11. Dharmarajan K, Hsieh AF, Lin Z, et al. Diagnoses and timing of 30-day readmissions after hospitalization for heart failure, acute myocardial infarction, or pneumonia. *JAMA.* 2013;309(4):355-363.

12. Redfield MM, Jacobsen SJ, Burnett JC Jr, Mahoney DW, Bailey KR, Rodeheffer RJ. Burden of systolic and diastolic ventricular dysfunction in the community: appreciating the scope of the heart failure epidemic. *JAMA.* 2003;289(2):194-202.

13. Universal health outcome measures for older persons with multiple chronic conditions. *J Am Geriatr Soc.* 2012;60(12):2333-2341.

14. Kitzman DW, Brubaker P, Morgan T, et al. Effect of caloric restriction or aerobic exercise training on peak oxygen consumption and quality of life in obese older patients with heart failure with preserved ejection fraction: a randomized clinical trial. *JAMA.* 2016;315(1):36-46.

15. Brown RS, Peikes D, Peterson G, Schore J, Razafindrakoto CM. Six features of Medicare coordinated care demonstration programs that cut hospital admissions of high-risk patients. *Health Aff (Millwood).* 2012;31(6):1156-1166.

16. Bradley EH, Curry L, Horwitz LI, et al. Hospital strategies associated with 30-day readmission rates for patients with heart failure. *Circ Cardiovasc Qual Outcomes.* 2013;6(4):444-450.

17. Feltner C, Jones CD, Cene CW, et al. Transitional care interventions to prevent readmissions for persons with heart failure: a systematic review and meta-analysis. *Ann Intern Med.* 2014;160(11):774-784.

18. Redfield MM, Anstrom KJ, Levine JA, et al. Isosorbide mononitrate in heart failure with preserved ejection fraction. *N Engl J Med.* 2015;373(24):2314-2324.

19. Santangeli P, Di Biase L, Dello Russo A, et al. Meta-analysis: age and effectiveness of prophylactic implantable cardioverter-defibrillators. *Ann Intern Med.* 2010;153(9):592-599.

20. Healey JS, Hallstrom AP, Kuck KH, et al. Role of the implantable defibrillator among elderly patients with a history of life-threatening ventricular arrhythmias. *Eur Heart J.* 2007;28(14):1746-1749.

21. Dharmarajan K, Hsieh AF, Kulkarni VT, et al. Trajectories of risk after hospitalization for heart failure, acute myocardial infarction, or pneumonia: retrospective cohort study. *BMJ.* 2015;350:h411.

22. Allen LA, Hernandez AF, Peterson ED, et al. Discharge to a skilled nursing facility and subsequent clinical outcomes among older patients hospitalized for heart failure. *Circ Heart Fail.* 2011;4(3):293-300.

23. Henkel DM, Redfield MM, Weston SA, Gerber Y, Roger VL. Death in heart failure: a community perspective. *Circ Heart Fail.* 2008;1(2):91-97.

24. Lee DS, Austin PC, Rouleau JL, Liu PP, Naimark D, Tu JV. Predicting mortality among patients hospitalized for heart failure: derivation and validation of a clinical model. *JAMA.* 2003;290(19):2581-2587.

25. Brunner-La Rocca HP, Rickenbacher P, Muzzarelli S, et al. End-of-life preferences of elderly patients with chronic heart failure. *Eur Heart J.* 2012;33(6):752-759.

15 VALVULAR HEART DISEASE

Zeina Ibrahim, MD, FASE, FACC, FAHA
Vera H. Rigolin, MD, FASE, FACC, FAHA

PATIENT CASE: AORTIC STENOSIS

Mrs. R is a 92-year-old woman with history of severe aortic stenosis (AS), hypertension (HTN), atrial flutter, and nonobstructive coronary artery disease (CAD). She first developed symptoms around 2 years ago that were characterized by mild dyspnea on exertion and fatigue, and was appropriately referred for further therapy with either a surgical or transcatheter aortic valve replacement (TAVR). However, the patient at the time refused any further intervention for fear of complications given her advanced age.

She returned to the clinic 2 years later with now severe dyspnea even on minimal exertion, significant fatigue, dizziness, lower extremity edema, and weight loss. Physical examination revealed a frail elderly woman. The carotid pulse was slow and decreased in amplitude. On cardiac auscultation a soft S_2 was heard along with a late-peaking systolic murmur that was best heard at the right upper sternal border and radiated to the carotids.

Repeat echocardiography revealed a heavily calcified aortic valve with limited mobility (Figure 15-1). Doppler assessment of the aortic valve yielded a peak velocity of 5.4 m/sec, a mean gradient of 62 mm Hg, and a calculated aortic area of 0.6 cm², making the diagnosis of critical AS (Figure 15-2). The left ventricle (LV) showed moderate concentric hypertrophy with preserved ejection fraction (EF), but with evidence of diastolic dysfunction. Because of her significant, activity-limiting symptoms, the patient agreed to undergo further therapy. She was deemed high surgical risk because of high frailty score. She was therefore, referred for transcatheter aortic implantation with an Edwards SAPIEN 3 prosthesis. The procedure was successfully completed. However, the patient experienced a prolonged hospital course because of her advanced disease, significantly delayed intervention since symptom onset, and frailty. She has since recovered with markedly improved symptoms, and the latest echocardiogram shows a normally functioning prosthetic valve with a peak velocity to 2.8 m/sec, and mean gradient of 16 mm Hg (Figure 15-3).

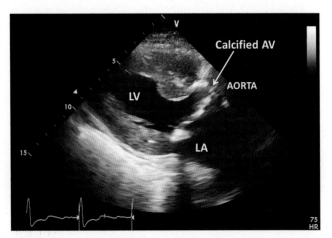

FIGURE 15-1 Parasternal long-axis echocardiographic view of a patient with severe aortic stenosis due to calcific degenerative disease. Note the heavily calcified aortic valve and the concentric hypertrophy of the left ventricle. Abbreviations: AV, aortic valve; LA, left atrium; LV, left ventricle.

ETIOLOGY AND PATHOPHYSIOLOGY

Aortic stenosis (AS) is the most frequent valvular heart disease. The prevalence of AS in the general population increases with age, and has been reported to occur in up to 9.8% of individuals aged 80 to 89 years.[1] The disease is usually caused by calcific degeneration of a trileaflet valve, or by progressive calcification of a congenitally abnormal valve, such as a bicuspid or unicuspid valve (Figure 15-4). Worldwide, however, rheumatic heart disease is still the most common etiology, and is usually accompanied by mitral

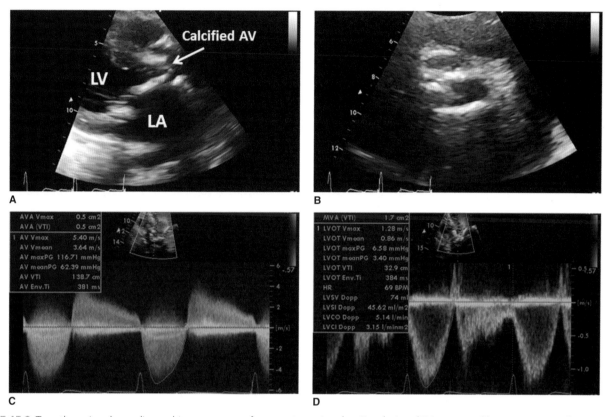

FIGURE 15-2 Transthoracic echocardiographic assessment of a stenotic aortic valve. Panels A and B (parasternal long-axis view and parasternal short-axis view) show the heavily calcified aortic valve with restricted opening in systole. Doppler hemodynamic assessment of the aortic valve (panels C and D) show significantly elevated velocity at 5.4 m/sec, mean pressure gradient of 62 mm Hg, and a calculated aortic valve of 0.6 cm^2. A diagnosis of critical aortic stenosis is made. Abbreviations: AV, aortic valve; LA, left atrium; LV, left ventricle.

disease. Traditional risk factors for atherosclerosis, such as HTN, smoking, and dyslipidemia, have been associated with the development of both calcific AS, and its predecessor, aortic sclerosis.[2]

A normal effective aortic valve area is about 3.0 to 4.0 cm^2 in adults. As the severity of the AS progresses, the valve area narrows, and the transvalvular pressure gradient increases. To compensate for the increased afterload obstruction, the LV undergoes concentric hypertrophy, and is thus able to maintain wall stress and cardiac

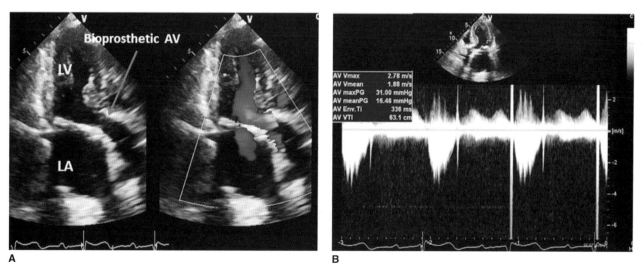

FIGURE 15-3 Transthoracic echocardiography of a patient post transcatheter aortic valve implantation. A normal functioning, well-seated bioprosthetic valve is seen in the aortic position in the 3-chamber view (panel A). Continuous-wave Doppler assessment across the aortic valve (panel B) shows a drop in the peak velocity to 2.7 m/sec (from a previous value of 5.4 m/sec). Abbreviations: AV, aortic valve; LA, left atrium; LV, left ventricle.

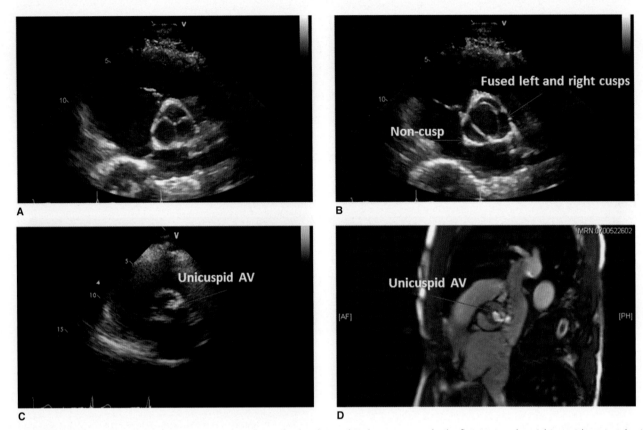

FIGURE 15-4 Short-axis echocardiographic view at the aortic valve level. Panel A shows a normal trileaflet aortic valve. A bicuspid aortic valve is seen in panel B. It opens as an ellipse in systole, and has fusion of the right and left cusps. Panels C and D are from a patient with a unicuspid valve; the echocardiogram shows an abnormal AV but no clear individual cusps. The MRI image in panel D, however, shows clearly the unicuspid valve.

output, at least for a while. Further progression of the stenosis severity and hypertrophy can lead to decreased compliance of the LV and the development of diastolic dysfunction. The progressive increase of LV hypertrophy and wall stress parallels an increase in oxygen demand, which cannot be met by the reduced coronary flow reserve. This supply-demand mismatch can result in angina, even if the epicardial coronary arteries are normal. Eventually, the compensatory mechanisms fail, and systolic dysfunction develops in the face of constant pressure overload.

CLINICAL FEATURES AND PHYSICAL EXAMINATION

Typically, patients with AS have a long latent period in which they are asymptomatic. There is a wide degree of variability in the actual degree of obstruction that would lead to symptoms in an individual patient, in part because of body size and physical fitness. In general, symptoms rarely develop until the AS is severe (defined as an area <1 cm^2, velocity >4 m/sec, and/or mean gradient >40 mm Hg), and even then, the patient might remain free of symptoms. In one series of asymptomatic patients with AS, survival free of death or valve replacement indicated by the development of symptoms was 5% at 2 years of follow-up.[3] On the other hand, other reports have shown a more aggressive progressive course of severe AS, with a high likelihood of developing symptoms within the following 3 to 5 years.[4] When symptoms do initially develop, they might be vague and nonspecific, such as decreased exercise tolerance, exertional dizziness, and dyspnea on exertion. The development of the classic clinical symptoms of AS, which include angina, syncope, and HF, signals a poor prognosis and decreased survival rate over the next 2 to 5 years, unless aortic valve replacement is performed.[5]

In asymptomatic patients, an abnormal physical examination might be the first clue to the presence of AS. A hallmark finding of severe AS is pulsus parvus et tardus, a carotid pulse that is diminished and delayed. This might be absent in the elderly, however, because of increased vasculature rigidity. The typical auscultatory findings include a systolic ejection murmur that is best heard over the right upper sternal border and radiates to the carotids. As the severity of the AS increases, the duration of the murmur becomes longer and peaks later. The intensity of the murmur is generally not a reflection of the severity of AS. Also, with severe AS, the aortic component of S_2 may become soft or even absent because the aortic valve is calcified and immobile.

DIAGNOSTIC TESTING

An electrocardiogram (ECG) of a patient with severe AS will often show LV hypertrophy (85% of patients). Chest radiography might be normal in these patients, or might show AV and aortic root calcifications, or cardiomegaly and pulmonary congestion if there is LV dysfunction.

The test of choice to establish the diagnosis of AS, determine the cause, and assess the severity, is a transthoracic echocardiogram (TTE). Two-dimensional echocardiography and M-mode can help determine the morphology of the aortic valve, and can often delineate if it is trileaflet or bicuspid. The aortic valve is usually thickened and calcified, with limited leaflet excursion during systole and reduced orifice size (Figures 15-1 through 15-4). In cases where TTE is equivocal or technically limited, a transesophageal echo may be useful (Figure 15-5). In the absence of HF, the LV cavity size is usually normal, and the LV wall is typically concentrically hypertrophied. Initially, the left ventricular ejection fraction (LVEF) is preserved, but as the disease progresses, systolic dysfunction and a drop in EF are seen.

Doppler echocardiography measures the velocity and pressure gradient across the diseased valve (Figure 15-6), and allows the calculation of the aortic area. The classification of the severity of the AS is dependent on the Doppler echo findings; the more severe the AS, the higher the velocity and pressure gradient, and the smaller the aortic area. In patients with low cardiac output, such as those secondary to LV dysfunction, the low flow across the valve might lead to low velocity and pressure gradient. This in turn will lead to an underestimation of the severity of the AS. On the other hand, the poor LV contraction can lead to poor leaflet mobility of a calcified aortic valve, and the illusion of a tight aortic area. This might be erroneously interpreted as severe AS, the so-called pseudo AS. In such cases of low-flow, low-gradient AS, the administration of low dose dobutamine may aid in the differentiation between true AS and pseudo AS, as well as the assessment of LV contractile reserve.

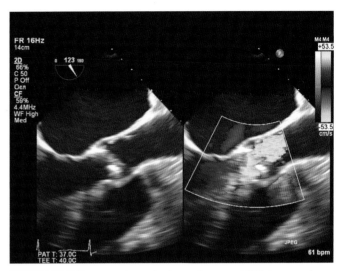

FIGURE 15-5 Transesophageal echocardiogram at 120 degrees showing the left ventricular outflow tract in a patient with severe aortic stenosis. The aortic valve appears calcified, thickened, and barely opens during systole. The color flow Doppler image on the right shows flow turbulence as the blood passes through the stenotic aortic valve.

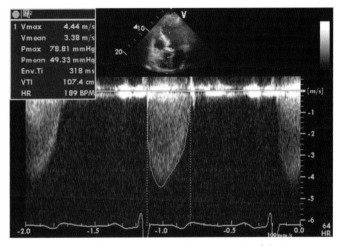

FIGURE 15-6 Continuous-wave Doppler assessment of the aortic valve in a patient with severe aortic stenosis secondary to degenerative calcific disease. The peak velocity across the valve is 4.4 m/sec, and the mean gradient is 50 mm Hg. The calculated valve area is 0.9 cm².

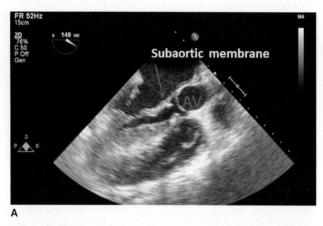
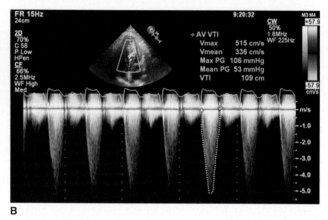

FIGURE 15-7 Transesophageal echocardiogram in a patient with high flow across the LV outflow tract but a normal aortic valve. Panel A shows a subaortic membrane (arrow) below the AV causing obstruction to outflow. Continuous-wave Doppler assessment of the LV outflow tract (panel B) reveals a peak velocity of 5 m/sec, and a mean gradient of 53 mm Hg.

DIFFERENTIAL DIAGNOSIS

AS remains the most common cause of LV outflow tract obstruction. Other causes include stenosis at the supravalvular level, which is uncommon and usually a part of a congenital disorder such as Williams syndrome. Or it could be secondary to stenosis at the subvalvular level, such as a discrete fibromuscular membrane present below the aortic valve (Figure 15-7), or, in extreme cases, a tunnel-like obstruction of the LV outflow tract.

MANAGEMENT

Asymptomatic patients with AS should be followed closely with serial clinical examinations, and assessment of any developing symptoms. Serial echocardiograms should be done, the frequency of which is determined by the severity of the stenosis. Once the patient develops severe AS, then more frequent clinical follow-up is recommended. Aortic valve replacement (AVR) is usually kept on hold until the patient develops symptoms. However, in specific situations, early AVR might be reasonable in asymptomatic severe AS patients. Patients with very severe asymptomatic AS (velocity 5.0 m/sec or greater, or mean pressure gradient 60 mm Hg or higher) and low surgical mortality, might benefit from early surgical AVR.[5]

No medical therapies are currently recommended to halt the progression of AS. Medical treatment of concomitant HTN or dyslipidemia is recommended according to standard guideline-directed therapy.

In symptomatic severe AS, or asymptomatic severe AS with secondary LV dysfunction (EF <50%), AVR is the treatment of choice. Once symptoms secondary to severe AS develop, outcomes are extremely poor unless the outflow obstruction is relieved. Even in patients with a low LVEF and severe AS, survival is better in those who undergo AVR compared to those treated medically.[5,6] The choice of intervention includes surgical or transcatheter AVR (TAVR). Whenever intervention is recommended and the surgical risk is low, surgical AVR is recommended. The choice between mechanical or bioprosthetic valve depends on the patient's age, ability to take and maintain therapeutic anticoagulation, and the

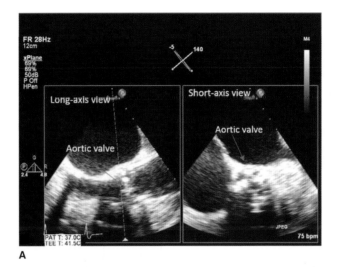

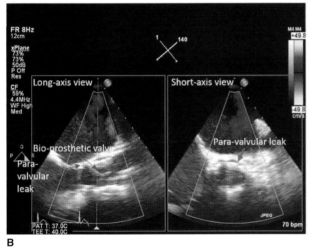

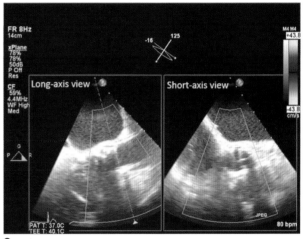

FIGURE 15-8 Transesophageal echocardiography showing transaortic valvular replacement (TAVR) in a patient with severe aortic stenosis. Panel A shows the stenosed and calcified aortic valve in the long- and short-axis views. Panel B shows the newly placed, bioprosthetic aortic valve with a mild paravalvular leak (arrows). Following another balloon inflation, the bioprosthetic valve is now fully deployed against the aortic annulus with resolution of the paravalvular leak.

patient's preference. In patients with severe symptomatic AS who are unable to undergo surgical AVR due to a prohibitive surgical risk or who have a high surgical risk, and who have an expected survival of >1 year after intervention, TAVR is recommended to improve survival and reduce symptoms (Figure 15-8).[7,8] Recently, TAVR has also been shown to be beneficial and comparable to open surgery in intermediate-risk patients.[9]

PROGNOSIS AND FOLLOW-UP

Frequency of follow-up for asymptomatic AS patients depends on the severity of the stenosis, and the presence of comorbidities. The more severe the AS, the closer the follow-up is scheduled, so that patients with severe AS should be evaluated every 6 months to 1 year with repeat TTE. It is hard to predict when patients with severe AS will develop symptoms, and thus the frequent clinical visits are geared to pick up insidious symptoms that might be missed by the patient.

In patients with severe symptomatic AS, treatment with surgical or TAVR results in improved survival rates, reduced symptoms, and improved exercise capacity. Thus, AVR is indicated in all symptomatic patients in the absence of serious comorbid conditions that limit life expectancy or quality of life.

Following the placement the prosthetic valve, regular clinical follow-up is indicated. A TTE is checked after the surgery, and repeated whenever there is a clinical change suggestive of valve dysfunction. Because of the high incidence of bioprosthetic valve dysfunction after 10 years, an annual TTE after that is recommended.[5]

PATIENT CASE: AORTIC REGURGITATION

Mr. P is a 51-year-old man with no significant past medical history, presented to the emergency department for evaluation of a few days history of dyspnea on minimal exertion that progressed to orthopnea. On presentation, he was found to be in florid HF with pulmonary edema. His symptoms rapidly improved upon diuresis. Mr. P admitted to a fairly sedentary lifestyle, and so previous symptoms such as exercise-induced dyspnea could not be elucidated. Physical examination revealed bounding peripheral pulses, a laterally displaced LV apical impulse, loud S_2, and a grade III/VI holodiastolic murmur heard best at the right upper sternal border while the patient was sitting up and leaning forward.

Workup revealed a large ascending aortic aneurysm extending from the root to the proximal transverse arch, measuring 6 cm in diameter (Figure 15-9). TTE revealed a significantly dilated LV cavity (LV end-diastolic diameter of 6.7 cm, and an LV end-diastolic volume of 263 mL) (Figure 15-10), severe systolic LV dysfunction (EF of 35%), and evidence of severe aortic regurgitation (AR). Further assessment of the aortic valve showed it to be trileaflet with no inherent evident disease. However, the dilated aortic root caused malcoaptation of the leaflets. Echocardiographic features of severe AR are noted (Figures 15-11 and 15-12).

Because of his severe, symptomatic AR with large ascending aneurysm, and detrimental cardiac sequelae, manifested by a dilated heart with depressed systolic function, Mr. P was referred for urgent

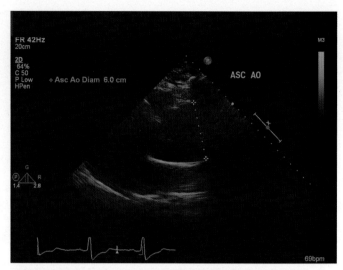

FIGURE 15-9 High parasternal long-axis view focused on the ascending aorta. The ascending aorta is significantly dilated and aneurysmal with a maximal measurement of 6 cm in diameter.

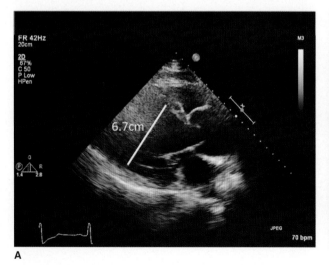
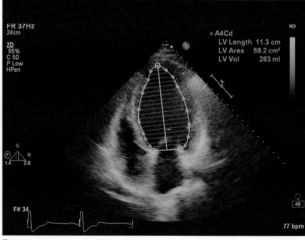

A   B

FIGURE 15-10 Parasternal long-axis and 4-chamber view of the left ventricle in a patient with severe aortic regurgitation. The left ventricle is severely dilated as assessed by both diameter and volume (internal diameter of 6.7 cm, and volume of 263 mL in end diastole).

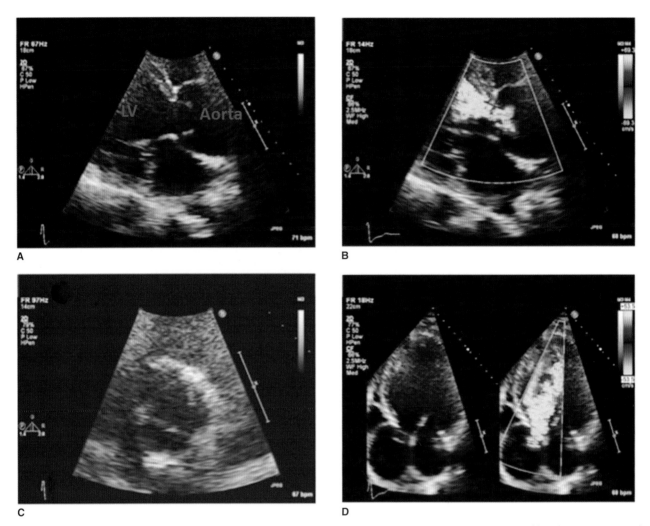

FIGURE 15-11 Transthoracic echocardiographic evaluation of a patient with severe aortic regurgitation secondary to dilated aortic root (panel A). The color Doppler in both panels B and D shows a large convergence zone and vena contracta suggestive of severe regurgitation. Panel C shows an intact trileaflet aortic valve in short axis that suggests that the etiology of the aortic regurgitation is secondary to the dilated aorta.

cardiac surgery. He underwent aortic root and valve replacement using a 27-mm mechanical valve within a 30-mm Valsalva graft, and replacement of the ascending aorta and proximal transverse arch with a 26-mm Dacron graft. Postoperative echocardiography shows a well-seated, mechanical valve in the aortic position with a peak velocity of 1.6 m/sec, mean gradient of 5 mm Hg, and no evidence of AR. Mr. P is out of the hospital now and continues to recover at home.

ETIOLOGY AND PATHOPHYSIOLOGY

Aortic regurgitation (AR) is caused by blood flow leaking back through the aortic leaflets due to an inadequate closure line. This could be due to a primary disease of the leaflets (Figures 15-13 and 15-14), or due to abnormalities of the aortic root or ascending aorta (Figure 15-9), or a combination of both (Figure 15-15) (Table 15-1). Worldwide, rheumatic heart disease remains the leading cause of AR. In the Western hemisphere, however, abnormalities of the aortic root and bicuspid aortic valves, are the more common causes of AR.[2,10]

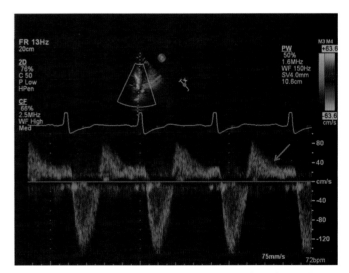

FIGURE 15-12 Pulsed-wave Doppler assessment of the descending aorta obtained from the suprasternal notch. Note the holodiastolic flow reversal (arrow) that signifies backward blood flow from the aorta into the left ventricular cavity. This is a marker of severe aortic regurgitation.

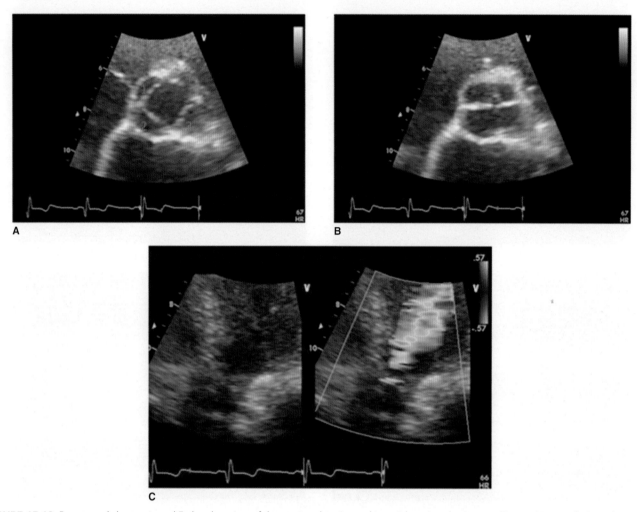

FIGURE 15-13 Parasternal short-axis and 5-chamber view of the aortic valve. A quadricuspid aortic valve is seen (4 cusps) in systole (open) in panel A, and diastole (closed) in panel B. Mild aortic regurgitation is seen secondary to malcoaptation of the leaflets (panel C).

Similarly, acute AR results from abnormalities of the valve itself, or from the aortic root. The clinical presentation and prognosis, though, varies greatly from that of chronic AR, and the list of causes is more limited. The major causes include endocarditis with valve destruction and leaflet perforation; aortic dissection that leads to aortic root dilation and can extend into the valve causing a flail leaflet; and traumatic (deceleration injury or blunt trauma), or iatrogenic (procedure-related) rupture of leaflets/root.

Regardless of the cause of AR, the hemodynamic consequence on the heart is the same. Due to the malcoaptation of the leaflets, a portion of the stroke volume leaks back into the LV in every diastolic cycle. This will lead to an increase in end diastolic volume and wall stress, which in turn cause the LV to dilate and undergo eccentric hypertrophy. These compensatory changes raise the stroke volume, and thus maintain the effective cardiac output initially. A combination of increased wall stress and elevation of systolic blood pressure due to increased stroke volume leads to an increased LV afterload. The net result is an increase in both LV preload and afterload. With progressive LV dilatation, preload reserve may be exhausted, leading to an afterload mismatch and deterioration of systolic function.[11] Initially the process is reversible, but with time, myocardial contractile dysfunction might develop leading to irreversible LV dysfunction.[12]

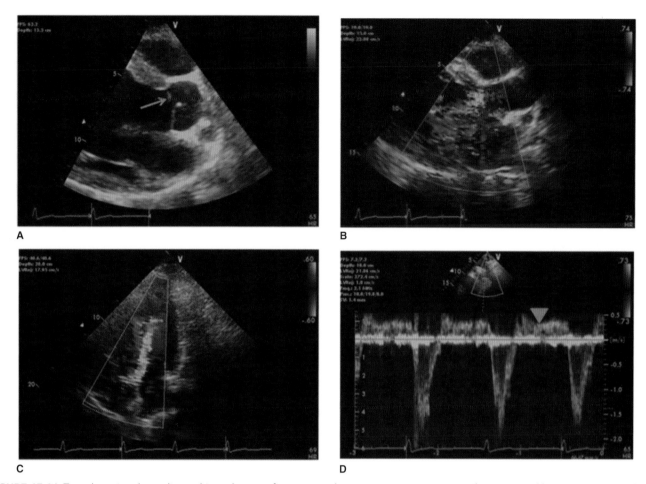

A   B

C   D

FIGURE 15-14 Transthoracic echocardiographic evaluation of a patient with severe aortic regurgitation. The parasternal long-axis view (panel A) shows flail right aortic cusps (arrow) secondary to a previous episode of endocarditis. Color-flow Doppler shows severe aortic regurgitation. Pulsed-wave Doppler in the suprasternal notch view (panel D) shows holodiastolic flow reversal (arrowhead) consistent with severe aortic regurgitation.

In contrast, acute AR is often a catastrophic event because the LV would not have enough time to adapt to the sudden increase in the LV volume. The effective forward stroke volume can abruptly fall with ensuing hypotension and cardiogenic shock. And the sudden increase in LV diastolic pressure can be transmitted to the pulmonary vasculature leading to pulmonary congestion and edema.

CLINICAL FEATURES AND PHYSICAL EXAMINATION

Patients with chronic AR typically remain asymptomatic for a long period of time. As the compensatory LV changes fail, LV dysfunction develops and with it patients gradually experience symptoms. Symptoms in patients with severe AR include exertional dyspnea, angina due to a reduction in coronary flow reserve, and ultimately symptoms of HF including dyspnea at rest, orthopnea, and paroxysmal nocturnal dyspnea. Because of the LV enlargement, patients may complain of an uncomfortable sensation in their chest that is worsened when lying supine.

There is a wide array of physical findings with chronic AR, primarily related to the increased stroke volume (leading to increased systolic pressure), and then the sudden drop of diastolic pressure (due to the regurgitant volume). This is manifested clinically in a

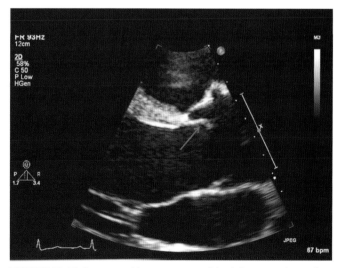

FIGURE 15-15 Parasternal long-axis view of the left ventricular outflow tract in a patient with a bicuspid aortic valve and aortic root aneurysm. Note the systolic doming of the aortic leaflets (red arrow) with incomplete opening. The aortic root is dilated at 4.4 cm in diameter. The combination of the dilated root and the bicuspid valve resulting in leaflet malcoaptation led to the development of moderate to severe aortic regurgitation.

wide pulse pressure, a bisferiens pulse (double systolic peaks with increased amplitude), or water hammer or Corrigan's pulse (rapid upstroke followed by rapid collapse). Many of the associated signs are related to increased capillary pulsations in the eyes (Becker's sign), uvula (Müller's sign), and nail bed (Quincke's sign).

Because of the dilated LV, the apical impulse is generally diffuse and displaced laterally. The intensity of the S_2 is variable depending on the etiology of the AR; it might be soft if the aortic leaflets are thickened and retracted, or loud in the presence of dilated aortic root. The classic murmur of AR is a blowing, decrescendo diastolic murmur, heard best at the left upper sternal border with the patient sitting up and leaning forward in deep expiration. Early in the disease, the murmur is confined to early diastole. The murmur lengthens to a holodiastolic murmur as the disease progresses. At end-stage disease, when the LV fails, the murmur shortens again because of the elevated LV end-diastolic pressure and rapid equalization of the gradient between the LV and aorta. Interestingly, another murmur might be audible at the apex in severe AR. The Austin Flint murmur is a mid-late diastolic, low-pitched murmur that is believed to be secondary to the vibration of the anterior mitral leaflet as it is struck by the regurgitant jet, or secondary to partial closure of the mitral valve (MV) by the elevated LV diastolic pressure.[10,11]

Signs and symptoms of cardiogenic shock typically dominate the clinical presentation of acute AR, including hypotension, tachycardia, diaphoresis, and pulmonary edema. Physical signs may be very nonspecific, or even absent, so a high degree of clinical suspicion is required to make a timely diagnosis.

DIAGNOSIS

Chest radiography may demonstrate an enlarged cardiac silhouette in patients with chronic AR. In end-stage disease, evidence of pulmonary congestion and edema may be seen. TTE is an essential imaging modality in the evaluation of AR, specifically in assessing the severity of the regurgitation, and the deleterious consequences of the disease on the LV size and function. The etiology of the AR can be assessed by 2-D echo. For example, thickened and retracted leaflets are suggestive of rheumatic heart disease. Leaflet perforation or a flail leaflet with a mobile mass is highly suggestive of bacterial endocarditis (Figure 15-14). A bicuspid valve with malcoaptation of the leaflets might be detected as the cause of the AR (Figure 15-15). Evaluation of the aortic root and ascending aorta is also essential and might lead to the diagnosis of the cause of the AR (Figure 15-9). Aortic root dilatation is often idiopathic, but could also be secondary to bicuspid disease, Marfan syndrome, or other aortitis disorders. Estimation of the LV volumes and function using 2-D echo is essential for determining prognosis, and for clinical treatment decisions (Figure 15-10). Three-dimensional echo can also be useful to accurately measure LV volumes and EF.

Color-flow and spectral Doppler echocardiography are used to detect AR and assess its severity by a mixture of qualitative and quantitative measurements. Cutoff values for the width of the jet in the LVOT, the vena contracta width (narrowest segment of the color flow jet), the regurgitant volume and fraction exist to help

Table 15-1 Causes of Chronic Aortic Regurgitation Divided into 2 Broad Categories: Primary Disease of the Valve Leaflets, and Abnormalities of the Aortic Root and Ascending Aorta

Valve/Leaflet Abnormalities	Aortic Root or Ascending Aortic Abnormalities
Rheumatic heart disease	Idiopathic or age-related aortic dilation
Congenital valve disease (bicuspid, unicuspid)	Isolated cystic medial necrosis of the aorta
Infective endocarditis	Cystic medial necrosis associated with bicuspid valve or Marfan syndrome
Myxomatous infiltration of aortic valve	Aortic dissection
Drug-induced valvulopathy (ergot-derived, anorectic)	Syphilitic aortitis
Trauma	Giant cell arteritis
Systemic disorders (lupus erythematosus, antiphospholipid syndrome, Whipple disease, Crohn disease, Takayasu arteritis, rheumatic arthritis)	Other aortitis (ankylosing spondylitis, Behcet syndrome, psoriatic arthritis, Reiter syndrome, relapsing polychondritis)

quantify the severity of AR. Unfortunately, no single method is sufficient to provide an accurate assessment of AR severity, and it is usually a combination of different parameters that succeeds in making an accurate diagnosis (Figure 15-11). The finding of holo-diastolic flow reversal in the abdominal aorta is usually indicative of severe AR. If there is a high clinical suspicion for endocarditis and a TTE is nondiagnostic, then transesophageal echocardiography (TEE) is indicated to rule out vegetations or aortic root abscesses.

In acute AR, the color flow assessment might be underwhelming because of the rapid equilibration of pressure gradient across the 2 chambers. However, a continuous Doppler signal across the valve will show a dense and steep diastolic slope. Premature mitral closure, and holodiastolic flow reversal of the abdominal aorta may also be seen. TEE may also be required to assess the etiology of acute AR, including aortic dissection, flail aortic leaflet, or endocarditis.

MANAGEMENT

Intervention for AR, when indicated, generally involves surgical AVR, with or without aortic root repair/replacement. Asymptomatic patients with severe AR and normal LV size and function usually require no immediate intervention, but will need close follow-up to detect symptoms as early as possible. In patients with asymptomatic AR and preserved systolic function, published data report that the rate of progression to asymptomatic LV dysfunction is <3.5% per year; the development of symptoms or LV dysfunction is less than 6% per year; and the risk of sudden cardiac death is <0.2% per year.[12,13]

Symptom development signals a high risk of death if AVR is not performed.[5] In a series of 246 patients with advanced HF symptoms secondary to AR, the mortality was as high as 24.6% per year without surgery.[14] Therefore, AVR is indicated for symptomatic patients with severe AR regardless of LV systolic function. AVR is also indicated for patients with severe AR with LV systolic dysfunction (EF <50%), even if the patient remains asymptomatic. Outcomes with surgery are better with immediate referral, rather than waiting for symptoms to develop or for further LV dysfunction to occur.[5] Severe LV dilation indicates a significant degree of LV remodeling and is associated with subsequent development of symptoms and/or LV systolic dysfunction.[5] Thus AVR is a reasonable option for patients with severe AR and severe LV dilatation (defined as LV end-systolic dimensions >50 mm, or LV end-diastolic dimension >65 mm), even if they are asymptomatic with preserved systolic function.[5]

Patients who are candidates for surgery with appropriate indications for intervention should undergo surgical AVR with either a mechanical or bioprosthetic aortic valve. However, in patients who have a prohibitive or very high surgical risk because of comorbidities, then medical therapy can be used to alleviate symptoms. Medical therapy with vasodilating drugs including angiotensin-converting enzyme (ACE) inhibitors or angiotensin II receptor blockers (ARBs) improves hemodynamic abnormalities in patients with AR and improves forward cardiac output. The data, however, are not supportive of the use of vasodilator therapy routinely in patients with chronic asymptomatic AR and normal LV systolic function.

FOLLOW-UP

Patients with asymptomatic severe AR with normal LV systolic function, who do not fulfill the criteria for AVR, should be followed closely with clinical exams and serial imaging. Such a strategy helps identify early on those patients who are progressing toward the threshold for surgery. Symptom development signals the need for surgical intervention. Consideration for surgery is also discussed if LV systolic function declines or the LV becomes severely dilated, even if the patient remains asymptomatic.

Routine postoperative care with close clinical follow-up and serial echocardiograms as clinically indicated is performed after AVR.

PATIENT CASE: MITRAL STENOSIS

Ms. R is a 35-year-old woman with history of moderate mitral stenosis secondary to rheumatic heart disease, and paroxysmal atrial fibrillation, who presented to the emergency department with 2 to 3 days history of fever, headache, palpitations, and mild shortness of breath. She was found to be febrile and tachycardic. ECG confirmed atrial fibrillation with rapid ventricular rate at 150 beats per minute. Her symptoms rapidly resolved with IV hydration, antipyretics and beta blockers, and her heart rate came down to 80 to 90 bpm. She was later diagnosed with influenza infection. Physical examination was noticeable for an irregular S_1S_2, loud S_1, and opening snap followed by a grade II/VI low-pitched diastolic murmur heard best at the apex while the patient was in the lateral decubitus position.

The issue of intervention on her MV was brought up during her hospitalization because of her presenting symptoms. When questioned further, Ms. R reported no symptoms of dyspnea on exertion or any other exercise-limiting symptom prior to her current presentation. Further testing included an echocardiogram that showed thickened and rheumatically deformed mitral leaflets with a hockey-stick deformity of the anterior leaflet (Figure 15-16), severe calcification of the subvalvular apparatus, and a mean pressure gradient across the valve of 5 mm Hg at a heart rate of 80 bpm. Several quantitative measures, including planimetry of the valve at the parasternal short-axis view (Figures 15-17 and 15-18), placed the valve area at 1.5 cm². All these measures are consistent with moderate mitral stenosis.

So if it is only moderate mitral stenosis, why did the patient have symptoms of dyspnea? It is important to note that conditions that increase cardiac output and blood flow through the heart (such as an infection), or shorten the diastolic emptying time (such as tachycardia from atrial fibrillation or fever) can raise the transmitral pressure gradient, increase the left atrial pressure, and cause pulmonary congestion even if the MV is not severely stenotic.

Because the patient is asymptomatic at baseline with no activity limitation, and the mitral stenosis is only moderate, a watchful waiting approach is recommended with serial imaging. Heart rate control for atrial fibrillation is also an integral part of her management. It is also entirely reasonable to refer for stress testing with hemodynamic evaluation to assess for true symptoms, functional capacity, and transvalvular gradient during exercise.

ETIOLOGY AND PATHOPHYSIOLOGY

Worldwide, rheumatic heart disease (RHD) remains the predominant cause of mitral stenosis (Figures 15-16 and 15-17), and the disease is more common in women compared to men.[15,16] Interestingly, up to 50% of patients with RHD are not aware of a history of rheumatic fever.[17] Much less common causes include radiation-induced valvular disease, congenital mitral abnormalities such as a parachute MV, and severe mitral annular calcification. It could also be a part of a systemic disease such as rheumatoid arthritis, systemic lupus erythematosus, Fabry disease, or carcinoid valve disease.

RHD causes an inflammatory process in the MV with progressive thickening, fibrosis, and calcification of the leaflet cusps, fusion of the leaflet commissures (Figure 15-17), and chordal shortening. Development of stenosis and clinical symptoms may take anywhere from 2 to 20 years.[18] A normal MV area is around 4.0 to 6.0 cm^2. In general, exertional symptoms start to develop when the area becomes <2.5 cm^2, and rest symptoms develop when the area is <1.5 cm^2.

As the MV area narrows, the transmitral pressure gradient and the left atrial pressure increase. The chronic elevation in left atrial pressure eventually leads to atrial remodeling with significant dilatation and fibrosis (Figure 15-19). In turn these changes increase the risk of development of atrial fibrillation and thrombus in situ formation.[19] Chronic exposure of the pulmonary vasculature to elevated pressures results in development of pulmonary congestion, reactive pulmonary HTN, and eventually, irreversible pulmonary HTN.

CLINICAL FEATURES AND PHYSICAL EXAMINATION

The duration of the asymptomatic phase varies by geographical location and can last anywhere from 2 to 44 years.[15,20] In a North American series, the rate of valve narrowing was about 0.1 cm^2/year.[21] Once symptoms develop, the prognosis significantly worsens, and the overall mortality increases unless the stenosis is corrected.[5]

Symptoms of mitral stenosis usually start with exertional dyspnea and decreased exercise tolerance. It is noteworthy that many patients fail to recognize their symptoms initially because the slow progression of the mitral stenosis is accompanied by a gradual reduction in activity. Other symptoms include hoarseness from the left atrial dilatation, palpitations secondary to the development of atrial fibrillation, or hemoptysis due to increased pulmonary pressure and vascular congestion. An embolic event may also develop secondary to the development of a thrombus within the left atrium. Of note, any condition that increases blood flow across the MV (such as fever or pregnancy), or shortens the diastolic filling time (such as tachycardia due to exertion or infection), can precipitate symptoms.

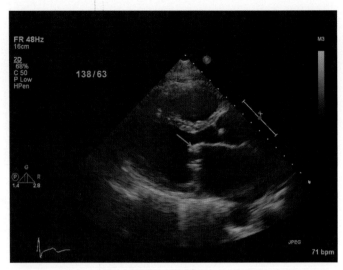

FIGURE 15-16 Parasternal long-axis view in a patient with mitral stenosis secondary to rheumatic valve disease. Rheumatic changes of the mitral valve are seen as thickened mitral leaflets, restricted motion, and diastolic doming due to the commissural fusion; the so-called hockey-stick deformity of the anterior leaflet (arrow).

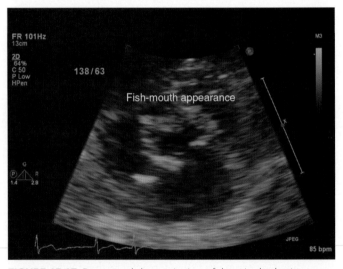

FIGURE 15-17 Parasternal short-axis view of the mitral valve in a patient with mitral stenosis secondary to rheumatic heart disease. The mitral leaflets are thickened with restricted opening, and the commissures are fused resulting in fish-mouth appearance of the mitral valve.

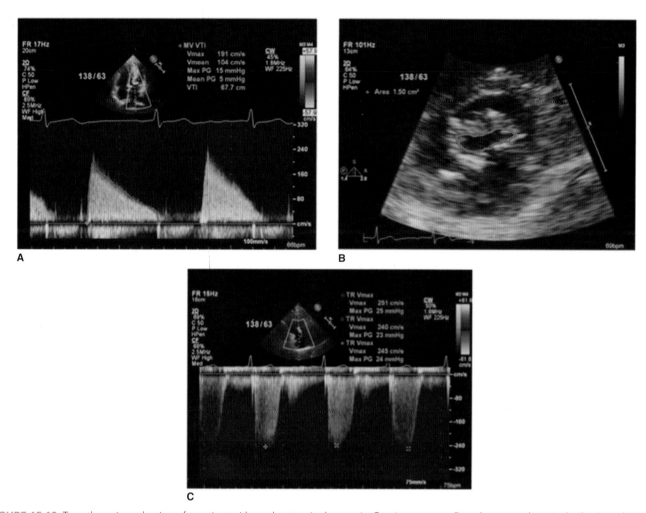

FIGURE 15-18 Transthoracic evaluation of a patient with moderate mitral stenosis. Continuous-wave Doppler across the mitral valve (panel A) shows the gradient to be 5 mm Hg. Planimetry of the mitral valve (panel B) in the short-axis view reveals the area to be 1.5 cm^2. Panel C allows the calculation of the systolic pulmonary pressure from the tricuspid regurgitation jet (25 mm Hg plus the right atrial pressure). All of this is consistent with moderate mitral stenosis.

Classic physical examination findings in patients with mitral stenosis include a normal apical LV impulse, a loud S_1 (this later becomes soft as the valve becomes more calcified and immobile), and an opening snap followed by a low-pitched diastolic rumble. The murmur is heard best at the apex in the left lateral decubitus position. The length of the murmur correlates with the severity of the stenosis. The shorter the time interval from S_2 to the opening snap, and the longer the murmur, the more severe the mitral stenosis; this reflects a significantly elevated left atrial pressure that forced the MV open early in diastole.

DIAGNOSIS

Left atrial enlargement is the most common finding on chest radiography in patients with severe mitral stenosis. As the disease progresses, findings of pulmonary congestion or edema or right atrial or right ventricular chamber enlargement might be seen. ECG often shows left atrial enlargement. Atrial fibrillation may also be seen.

Echocardiography is the main imaging tool for diagnosis and assessment of severity of mitral stenosis. Rheumatic changes of

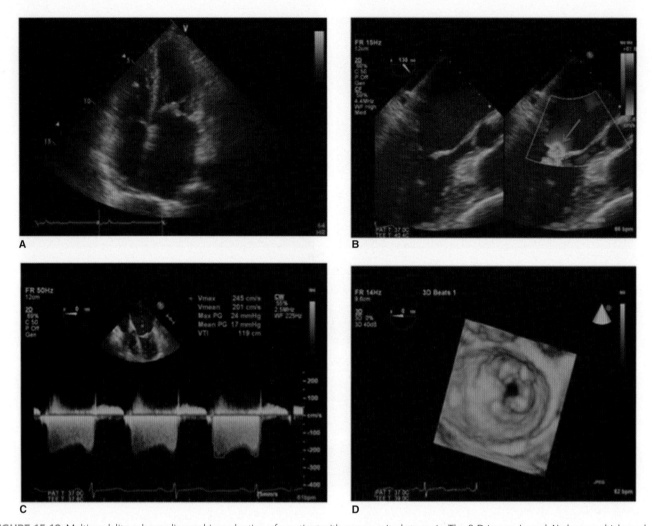

FIGURE 15-19 Multimodality echocardiographic evaluation of a patient with severe mitral stenosis. The 2-D image (panel A) shows a thickened and restricted mitral valve with secondary severely dilated atrium. The transesophageal echo image (panel B) shows restricted flow into the left ventricle (flow convergence zone). The transmitral gradient is significantly elevated at 17 mm Hg (panel C). The 3-D evaluation of the mitral valve (panel D) shows a significantly narrowed orifice with commissural fusion. The relative mobility of the leaflets, and lack of severe calcifications on the leaflets and submitral apparatus make this a favorable valve for percutaneous balloon valvotomy.

the MV are seen as thickened mitral leaflets, restricted motion, and diastolic doming due to the commissural fusion; the so-called hockey-stick deformity (Figure 15-16). The posterior leaflet is often more affected, and leaflet restriction is seen in both systole and diastole. Two-dimensional echo also evaluates the left atrial size, the LV size and function, and the right-sided cardiac chamber size and function (Figure 15-19). Hemodynamic severity is assessed by Doppler examination across the MV to measure the mean gradient and calculation of the MV area (Figures 15-18 and 15-19).[22] Guidelines also advocate the measurement of the MV area by planimetry if the valve is not too heavily calcified and obscured.[5] The short-axis view on the TTE demonstrates commissural fusion and allows planimetry of the mitral orifice (Figures 15-17 and 15-18). A MV area ≤1.5 cm^2 is considered severe. This usually corresponds to a transmitral mean gradient of >5 mm Hg to 10 mm Hg at a normal heart rate. However, the mean pressure gradient will vary greatly with changes in transvalvular flow and diastolic filling time.

Echocardiography also assesses the feasibility for percutaneous mitral balloon commissurotomy. One way to assess this is through the Wilkins score, which combines valve thickening, mobility, and calcification with subvalvular scarring in a 16-point scale; optimal results with balloon valvuloplasty are usually achieved with a score of 8 or less.

Exercise stress echocardiography is indicated if there is a discrepancy between the severity of mitral stenosis as assessed by echocardiography, and patient's symptoms. Resting and post exercise hemodynamic evaluation of the transvalvular gradient and pulmonary pressure is performed.[23]

DIFFERENTIAL DIAGNOSIS

Certain conditions, although uncommon, can mimic the hemodynamic abnormalities seen in mitral stenosis. These include a vegetation on the MV large enough to cause obstruction of flow, a large atrial myxoma, cor triatriatum sinistrum (a thick, fenestrated ridge that divides the left atrium), a degenerative stenotic mitral prosthetic valve, or a supravalvular mitral ring that is usually a part of the Shone complex.

MANAGEMENT

Valvular intervention is indicated in patients with severe mitral stenosis who develop symptoms. The options of intervention include percutaneous mitral balloon commissurotomy (PMBC), surgical commissurotomy, surgical mitral valve replacement (MVR), and rarely MV repair. The choice of therapy depends on the favorability of the valve morphology. In general PMBC is preferred if the valve is mobile, relatively thin, and free of calcium (Figures 15-19 and 15-20). Symptomatic patients with severe mitral stenosis and who have either unfavorable MV morphology or have previously failed PMBC should undergo surgical treatment.

It is also reasonable to consider PMBC in patients with very severe mitral stenosis (area <1 cm^2), patients who develop atrial

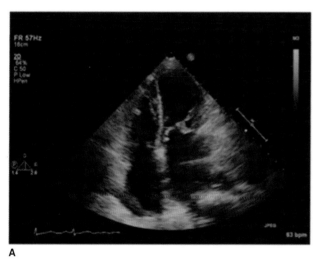
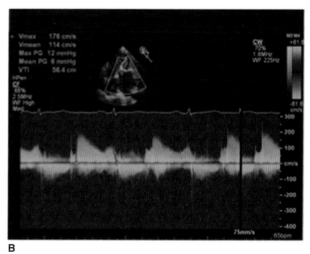

A   **B**

FIGURE 15-20 Echocardiographic evaluation of a patient with severe mitral stenosis post balloon valvotomy. The 4-chamber view shows improved opening of the mitral valve leaflets. Continuous-wave Doppler shows a significant drop in the transmitral pressure gradient to 6 mm Hg (from a previous mean gradient of 17 mm Hg).

fibrillation, or patients with exercise-induced hemodynamic abnormalities (mean gradient >15 mm Hg),[24] and favorable morphology for intervention, even if they are asymptomatic.[5]

Anticoagulation should be started for any patient who develops atrial fibrillation secondary to mitral stenosis.[25] Heart rate control is reasonable in patients with mitral stenosis and atrial fibrillation to control the heart rate, and in patients in normal sinus rhythm but with exercise-induced symptoms.

FOLLOW-UP

Rheumatic mitral stenosis is a slowly progressive disease, characterized by a prolonged latent phase between the initial rheumatic illness and the development of valve stenosis. The rate of progression is highly variable though, and thus when even mild stenosis develops, close clinical follow-up is recommended to assess development of symptoms with repeat TTE at intervals dictated by valve area. Less than severe mitral stenosis with an area of >1.5 cm^2 would require repeat imaging every 3 to 5 years, whereas very severe mitral stenosis with an area of <1 cm^2 would require yearly imaging.[5]

PATIENT CASE: MITRAL REGURGITATION

Mr. B, a 71-year-old man with a history of MV prolapse who was being followed at prolonged intervals for this problem, presented to the clinic for evaluation of a few weeks history of worsening dyspnea on exertion. He had been very active prior and would go biking several times a week. Physical examination revealed a laterally displaced LV apical impulse, loud P2, and a grade III/VI holosystolic murmur that radiates into the axilla. The murmur worsened with standing and with Valsalva maneuver.

TTE evaluation showed a mildly dilated LV with preserved systolic function, and severely dilated left atrium; a myxomatous MV with flail posterior valve (P2 scallop), and secondary severe mitral regurgitation (MR) (Figures 15-21 and 15-22). The systolic pulmonary pressure was also severely elevated in excess of 90 mm Hg. Due to his overall progressive symptoms, severe mitral regurgitation with leaflet prolapse and severe pulmonary HTN, Mr. B was referred to urgent surgery.

Because of the valve favorability, and the hospital expertise, Mr. B underwent MV repair rather than replacement. Trapezoid resection of the P2 flail segment was done with insertion of a 36 mm Physio II ring. Mr. B had a very smooth postoperative course and was discharged home a few days later. A repeat echocardiogram showed a well-seated mitral annuloplasty ring and a mean gradient of 2 mm Hg (Figure 15-23). Additionally, there was no mitral or periannular regurgitation, the EF dropped from 65% preoperatively to 51% postoperatively as expected (this is due to the increased afterload to the LV after removal of mitral regurgitation), and there was dramatic reverse remodeling of the LV (drop of the end diastolic volume from 178 to 125 mL and drop in the left atrial size to almost half). The patient feels almost back to normal now and is able to engage in any physical activity he wants with no limiting symptoms.

ETIOLOGY AND PATHOPHYSIOLOGY

Mitral regurgitation (MR) is a common valvular disorder that can arise from abnormalities of the MV or any of the surrounding structures. MR has many etiologies, which can be broadly divided into 2 categories. Primary MR, also termed organic MR, is secondary to abnormalities of 1 or more components of the valvular apparatus including the leaflets, chordae, papillary muscle, or mitral annulus. Degenerative MV disease (MV prolapse, flail leaflet) is the leading cause of primary MR in the United States, and ranges from myxomatous MV disease with redundant mitral leaflets and chordae (Figures 15-21, 15-24, and 15-25), to fibroelastic deficiency disease seen in older populations. Less common conditions include infective endocarditis, which may lead to leaflet perforation, deformity, and chordal rupture; congenital causes such as mitral cleft; drug-induced (anorectic drugs, ergotamine, bromocriptine); and mitral annular calcification. Rheumatic heart disease remains a common cause worldwide, but less so in the United States. Studies from North America show the prevalence of degenerative MV disease with mitral prolapse to be about 2% to 3%.[26]

Secondary or functional MR is due to significant LV dysfunction that is either caused by CAD, related MI (ischemic chronic secondary MR) (Figure 15-26), or idiopathic myocardial disease (nonischemic chronic secondary MR) (Figure 15-27). The MV itself is normal in these cases. The dilated LV causes papillary muscle displacement and leaflet tethering (especially if there are wall motion abnormalities involving the inferior or inferolateral wall), which in turn prevents mitral leaflet coaptation.

In acute MR, there is a sudden increase in the LV volume (preload). The LV compensates by enhanced inotropy. Effective cardiac output, however, drops because much of the flow is directed to the left atrium. This, in turn, might lead to pulmonary congestion and edema. If the patient tolerates the acute hemodynamic event, then he or she may progress to a chronic compensated state.

In chronic compensated MR, the LV dilates with development of eccentric hypertrophy, and the left atrium dilates to accommodate the increased preload at lower filling pressures.

CLINICAL FEATURES AND PHYSICAL EXAMINATION

Patients with compensated chronic severe MR might remain asymptomatic for years and it is still unclear what causes them to transition to a decompensated state with depressed myocardial contractility and low EF.[27] The most common symptoms that may develop include exertional dyspnea and fatigue, or palpitations secondary to the development of atrial fibrillation. With more advanced disease, the LV fails and patients may present with signs and symptoms of HF.

Physical exam cannot reliably distinguish primary from secondary causes of MR. The apical impulse may be enlarged and displaced laterally in patients with severe MR. The S$_1$ is usually soft, and a widely split S$_2$ is common. A diastolic rumble is sometimes heard and it reflects the increased blood flow across the MV. The systolic murmur of MR is usually heard best at the apex in the left

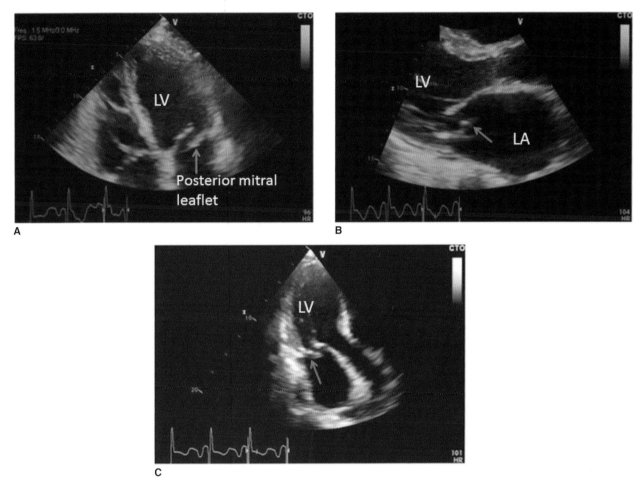

FIGURE 15-21 Echocardiographic evaluation of a patient with a flail mitral valve and secondary severe mitral regurgitation. Panels A-C show that the posterior leaflet tip (most likely the P2 scallop) prolapses and points into the left atrium (red arrow) leaving behind a large gap between the leaflets. Large left atrial size is also appreciated in panel B. Abbreviations: LA, left atrium; LV, left ventricle.

lateral decubitus position. With severe degenerative MR, the murmur is holosystolic and radiates into the axilla. Acute MR causes short, early systolic murmurs. MV prolapse might cause late onset of systolic murmur that changes in timing and loudness with various maneuvers that alter the preload and afterload. Signs of pulmonary HTN, such as a loud P2, are usually ominous and represent advanced disease.

DIAGNOSIS

Echocardiography is often enough to make a diagnosis of MR, determine its etiology (Figures 15-21, 15-24, and 15-25), assess its severity and possible deleterious sequelae on the cardiac chamber sizes and functions, and ultimately help build a treatment plan. It is important to note that due to the increased preload condition and normal or decreased afterload, the EF is higher in MR. Thus a normal LVEF is around 70%, and LV dysfunction is evident when it drops to below 60%.

Determination of the severity of MR is made on the basis of several qualitative and quantitative parameters including color jet area; vena contracta; continuous-wave Doppler intensity; and measurements of effective orifice area, regurgitant volume, and regurgitant

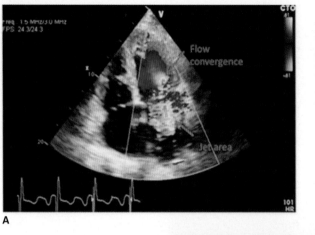

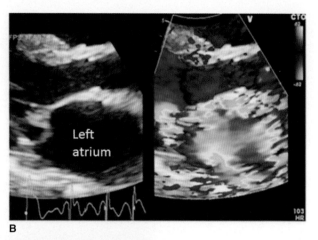

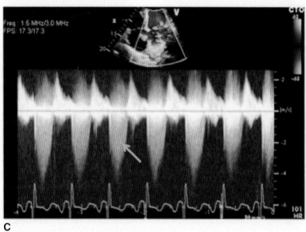

FIGURE 15-22 Doppler echocardiographic assessment in a patient with severe mitral regurgitation secondary to mitral valve prolapse. Panel A shows a large proximal convergence zone (seen in the left ventricle) and a large jet area seen in the left atrium. Panel B shows a large jet area in the left atrium. Panel C shows continuous-wave Doppler across the mitral valve; the regurgitation signal is dense and early peaking (green arrow). All of these findings are suggestive of severe mitral regurgitation.

fraction using the proximal isovelocity surface area or quantitative Doppler flow measurements (Figure 15-22 and Figure 15-28).[5,28] Flow reversal into the pulmonary veins during systole is also a sign of severe MR (Figure 15-29). TEE is invaluable to establish valvular anatomy and cause of MR before and during surgical repair (Figure 15-30)[29] or percutaneous intervention on the mitral valve.

Exercise testing with hemodynamic assessment is reasonable in patients with chronic MR when there is a discrepancy between clinical symptoms and echocardiographic findings. Exercise testing might also aid in determining functional capacity, and teasing out underlying symptoms.

MANAGEMENT

Treatment decisions are dependent on the severity of MR, the presence of symptoms, the possibility of successful valve repair rather than replacement, and the presence of LV systolic dysfunction. When surgical intervention is indicated, mitral repair is preferentially recommended over valve replacement if a successful and durable repair can be accomplished. Maintaining the native valve avoids the complications associated with prosthetic valves and the need for anticoagulation, and maintains the integrity of the mitral valve apparatus.[5,30,31]

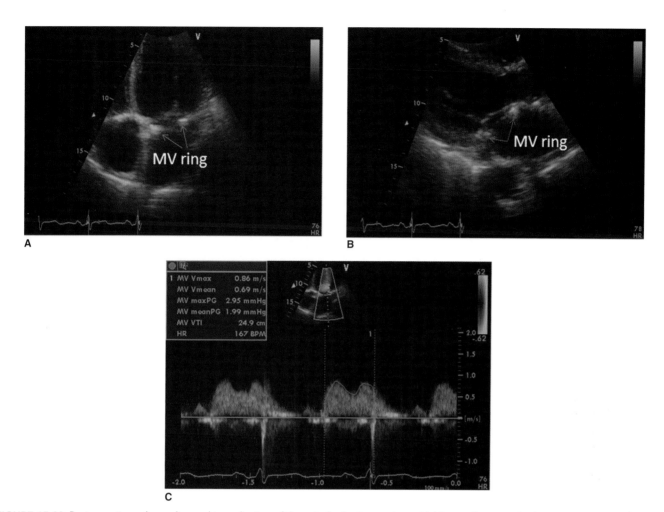

FIGURE 15-23 Postoperative echocardiographic evaluation of the mitral valve in a patient with history of severe mitral regurgitation. Mitral repair was done and a well-seated mitral ring is seen in the mitral annulus position. The transmitral gradient (panel C) shows normal pressure after surgery (mean gradient 2 mm Hg).

It is therefore critical that patients with severe MR who may require surgery are referred to experienced, high-volume surgical centers, where the chances of a successful repair are high. MR caused by nonrheumatic posterior MV prolapse can usually be repaired. On the other hand, involvement of the anterior mitral leaflet or both leaflets, or having a calcified or rheumatic mitral valve diminishes the likelihood of repair, even in experienced hands.[12]

Patients with symptomatic severe MR should be referred for surgical intervention. Even mild symptoms portend a worse outcome, and patients should be referred for treatment as early as possible. Mitral valve surgery is recommended for chronic severe primary MR and LV dysfunction (LVEF 30%-60% and/or LVESD ≥40 mm), even if the patient is asymptomatic. MV repair is also reasonable in asymptomatic patients with severe MR and preserved LV function if there is a high likelihood of surgical success (>90% success rate), or if the patient develops atrial fibrillation or resting pulmonary HTN.

For severely symptomatic patients (NYHA class III to IV) with chronic severe primary MR who have favorable anatomy and a reasonable life expectancy but who have a prohibitive surgical risk because of severe comorbidities, an alternative therapy is now available. Transcatheter mitral valve repair using the MitraClip device has been shown to reduce the severity of MR and improve symptoms (Figures 15-31 and 15-32).

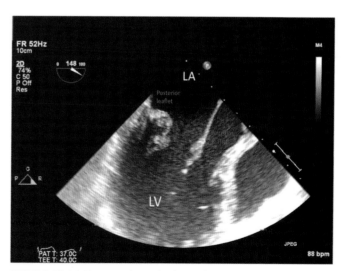

FIGURE 15-24 Transesophageal echocardiogram at the mid esophagus level; long-axis view showing myxomatous changes of the mitral valve with elongation of the anterior leaflet and focal thickening of the posterior leaflet. Abbreviations: LA, left atrium; LV, left ventricle.

PROGNOSIS AND FOLLOW-UP

Close clinical follow-up and serial imaging is indicated in patients with chronic MR to assess for the development of symptoms, and examine for changes in severity of MR and LV size and function. TTE follow-up every 3 to 5 years is recommended for mild MR, and every 1 to 2 years for moderate MR, unless clinical status suggests a worsening in severity.

In patients with severe asymptomatic MR, annual or semiannual surveillance of LV function (estimated by LVEF and end-systolic dimension) and pulmonary artery pressure should be carried out. Progression to symptomatic severe MR varies from patient to patient, but once symptoms develop the prognosis is considerably poorer. For this reason careful surveillance is mandatory.

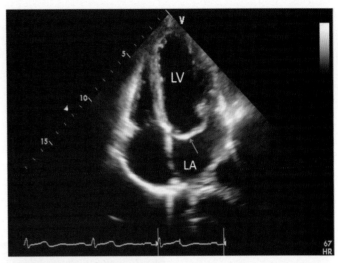

FIGURE 15-25 Transthoracic echocardiogram; 4-chamber view. There is prolapse of the anterior mitral valve leaflet (red arrow) in this patient with myxomatous mitral valve disease. Abbreviations: LA, left atrium; LV, left ventricle.

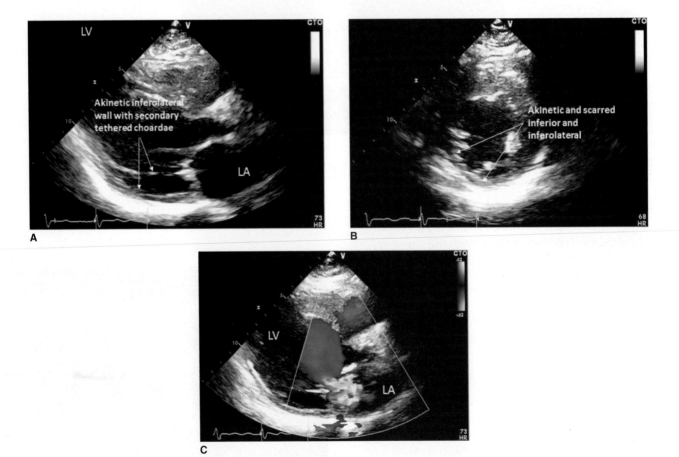

FIGURE 15-26 Transthoracic echocardiogram from a patient with ischemic cardiomyopathy. Panels A and B show the akinetic and scarred inferior and inferolateral left ventricular walls. The chordae and the posterior mitral leaflet become tethered and restricted secondary to ventricular remodeling and associated papillary muscle displacement. Posteriorly directed mitral regurgitation develops as a result (panel C). Abbreviations: LA, left atrium; LV, left ventricle.

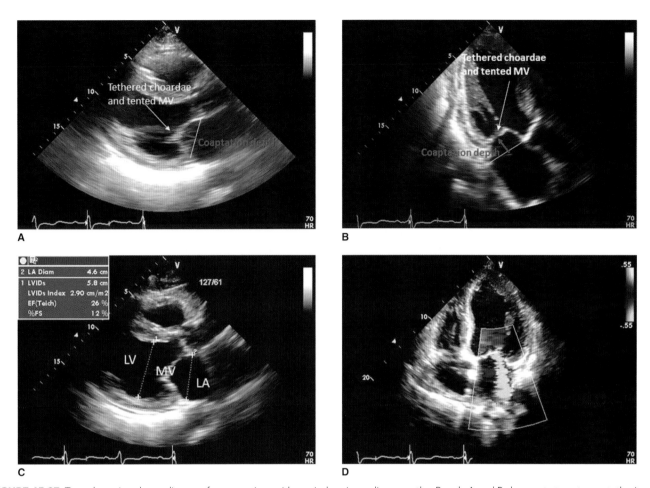

FIGURE 15-27 Transthoracic echocardiogram from a patient with nonischemic cardiomyopathy. Panels A and B demonstrate extreme tethering of the mitral valve leaflets. Because of the tethering, the mitral leaflets are tented into the LV cavity instead of coapting just below the mitral annulus. The extent of tethering can be measured by the coaptation depth, which is the distance from the mitral valve annulus to the coaptation point of the mitral valve leaflets. Panel C shows a significantly dilated left ventricle with secondary tethering of the mitral valve chordae and the mitral leaflets themselves. Leaflet tethering results in moderate to severe mitral regurgitation (panel D). Abbreviations: LA, left atrium; LV, left ventricle; MV, mitral valve.

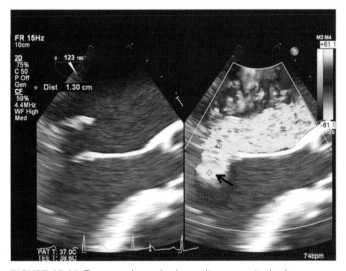

FIGURE 15-28 Transesophageal echocardiogram; mitral valve assessment at 120 degrees. Myxomatous changes of the mitral valve are present. A flail posterior mitral valve leaflet is present with associated severe mitral regurgitation. Quantitative measures of severity were determined by an effective regurgitant orifice (ERO) area = 1.2 cm^2, and a calculated regurgitant volume by PISA method = 100 cm^3.

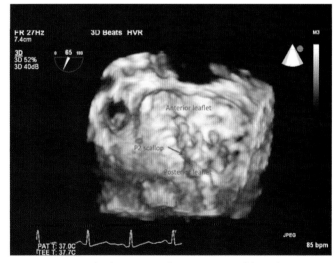

FIGURE 15-29 Pulsed-wave Doppler assessment of the pulmonary vein in a patient with severe mitral regurgitation. Note the backward flow of blood into the pulmonary veins (arrow) during systole (systolic flow reversal) due to the severity of the regurgitation flow.

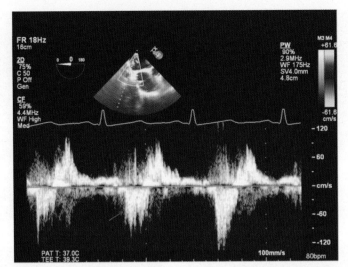

FIGURE 15-30 Three-dimensional assessment of the mitral valve on transesophageal echocardiogram. A bulging mass is seen in the middle of the lower leaflet of the mitral valve. This represents a flail P2 scallop (red arrow).

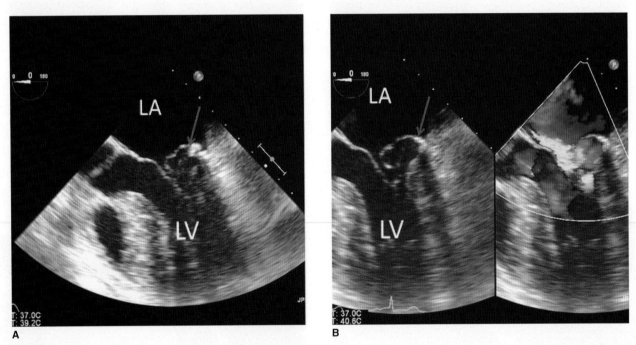

FIGURE 15-31 Transesophageal echocardiogram at the midesophageal level focusing on the mitral valve in a patient with severe mitral regurgitation. The mitral valve is myxomatous with prominent prolapse of the P2 scallop (red arrow). The color Doppler image (panel B) shows severe, anteriorly directed mitral regurgitation.

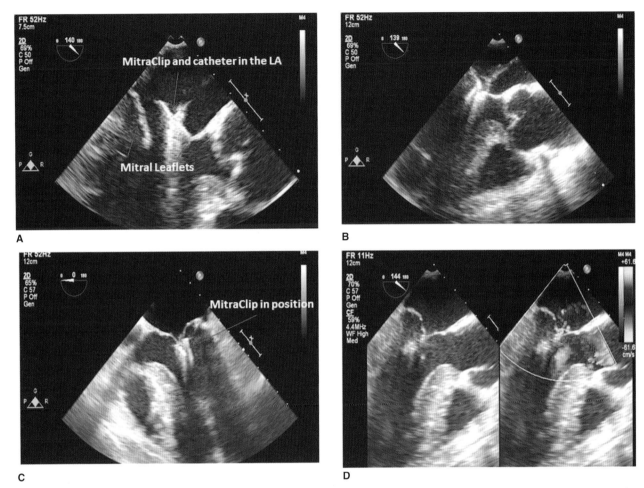

FIGURE 15-32 Echocardiogram during a transcatheter mitral repair procedure in a patient with severe myxomatous mitral regurgitation. Panels A and B show the catheter and the MitraClip as it enters the left atrium heading towards the mitral leaflets. The MitraClip attaches to the leaflet tips and is deployed. Panels C and D show the final result: the MitraClip is well attached to the leaflet tips and there is only trivial residual mitral regurgitation.

REFERENCES

1. Eveborn G, Schirmer H, Heggelund G. The evolving epidemiology of valvular aortic stenosis:. the Tromsø study. *Heart.* 2013;99:396.

2. Otto CM, Bonow RO. Valvular heart disease. In: Libby P, Bonow RO, Mann DL, Zipes DP, eds. *Braunwald's Heart Disease: A Textbook of Cardiovascular Medicine.* 8th ed. Philadelphia, PA: WB Saunders; 2007:1625-1712.

3. Rosenhek R, Binder T, Porenta G, et al. Predictors of outcome in severe, asymptomatic aortic stenosis. *N Engl J Med.* 2000;343:611-617.

4. Pellikka PA, Sarano ME, Nishimura RA, et al. Outcome of 622 adults with asymptomatic, hemodynamically significant aortic stenosis during prolonged follow-up. *Circulation.* 2005;111:3290-3295.

5. Nishimura RA, Otto CM, Bonow RO, et al. 2014 AHA/ACC guideline for the management of patients with valvular heart disease: a report of the American College of Cardiology/American Heart Association Task Force on Practice Guidelines. *Circulation.* 2014;129:2440-2492.

6. Clavel MA, Webb JG, Rodes-Cabau J, et al. Comparison between transcatheter and surgical prosthetic valve implantation in patients with severe aortic stenosis and reduced left ventricular ejection fraction. *Circulation*. 2010;122:1928-1936.

7. Kodali SK, Williams MR, Smith CR, et al. Two-year outcomes after transcatheter or surgical aortic-valve replacement. *N Engl J Med*. 2012;366:1686-1695.

8. Makkar RR, Fontana GP, Jilaihawi H, et al. Transcatheter aortic-valve replacement for inoperable severe aortic stenosis. *N Engl J Med*. 2012;366:1696-1704.

9. Leon MB, Smith CR, Mack MJ, et al. Transcatheter or surgical aortic-valve replacement in intermediate-risk patients. *N Engl J Med*. 2016;374(17):1609-1620.

10. Enriquez-Sarano M, Tajik AJ. Clinical practice. aortic regurgitation. *N Engl J Med*. 2004; 351:1539.

11. Rigolin VH, Bonow RO. Hemodynamic characteristics and progression to heart failure in regurgitant lesions. *Heart Fail Clin*. 2006;2:453-460.

12. Maganti K, Rigolin VH, Sarano ME, and Bonow RO. Valvular heart disease: diagnosis and management. *Mayo Clin Proc*. 2010;85(5):483-500.

13. Borer JS, Bonow RO. Contemporary approach to aortic and mitral regurgitation. *Circulation*. 2003;108:2432-2438.

14. Dujardin KS, Enriquez-Sarano M, Schaff HV, et al. Mortality and morbidity of aortic regurgitation in clinical practice: a long-term follow-up study. *Circulation*. 1999;99:1851-1857.

15. Horstkotte D, Niehues R, Strauer BE. Pathomorphological aspects, aetiology and natural history of acquired mitral valve stenosis. *Eur Heart J*. 1991;12:55-60.

16. Zühlke L, Engel ME, Karthikeyan G, et al. Characteristics, complications, and gaps in evidence-based interventions in rheumatic heart disease: the Global Rheumatic Heart Disease Registry (the REMEDY study). *Eur Heart J*. 2015;36:1115.

17. Selzer A, Cohn KE. Natural history of mitral stenosis: a review. *Circulation*. 1972;45:878.

18. Marcus R, Sareli P, Pocock W, Barlow J. The spectrum of severe rheumatic mitral valve disease in a developing country. Correlations among clinical presentation, surgical pathologic findings, and hemodynamic sequelae. *Ann Intern Med*. 1994;120:177.

19. Nunes MC, Handschumacher MD, Levine RA, et al. Role of LA shape in predicting embolic cerebrovascular events in mitral stenosis: mechanistic insights from 3D echocardiography. *JACC Cardiovasc Imaging*. 2014;7:453.

20. World Health Organization. *Rheumatic Fever and Rheumatic Heart Disease: Report of a WHO Expert Panel*. October 29-November 1, 2001. Geneva: WHO; 2004.

21. Sagie A, Freitas N, Padial LR, et al. Doppler echocardiographic assessment of long-term progression of mitral stenosis in 103 patients: valve area and right heart disease. *J Am Coll Cardiol*. 1996;28:472.

22. Baumgartner H, Hung J, Bermejo J. Echocardiographic assessment of valve stenosis: EAE/ASE recommendations for clinical practice. *Eur J Echocardiogr*. 2009;10:1-25.

23. Reis G, Motta MS, Barbosa MM, et al. Dobutamine stress echocardiography for noninvasive assessment and risk stratification of patients with rheumatic mitral stenosis. *J Am Coll Cardiol*. 2004;43:393-401.

24. Otto CM, Davis KB, Reid CL, et al. Relation between pulmonary artery pressure and mitral stenosis severity in patients undergoing balloon mitral commissurotomy. *Am J Cardiol*. 1993;71:874-878.

25. Perez-Gomez F, Alegria E, Berjon J, et al. Comparative effects of antiplatelet, anticoagulant, or combined therapy in patients with valvular and nonvalvular atrial fibrillation: a randomized multicenter study. *J Am Coll Cardiol*. 2004;44:1557-1566.

26. Singh JP, Evans JC, Levy D, et al. Prevalence and clinical determinants of mitral, tricuspid, and aortic regurgitation (the Framingham Heart Study). *Am J Cardiol*. 1999;83:897.

27. Gaasch W, Meyer T. Left ventricular response to mitral regurgitation: implications for management. *Circulation*. 2008;118:2298.

28. Zoghbi WA, Enriquez-Sarano M, Foster E, et al. Recommendations for evaluation of the severity of native valvular regurgitation with two-dimensional and Doppler echocardiography. *J Am Soc Echocardiogr*. 2003;16:777-802.

29. Saiki Y, Kasegawa H, Kawase M, et al. Intraoperative TEE during mitral valve repair: does it predict early and late postoperative mitral valve dysfunction? *Ann Thorac Surg*. 1998;66:1277-1281.

30. Goldman ME, Mora F, Guarino T, et al. Mitral valvuloplasty is superior to valve replacement for preservation of left ventricular function: an intraoperative two-dimensional echocardiographic study. *J Am Coll Cardiol*. 1987;10:568-575.

31. David TE, Ivanov J, Armstrong S, et al. A comparison of outcomes of mitral valve repair for degenerative disease with posterior, anterior, and bileaflet prolapse. *J Thorac Cardiovasc Surg*. 2005;130:1242-1249.

16 CARDIOTOXICITY

Daniel Lenihan, MD, FACC
Jai Singh, MD

PATIENT CASES

CASE 1

A 51-year-old woman presents to the emergency department with dyspnea on exertion, orthopnea, and paroxysmal nocturnal dyspnea. She has a history of newly diagnosed breast cancer having recently completed treatment with anthracycline followed by trastuzumab. An echocardiogram was ordered, which revealed moderately dilated left ventricle (LV) and severely depressed LV systolic function (left ventricular ejection fraction; LVEF 25%) with global hypokinesis (Figure 16-1).

CASE 2

An 82-year-old man with a history of advanced renal cell cancer presents with asymmetric left leg swelling and pain. He has been receiving cancer treatment with a vascular endothelial growth factor (VEGF) signaling pathway inhibitor (pazopanib). A venous duplex ultrasound of the lower extremities was ordered, which confirmed a deep vein thrombosis (DVT) in the left leg from the proximal femoral vein to the calf veins (Figure 16-2). He was placed on lifelong anticoagulation with Warfarin.

CASE 3

A 70-year-old man with a history of metastatic prostate cancer on chronic androgen-deprivation therapy presents complaining of shortness of breath with exertion and fatigue. Workup was notable for an electrocardiogram (ECG) with ischemic ST-T wave changes in the anterior leads and blood testing revealing an elevated cardiac troponin I. He underwent coronary angiography that demonstrated a significant stenosis in the proximal left anterior descending artery (Figure 16-3). He underwent a stenting procedure and was placed on aspirin, clopidogrel, and atorvastatin.

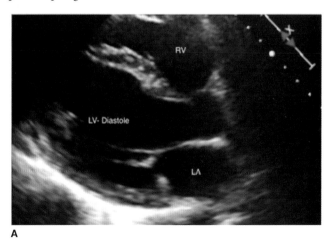
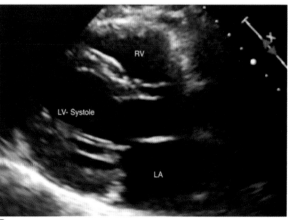

A   **B**

FIGURE 16-1 Severe systolic dysfunction with global hypokinesis and left ventricular dilation in a patient with anthracycline ± trastuzumab related cardiomyopathy. Images are similar with image A in diastole and image B in systole representing severe cardiomyopathy.

INTRODUCTION

There are approximately 15.5 million cancer survivors in the United States and that number is expected to increase to more than 20 million by 2026.[1] As a result, cardiovascular disease (CVD) has become the second leading cause of long-term morbidity and mortality among cancer survivors.[2,3] Understanding the cardiac toxic effects of contemporary cancer therapies and the cancer itself has become of paramount importance and has been the impetus for the discipline of cardio-oncology.

EPIDEMIOLOGY

- Current anticancer therapies are associated with unique and various degrees of direct as well as indirect cardiovascular (CV) insults.

- The true incidence of cancer treatment-induced CV injury is likely underreported and varies widely, depending on the type and duration of therapy, and underlying patient comorbidities.

- Among older cancer survivors, CVD is a more common contributor than cancer to mortality.[1,4]

- Survivors of childhood cancers are at a 15-fold increased risk of developing congestive heart failure (CHF) and at a 7-fold increased risk of premature death due to cardiac causes when compared to the general population.[5]

- The U.S. National Health and Nutrition Examination Survey reported adult cancer survivors, compared to noncancer controls, were more likely to report ischemic heart disease (13.7% vs 5.2%) and CHF (7.9% vs 2.1%).[6]

- Anthracyclines and mediastinal radiation therapy reveal a dose-dependent increased risk of cardiotoxicity (LV systolic dysfunction).

- A contemporary large population-based cohort study with a median follow-up of 20 years revealed a 4.5-fold increased risk of CHF in Hodgkin lymphoma survivors treated with ≥250 mg/m^2 of doxorubicin compared to those not treated with doxorubicin or mediastinal radiation therapy.[7]

- Mediastinal radiation therapy ≥30 Gy was associated with a 2.8- to 4.7-fold increase in CHF.[7]

- A combination of lower dose anthracyclines (≤250 mg/m^2 doxorubicin) plus mediastinal radiation therapy resulted in a 5.4-fold increased risk of CHF.[7]

- In contemporary randomized controlled breast cancer trials for trastuzumab, there appears to be an increase in symptomatic heart failure (HF; 0.6%-4.1%) and a significant increase in asymptomatic LV systolic dysfunction (3%-19%), with about one-third having persistent LV systolic dysfunction.[8,9]

- Of note, roughly 80% of those enrolled in clinical trials for trastuzumab, similar to most cancer trials, did not have a history of CVD or HF, and as such real-world registry data suggest a higher rate of trastuzumab-associated cardiotoxicity.[10,11]

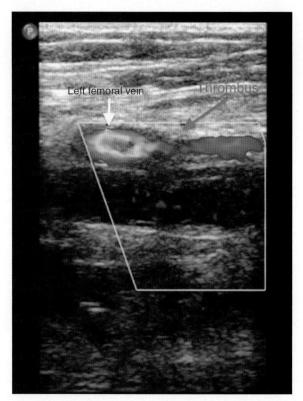

FIGURE 16-2 Thrombus causing turbulent flow in the left proximal femoral vein and extending to the calf veins in a patient receiving a VEGF signaling pathway inhibitor (pazopanib) for advanced renal cell carcinoma.

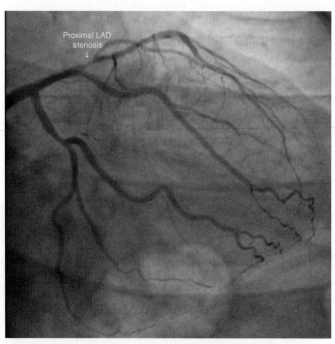

FIGURE 16-3 Patient with the development of a symptomatic high-grade severe stenosis of the proximal left anterior descending (LAD) artery while receiving chronic androgen-deprivation therapy (ADT) for metastatic prostate cancer.

ETIOLOGY AND PATHOPHYSIOLOGY

- CVD and cancer are intricately linked due to shared common risk factors, coexistence of both diseases in an aging population, and direct adverse effects of cancer treatments on CV health.
- There are several purported mechanisms of anthracycline toxicity including: DNA damage caused by disruption of the normal catalytic cycle of topoisomerase 2β causing DNA double-strand breaks and activation of apoptosis, as well as changes in the transcriptome causing mitochondrial dysfunction and generation of reactive oxygen species.[12,13]
- Trastuzumab blocks the ErB2 (aka Her2) pathway, which normally acts as a response/repair mechanism to myocardial injury.[14]
- Radiation therapy increases the risk of early and complex atherosclerosis in any vascular bed within the radiation field.[15]
- Inhibitors of VEGF affect angiogenesis, endothelial cell survival, vasodilatation, and cardiac contractile function with resulting hypertension (HTN), the most common on-target CV effect.[16]
- Table 16-1 provides a more comprehensive list of treatment-related cardiac effects by class of therapy.

RISK FACTORS

Non-treatment-related modifiers of CV risk include:

- Older age
- Traditional CV risk factors: Smoking, HTN, diabetes mellitus, and dyslipidemia
- Borderline low baseline LVEF 50% to 54%
- History of atherosclerotic CVD (myocardial infarction, cerebrovascular disease, peripheral vascular disease)
- History of recovery from HF
- Valvular heart disease
- Frailty
- Poor cardiorespiratory fitness

DIAGNOSIS

A comprehensive history and physical examination should be performed in all cancer patients prior to initiating potentially cardiotoxic therapy with serial CV assessment during and after treatment completion.

BEFORE CANCER THERAPY

- Screen for traditional CV risk factors (smoking, HTN, diabetes mellitus, dyslipidemia, physical activity, diet, and body mass index [BMI]).
- Screen for a history of cardiomyopathy, CHF, and CAD.

- Screen for history of arrhythmias/syncope, or QT interval >500 ms.
- Obtain baseline ECG to monitor for any conduction abnormalities, arrhythmias, or suggestion of prior myocardial infarction.
- Identify the planned type of therapy and the associated potential cardiotoxic effects (Table 16-1), in particular, the cumulative dose of anthracyclines, and dose/location of mediastinal radiation.

DURING CANCER THERAPY

- Screen for cardiac complications and continue to screen for traditional CV risk factors (smoking, HTN, diabetes mellitus, dyslipidemia, physical activity, diet, and BMI).
- Monitor for syncope or hypotension.
- Surveillance ECG to monitor QT interval and development of any conduction disease or ischemic injury.
- In individuals with clinical signs (ie, elevated jugular venous pressure) or symptoms (ie, orthopnea, paroxysmal nocturnal dyspnea, lower extremity edema, dyspnea on exertion) of cardiac compromise, a 2-dimensional echocardiogram (2D echo) should be performed.
  - If an echocardiogram is not technically feasible, then a cardiac magnetic resonance imaging (MRI) or a multigated acquisition (MUGA) scan should be performed.
- In asymptomatic individuals considered at moderate to high risk for LV systolic dysfunction (ie, history of cardiac risk factors or disease plus anthracycline/mediastinal radiation at any dose, doxorubicin dose ≥250 mg/m², mediastinal radiation ≥30 Gy, or low-dose anthracycline plus mediastinal radiation), a 2D echo should be considered for routine surveillance.
- Periodic 2D echo surveillance may be considered in patients with metastatic breast cancer continuing to receive trastuzumab indefinitely.
- Measurement of circulating natriuretic peptides, cardiac troponins, or echocardiographic strain can provide some diagnostic and prognostic utility in asymptomatic cancer patients receiving cardiotoxic therapies.[17-19]

AFTER CANCER THERAPY

- Continue to screen for cardiac disease and traditional CV risk factors (smoking, diabetes mellitus, HTN, dyslipidemia, BMI).
- In individuals with signs or symptoms of cardiac compromise, a complete 2D echo should be performed in addition to checking serum cardiac biomarkers (eg, troponin I, BNP, NT-proBNP).
  - Cardiac MRI or MUGA if 2D echo is not technically feasible.
- In asymptomatic patients considered at moderate to high risk of LV systolic dysfunction, a screening 2D echo may be considered 6 to 12 months after completion of cancer therapy.

Table 16-1 Common Cancer Therapies and Associated Cardiotoxicities

Class	Examples	Cardiotoxicity	Comments
Traditional Therapies			
Anthracyclines	Doxorubicin	LV systolic dysfunction	Highest risk:
	Daunorubicin	CHF	$\geq$250 mg/m^2 doxorubicin
	Epirubicin		$\geq$600 mg/m^2 epirubicin
Radiation		Premature CAD	$\geq$30 Gy
		Valvular heart disease	Field of exposure
		Myocarditis/pericarditis	
		Arrhythmia	
Alkylating agents	Cyclophosphamide	CHF	With higher dose
		Myocarditis/pericarditis	
Platinum	Cisplatin	HTN	
	Carboplatin	Myocardial ischemia	
	Oxaliplatin	LV hypertrophy	
Antimetabolites	5-fluorouracil	Myocardial ischemia	
		Vasospasm	
Antimicrotubules	Paclitaxel	Arrhythmias	
		Thrombosis	
Novel Therapies			
HER-2 inhibitors	Trastuzumab	LV systolic dysfunction	
		CHF	
VEGF signaling pathway (VSP) inhibitors	Bevacizumab	HTN	
	Sunitinib	Proteinuria	Similar to
	Sorafenib	Thromboembolic (arterial and venous)	preeclampsia
	Pazopanib		
	Axitinib	Cardiomyopathy	
Tyrosine kinase inhibitors	Imatinib	Rare	
	Dasatinib	Pulmonary HTN	
	Nilotinib	Peripheral arterial disease	
	Ponatinib	Vascular events	Not a class effect
	Ibrutinib	Atrial fibrillation	
	Everolimus	Hypercholesterolemia	
	(mTOR inhibitor)	Hypertriglyceridemia	
		Hyperglycemia	

(Continued)

Table 16-1 Common Cancer Therapies and Associated Cardiotoxicities (Continued)

Class	Examples	Cardiotoxicity	Comments
Immunomodulators	Thalidomide	Venous thromboembolic	Thromboprophylaxis with aspirin or anticoagulation
	Lenalidomide	Arterial thromboembolic	
	Pomalidomide		
Proteasome inhibitors	Bortezomib	Rare	
	Carfilzomib	HTN	
		CHF	
		Venous thromboembolic	
		Arrhythmia	
Immune checkpoint inhibitors	Nivolumab (PD-1)	Autoimmune myocarditis	Case reports
	Pembrolizumab (PD-1)		
Androgen-deprivation therapy	Leuprolide	Hypercholesterolemia	CV risk greater in those with prior CV events
	Goserelin	Hyperglycemia	
	Bicalutamide	Increase in subcutaneous fat	
	Enzalutamide	CVD	

DIFFERENTIAL DIAGNOSIS

- Figure 16-4 provides a breakdown of the broad spectrum of potential CV effects from cancer therapy and the cancer itself by categories including vascular, metabolic, electrical, structural, and myocardial.
- Direct CV involvement from a primary cancer
  - Cardiac amyloidosis from plasma cell dyscrasia
  - Cardiac metastasis
  - Tricuspid valve disease resulting from carcinoid tumors
- Age-related progression of known CVD and/or structural heart disease
- Uncontrolled traditional CV risk factors (smoking, HTN, diabetes mellitus, dyslipidemia)
- Viral-induced myocarditis/pericarditis
- Cardiac tumors
  - Myxoma
  - Papillary fibroelastoma
  - Rhabdomyoma
  - Angiosarcoma

MANAGEMENT

NONPHARMACOLOGIC

- In addition to close monitoring for early detection of cardiotoxicity, as mentioned above, early treatment of any CV dysfunction is vital. Appreciating the common CV effects by therapy type (Table 16-1) will assist in remaining vigilant.

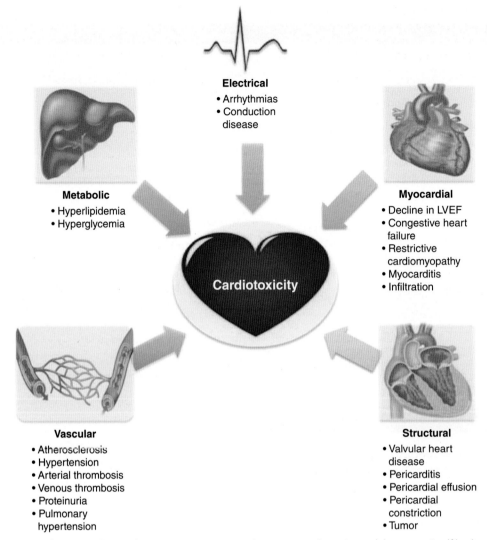

Electrical
- Arrhythmias
- Conduction disease

Metabolic
- Hyperlipidemia
- Hyperglycemia

Myocardial
- Decline in LVEF
- Congestive heart failure
- Restrictive cardiomyopathy
- Myocarditis
- Infiltration

Cardiotoxicity

Vascular
- Atherosclerosis
- Hypertension
- Arterial thrombosis
- Venous thrombosis
- Proteinuria
- Pulmonary hypertension

Structural
- Valvular heart disease
- Pericarditis
- Pericardial effusion
- Pericardial constriction
- Tumor

FIGURE 16-4 The spectrum of common CV conditions in cancer survivors due to cancer therapies and the cancer itself broken down by 5 broad categories including vascular, metabolic, electrical, structural, and myocardial.

MEDICATIONS

- Maintain adherence to standard guidelines for management of HTN, hyperlipidemia, diabetes mellitus, HF, ischemic heart disease, and valvular heart disease, which also underscores the expanded spectrum of cardiotoxicities beyond LV systolic dysfunction.[20-25]

- Additional management considerations with regards to certain cancer therapies include:
  - Daily blood pressure checks in individuals undergoing VEGF inhibitor therapy.
  - Early and aggressive treatment of HTN to a goal of at least <140/90 mm Hg per the guidelines.[22]
  - Given a signal for potential prevention of chemotherapy-induced LV dysfunction, renin-angiotensin system inhibitors and beta blockers should be considered first-line therapy options.[26]

- Caution using nondihydropyridines (verapamil, diltiazem) in tyrosine kinase inhibitor (TKI) induced HTN as they inhibit cytochrome P450, which can delay the metabolism of TKIs.[27]

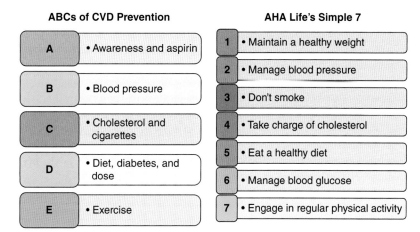

FIGURE 16-5 The ABCs of cardiovascular disease (CVD) prevention developed and applied to cancer patients at Vanderbilt University Medical Center, similar to the AHA Life's Simple 7 campaign.

- Once a patient develops HF or asymptomatic LV systolic dysfunction due to chemotherapy, guideline-directed medical therapy (GDMT) for HF should be intiated.[25]
- Early discontinuation of HF therapy is not recommended.

REFERRAL OR HOSPITALIZATION

- Any signs of ischemic heart disease, LV systolic dysfunction, HF, or structural heart disease should be referred to a cardiologist or cardio-oncologist.

PREVENTION

Among all cancer patients, rapid identification and treatment of CV risk factors is vital to reduce cardiotoxicity. The American Heart Association recently introduced the concept of promoting "ideal cardiovascular health" and recommending the following strategic impact goals: "By 2020, to improve the cardiovascular health of all Americans by 20% while reducing deaths from cardiovascular diseases and stroke by 20%."[28] This has been endorsed by the American Cancer Society as well and includes the following 7 metrics (Life's Simple 7), which should be evaluated and managed at each visit. Four of the metrics (smoking, weight, physical activity, and diet) are health behaviors and 3 of the metrics (blood pressure, cholesterol, and glucose) are health factors. Figure 16-5 lists a practical ABCDE algorithm for CVD prevention, which can be applied to all cancer patients with notable parallel to the goals of the Life's Simple 7 campaign.[29]

- **Smoking:** Never smoker or quit >12 months ago
  - Current smoking is similar in cancer survivors compared to the general population and is associated with increased risk of all cause mortality, cancer-related and CV-related mortality, secondary malignancies, and treatment-related cardiotoxicities.[30,31]
- **Body mass index:** BMI <25 kg/m^2
  - Among cancer survivors focus should be on weight maintenance and avoidance of weight gain especially in cancer patients with multiple comorbidities.

- **Physical activity:** ≥150 minutes/week of moderate intensity physical activity or ≥75 minutes/week of vigorous intensity activity or combination
  - Adherence to guideline recommendations for physical activity has been associated with improved overall mortality among colorectal, breast, and prostate cancer survivors, and reduction of CV events independent of BMI among nonmetastatic breast cancer survivors.[32-34]
  - Current ongoing exercise trials are investigating the preventative efficacy of exercise 24 hours before every chemotherapy cycle (ClinicalTrials.gov identifier: NCT02006979).
- **Diet:** Four to five components of a healthy dietary pattern
  - 4.5 cups of fruit and vegetables daily
  - 3.5 cups of whole grains daily
  - 2.5 servings of fish per week
  - Avoid salt
  - Avoid sugar
  - Among survivors of colorectal and breast cancer, adherence to a healthy dietary pattern has been associated with reduced all-cause mortality.[35,36]
- **Blood pressure:** BP <120/80 mm Hg untreated
  - HTN is more prevalent in cancer survivors compared to the general population.[37]
- **Cholesterol:** Total cholesterol <200 mg/dL untreated
  - Four statin benefit groups per the new 2013 guidelines:[24]
    - Established atherosclerotic cardiovascular disease (ASCVD)
    - LDL ≥190 mg/dL
    - 40 to 75 years of age with diabetes mellitus and LDL 70 to 189 mg/dL
    - Any individual not in the previous 3 categories with an estimated 10-year risk of CVD ≥7.5% by the new ASCVD risk calculator
  - Small clinical trial of 40 patients undergoing anthracycline-containing chemotherapy showed atorvastatin use appeared to be protective at 6-month follow-up for LV systolic dysfunction compared to controls.[38]
- **Glucose:** Fasting plasma glucose <100 mg/dL untreated
  - Having diabetes mellitus increases all-cause mortality among cancer patients.[39]
  - Adherence to the American Diabetes Association (ADA) guidelines is important including screening all cancer patients for type 2 diabetes mellitus and for prediabetes, ie, fasting plasma glucose of 100 mg/dL to 125 mg/dL or a HgA1c 5.7% to 6.4%.[20]
- Aspirin use for primary prevention is controversial with a recent meta-analysis yielding a modest benefit of reducing CVD events closely matched by increased major bleeding risks.[40] Suggest individual shared decision-making with the patient weighing the CV benefits (ie, higher ASCVD risk score) with the risk of bleeding.
- Modifying chemotherapy administration has become an early strategy to reduce cardiotoxicity especially with anthracyclines and trastuzumab.
  - Dose limitations of anthracyclines applied to most protocols.
  - Doxorubicin analogs (ie, epirubicin, idarubicin) may be less cardiotoxic.
  - Liposomal encapsulation of anthracyclines theoretically reduces myocardial endothelial absorption.
  - Protocols with drug-free intervals between 2 potentially cardiotoxic therapies such as anthracycline followed by trastuzumab.
- One FDA-approved cardioprotective agent is dexrazoxane, which appears to prevent anthracyclines from binding to the topoisomerase-2β-DNA complex and has shown reductions in HF and LVEF decline although no difference in survival.
  - Due to concerns of acute myeloid leukemia and myelodysplastic syndrome in children, the FDA has limited its indication to women with metastatic breast cancer who have already received > 300 mg/m² of doxorubicin and would benefit from additional doxorubicin treatment.
- Based on small, heterogeneous studies, there does appear to be a promising signal with the administration of beta blockers or angiotensin-converting enzyme (ACE) inhibitors to prevent HF or LVEF decline, with the largest benefit seen in those at the highest baseline risk once again highlighting the importance of CV risk assessment.[41]
- International Myeloma Working Group has recommended thromboprophylaxis with either aspirin or anticoagulation for high-risk myeloma patients undergoing immunomodulator therapies (thalidomide, lenalidomide, pomalidomide).[42,43]
- Early recognition and prevention of HF in patients receiving anthracyclines or trastuzumab has been the main focus for traditional cancer therapies, and this concept can be applied broadly to early recognition and prevention of CV risk factors and CVD to all cancer patients with special attention to common cardiotoxicities by therapy.

PROGNOSIS

Delay in recognition or treatment of traditional CV risk factors and/or cancer therapy-associated cardiotoxicities significantly worsens morbidity and mortality.

FOLLOW-UP

Follow-up frequency is based on the extent of illness and comorbidities in addition to symptoms and may include primary care physicians, oncologists, cardiologists, and cardio-oncologists. Patients should have ongoing evaluation of risk factors and symptoms every 4 to 12 months.

PATIENT EDUCATION

Advise patients on the vital importance of attaining ideal CV health to reduce long-term cardiotoxicity. Additional emphasis should be placed on increased awareness of risk associated with cancer therapies they have received and what signs and symptoms they should be monitoring.

PATIENT RESOURCES

American Heart Association Life's Simple 7 Success Plan: http://www.heart.org/HEARTORG/Conditions/My-Life-Check—Lifes-Simple-7_UCM_471453_Article.jsp#.Wr1gz2aZPUI?

The National Comprehensive Cancer Network (NCCN) Patient and Caregiver Resources on Cardiotoxicity: https://www.nccn.org/patients/resources/life_with_cancer/managing_symptoms/cardiac_toxicity.aspx

PROVIDER RESOURCES

2013 Atherosclerotic Cardiovascular Disease (ASCVD) pooled cohort risk equation: http://tools.acc.org/ASCVD-Risk-Estimator/

2013 American Heart Association (AHA) Heart Failure Guidelines: http://circ.ahajournals.org/content/128/16/1810

REFERENCES

1. Miller KD, Siegel RL, Lin CC, et al. Cancer treatment and survivorship statistics, 2016. *CA Cancer J Clin.* 2016;66:271-289.

2. Oeffinger KC, Mertens AC, Sklar CA, et al. Chronic health conditions in adult survivors of childhood cancer. *N Engl J Med.* 2006;355:1572-1582.

3. Armenian SH, Xu L, Ky B, et al. Cardiovascular disease among survivors of adult-onset cancer: a community-based retrospective cohort study. *J Clin Oncol.* 2016;34:1122-1130.

4. Bodai BI, Tuso P. Breast cancer survivorship: a comprehensive review of long-term medical issues and lifestyle recommendations. *Perm J.* 2015;19:48-79.

5. Armstrong GT, Liu Q, Yasui Y, et al. Late mortality among 5-year survivors of childhood cancer: a summary from the Childhood Cancer Survivor Study. *J Clin Oncol.* 2009;27:2328-2338.

6. Tashakkor AY, Moghaddamjou A, Chen L, et al. Predicting the risk of cardiovascular comorbidities in adult cancer survivors. *Curr Oncol.* 2013;20:e360-e370.

7. van Nimwegen FA, Schaapveld M, Janus CP, et al. Cardiovascular disease after Hodgkin lymphoma treatment: 40-year disease risk. *JAMA Intern Med.* 2015;175:1007-1017.

8. Slamon D, Eiermann W, Robert N, et al. Adjuvant trastuzumab in HER2-positive breast cancer. *N Engl J Med.* 2011;365:1273-1283.

9. Suter TM, Procter M, van Veldhuisen DJ, et al. Trastuzumab-associated cardiac adverse effects in the herceptin adjuvant trial. *J Clin Oncol.* 2007;25:3859-3865.

10. Bowles EJ, Wellman R, Feigelson HS, et al. Risk of heart failure in breast cancer patients after anthracycline and trastuzumab treatment: a retrospective cohort study. *J Natl Cancer Inst.* 2012;104:1293-1305.

11. Thavendiranathan P, Abdel-Qadir H, Fischer HD, et al. Breast cancer therapy-related cardiac dysfunction in adult women treated in routine clinical practice: a population-based cohort study. *J Clin Oncol.* 2016;34:2239-2246.

12. Zhang S, Liu X, Bawa-Khalfe T, et al. Identification of the molecular basis of doxorubicin-induced cardiotoxicity. *Nat Med.* 2012;18:1639-1642.

13. Gianni L, Herman EH, Lipshultz SE, et al. Anthracycline cardiotoxicity: from bench to bedside. *J Clin Oncol.* 2008;26:3777-3784.

14. Wadugu B, Kuhn B. The role of neuregulin/ErbB2/ErbB4 signaling in the heart with special focus on effects on cardiomyocyte proliferation. *Am J Physiol Heart Circ Physiol.* 2012;302:H2139-H2147.

15. Correa CR, Litt HI, Hwang WT, et al. Coronary artery findings after left-sided compared with right-sided radiation treatment for early-stage breast cancer. *J Clin Oncol.* 2007;25:3031-3037.

16. Yla-Herttuala S, Rissanen TT, Vajanto I, et al. Vascular endothelial growth factors: biology and current status of clinical applications in cardiovascular medicine. *J Am Coll Cardiol.* 2007;49:1015-1026.

17. Thavendiranathan P, Poulin F, Lim KD, et al. Use of myocardial strain imaging by echocardiography for the early detection of cardiotoxicity in patients during and after cancer chemotherapy: a systematic review. *J Am Coll Cardiol.* 2014;63:2751-2768.

18. Ky B, Putt M, Sawaya H, et al. Early increases in multiple biomarkers predict subsequent cardiotoxicity in patients with breast cancer treated with doxorubicin, taxanes, and trastuzumab. *J Am Coll Cardiol.* 2014;63:809-816.

19. Cardinale D, Colombo A, Torrisi R, et al. Trastuzumab-induced cardiotoxicity: clinical and prognostic implications of troponin I evaluation. *J Clin Oncol.* 2010;28:3910-3916.

20. American Diabetes Association. Standards of medical care in diabetes-2016 abridged for primary care providers. *Clin Diabetes.* 2016;34:3-21.

21. Fihn SD, Blankenship JC, Alexander KP, et al. 2014 ACC/AHA/AATS/PCNA/SCAI/STS focused update of the guideline for the diagnosis and management of patients with stable ischemic heart disease: a report of the American College of Cardiology/American Heart Association Task Force on Practice Guidelines, and the American Association for Thoracic Surgery, Preventive Cardiovascular Nurses Association, Society for Cardiovascular Angiography and Interventions, and Society of Thoracic Surgeons. *Circulation.* 2014;130:1749-1767.

22. James PA, Oparil S, Carter BL, et al. 2014 evidence-based guideline for the management of high blood pressure in adults: report from the panel members appointed to the Eighth Joint National Committee (JNC 8). *JAMA.* 2014;311:507-520.

23. Nishimura RA, Otto CM, Bonow RO, et al. 2014 AHA/ACC guideline for the management of patients with valvular heart disease: a report of the American College of Cardiology/

American Heart Association Task Force on Practice Guidelines. *Circulation.* 2014;129:e521-e643.

24. Stone NJ, Robinson JG, Lichtenstein AH, et al. 2013 ACC/AHA guideline on the treatment of blood cholesterol to reduce atherosclerotic cardiovascular risk in adults: a report of the American College of Cardiology/American Heart Association Task Force on Practice Guidelines. *Circulation.* 2014;129:S1-S45.

25. Yancy CW, Jessup M, Bozkurt B, et al. 2013 ACCF/AHA guideline for the management of heart failure: a report of the American College of Cardiology Foundation/American Heart Association Task Force on Practice Guidelines. *J Am Coll Cardiol.* 2013;62:e147-e239.

26. McKay RR, Rodriguez GE, Lin X, et al. Angiotensin system inhibitors and survival outcomes in patients with metastatic renal cell carcinoma. *Clin Cancer Res.* 2015;21:2471-2479.

27. Haouala A, Widmer N, Duchosal MA, et al. Drug interactions with the tyrosine kinase inhibitors imatinib, dasatinib, and nilotinib. *Blood.* 2011;117:e75-e87.

28. Lloyd-Jones DM, Hong Y, Labarthe D, et al. Defining and setting national goals for cardiovascular health promotion and disease reduction: the American Heart Association's strategic impact goal through 2020 and beyond. *Circulation.* 2010;121:586-613.

29. Guan J, Khambhati J, Jones LW, et al. Cardiology patient page. ABCDE steps for heart and vascular wellness following a prostate cancer diagnosis. *Circulation.* 2015;132:e218-e220.

30. Warren GW, Alberg AJ, Kraft AS, et al. The 2014 Surgeon General's report: "The health consequences of smoking--50 years of progress": a paradigm shift in cancer care. *Cancer.* 2014;120:1914-1916.

31. Shields PG. New NCCN guidelines: smoking cessation for patients with cancer. *J Natl Compr Canc Netw.* 2015;13:643-645.

32. Kenfield SA, Stampfer MJ, Giovannucci E, et al. Physical activity and survival after prostate cancer diagnosis in the health professionals follow-up study. *J Clin Oncol.* 2011;29:726-732.

33. Schmid D, Leitzmann MF. Association between physical activity and mortality among breast cancer and colorectal cancer survivors: a systematic review and meta-analysis. *Ann Oncol.* 2014;25:1293-1311.

34. Jones LW, Habel LA, Weltzien E, et al. Exercise and risk of cardiovascular events in women with nonmetastatic breast cancer. *J Clin Oncol.* 2016;34:2743-2749.

35. Meyerhardt JA, Niedzwiecki D, Hollis D, et al. Association of dietary patterns with cancer recurrence and survival in patients with stage III colon cancer. *JAMA.* 2007;298:754-764.

36. Kwan ML, Weltzien E, Kushi LH, et al. Dietary patterns and breast cancer recurrence and survival among women with early-stage breast cancer. *J Clin Oncol.* 2009;27:919-926.

37. Weaver KE, Foraker RE, Alfano CM, et al. Cardiovascular risk factors among long-term survivors of breast, prostate, colorectal, and gynecologic cancers: a gap in survivorship care? *J Cancer Surviv.* 2013;7:253-261.

38. Acar Z, Kale A, Turgut M, et al. Efficiency of atorvastatin in the protection of anthracycline-induced cardiomyopathy. *J Am Coll Cardiol.* 2011;58:988-989.

39. Barone BB, Yeh HC, Snyder CF, et al. Long-term all-cause mortality in cancer patients with preexisting diabetes mellitus: a systematic review and meta-analysis. *JAMA.* 2008;300:2754-2764.

40. Guirguis-Blake JM, Evans CV, Senger CA, et al. Aspirin for the primary prevention of cardiovascular events: a systematic evidence review for the U.S. Preventive Services Task Force. Rockville (MD): U.S. Preventive Services Task Force Evidence Syntheses, formerly Systematic Evidence Reviews; 2015.

41. Kalam K, Marwick TH. Role of cardioprotective therapy for prevention of cardiotoxicity with chemotherapy: a systematic review and meta-analysis. *Eur J Cancer.* 2013;49:2900-2909.

42. Palumbo A, Rajkumar SV, San Miguel JF, et al. International Myeloma Working Group consensus statement for the management, treatment, and supportive care of patients with myeloma not eligible for standard autologous stem-cell transplantation. *J Clin Oncol.* 2014;32:587-600.

43. Li W, Croce K, Steensma DP, et al. Vascular and metabolic implications of novel targeted cancer therapies: focus on kinase inhibitors. *J Am Coll Cardiol.* 2015;66:1160-1178.

17 ADULT CONGENITAL HEART DISEASE

Lauren J. Hassen, MD, MPH
William H. Marshall V, MD
Elisa Bradley, MD

INTRODUCTION: GENERAL PRINCIPLES IN ADULT CONGENITAL HEART DISEASE

Congenital heart disease (CHD) is a term used to describe a malformation of the heart or great vessels present since birth. In adults with congenital heart disease (ACHD), one must consider not only the original CHD anatomy, but also the type of surgical repair(s), as well as understand the natural history of both the underlying anatomy and surgical palliation.

The overall profile of CHD in the United States has shifted strikingly in the last decade whereby there has been an increase in those living with CHD, and now greater proportion of adults versus children (Figure 17-1). This observation foreshadows the future growth of the ACHD population in the United States. In fact, by current estimates, the number of adults living with CHD is substantial. Canadian data reported that 40,000 ACHD patients comprised 66% of CHD care nationally in Canada in 2010 (Figure 17-2).[2] If these data are extrapolated and applied to the U.S. population, the number of potential ACHD patients seeking care in 2010 is on the order of 1.5 million. Not only have overall numbers of ACHD patients increased, but there has also been a marked jump in adults with severe forms of CHD. In adults the overall prevalence of severe CHD increased 85% versus 22% for children.[3] For the first time ever, data were released in late 2014 showing that patients who received their care at a specialized ACHD center had an independent reduction in mortality.[4] This shift in mortality benefit occurred after the release of national consensus guidelines, indicating that both expert opinion and evidence-based medicine in ACHD had an impact on overall survival. With increasing numbers of adults surviving CHD, there is a substantial need for better understanding of CHD in the adult population as they continue to age.[5] Ultimately, this calls for better understanding and recognition of CHD, surgical repair(s), and late sequelae related to underlying anatomy and palliation. Here we review the *most common ACHD lesions* that present to adult cardiology clinics, along with exam findings, special testing, and considerations for expected management in the setting of underlying anatomy and prior surgical repair. Several practice management guidelines are outlined as part of this review.[6-11]

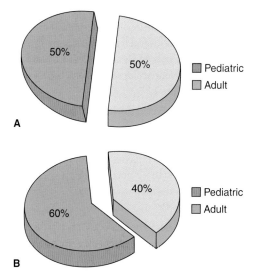

FIGURE 17-1 Proportion of adults with congenital heart disease. The adult population with congenital heart disease is expanding at a greater rate than the pediatric population with congenital heart disease. Proportion of adults with congenital heart disease as compared to children with congenital heart disease in 2000 (A) and in 2010 (B). (Data from Williams RG, Person GD, Barst RJ, et al. Report of the national heart blood lung institute working group on research in adult congenital heart disease. *J Am Coll Cardiol.* 2006;47:701-707.)

SEPTAL DEFECTS

ATRIAL SEPTAL DEFECT

Overview

- Secundum atrial septal defect (ASD): Defect of the fossa ovalis due to enlarged ostium secundum or inadequate septal tissue. It is the most common type of ASD (75%), and occurs more frequently in women (Figure 17-3).

- Primum ASD: Defect in the lower atrial septum due to lack of septum primum and endocardial cushion fusion. Primum defects account for 15% of overall ASDs and are commonly associated with trisomy 21, atrioventricular septal defects (AVSDs), and cleft mitral valve (Figure 17-3).

- Sinus venosus ASD: Defect at the level of the superior vena cava (SVC) or inferior vena cava (IVC) as they enter the right atrium at the intra-atrial septum. Typically occurs as a result of unroofing of a pulmonary vein as it passes behind the right atrium en route to the left atrium. This defect accounts for 10% of ASDs and is highly associated with partial anomalous venous return (PAPVR) (Figure 17-3).

- Unroofed coronary sinus: The least common type of ASD (1%); associated with persistent left superior vena cava (L-SVC) (Figure 17-3).

Associated Defects and Physiology

- Associated defects: Valvular pulmonic stenosis (PS), mitral valve prolapse

- Physiology:
  - Typically there is a left-to-right shunt at the level of the ASD due to the increased compliance of the right ventricle as compared to the left ventricle.

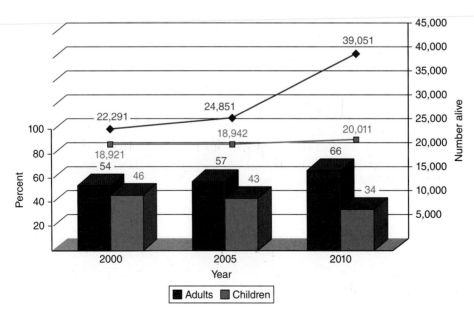

FIGURE 17-2 Number of people living with congenital heart disease. Data from Canada showing the number of adults (*red*) and number of children (*purple*) currently living with congenital heart disease from years 2000 to 2010. (Reproduced with permission from Marelli AJ, Ionescu-Ittu R, Mackie AS, Guo L, Dendukuri N, Kaouach M. The prevalence of congenital heart disease in the general population from 2000 to 2010. *Circulation.* 2014:130:749-756.)

○ Late findings include right heart (atrium/RA and ventricle/RV) enlargement due to overcirculation at the level of the shunt. The volume load and resultant chamber enlargement can precipitate atrial arrhythmias, which increase in frequency with age.

○ About 10% of patients with an ASD develop pulmonary hypertension (HTN). This has been reported in unrepaired defects and also late after ASD closure.

Clinical Findings, Diagnosis, and Management

• Clinical presentation: Most patients are asymptomatic; however, symptoms can range from dyspnea on exertion, fatigue, palpitations due to arrhythmias, or in rare cases, hypoxia and cyanosis from Eisenmenger syndrome (ES, see further).

• Examination findings: Fixed split S_2, loud P_2 (if pulmonary HTN present), soft systolic murmur may be heard due to increased flow across the PV. Rarely, a large shunt may produce a diastolic rumble.

• Electrocardiogram: Incomplete right bundle-branch block (rSR') (Figure 17-4) and atrioventricular block (AVB). Right axis deviation can be seen in an ASD where right heart chamber enlargement is present; however, in the case of a primum defect left axis deviation is almost always present.

• Chest x-ray: Enlarged right heart and increased pulmonary vasculature.

• Echocardiogram: Echo "drop-out" at the interatrial septum may be seen in adults with adequate image quality (Figure 17-5). Saline contrast bubble study may be used to confirm the presence of an interatrial shunt when 2-dimensional and color Doppler evaluation are inconclusive. Transesophageal echocardiogram (TEE) is particularly useful for evaluation of sinus venosus and coronary sinus defects.

• Advanced imaging: Cardiac computed tomography (CT) and magnetic resonance imaging (MRI) are typically not required for diagnosis unless there are inconclusive echocardiogram results.

• Cardiac catheterization: Generally not required for diagnosis, but useful to evaluate pulmonary vascular resistance, pulmonary to systemic flow, and for coronary evaluation in patients considered for closure.

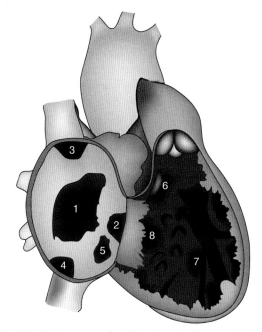

FIGURE 17-3 Various types of atrial and ventricular septal defects (ASD and VSD, respectively). The heart is viewed from a right anterior oblique projection, and the right ventricular and right atrial free walls have been removed. **1.** Secundum-type ASD. **2.** Primum-type ASD. **3.** Superior sinus venosus ASD. **4.** Inferior sinus venosus ASD. **5.** Coronary sinus ASD. **6.** Perimembranous VSD. **7.** Muscular VSD. **8.** Inlet VSD. (Reproduced with permission from Fuster V, Walsh RA, Harrington RA. *Hurst's the Heart*. 13th ed. New York, NY: McGraw-Hill Education; 2011. Figure 84-17.)

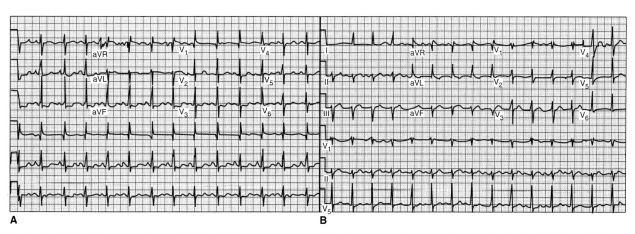

FIGURE 17-4 A. 12-lead electrocardiogram (ECG) of a 30-year-old woman with a large secundum-type atrial septal defect (ASD; 42 mm in diameter by transesophageal echocardiography) and moderate pulmonary hypertension. Note the right-axis deviation and tall precordial R waves consistent with right ventricular enlargement or hypertrophy. There is evidence of right atrial abnormality. **B.** An ECG of a 33-year-old man with a primum-type ASD surgically repaired at 3 years of age. Note the continued presence of a characteristic RSR complex in lead V1 and QRS left-axis deviation. (Reproduced with permission from Fuster V, Walsh RA, Harrington RA. *Hurst's the Heart*. 13th ed. New York, NY: McGraw-Hill Education; 2011. Figure 84-16.)

- Management:
  - *Closure indicated:* Evidence of RA or RV enlargement (± symptoms) if pulmonary to systemic flow (Qp:Qs) is >1.5, ASD >10 mm on echo, presence of paradoxical embolism, platypnea-othodeoxia, those undergoing other cardiac surgery, and in patients with pulmonary HTN only if pulmonary vascular resistance is <2/3 systemic resistance or who are responsive to test occlusion or pulmonary vasodilators. Catheter-based closure is indicated in secundum defects if size permits. Remainder of ASD types are closed surgically.
  - *Closure contraindicated:* Irreversible severe pulmonary arterial HTN with a bidirectional or right-to-left shunt.
  - *Atrial arrhythmias:* Rate and rhythm control strategies are reasonable with anticoagulation if the patient meets clinical criteria for high risk of stroke.

VENTRICULAR SEPTAL DEFECT

Overview

Ventricular septal defects (VSDs) are the most common CHD in infants (0.5%-5%) with the majority (80%) closing spontaneously.

- Type 1 (subpulmonary, infundibular, supracristal, conal, doubly committed juxta-arterial): Accounts for ~6% of VSDs (33% in Asian populations) and is located near the RV outflow tract. Frequently causes aortic insufficiency (Figures 17-3 and 17-6A).

- Type 2 (perimembranous, conoventricular): The most common type of VSD (80%) located in the membranous portion of the LV septum (Figures 17-3 and 17-6B). May be associated with aortic insufficiency. Can frequently be seen with a "septal aneurysm," which is the result of partial closure of the defect by tricuspid leaflet tissue (Figure 17-6). Can rarely be a cause of a Gerbode defect (connection between RA and LV).

- Type 3 (AV canal type, inlet): Accounts for 5% to 8% of VSDs and is commonly associated with trisomy 21. Defect occurs in the lower RV adjacent to the tricuspid valve (Figures 17-3 and 17-6C).

- Type 4 (muscular): In infants this type of VSD accounts for 20% of VSDs, but less common in adults. Can occur in the central, apical, or marginal portions of the septum. The usual course is spontaneous closure (Figures 17-3 and 17-6D).

Associated Defects and Physiology

- Associated defects: Frequently seen with other types of CHD, in particular tetralogy of Fallot (ToF) and transposition of the great arteries.

- Physiology:
  - In the usual situation blood flows from the higher pressure LV to the RV across the VSD. This can lead to LV volume overload and left heart chamber enlargement. Over time, if uncorrected, a large shunt may reverse such that flow is from RV to LV when pulmonary vascular remodeling and pulmonary HTN develop (a condition called Eisenmenger syndrome [ES]).
    - Size of VSD and physiology (non-ES):
      - Small: <1/3 size of aortic annulus with no LV volume overload or pulmonary HTN (small net left-to-right shunt)

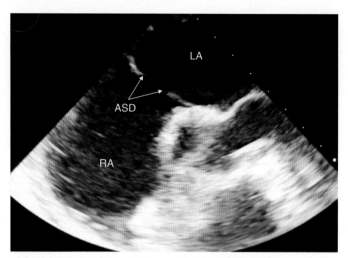

FIGURE 17-5 Atrial septal defect. Transesophageal echocardiogram demonstrating a right atrial enlargement and a 1-cm secundum-type atrial septal defect. Abbreviations: ASD, atrial septal defect; LA, left atrium; RA, right atrium. (Reproduced with permission from Pahlm O, Wagner GS. *Multimodal Cardiovascular Imaging: Principles and Clinical Applications.* New York, NY: McGraw-Hill Education; 2011. Figure 1-43.)

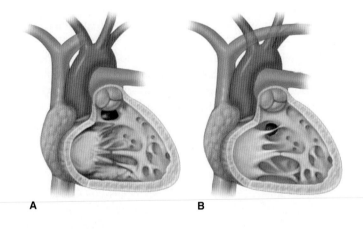

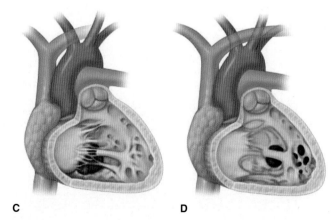

FIGURE 17-6 Classic anatomic types of VSD. **A,** Type I (conal, supracristal, infundibular, doubly committed, and juxta-arterial) VSD; **B,** Type II or perimembranous VSD; **C,** Type III VSD (atrioventricular canal type or inlet septum type); and **D,** Type IV VSD (single or multiple), also called muscular VSDs. (Reproduced with permission from Ventricular septal defect. In: Mavroudis C, Backer CL, eds. *Pediatric Cardiac Surgery.* 4th ed. Wiley-Blackwell, 2013.)

○ Moderate: 1/3 to 2/3 size of aortic annulus with mild-moderate LV volume overload and no/mild pulmonary HTN (moderate left-to-right shunt; Qp:Qs 1.5-1.9)

○ Large: 2/3 size of aortic diameter and large left-to-right shunt. Pulmonary HTN is typical and the LV is volume overloaded (Qp:Qs usually >2.0)

Clinical Findings, Diagnosis, and Management

- Clinical presentation: Varies from asymptomatic murmur to HF.

- Examination findings: Harsh loud holosystolic murmur. Murmur can become quieter over time if RV pressure approaches LV pressure.

- Electrocardiogram: May show LA and LV enlargement. If right ventricular hypertrophy (RVH) is seen, consider ES.

- Chest x-ray: Cardiomegaly will be evident if the defect is moderate or large in size. Increased pulmonary vascular markings.

- Echocardiogram: This is the preferred study for diagnosis including evaluation of anatomy but also physiologic shunt (Figure 17-7).

- Advanced imaging: May be helpful if there is concern about concomitant CHD.

- Catheterization: The most accurate way to assess shunt flow and pulmonary vascular resistance (Figure 17-8).

- Management:

  ○ *Closure indicated:* Evidence of LV volume overload (with Qp:Qs >2) OR history of endocarditis are absolute indications for closure. It is reasonable to consider closure if pulmonary HTN is present and pulmonary pressures are <2/3 systemic pressure and pulmonary vascular resistance is <2/3 systemic vascular resistance (if Qp:Qs is >1.5). It is also reasonable to consider closure if the shunt Qp:Qs is >1.5 and there is diastolic dysfunction present. Catheter-based closures can be considered with type 4 defects where there is significant left heart enlargement and the VSD is remote from the tricuspid valve.

  ○ *Closure contraindicated:* Closure is not indicated if there is severe, irreversible pulmonary HTN.

ATRIOVENTRICULAR SEPTAL DEFECT

Overview

Atrioventricular septal defect (AVSD) is also known as "AV canal defect/AVCD," "endocardial cushion defect," or "common atrioventricular canal/CAVC" (Figure 17-9). This defect is the result of fusion abnormalities between the septum primum and endocardial cushions, and presents in 3 broad variations:

- Complete AVSD: Combination of primum ASD, type 3 VSD, and common atrioventricular (AV) valve.

- Incomplete AVSD: Primum ASD, no VSD, and cleft anterior mitral leaflet.

- Partial AVSD: Cleft anterior mitral leaflet.

Associated Defects and Physiology

- Associated defects: About 30% of AVSD occurs in patients with trisomy 21 (although partial AVSD is NOT associated with trisomy 21). Other common associated lesions are ToF,

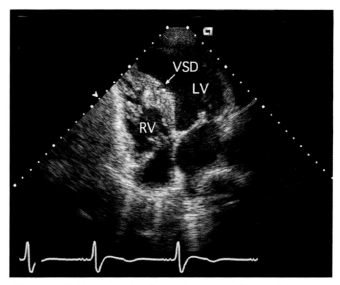

FIGURE 17-7 Transthoracic echocardiogram in a 45-year-old woman with a small muscular ventricular septal defect (VSD). Abbreviations: LV, left ventricle; RV, right ventricle. (Reproduced with permission from Crawford MH. *Current Diagnosis & Treatment: Cardiology.* 4th ed. New York, NY: McGraw-Hill Education; 2014. Figure 31-12.)

conotruncal anomalies, subaortic stenosis, and heterotaxy syndromes.

- Physiology: The unrestricted septal defects allow deoxygenated and oxygenated blood from the right and left sides of the heart to mix. As a result, children present cyanotic. Over time, if unrepaired, unrestricted pulmonary blood flow leads to increase pulmonary vascular resistance and ES. Adults presenting with an unrepaired AVCD are typically in this stage (ES).

Clinical Findings, Diagnosis, and Management

- Clinical presentation: Children are typically cyanotic, and so it is common to undergo repair in childhood. Adults that present with an unrepaired defect typically have findings consistent with ES (HF, cyanosis, arrhythmia).

- Examination findings: In those repaired, there may be a soft systolic murmur of mitral regurgitation. In the unrepaired patient, the exam is more significant, reflecting underlying Eisenmenger physiology (acrocyanosis) (Figure 17-10).

- Electrocardiogram: Signs of chamber enlargement. In an unrepaired adult, most typically this is RVH. AV node dysfunction is common late after surgery, and so frequent monitoring for conduction system disease is recommended.

- Chest x-ray: Unrepaired patients typically have cardiomegaly.

- Echocardiogram: The study of choice to diagnose and evaluate shunt physiology (Figure 17-11).

- Advanced imaging: Typically only helpful to evaluate for associated lesions or if echo images are suboptimal.

- Catheterization: May be used to evaluate shunt flow and pulmonary artery pressure when considering surgery/reoperation.

- Management: Initial repair is completed in infancy. However, reoperation is often required in the adult population and can be considered reasonable if:

  - Left-sided AV valve regurgitation or stenosis leads to symptoms, arrhythmias, or there is increase in left heart size or reduction in function.
  - LV outflow tract obstruction if the mean/peak gradients are >50/70 mm Hg or lower gradients with concomitant mitral regurgitation or aortic insufficiency.
  - Residual AS or VSD with a significant left-to-right shunt (see ASD and VSD above).

PATENT DUCTUS ARTERIOSIS
Overview

The patent ductus arteriosis (PDA) is a persistent connection between the proximal descending aorta and the roof of the pulmonary artery.

Associated Defects and Physiology

- Associated defects: Associated with multiple conditions including ASD, VSD, maternal rubella infection, fetal valproate syndrome, and other chromosomal abnormalities.

- Physiology: The patent ductus permits left-to-right shunting of blood from the aorta to the pulmonary bed. If left unrepaired,

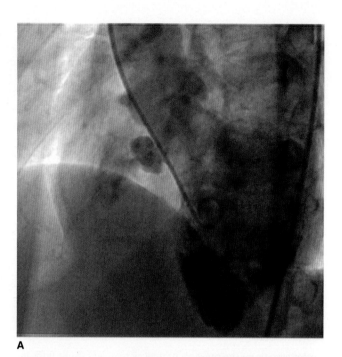

A

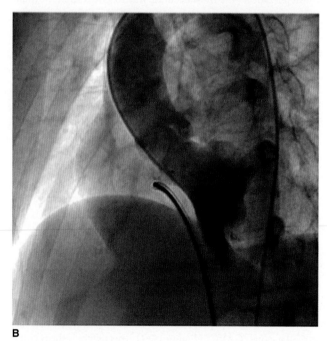

B

FIGURE 17-8 As captured by left ventriculography in a single plane (45° left anterior oblique/10° cranial). A. Perimembranous ventricular septal defect with aneurysm. B. The occluder was used to close, at the inlet, the perimembranous ventricular septal defect with aneurysm. The entire aneurysm was compressed between the left and right discs of the device. (Reproduced with permission Bian C, Ma J, Wang J, et al. Perimembranous ventricular septal defect with aneurysm two options for transcatheter closure. *Tex Heart Inst J.* 2011;38(5):528-532.)

this may cause LA and LV dilatation and volume overload. Large PDAs with unrestricted flow may result in Eisenmenger physiology (Figure 17-12).

Clinical Findings, Diagnosis, and Management

- Clinical presentation: Varies with the size of the PDA. May range from asymptomatic to dyspnea, fatigue, or cyanosis (with ES).

- Examination findings: Classically, a continuous machinery-type murmur is described below the left clavicle. In large lesions, there may be a widened pulse pressure. Differential cyanosis and clubbing (between hands and feet) (Figure 17-12B) can be seen when the shunt becomes right-to-left and deoxygenated blood is preferentially directed to the lower extremities.

- Electrocardiogram: May be normal or with LA or LV enlargement. If pulmonary HTN is present as in ES, then RVH may also be seen.

- Chest x-ray: Normal to cardiomegaly.

- Echocardiogram: Echo is reasonable to evaluate the size of the PDA, net shunt direction, and to estimate pulmonary artery pressures.

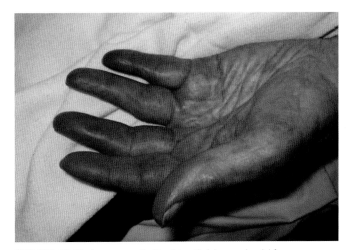

FIGURE 17-10 Acrocyanosis. Persistently blue and cold fingers. (Reproduced with permission from Knoop KJ, Stack LB, Storrow AB, Thurman RJ. *The Atlas of Emergency Medicine.* 4th ed. New York, NY: McGraw-Hill Education; 2016. Photographer: Lawrence B. Stack, MD. Figure 12.56.)

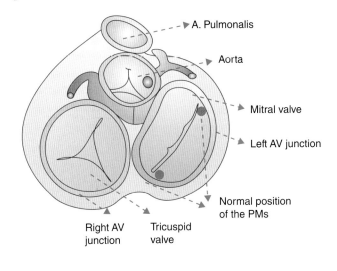

(a)

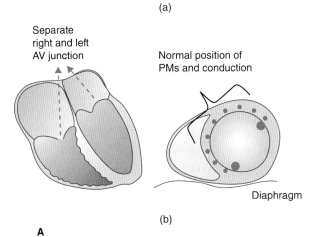

A   (b)

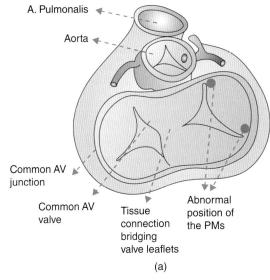

(a)

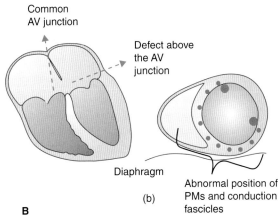

B   (b)

FIGURE 17-9 Differences in anatomic characteristics between normal (A) and primum atrioventricular septal defect (AVSD). (B) Both the normal and primum AVSD hearts are first shown from modified left anterior oblique view at the level of the valves (a). The apical 4-chamber view and short-axis view of the heart at the level of papillary muscles are also presented (b). Abbreviations: A, arteria; AV, atrioventricular; PMs, papillary muscles. (Modified with permission from Adachi I, Uemura H, McCarthy KP, et al. Surgical anatomy of atrioventricular septal defect. *Asian Cardiovasc Thorac Ann.* 2008;16:497-502.)

- Advanced imaging: May be used if not visible on standard echo images.

- Catheterization: Preferred method of determining degree of shunt present and direction of shunt in hemodynamically significant lesions (Figures 17-12C and D).

- Management: Small defects with no evidence of overcirculation can be followed every 3 years.

  ○ *Closure indicated:* Consider closure when there is LA or LV enlargement, prior endocarditis, pulmonary HTN is present with net left-to-right shunt, patient is asymptomatic but PDA is small and can be closed via catheter.

  ○ *Closure contraindicated:* No closure if there is evidence of pulmonary arterial HTN and net right-to-left shunt.

ABNORMALITIES OF PULMONARY VENOUS RETURN

PARTIAL ANOMALOUS PULMONARY VENOUS RETURN

Overview

In PAPVR, one or more of the pulmonary veins drains to the systemic venous system or RA. Although the systemic venous connection can occur at any level, some typical forms include right upper pulmonary vein to RA, left sided pulmonary vein to the innominate vein, right-sided pulmonary vein to the SVC or IVC.

Associated Defects and Physiology

- Associated defects: Anomalous veins can be associated with pulmonary sequestration and aortopulmonary collaterals (AP collaterals) to the lungs. Although the defect is typically isolated, it may be seen infrequently with other types of CHD. It is common in cases of polysplenia-type heterotaxy.

- Physiology: Similar to an ASD, this leads to left-to-right shunting of blood. If ES develops, however, this will not result in reversal of the shunt.

Clinical Findings, Diagnosis, and Management

- Clinical presentation: Most patients are asymptomatic; however, with larger shunts (>1 anomalous vein), there may be dyspnea on exertion, exercise intolerance, and if RV is significantly involved, there could be signs of right HF.

- Examination findings: Physical findings are highly variable. The examination may be completely normal if the shunt is small. If the shunt is large, then there may be evidence of RV enlargement and an RV heave may be appreciated. If severe tricuspid regurgitation (TR) is present or RV failure, there may be peripheral edema, liver congestion, and elevated jugular venous distention.

- Electrocardiogram: Usually unremarkable, but with right heart enlargement/dysfunction, there may be RVH.

- Chest x-ray: Right heart enlargement and increased pulmonary vascular markings. Scimitar syndrome is the case where PAPVR

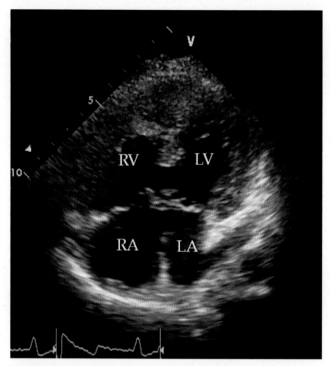

FIGURE 17-11 Apical 4-chamber image of an inlet ventricular septal defect and an ostium primum atrial septal defect (complete AV canal defect). The ventricular septal defect (VSD) is situated more inferiorly than the typical position of a perimembranous VSD. (Reproduced with permission from Fuster V, Walsh RA, Harrington RA. *Hurst's the Heart.* 13th ed. New York, NY: McGraw-Hill Education; 2011. Figure 18-113A.)

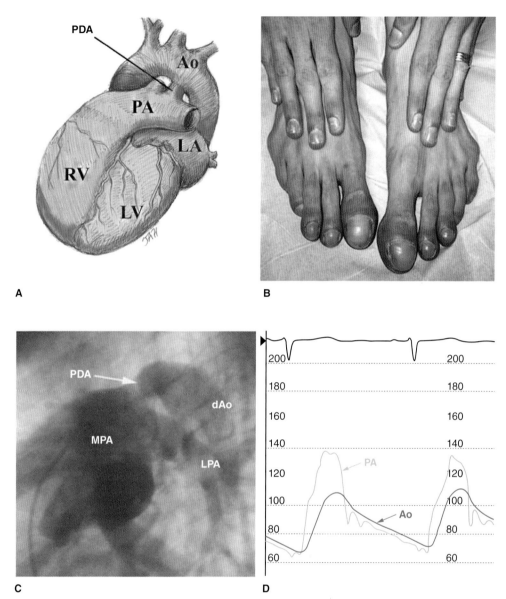

FIGURE 17-12 A. Patent ductus arteriosus (PDA) in a patient with severe pulmonary hypertension (Eisenmenger syndrome). Due to the suprasystemic pulmonary arterial resistance, deoxygenated (cyanotic) blood from the right ventricle (RV) and pulmonary artery (PA) is shunted across the PDA to the aorta (Ao). The left atrium (LA) and left ventricle (LV) are labeled. **B.** Differential clubbing and cyanosis of the toes due to lower extremity perfusion by the deoxygenated blood crossing the PDA. **C.** Angiogram in a dilated main pulmonary artery (MPA) with shunting noted across the PDA to the descending aorta (dAo). The left pulmonary artery (LPA) is labeled. **D.** Direct pressure recordings in the Ao and PA demonstrating suprasystemic PA systolic pressure. (Reproduced with permission from Kasper D, Fauci A, Hauser S, Longo D, Jameson JL, Loscalzo J. *Harrison's Principles of Internal Medicine.* 19th ed. New York, NY: McGraw-Hill Education; 2015. Figure 282-3.)

returns to the IVC, hepatic veins, or subdiaphragmatic veins (Figure 17-13).

- Echocardiogram: RA and RV enlargement. Occasionally the anomalous vein can be identified. This is more common on transesophageal imaging.

- Advanced imaging: Frequently required to identify the anatomy of pulmonary venous drainage (Figure 17-14).

- Catheterization: Important to quantify the degree of shunt, location, and determine whether or not pulmonary HTN is present.

- Management:
  - Surgical repair is indicated if the shunt is significant (see ASD management) similar to management of ASD. Post repair, about 10% of patients can develop pulmonary venous stenosis at the anastomosis site. This is highly variable based upon center and surgeon experience.

TOTAL ANOMALOUS PULMONARY VENOUS RETURN

Overview

Total anomalous pulmonary venous return (TAPVR) is failure of the pulmonary venous confluence to fuse with the posterior wall of the left atrium. Typically this confluence is behind the RA and a decompressing vein drains to the systemic venous system (SVC, IVC, etc.).

Associated Defects and Physiology

- Associated defects: If there is partial fusion of the pulmonary venous confluence, a residual perforated membrane between this confluence and the left atrium results in cor triatriatum (Figure 17-15). Asplenia-type heterotaxy is seen with TAPVR in ~90% of patients.
- Physiology: Because all 4 of the pulmonary veins drain to the systemic venous system (and RA, RV), these patients are dependent on shunts at the atrial, ventricular, or PDA level. Repair must be completed in childhood, as most cases are incompatible with life if there is not sufficient mixing of deoxygenated and oxygenated blood.

Clinical Findings, Diagnosis, and Management

- Clinical presentation: This condition is nearly 100% identified at or prior to birth. Patients without any pulmonary vein obstruction and adequate shunting present with cyanosis, whereas those with pulmonary vein anastomotic stenosis or insufficient shunt, typically present in cardiogenic shock. Adult patients present late after repair, and it would be highly unusual to survive to adulthood and present without repair.
- Examination findings: There may be no symptoms late after repair. If there is obstruction at the repair site then there may be findings consistent with pulmonary HTN.
- Electrocardiogram: Repaired patient ECG will be normal.
- Chest x-ray: Repaired patient will be normal.
- Echocardiogram: Repaired patient will be normal, unless there is stenosis at the anastomosis, then there may be right heart enlargement and/or dysfunction.
- Advanced imaging: Can be used to identify the anastomosis/prior surgical repair site.
- Catheterization: Most frequently used to determine if there is pulmonary vein stenosis post repair.
- Management: The majority of adults will have received surgical repair in childhood. Postoperatively they are followed to monitor for stenosis of the pulmonary veins/anastomosis. A workup for this should be undertaken if there is poor exercise tolerance or pulmonary HTN. Percutaneous stenting or surgery may be undertaken to treat stenosis in a repaired patient.

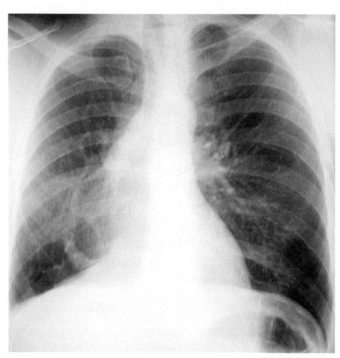

FIGURE 17-13 This case shows the characteristic appearance of venolobar (scimitar) syndrome. The scimitar vein is the result of partial anomalous pulmonary venous return. (Reproduced with permission from Chen MYM, Pope TL, Ott DJ. *Basic Radiology.* 2nd ed. New York, NY: McGraw-Hill Education; 2011. Figure 3-43.)

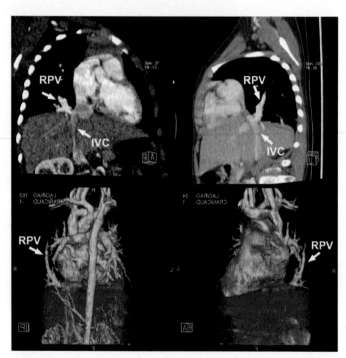

FIGURE 17-14 Multiplanar reformatted (top row) and 3-dimensional volume-rendered (bottom row) computed tomography images demonstrating partial anomalous pulmonary venous return of the right-sided pulmonary veins (RPV) into the subdiaphragmatic inferior vena cava (IVC) with some narrowing noted at the ostium (red arrow). (Reproduced with permission from Pahlm O, Wagner GS. *Multimodal Cardiovascular Imaging: Principles and Clinical Applications.* New York, NY: McGraw-Hill Education; 2011. Figure 5-15.)

LEFT HEART OBSTRUCTIVE LESIONS

BICUSPID AORTIC VALVE

Overview

A bicuspid aortic valve (BAV) is an aortic valve with 2 leaflets or cusps, instead of the usual 3 (Figure 17-16). This may occur due to the congenital presence of only 2 cusps, or secondary to a raphe between 2 of the 3 cusps (failure to delaminate). BAV is the most common congenital cardiac malformation, present in 1 in 80 adults. Men are affected more than women, with a male vs female prevalence ratio of 4 to 1. The condition is heritable (autosomal dominant with reduced penetrance). Left coronary cusp and noncoronary cusp fusion is rare, and so typically BAV is classified as either type 1 or type 2.

- Type 1: Fusion of the right and left coronary cusps (80%)

- Type 2: Fusion of the right and noncoronary cusps

Associated Defects and Physiology

- Associated defects: 10% of patients also have coarctation of the aorta (CoA). Other associations include subaortic stenosis, parachute mitral valve, VSD, PDA. There is at least 1 study that suggests BAV patients have increased risk of cerebral aneurysms (up to 10%).[17]

- Physiology: Right-noncoronary cusp fusion is associated with higher risk of developing aortic stenosis and regurgitation. The tissue of the aorta is abnormal in patients with a BAV, and is similar to the cystic medial necrosis of Marfan syndrome (MFS), which increases risk of aortic dilation and dissection, although is felt to do so to less of a degree than typical connective tissue diseases such as MFS.

Clinical Findings, Diagnosis, and Management

- Clinical presentation: Two-thirds of patients develop symptoms of aortic stenosis (AS) by the fifth decade (ie, angina, dyspnea, syncope). Consider this diagnosis in a young (40- to 60-year-old) patient with AS. Patients with calcific AS typically present after age 70 years.

- Examination findings: Patients typically have a systolic ejection sound due to valve opening, which usually disappears by the fourth decade due to calcification. In the presence of associated AS, they may have a crescendo-decrescendo midsystolic murmur at the upper sternal border with radiation to the neck. With more significant AS, the murmur peaks later and peripheral pulses are diminished and delayed (pulsus parvus et tardus).

- Electrocardiogram: There may be signs of LV hypertrophy, left atrial enlargement, or ST-T repolarization.

- Chest x-ray: The chest x-ray is typically normal, although may show cardiomegaly if LV hypertrophy or dilation is present, or signs of calcification of the valve if the patient has developed AS.

- Echocardiogram: TTE is used to qualify the lesion (anatomy of cusp fusion), to quantify degree of AS or aortic insufficiency if present, and to assess the aortic root. May require TEE if difficult to visualize via transthoracic (Figure 17-17).

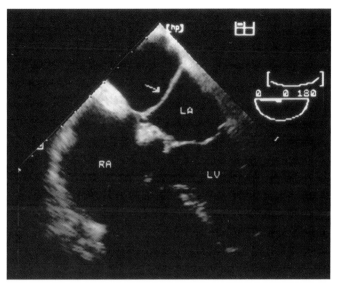

FIGURE 17-15 Transverse transesophageal image of cor triatriatum. A membrane (*arrow*) is present in the left atrium. Abbreviations: LA, left atrium; LV, left ventricle; RA, right atrium. (Reproduced with permission from Fuster V, Walsh RA, Harrington RA. *Hurst's the Heart*. 13th ed. New York, NY: McGraw-Hill Education; 2011. Figure 18-116.)

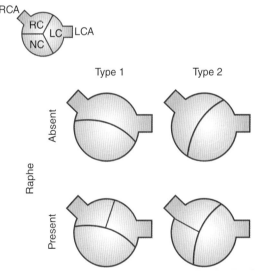

FIGURE 17-16 Schematic of bicuspid aortic valve (BAV) leaflet phenotypes from a parasternal short-axis view on echocardiography. Small inset top left depicts a normal trileaflet aortic valve in a similar orientation with right coronary cusp (RC), left coronary cusp (LC), noncoronary cusp (NC), and ostia of the coronary arteries. Type 1 shows congenital fusion of the right and left coronary cusps, the most common BAV phenotype, which occurs in approximately 80% of patients. The remainder of patients have the type 2 phenotype with congenital fusion of the right and noncoronary cusps. In both types, there may be a raphe, or ridge, in the larger cusp where a commissural separation would normally occur. (Reproduced, with permission, from Schaefer BM, Lewin MB, Stout KK, et al. The bicuspid aortic valve: an integrated phenotypic classification of leaflet morphology and aortic root shape. *Heart*. 2008;94(12):1634-1638.)

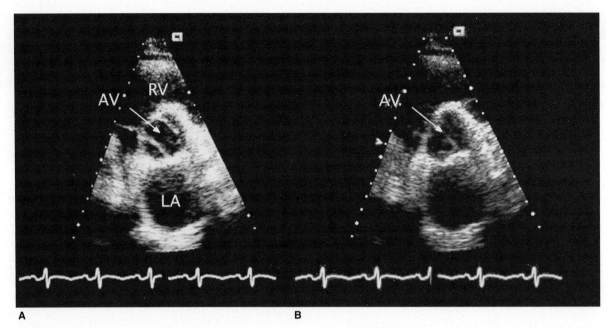

FIGURE 17-17 Transesophageal echocardiographic views of a patient with bicuspid aortic valve. A. Systolic frame showing 2 leaflets of the aortic valve (AV) with an ovoid opening (*arrow*). **B.** Diastolic frame showing the single line of coaptation (*arrow*). Abbreviations: LA, left atrium; RV, right ventricle. (Reproduced with permission from Crawford MH. *Current Diagnosis & Treatment: Cardiology.* 4th ed. New York, NY: McGraw-Hill Education; 2014. Figure 31-1.)

- Advanced imaging: MRI or CT may be useful to evaluate the thoracic aorta, particularly if concomitant aortopathy is present.

- Catheterization: Cardiac catheterization is recommended if there is discordance between patient symptoms and diagnostic imaging studies. However, if symptoms and surface echocardiogram findings are concordant, cardiac catheterization is not required for diagnosis of this condition or evaluation of the degree of stenosis (AS)/regurgitation (AR).

- Management:

  o *Medical therapy*: Beta blockers are indicated for patients with BAV and aortic dilatation (class IIa indication). Statins can be used to delay valve sclerosis (class IIb indication). Angiotensin II receptor blockers (ARBs) are currently under study to determine if they reduce rates of aortic dilatation. Endocarditis prophylaxis is not required unless there has been replacement of the valve.

  o *Serial imaging*: TTE should be done yearly (as well as ECG) for AS when mean Doppler gradient >30 mm Hg or peak gradient >50 mm Hg, and every 2 years if gradients are less (with ECG) (class I indication). The aorta should be imaged with CT or MRI annually if >40 mm, or every 2 years if <40 mm; however, some studies indicate that imaging can be as infrequent as every 5 years if the aorta is normal in size.

  o *Invasive therapies*:

    o Balloon valvuloplasty: In older adults, this can be considered as a bridge to aortic valve replacement (class IIb indication), but is otherwise generally contraindicated. It is, however, indicated in the following groups of young adults or adolescents:

      o Class I indications: No calcification of the valve and no AR AND the patient has symptoms (angina, dyspnea, syncope) AND peak-to-peak gradient >50 mm Hg; ST or

T wave abnormalities with rest or exercise AND peak-to-peak gradient >60 mm Hg.

- Class IIa indications: Peak-to-peak gradient >50 mm Hg in preparation for pregnancy or activity in competitive sport.
- Surgical repair/replacement: Indications are similar to those for AS or AR with a normal valve:
  - Class I indications: Patient with severe AS and symptoms or with LV dysfunction (LVEF <50%); adolescent/young adult with severe AR, symptoms, and LVEF <50% or LV end-diastolic diameter (LVEDD) >4 standard deviations above normal; at the time of ascending aorta repair when the ascending aorta is >5.0 cm or dilatation ≥5 mm/year.
  - Class IIa indications: Asymptomatic patient with severe AR, normal LVEF, but severe LV dilatation (LVEDD >75 mm; or LV end-systolic diameter >55 mm).
  - Several class IIb indications exist, but are not discussed further here.

SUBAORTIC STENOSIS

Overview

Subaortic stenosis is a fibrous or fibromuscular ring in the LV outflow tract. Subaortic stenosis has a male predominance (2 to 1).

Associated Defects and Physiology

- Associated defects: Usually a solitary lesion; however, can occur with other abnormalities including VSD (37%), BAV (23%), or with AVSD as indicated above. May be a part of Shone's complex (CoA, valvular or subvalvular aortic stenosis, parachute mitral valve, supravalvular mitral ring/membrane).
- Physiology: Subvalvular accelerated turbulent flow causes aortic valvular damage in the form of obstruction or aortic regurgitation. Physiology may be similar to valvular AS if severe.

Clinical Findings, Diagnosis, and Management

- Clinical presentation: Often presents asymptomatically with murmur on examination. As it progresses, symptoms of AS (valvular or subvalvular) or AR may be present.
- Examination findings: A crescendo-decrescendo murmur may be auscultated at the left parasternal apical border. A murmur representing AR may also be appreciated.
- Electrocardiogram: May be normal, but watch for signs of LV hypertrophy, left atrial enlargement, or ST-T repolarization.
- Chest x-ray: Chest imaging may show cardiomegaly if LV hypertrophy or dilation is present.
- Echocardiogram: Diagnostic study of choice to illustrate the anatomy, gradient, and associated findings (ie, AR, mitral involvement, systolic function) (Figure 17-18). In the case where there is a subaortic membrane AND stenotic aortic valve disease, TEE is useful to determine the site of stenosis that is most severe.
- Advanced imaging: May be useful to accurately define the anatomy, depending on the quality of TTE or TEE images.

- Catheterization: Cardiac catheterization is recommended if there is discordance between patient symptoms and diagnostic imaging studies. However, if symptoms and surface echocardiogram findings are concordant, cardiac catheterization is not required for diagnosis of this condition or the degree of stenosis/insufficiency.
- Management: Surgical repair may be considered for some patients, although there is recurrence of the fibromuscular band after surgery is present in at least one-third of patients.
  - Class I indications for surgery:
    - Mean gradient >30 mm Hg or peak gradient >50 mm Hg
    - Progressive AR and LVEDD >50 mm or LVEF <55%
  - Class IIb indications for surgery:
    - Mean gradient 30 mm Hg with progressive AR or AS.
    - Peak gradient <50 mm Hg and mean <30 mm Hg AND either LV hypertrophy, a planned pregnancy, or plans to engage in competitive sport.

SUPRAVALVULAR AORTIC STENOSIS

Overview

Supravalvular aortic stenosis is a fixed obstruction immediately distal to the sinus of Valsalva. The coronary arteries arise proximal to the obstruction; therefore, they are exposed to high pressures during systole, but receive low pressure flow during diastole.

Associated Defects and Physiology

- Associated defects: About half of patients with supravalvular AS have aortic valve abnormalities, and a minority may have concomitant disease in the pulmonary arterial (PA) system, such as peripheral PA stenosis. Williams syndrome, caused by an autosomal dominant mutation on chromosome 7, which includes the elastin gene, is associated with supravalvular AS. Other characteristics associated with Williams syndrome include elfin facies, cognitive disorders, joint abnormalities, and behavioral problems.
- Physiology: Similar to AS, except that there is sometimes coronary artery involvement.

Clinical Findings, Diagnosis, and Management

- Clinical presentation: Patients have symptoms of outflow obstruction including dyspnea, angina, and syncope. Signs include HTN and findings of coronary ischemia.
- Examination findings: The Coanda effect, which describes discordant amplitude of carotid and upper extremity arterial pulses, is a classic exam finding caused by preferential flow up the right-sided portion of the ascending aorta. There may also be a differential blood pressure in the upper extremities, a thrill over the suprasternal notch, and a crescendo/decrescendo murmur at the left upper sternal border with radiation to the right neck.
- Electrocardiogram: Usually normal.
- Chest x-ray: Usually normal.
- Echocardiogram: Used to characterize the anatomy of the proximal aorta, obstruction, and associated defects (Figure 17-19).

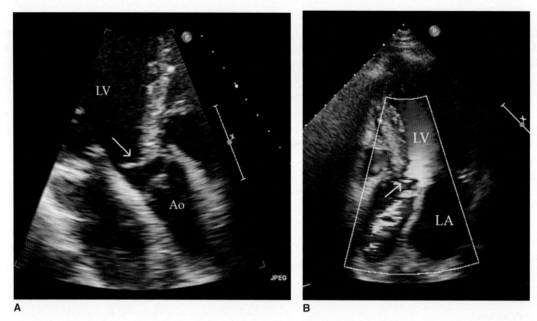

A   B

FIGURE 17-18 A. Apical 3-chamber view of discrete subaortic stenosis (SAS). A fibrous ridge (*arrow*) is present in the left ventricular outflow tract. **B.** Apical 5-chamber view of discrete SAS with color-flow Doppler, demonstrating aliasing and proximal flow convergence in the LV outflow tract. (Reproduced with permission from Fuster V, Walsh RA, Harrington RA. *Hurst's the Heart.* 13th ed. New York, NY: McGraw-Hill Education; 2011. Figure 18-122AB.)

- Advanced imaging: MRI or CT imaging is often required to accurately define the anatomy and look for associated defects. Additionally, myocardial perfusion imaging should be used if there is suspicion for ischemia due to coronary involvement.

- Catheterization: As indicated to investigate for myocardial ischemia. Typically level of stenosis can be differentiated on non-invasive imaging studies.

- Management:

  ○ *Serial imaging:* Proximal renal arteries and main and branch pulmonary artery flow should be evaluated at time of diagnosis. TTE and MRI or CT should be performed serially to assess anatomy of left ventricular outflow tract (LVOT), systolic/diastolic function, and valvular evaluation.

  ○ *Screening:* Periodic screening for myocardial ischemia is recommended. Additionally, all first-degree relatives should have screening for this heritable condition.

  ○ *Invasive therapies:* Surgical repair may be warranted in the following groups (class I indications):

    ○ Symptoms AND/OR mean gradient >50 mm Hg and peak gradient >70 mm Hg

    ○ Lesser gradients AND symptoms, LV hypertrophy, planned pregnancy or competitive sport, or LV systolic dysfunction

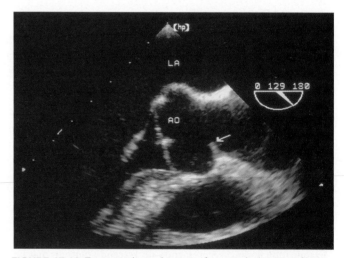

FIGURE 17-19 Transesophageal image of supravalvular AS. A fibrous ridge extends into the aortic lumen just above the sinus of Valsalva. Abbreviations: aorta, Ao; left atrium, LA. (Reproduced with permission from Fuster V, Walsh RA, Harrington RA. *Hurst's the Heart.* 13th ed. New York, NY: McGraw-Hill Education; 2011. Figure 18-122E).

COARCTATION OF THE AORTA

Overview

Coarctation of the aorta (CoA) is a narrowing of the aorta near the level of the ligamentum arteriosum (the remnant of the ductus arteriosus). The narrowing may be preductal or postductal (Figure 17-20). This causes an obstruction in blood flow to the thoracic descending aorta, which is then perfused in part by collateral flow from the axillary

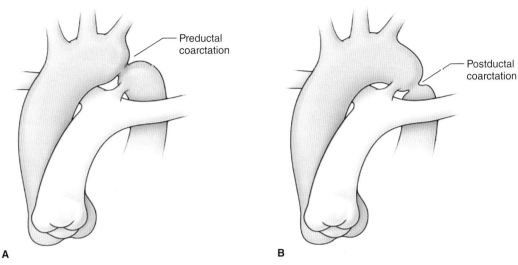

FIGURE 17-20 Anatomic features of aortic coarctation. **A.** Preductal coarctation, in which differential cyanosis may occur. **B.** Postductal coarctation. (Reproduced with permission from Crawford MH. *Current Diagnosis & Treatment: Cardiology.* 4th ed. New York, NY: McGraw-Hill Education; 2014. Figure 31-14.)

and internal thoracic arteries. The most severe form of CoA is complete interruption of the aortic arch (Figure 17-21).

Associated Defects and Physiology

- Associated defects: BAV (85%), brachiocephalic vessel anomalies, subaortic stenosis, VSD, arch hypoplasia, circle of Willis cerebral artery aneurysm (10%). One-third of patients with Turner syndrome have CoA.

- Physiology: Depends on the degree of narrowing and anticipated evidence of hypoperfusion distal to the site of obstruction. These patients also have an intrinsic aortic wall abnormality similar to the aorta of patients with BAV. This predisposes to aortic dilatation and dissection.

Clinical Findings, Diagnosis, and Management

- Clinical presentation: Patients may present asymptomatically with only signs of systemic HTN. However, symptoms may include headache, epistaxis, and claudication.

- Examination findings: A brachial-femoral delay is often noted; the term denotes a delayed pulse with lower amplitude in the lower extremities when compared with upper extremities. A left intrascapular murmur may also be appreciated.

- Electrocardiogram: Typically normal, except in the case where it causes long-standing HTN and LV hypertrophy, in which case LV hypertrophy is seen.

- Chest x-ray: Classic signs include rib notching, present on the inferior rib borders (Figure 17-22-B) as well as the reverse figure-of-3 sign, due to indentation at the CoA. Similarly, if a barium swallow is obtained, an E sign can be seen as a mirror image of the 3 sign, also due to the preductal and postductal regions of the aorta (Figure 17-23).

- Echocardiogram: The suprasternal notch window with color flow and continuous wave may show turbulence in the descending aorta and continuous forward diastolic flow.

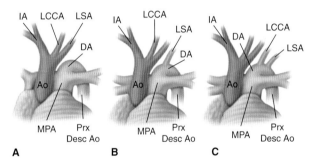

FIGURE 17-21 Anatomic types of interrupted aortic arch. **A,** Type A, interruption distal to the left subclavian artery. **B,** Type B, interruption between the left subclavian and left carotid arteries. **C,** Type C, interruption between the left carotid and innominate artery. (Ao, aorta; DA, ductus arteriosus, IA, innominate artery; LCCA, left common carotid artery; LSA, left subclavian artery; MPA, main pulmonary artery; Prx Desc Ao, proximal descending aorta.) (Reproduced with permission from Jonas RA. Interrupted aortic arch. In: Mavroudis C, Backer CL, eds. *Pediatric Cardiac Surgery.* 4th ed. Wiley-Blackwell, 2013.)

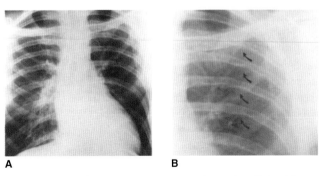

FIGURE 17-22 A. Coarctation causes severe obstruction of blood flow in the descending thoracic aorta. The descending aorta and its branches are perfused by collateral channels from the axillary and internal thoracic arteries through the intercostal arteries (*arrows*). (Reproduced with permission from Brickner ME, et al. Congenital heart disease in adults. First of two parts. *N Engl J Med.* 2000;342:256-263. Copyright © 2000 Massachusetts Medical Society. All rights reserved.) **B.** The chest radiogram from a patient with aortic coarctation showing marked rib notching (*arrows*). (Reproduced with permission from Bruce CJ, et al. Images in clinical medicine. Aortic coarctation and bicuspid aortic valve. *N Engl J Med.* 2000;342:249. Copyright © 2000 Massachusetts Medical Society. All rights reserved.)

- Advanced imaging: All patients with CoA should have 1 MRI or CT of the thoracic aorta and cerebral vasculature at the time of diagnosis. Stress testing may be helpful to determine the rest and exercise gradient as well as rest/exercise HTN.

- Catheterization: Particularly in adults, catheterization is employed for percutaneous intervention, as noted below.

- Management:

  ○ *Invasive therapies:*

  ○ Initial therapy: Surgical repair/replacement, balloon angioplasty, and/or covered stent placement to the coarctation segment should be performed when peak-to-peak CoA gradient ≥20 mm Hg OR peak-to-peak CoA gradient <20 mm Hg when there is anatomic or radiological evidence of significant collateral flow (class I indication). The type of surgical repair is dependent on both the anatomy of the lesion and the surgeon's preference (Figure 17-24). Recurrence rate after balloon angioplasty is 7%. It should be noted that the preferred treatment in an adult patient (due to well-developed spinal arteries) is percutaneous, as surgical intervention involves cross-clamping of the aorta, which may compromise the spinal arteries.

  ○ Therapies for recurrence: Percutaneous catheter therapies, such as covered stent placement, may be utilized in the setting of recurrent discreet CoA and peak-to-peak gradient of ≥20 mm Hg (class I indication). Stent placement for long-segment CoA may be considered as well (class IIb indication). Covered stents are also used to treat late sequelae of initial CoA repair such as pseudoaneurysm and aneurysm.

  ○ *Serial imaging:* CoA repair site should be evaluated at least every 5 years (irrespective of repair status) by MRI or CT.

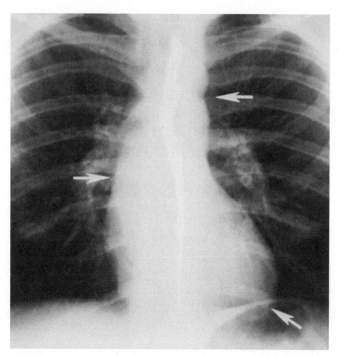

FIGURE 17-23 PA view of another patient with aortic coarctation showing the 3 sign of the deformed descending aorta and E sign on the barium-filled esophagus. The *upper arrow* points to the level of coarctation, and the *lower arrow* marks the apex of the enlarged LV. The *arrow* on the patient's right indicates the dilated ascending aorta. (Reproduced with permission from Fuster V, Walsh RA, Harrington RA. *Hurst's the Heart.* 13th ed. New York, NY: McGraw-Hill Education; 2011. Figure 17-1C.)

RIGHT VENTRICULAR OUTFLOW TRACT OBSTRUCTION

PULMONARY STENOSIS

Overview

Pulmonary stenosis (PS) can occur at the level of the valve or infundibulum (Figure 17-25B), or may be supravalvular. Stenosis may also exist at any level of the pulmonary tree, including within the branch pulmonary arteries. Symptoms typically are driven by the degree of involvement of the pulmonary vasculature when peripheral pulmonary stenosis is present. The most common site of stenosis, however, is at the level of the pulmonic valve (80%-90%). Three types of valvular PS exist:

- Dome-shaped pulmonary valve/commissural fusion, with a narrow central opening and a dilated pulmonary trunk (Figure 17-25A).

- Dysplastic valve with myxomatous thickening of leaflets and no commissural fusion. With this anatomy, the leaflets have little mobility. However, there is typically no pulmonary trunk dilatation.

- Unicuspid/bicuspid valve.

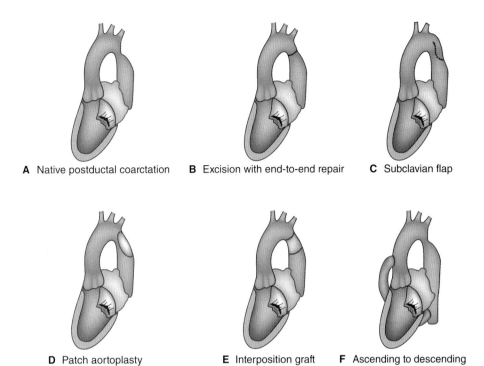

A Native postductal coarctation   **B** Excision with end-to-end repair   **C** Subclavian flap

D Patch aortoplasty   **E** Interposition graft   **F** Ascending to descending aorta interposition graft

FIGURE 17-24 Surgical techniques for repair of coarctation of the aorta. **A.** Unrepaired coarctation of the aorta. **B.** Excision of the narrowed segment with end-to-end anastomosis. **C.** Subclavian flap repair. **D.** Prosthetic patch aortoplasty. **E.** Excision of the narrowed segment and placement of a prosthetic conduit. **F.** Prosthetic conduit placement from the ascending to the descending aorta. (Reproduced with permission from Fuster V, Walsh RA, Harrington RA. *Hurst's the Heart.* 13th ed. New York, NY: McGraw-Hill Education; 2011. Figure 84-21.)

Associated Defects and Physiology

- Associated defects: Valvular PS occurs in 7% to 12% of all congenital heart disease. The dome-shaped type is often seen with Noonan syndrome (Figure 17-26), and the unicuspid/bicuspid type is often seen as part of ToF. Alagille and Rubinstein syndromes are also associated with PS.

- Physiology: Based on the degree of outflow tract obstruction and, after repair, on the presence/absence of pulmonic insufficiency (PI).

Clinical Findings, Diagnosis, and Management

- Clinical presentation: Patients are often asymptomatic with a systolic murmur. However, they may have progressive exercise intolerance, peripheral edema, syncope, or angina. There may be cyanosis in the setting of a patent foramen ovale (PFO).

- Examination findings:
  - A systolic ejection murmur is typically appreciated, increasing with inspiration in midsystole. An ejection sound may be heard due to the valve opening. Signs of increasing right-sided pressures and volume overload may be present, such as elevated jugular venous pressure (JVP) with increased A wave, RV lift or heave, soft P_2, split S_2, or right-sided S_4.
  - In patients with Noonan syndrome findings may include short stature, web neck, hypertelorism, lymphedema, low-set ears, low-set hairline, hyperelastic skin, chest deformities, cryptorchidism and micrognathia. One-third are developmentally delayed.

- Electrocardiogram: Right atrial enlargement, RVH, and right axis deviation (Figure 17-27).

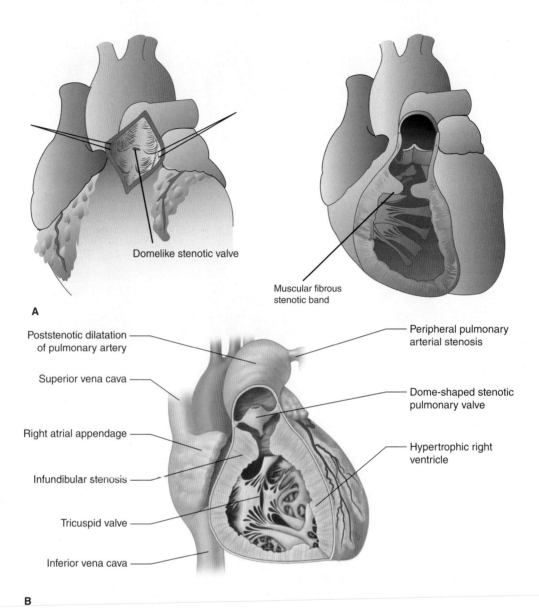

A

Domelike stenotic valve

Muscular fibrous stenotic band

Poststenotic dilatation of pulmonary artery

Peripheral pulmonary arterial stenosis

Superior vena cava

Dome-shaped stenotic pulmonary valve

Right atrial appendage

Hypertrophic right ventricle

Infundibular stenosis

Tricuspid valve

Inferior vena cava

B

FIGURE 17-25 Anatomic features of pulmonary stenosis. **A.** Pulmonary stenosis. Top: Valvular pulmonary stenosis. Bottom: Infundibular pulmonary stenosis. (Reproduced with permission from Doherty GM. *Current Diagnosis & Treatment: Surgery.* 14th ed. New York, NY: McGraw-Hill Education; 2015. Figure 19-34.) **B.** Pulmonary stenosis. Structures enlarged: right ventricle and sometimes pulmonary artery (poststenotic dilation).

- Chest x-ray: May show enlarged right or left pulmonary arteries, or pulmonary congestion (Figure 17-28).

- Echocardiogram: Diagnostic in most cases (Figure 17-29). Doppler should be used to look for degree of PS and presence and degree of PI.

- Advanced imaging: Generally not required

- Catheterization: Catheterization is generally required for treatment of PS via percutaneous intervention as noted below. It is rarely required to confirm findings, as noninvasive imaging is quite good at making the diagnosis and determining the degree of stenosis.

- Management:

  ○ *Serial imaging*: Frequency of examinations and TTEs is based on gradient. For a gradient <30 mm Hg, there is little risk of progression; the patient may be followed every 5 years with an examination and TTE. Patients with higher gradients should be followed more frequently.

○ *Invasive therapies*: The decision to intervene is based on symptoms and gradient. At >50 mm Hg, the lesion is often causing symptoms and may necessitate intervention. Balloon valvotomy and surgical replacement/repair are the current treatment options for valvular PS, with percutaneous valve replacement still under investigation.

   ○ Class I indications for balloon valvotomy:
      ○ Asymptomatic patients with domed pulmonary valve and peak gradient >60 mm Hg or mean >40 mm Hg with less than moderate PI.
      ○ Symptomatic patients with domed pulmonary valve and peak >50 mm Hg or mean >30 mm Hg with less than moderate PI.
   ○ Class I indications for surgical treatment (commissurotomy or valve replacement):
      ○ Severe PS and associated hypoplastic pulmonary annulus, severe PI, subvalvular PS, or supravalvular PS.
      ○ Dysplastic pulmonary valve.
      ○ Associated severe TR and the need for a maze procedure.
   ○ A surgical approach is preferred for dysplastic pulmonary valves, due to poor outcomes after balloon valvotomy. However, a balloon valvotomy may be reasonable to consider in an asymptomatic patient with peak gradient >60 mm Hg or mean >40 mm Hg.
   ○ Indications for repair of supravalvular PS include RV systolic pressure >50 mm Hg and affected PA segments <50% the diameter of the adjacent vessel. Percutaneous therapy is preferred.

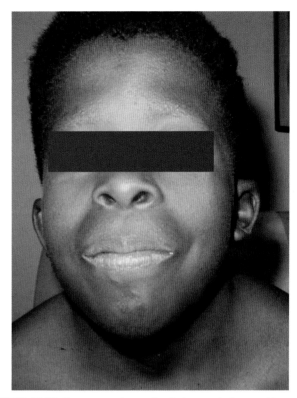

FIGURE 17-26 Noonan syndrome: Ptosis, hypertelorism, and low-set ears associated with valvular pulmonic stenosis. (Reproduced with permission from Fuster V, Walsh RA, Harrington RA. *Hurst's the Heart.* 13th ed. New York, NY: McGraw-Hill Education; 2011. Figure 14-17.)

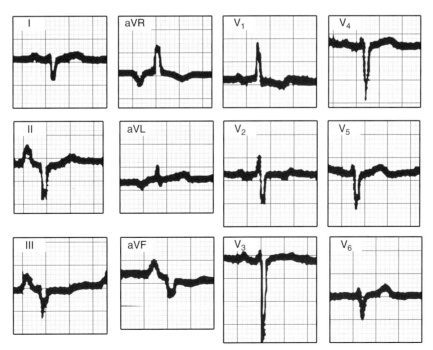

FIGURE 17-27 Right atrial and right ventricular hypertrophy. The P waves are abnormally tall in leads II, III, and aVF, indicating right atrial abnormality. The frontal plane QRS axis is oriented rightward (deep S in I) and superiorly (QS complexes in II, III, and aVF); the axis is −110 degrees. A tall R wave is present in V_1. The rightward axis and tall R wave in V_1 indicate right ventricular hypertrophy. In the presence of right ventricular hypertrophy, QS complexes need not indicate myocardial infarction.

○ Surgical treatment of infundibular stenosis/subvalvular PS includes resection of the hypertrophied muscle bundles in cases of >60 mm Hg peak or >40 mm Hg mean intraventricular gradient without symptoms, or >50 mm Hg peak or >30 mm Hg mean gradient with symptoms.

EISENMENGER SYNDROME

Overview

Patients with pulmonary arterial hypertension (PAH) who have a left-to-right shunt may ultimately develop an end-stage disease termed *Eisenmenger syndrome (ES)*. This refers to the reversal of blood flow across a defect at the level of the pulmonary and systemic ventricles or arteries, resulting in pulmonary to systemic shunting of blood. In other words, the left-to-right shunt becomes right-to-left. This occurs when pulmonary blood pressures have risen to meet or exceed systemic blood pressures.

Clinical Findings, Diagnosis, and Management

- Clinical presentation: Dyspnea on exertion is most common, but other symptoms may include palpitations, edema, hemoptysis, and cyanosis.

- Examination findings: Central cyanosis, clubbing, signs of right heart failure (JVP, increased A wave, ascites, RV impulse, PA impulse, palpable P_2, cessation of previous shunt murmur). Tophaceous deposits may be evident due to decreased clearance of urate (Figure 17-30).

- Electrocardiogram: Right atrial enlargement, RVH, right axis deviation. Other findings may relate to the underlying lesion or condition.

- Chest x-ray: Findings of pulmonary vessel congestion may be evident (Figure 17-31).

- Echocardiogram: Demonstrates defect with bidirectional or pulmonary to systemic shunting and increased pulmonary artery pressure. Agitated saline bubble study is contraindicated, as it can result in air embolism.

- Advanced imaging: Advanced imaging is not required to make the diagnosis of ES; however, it can be useful to follow biventricular size and function over time.

- Catheterization: While cardiac catheterization is not required to diagnose ES, it may be useful to measure pulmonary artery pressures, particularly when advanced pulmonary arterial HTN-specific medications are considered/used.

- Management:
  ○ Much of the management of ES involves prevention, recognition, and treatment of these frequently associated conditions, which will not be discussed in detail here:
    ○ Ventricular arrhythmias in 50%
    ○ Hemoptysis in 20%
    ○ Pulmonary embolism in 10%
    ○ Syncope in 10%
    ○ Endocarditis in 10%
    ○ Neurovascular disease and infection (cerebral hemorrhage, emboli, abscess)

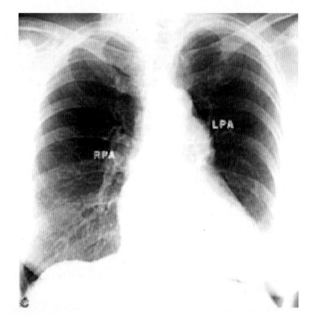

FIGURE 17-28 Pulmonary stenosis. Structures enlarged: right ventricle and sometimes pulmonary artery (poststenotic dilation). (Reproduced from Bashore TM, Granger CB, Jackson KP, Patel MR. *Heart Disease.* In: Papadakis MA, McPhee SJ, Rabow MW, eds. Current Medical Diagnosis & Treatment 2018 New York, NY: McGraw-Hill.)

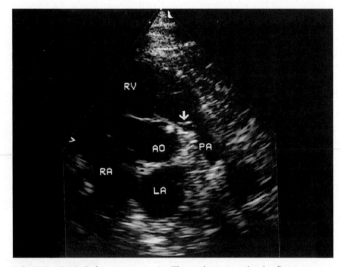

FIGURE 17-29 Pulmonic stenosis. The pulmonic valve leaflet is thickened and echo-reflective, and does not open completely during systole (*arrow*). (Reproduced with permission from Fuster V, Walsh RA, Harrington RA. *Hurst's the Heart.* 13th ed. New York, NY: McGraw-Hill Education; 2011. Figure 18-85A.)

○ Hypoxemia and associated hypoxia, which lead to poly-cythemia and increased cell turnover, causing pigmented gallstones, gout, renal disease, and hyperviscosity syndrome with fatigue, headache, dizziness.

○ *Medical therapy:*
  ○ Class I indications:
    ○ Avoid the following activities/conditions: Dehydration, strenuous exercise and isometric exercise, acute exposure to excessive heat (ie, hot tub), iron deficiency.
    ○ Annual blood counts, iron level, creatinine, and uric acid.
    ○ Annual digital oximetry and appropriate treatment with oxygen.
    ○ Pulmonary vasodilators can improve quality of life.
    ○ Warfarin should be considered for prevention of pulmonary emboli/cerebral emboli; however, if there is active hemopty-sis, this is contraindicated.
    ○ In general, therapeutic phlebotomy for erythrocytosis should not be done, but can be considered if hematocrit is >65% and there is evidence of hyperviscosity in the absence of dehydration.
  ○ *Endocarditis prophylaxis:* Should be considered given the cyanotic nature of this lesion (class IIa indication).
  ○ *Reproduction:* In general, pregnancy should be avoided. Early pregnancy termination is recommended (class I indication).

TETRALOGY OF FALLOT

Overview

Tetralogy of Fallot (ToF) is the most common cyanotic type of congenital heart disease, representing 5% to 10% of all congenital heart defects. It consists of 4 major defects: subpulmonary infun-dibular stenosis, aorta overriding (posterior malalignment) VSD, and RV hypertrophy (Figure 17-32).

Associated Defects and Physiology

• Associated defects: 5% of patients have an ASD (pentology of Fallot). Patients can also have a right-sided aortic arch and coro-nary artery anomalies. It is commonly associated with 22q11 deletion, Alagille syndrome, CHARGE syndrome, and as part of the VATER/VACTERL associations.

• Physiology: The RVOT is narrowed, restricting systemic venous blood flow into the pulmonary vasculature. A cyanotic tet spell can be caused by periods of increased myocardial contractil-ity, which cause dynamic infundibular subpulmonic stenosis to become exacerbated, leading to worsening resistance to pulmo-nary blood flow and causing the preferential shunting of blood from the RV to the LV across the VSD.

Clinical Findings, Diagnosis, and Management

• Clinical presentation: Most patients undergo repair in the first year of life; however, adults can present unrepaired similar to patients with a nonrestrictive VSD without pulmonary HTN, as the subpulmonic stenosis protects the pulmonary vasculature from overcirculation, and ultimately from pulmonary HTN. Pal-liative repair in the first year of life varies depending on where and when (year) it was completed. Typically it involves patching

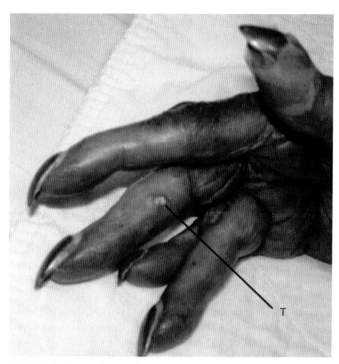

FIGURE 17-30 The hand of a 59-year-old woman with pulmonary hypertension, a large atrial septal defect, cyanosis, and hyperuricemia. Note the cyanosis and clubbing of the digits. A tophaceous urate deposit (T) is noted on the middle phalanx of the second digit. (Repro-duced with permission from Fuster V, Walsh RA, Harrington RA. *Hurst's the Heart.* 13th ed. New York, NY: McGraw-Hill Education; 2011. Figure 84-6.)

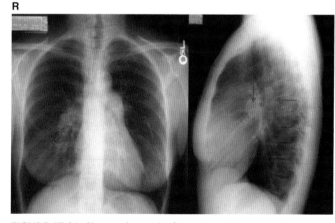

FIGURE 17-31 Chest radiograph of a patient with severe pulmonary hypertension. Note the enlarged pulmonary arteries (*red arrows*) visible on both PA and lateral films. (Reproduced with permission from Kasper D, Fauci A, Hauser S, Longo D, Jameson JL, Loscalzo J. *Harrison's Principles of Internal Medicine.* 19th ed. New York, NY: McGraw-Hill Education; 2015. Figure 308E-52.)

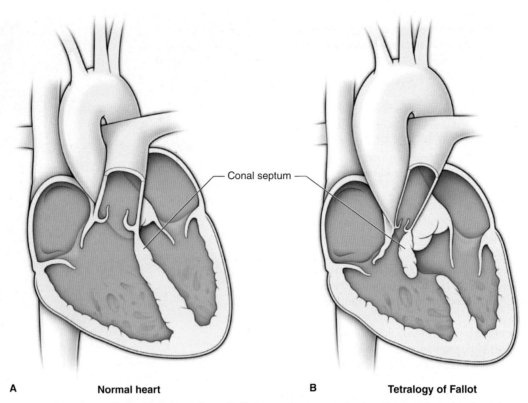

A   **Normal heart**   **B**   **Tetralogy of Fallot**

FIGURE 17-32 Anatomy of tetralogy of Fallot (ToF). Note that in ToF, the conal septum is displaced anteriorly and to the right, resulting in a smaller pulmonary artery orifice and subpulmonic obstruction. (Reproduced with permission from Crawford MH. *Current Diagnosis & Treatment: Cardiology.* 4th ed. New York, NY: McGraw-Hill Education; 2014. Figure 31-23.)

the VSD (and ASD, if present) with enlargement of the RVOT. Patients can be left with severe PI or residual PS, leading to signs of RV failure such as dyspnea with exertion and edema.

- Examination findings: Post repair, patients typically can have a soft systolic murmur from flow across the RVOT. They may or may not have a diastolic murmur of PI. A pansystolic murmur post repair may indicate a residual VSD or patch leak at the VSD repair site. Patients with a history of arterial-to-pulmonary shunt (Blalock-Taussig-Thomas shunt) may lead to reduced or absent pulses on the ipsilateral upper extremity.

- Electrocardiogram: RVH and right bundle-branch block (RBBB) common in patients with repair prior to the 1990s. If the QRS is >180 ms, there are some data that suggest there is increased risk for sustained ventricular arrhythmias and sudden death.[13]

- Chest x-ray: A boot-shaped horizontal heart is classic in unrepaired ToF (Figure 17-33). A right-sided aortic arch may be seen. In repaired ToF, there will be evidence of RA and RV enlargement.

- Echocardiogram: TTE is useful for routine follow-up of PI, RVH/RVE, systolic function, and to assess for degeneration of repair (Figure 17-34, unrepaired defect; Figure 17-35, Doppler interrogation of pulmonary valve in a patient with PI). This is indicated as a part of yearly follow-up (class I indication).

- Advanced imaging: Cardiac MRI or CT can be useful to evaluate RV size and function, particularly as it relates to PS or PI, which can occur late after repair.

- Catheterization: In the adult patient, catheterization may be useful to determine the degree of stenosis or regurgitation at the level of

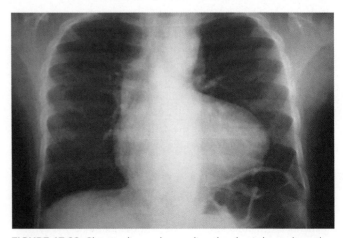

FIGURE 17-33 Chest radiograph revealing the classic boot-shaped heart of tetralogy of Fallot. (Reproduced with permission from Shah BR, Lucchesi M, eds. *Atlas of Pediatric Emergency Medicine.* New York, NY: McGraw-Hill; 2006.)

the pulmonary valve, if imaging studies are compromised by calcification from prior repair. Additionally, catheterization is frequently used to deliver percutaneous pulmonary valve, when indicated. In patients with a prior annuloplasty, the most common indication is for pulmonary insufficiency, and in those with a prior homograft, PS is the most common indication for this procedure.

- Management:

  - *Surgical treatment:* Indicated for severe symptomatic PI and symptoms (class I indication). Pulmonary valve replacement with severe PI is a class II indication if the patient has any of the following: moderate to severe RV dysfunction, moderate to severe RV enlargement, symptomatic or sustained atrial or ventricular arrhythmias, and moderate to severe TR. It is a class II indication for patients with residual RVOT obstruction and any of the following: peak gradient >50 mm Hg, RV/LV pressure ratio >0.7, progressive or severe dilation of the RV with dysfunction, residual VSD with left-to-right shunt >1.5:1, severe AR with symptoms or more than mild LV dysfunction, or a combination of multiple remaining lesions leading to RV enlargement or reduced function.

  - *Arrhythmia prevention:* In patients at high risk, referral to an EP specialist is recommended. Risk factors include prior palliative shunt, infundibulotomy/RV scar, QRS duration >180 ms, inducible VT at EP study, NSVT on monitor, LVEDP of >12 mm Hg, cardiothoracic ratio of >0.6 on chest x-ray, and age >18. Patients should have an annual ECG to assess rhythm and QRS duration.[8,14]

TRANSPOSITION OF THE GREAT ARTERIES

DEXTRO-TRANSPOSITION OF THE GREAT ARTERIES

Overview

In patients born with dextro-transposition of the great arteries (d-TGA), the aorta arises from the morphologic right ventricle rather than the left; similarly, the pulmonary trunk originates in the morphologic left ventricle rather than the right. Therefore, deoxygenated blood return from the body flows from the right atrium to the right ventricle and then back out to the body through the aorta. In a parallel circuit, oxygenated blood flows from the lungs to the left atrium to the left ventricle and then back to the lungs via the pulmonary artery. Prior to intervention, a septal defect and/or intact PDA allows for the mixing of deoxygenated and oxygenated blood for survival (Figures 17-36 and 17-37).

Associated Defects and Physiology

- Associated defects: In patients with d-TGA, 45% have a VSD and 25% have some type of LV outflow tract obstruction. Many have a PDA and coronary anomalies.

- Physiology: Cyanosis occurs in infancy due to inadequate mixing. Without intervention, one-third of infants die in the first week of life, and 90% die before 1 year of life. Physiology after intervention depends on the type of repair done in infancy:

  - Atrial switch (Figures 17-38 and 17-39): These procedures are commonly known as the Mustard and Senning repairs,

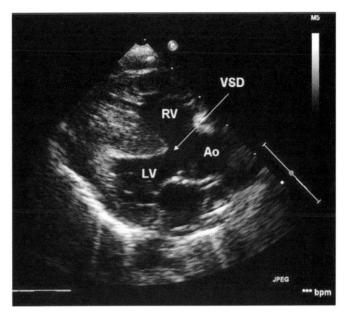

FIGURE 17-34 Parasternal long-axis image of tetalogy of Fallot. The right ventricle (RV) is enlarged, and a large VSD is present . (Reproduced with permission from Jonas RA. Interrupted aortic arch. In: Mavroudis C, Backer CL, eds. *Pediatric Cardiac Surgery.* 4th ed. Wiley-Blackwell, 2013.)

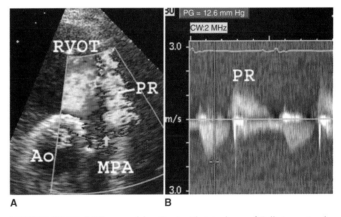

FIGURE 17-35 A 28-year-old patient with tetralogy of Fallot repaired during childhood with transannular patch placement. **A.** Transthoracic 2-dimensional and color-flow Doppler in the parasternal short-axis projection demonstrating severe pulmonary regurgitation (PR) from the main pulmonary artery (MPA) to the right ventricular outflow tract (RVOT). The aortic valve is labeled (Ao). The *blue vertical arrow* points to a flail portion of the remaining pulmonary valve. **B.** Continuous-wave Doppler interrogation of the RVOT and MPA in the parasternal short-axis projection demonstrates a low-velocity (< 2 m/s) jet of pulmonary regurgitation (PR) that ends before the onset of systole, consistent with elevated right ventricular diastolic pressure and restrictive right ventricular physiology. There is mild residual pulmonary stenosis. (Reproduced with permission from Fuster V, Walsh RA, Harrington RA. *Hurst's the Heart.* 13th ed. New York, NY: McGraw-Hill Education; 2011. Figure 84-9.)

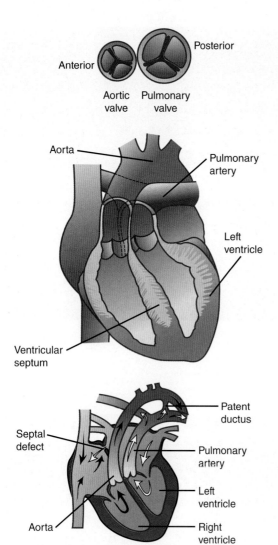

FIGURE 17-36 Typical transposition of the great arteries. The aorta arises from the morphologic right ventricle and is anterior and slightly to the right of the pulmonary artery, which originates from the morphologic left ventricle. Inset at bottom illustrates the independent systemic and pulmonary circulations, which may be connected by a patent ductus arteriosus or atrial septal defect. Inset at top illustrates a common relationship of the 2 great arteries in typical transposition. (Reproduced with permission from Doherty GM. *Current Diagnosis & Treatment: Surgery.* 14th ed. New York, NY: McGraw-Hill Education; 2015. Figure 19-28.)

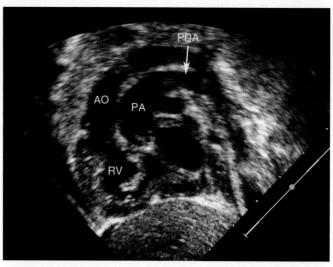

FIGURE 17-37 D-loop transposition of the great arteries. Subxiphoid short-axis echocardiogram image demonstrates the aorta (AO) arising anteriorly from the right ventricle (RV). Note the large patent ductus arteriosus (PDA) between the pulmonary artery (PA) and the descending aorta, which allows for mixing of the 2 parallel circulations. (Reproduced with permission from Fuster V, Walsh RA, Harrington RA. *Hurst's the Heart.* 13th ed. New York, NY: McGraw-Hill Education; 2011. Figure 83-33.)

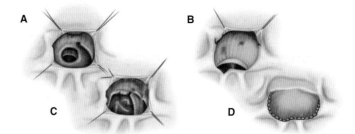

FIGURE 17-38 The Senning operation. **A,** The atrial septum is cut near the tricuspid valve, creating a flap attached posteriorly between the caval veins. **B,** The flap of atrial septum is sutured to the anterior lip of the orifices of the left pulmonary veins, effectively separating the pulmonary and systemic venous channels. **C,** The posterior edge of the right atrial incision is sutured to the remnant of atrial septum, diverting the systemic venous channel to the mitral valve. **D,** The anterior edge of the right atrial incision, lengthened by short incisions at each corner, is sutured around the cava above and below and to the lateral edge of the left atrial incision, completing the pulmonary channel and diversion of pulmonary venous blood to the tricuspid valve area. (Reproduced with permission from D-transposition of the great arteries. In: Mavroudis C, Backer CL, eds. *Pediatric Cardiac Surgery.* 4th ed. Wiley-Blackwell, 2013.)

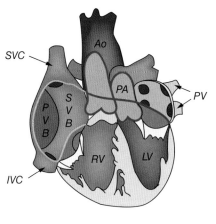
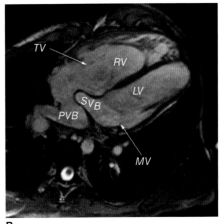

A   B

FIGURE 17-39 **A.** Valentine diagram of the cardiac anatomy in a patient with D-transposition of the great arteries who has undergone the Mustard or Senning atrial switch operation. Deoxygenated blood (*blue*) returning from the superior and inferior vena cava (SVC and IVC, respectively) is redirected via a systemic venous baffle (SVB) to the left ventricle (LV) and thereafter into the transposed pulmonary artery (PA). Oxygenated blood (*red*) returning from the lungs via the pulmonary veins (PVs) is redirected via a pulmonary venous baffle (PVB) to the systemic right ventricle (RV) and then to an anterior and rightward aorta (Ao). **B.** Cinecardiac magnetic resonance imaging scan (axial plane) demonstrating the SVB directing deoxygenated blood via the mitral valve (MV) to the subpulmonic LV and PVB directing oxygenated blood via the tricuspid valve (TV) to the systemic RV. (Reproduced with permission from Fuster V, Walsh RA, Harrington RA. *Hurst's the Heart.* 13th ed. New York, NY: McGraw-Hill Education; 2011. Figure 84-2.)

after the surgeons who originally performed them. In either, an intra-atrial baffle is used to redirect blood across the atrium from the SVC and IVC to the mitral valve. In a Mustard, a Dacron graft or section of pericardium is used to create the baffle. Conversely, in the Senning, the atrial septum itself is utilized for the baffle.

○ Rastelli procedure: Indicated for those with d-TGA, a VSD, and an RVOT obstruction. This procedure involves using a Teflon baffle to both occlude the VSD and direct blood from the left ventricle to the aorta. The pulmonary valve is replaced with a valved homograft conduit connecting the pulmonary artery to the right ventricle.

○ Arterial switch (Figure 17-40): Also known as the Jatene procedure, again after the surgeon who performed and first reported successful arterial switch. The great artery trunks are transected and sewn to the contralateral root with transposition of the coronary arteries to the neoaorta. This is the preferred procedure, as it allows the LV to act as the systemic ventricle.

Clinical Findings, Diagnosis, and Management

• Clinical presentation: Quite variable depending on type of repair

○ Atrial switch: Patients often present with symptoms of systemic ventricular failure, such as dyspnea and orthopnea. An obstruction or leak in the baffle, which occurs in 25% of patients, may cause paradoxical emboli or exercise-induced oxygen desaturation. Arrhythmias are also a common presentation, with 50% of patients experiencing sinus node dysfunction and 30% having intra-atrial reentry tachycardia by age 20 years.

○ Arterial switch: Aortic insufficiency may develop due to dilation of the neoaortic root, or stenosis near anastomosis sites causing AS or PS. Coronary ostia stenosis may cause symptoms of ischemia.

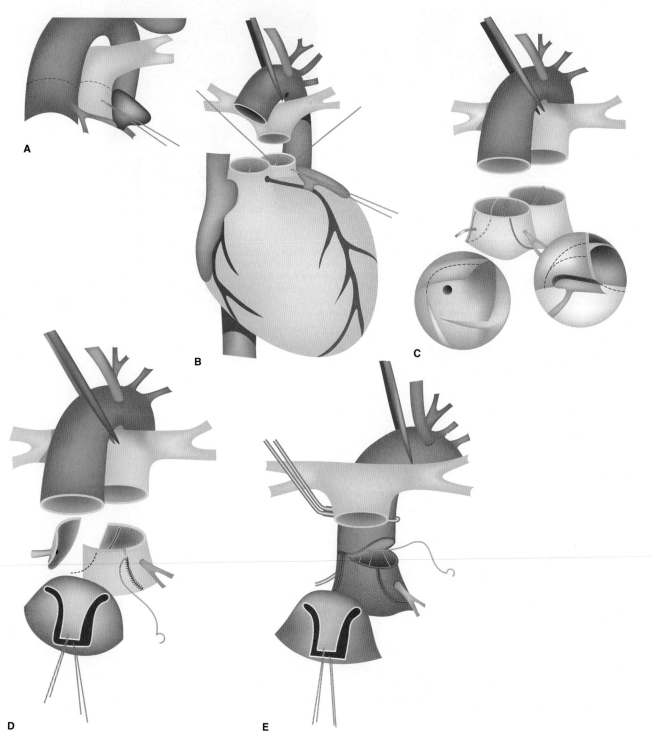

FIGURE 17-40 Surgical technique of the arterial switch operation. **A.** Aortic cannula is positioned distally in the ascending aorta, the ductus arteriosus is divided between suture ligatures, and the branch pulmonary arteries are dissected out to the hilum to provide adequate mobility for anterior translocation. The broken lines represent the levels of transection of the aorta and the main pulmonary artery. Marking sutures are placed in the anticipated sites of coronary transfer. **B.** Transection of the great arteries. The left ventricular outflow tract, neoaortic valve, and coronary arteries are inspected thoroughly. **C.** The coronary arterial buttons are excised from the free edge of the aorta to the base of the sinus of Valsalva. **D.** The coronary buttons are anastomosed to V-shaped excisions made in the neoaorta. **E.** The pulmonary artery is brought anterior to the aorta (Lecompte maneuver). Anastomosis of the proximal neoaorta is shown. **F.** and **G.** The coronary donor sites are filled with autologous pericardial patches. A single U-shaped patch (**F**) or 2 separate patches (**G**) may be used. **H.** Completed anastomosis of the proximal neopulmonary artery and the distal pulmonary artery. (Modified with permission from Castaneda AR. Anatomic correction of transposition of the great arteries at the arterial level. In: Sabiston DC Jr, Spencer FC, eds. *Surgery of the Chest*. 5th ed. Philadelphia, PA: WB Saunders; 1990.)

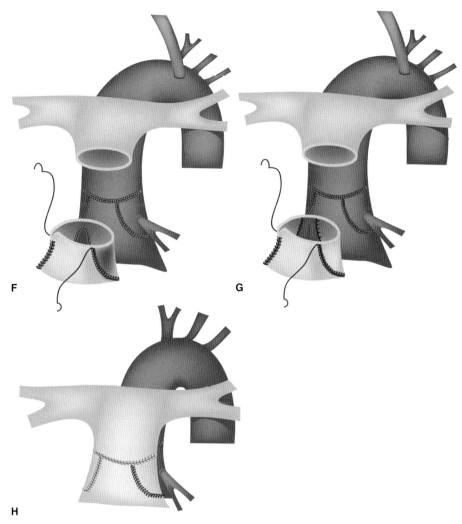

F   G

H

FIGURE 17-40 (Continued)

- Examination findings:
  - Atrial switch: Loud A_2. If there is RV failure there may be TR and RV heave.
  - Arterial switch: Usually unremarkable.

- Electrocardiogram:
  - Atrial switch: RVH, sinus bradycardia or junctional escape rhythms may be apparent.
  - Arterial switch: Typically normal.

- Chest x-ray: Uncorrected patients will have a classic "egg on a string" appearance. The adult repaired patient, if having undergone an atrial level switch, will typically have RV enlargement.
  - Atrial switch: Cardiomegaly.
  - Arterial switch: Typically normal.

- Echocardiogram: On TTE in an uncorrected patient, parallel great arteries with the aorta found anterior and rightward is typical. For patients who have had an arterial switch, suture lines for the great vessels or coronary buttons may be identifiable. It may be difficult to identify the morphologic ventricle, but the following landmarks may be helpful:
  - RV has a trabeculated apex and a moderator band.
  - Tricuspid valve (TV) is displaced apically in the RV.
  - LV is attached to a bileaflet AV valve.
- Advanced imaging: MRI (or CT, particularly if the patient has a pacemaker or metallic hardware) is the standard for assessment of ventricular function.
- Catheterization: Diagnostic catheterization can be used to further assess baffle leaks, presumed stenosis in conduits/baffles/great vessels, or unanticipated sources for ventricular dysfunction if these have been suggested by noninvasive means. It is also indicated to assess coronary anatomy after the arterial switch operation.
- Management:
  - *Medical therapies:* There are little data regarding the use of beta blockers or ACE inhibitors in this population.
  - *Serial imaging:* Patients should have a TTE and/or MRI yearly (class I indication).
  - *Electrophysiology:* Symptomatic sinus bradycardia or sick sinus syndrome warrants pacemaker (PPM) implantation (class I indication).
  - *Invasive therapies:*
    - Interventional catheterization (class IIa indications):
      - Atrial switch: Occlusion of baffle leak, dilation or stenting of obstruction at SVC or IVC, dilation or stenting of pulmonary obstruction.
      - Rastelli procedure: Can be used to dilate or stent conduit obstruction if RV pressure >50% systemic pressure or peak-to-peak gradient >30 mm Hg.
      - Arterial switch: Dilation or stenting of pulmonary arterial stenoses or coronary arterial stenoses
    - Surgical intervention:
      - Atrial switch (class I indications):
        - Moderate to severe systemic atrioventricular valve regurgitation (morphologic TV).
        - Baffle leak with left-to-right shunt >1.5:1, right-to-left shunt with arterial desaturation rest/exercise, symptoms, and progressive LV enlargement.
        - SVC or IVC baffle stenosis not amenable to percutaneous treatment.
        - Pulmonary obstruction not amenable to percutaneous intervention.
        - Symptomatic severe subpulmonary stenosis.
      - Rastelli procedure:
        - Conduit stenosis meeting criteria for surgery for PS.
        - Conduit regurgitation meeting criteria for surgery for PI.
        - Residual VSD meeting criteria for surgery for VSD.
        - Subaortic baffle stenosis with mean gradient of 50 mm Hg or less in the presence of AI.
      - Arterial switch (class I indications):
        - RVOT obstruction peak-to-peak gradient >50 mm Hg or RV/LV pressure ratio >0.7 not amenable to percutaneous intervention.
        - Coronary artery abnormality with myocardial ischemia not amenable to percutaneous treatment.
        - Severe neoaortic valve regurgitation.
        - Severe neoaortic root dilatation (>55 mm).

LEVO-TRANSPOSITION OF THE GREAT ARTERIES/CONGENITALLY CORRECTED TGA

Overview

Similar to d-TGA, in patients with levo-transposition of the great arteries (l-TGA), the aorta arises from the morphologic right ventricle and the pulmonary trunk originates in the morphologic left ventricle. However, the path of blood flow does not occur in a parallel circuit. Deoxygenated blood flows from the body into the right atrium, to the morphologic left ventricle, and then to the lungs through the pulmonary artery. Oxygenated blood flows from the lungs to the left atrium, to the morphologic right ventricle, and then out to the body through the aorta (Figure 17-41).

Associated Defects and Physiology

- Associated defects: Almost all (90%) have regurgitation of the systemic atrioventricular valve. VSD, most commonly perimembranous, will occur in 70% of patients. Also, 40% of patients have subvalvular or valvular PS. An Ebstein-like TV may occur as well.
- Physiology: Because the morphologic right ventricle acts as a systemic LV, pumping against systemic pressures, ventricular dysfunction is nearly universal by adulthood. This in combination with systemic atrioventricular valve regurgitation can lead to significant HF.

Clinical Findings, Diagnosis, and Management

- Clinical presentation: The majority of these patients are diagnosed either in childhood or adulthood (do not typically present in infancy). Presentation can vary from asymptomatic patients to those with signs of HF and arrhythmias.

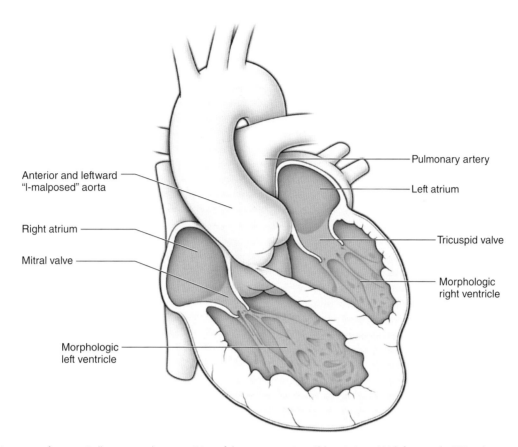

FIGURE 17-41 Anatomy of congenitally corrected transposition of the great arteries. Abbreviations: LV, left ventricle; RV, right ventricle. (Reproduced with permission from Crawford MH. *Current Diagnosis & Treatment: Cardiology.* 4th ed. New York, NY: McGraw-Hill Education; 2014. Figure 31-19.)

- Examination findings: The LV point of maximal impulse is shifted medially on examination, and there is a single S$_2$. A holosystolic murmur (VSD), a systolic ejection murmur (PS), and/or a diastolic murmur (AR) may be audible.

- Electrocardiogram: 50% of patients with l-TGA will have first-degree AV block. Another common finding is reversal of the precordial Q-wave pattern due to reversed septal activation. Complete heart block develops in 2% of these patients each year.

- Chest x-ray: Cardiomegaly due to left-sided RV enlargement may be present.

- Echocardiogram: On surface echocardiogram, parallel great arteries and an aorta that is anterior and leftward may be seen. See above for landmarks helpful in identifying morphological ventricles (Figure 17-42).

- Advanced imaging: MRI is the standard for assessment of ventricular function in this group of patients.

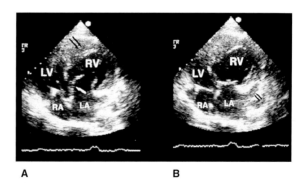

A   B

FIGURE 17-42 Apical transthoracic echocardiographic views in a patient with congenitally corrected transposition of the great arteries. **A.** The moderator band is clearly visualized (*double arrow*) in the left-sided morphologic right ventricle (RV). **B.** The narrow-based atrial appendage (*double arrow*) clearly identifies this as a left atrium (LA). The RV is spherically dilated, reflecting the pressure overload of this chamber. The left ventricle (LV) is small and compressed. Abbreviation: RA, right atrium. The left-sided atrioventricular (AV) valve is a morphologic tricuspid valve and the right-sided AV valve is a morphologic mitral valve. (Reproduced with permission from Crawford MH. *Current Diagnosis & Treatment: Cardiology.* 4th ed. New York, NY: McGraw-Hill Education; 2014. Figure 31-21.)

- Catheterization: Not typically indicated.
- Management:
  - *Medical therapies:* There are little data regarding the use of beta blockers or ACE inhibitors, although they may be beneficial in the setting of ventricular failure.
  - *Serial imaging:* TTE and/or MRI are recommended annually to evaluate heart size, function, and systemic atrioventricular valve function (class I indication).
  - *Electrophysiology:* Regular ECG monitoring for evidence of heart block, and PPM implantation in patients with symptomatic bradycardia is indicated.
  - *Invasive therapies:*
    - Surgical treatment (class I indications):
      - Severe AV valve regurgitation
      - Anatomic repair (arterial and atrial switch) when LV has been functioning at systemic pressures
      - VSD closure when LV-to-Ao baffle is not possible
      - LV-to-pulmonary artery conduit in cases of LV dysfunction and severe LV outflow obstruction
      - Moderate to progressive AV valve regurgitation
      - Conduit obstruction with high RV pressures or RV dysfunction after anatomic repair
      - Conduit obstruction and high LV pressures in patient with nonanatomic correction
      - Moderate to severe AR/neo-AR and ventricular dysfunction

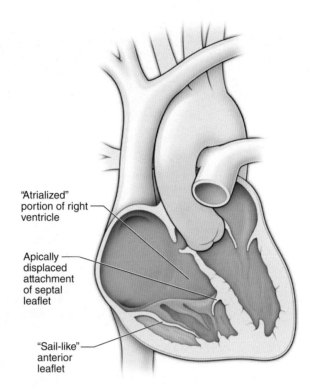

FIGURE 17-43 Anatomy of Ebstein anomaly. (Reproduced with permission from Crawford MH. *Current Diagnosis & Treatment: Cardiology.* 4th ed. New York, NY: McGraw-Hill Education; 2014. Figure 31-16.)

EBSTEIN ANOMALY

Overview

Ebstein anomaly refers to an apically displaced malformation of the TV with an atrialized portion of the RV and a large anterior leaflet due to failure of delamination of the TV tissue (Figure 17-43). This condition can be highly variable anatomically and therefore in the resultant degree of TV involvement and function. Ebstein anomaly accounts for 1% of congenital heart defects, and has been linked to maternal lithium use. There are 4 surgically recognized subtypes:

- Type I: Anterior TV leaflet large and mobile. Posterior and septal leaflets are apically displaced, dysplastic, or absent. Ventricular chamber size varies.

- Type II: Anterior, posterior, and often septal leaflets are present, but are small and apically displaced in a spiral pattern. Atrialized ventricle is large.

- Type III: Anterior leaflet is restricted, shortened, fused, and chordae are tethered. Frequently, papillary muscles directly insert into the anterior leaflet. Posterior and septal leaflets are displaced, dysplastic, not reconstructable. Large atrialized RV.

- Type IV: Anterior leaflet is deformed and displaced into the RVOT. Few to no chordae. Direct insertion of papillary muscle into valve is common. Posterior leaflet is absent or dysplastic. Septal leaflet is a ridge of fibrous material. Small atrialized RV.

Associated Defects and Physiology:

- Associated defects: Most common associations with Ebstein anomaly are atrial level shunts (ASD or PFO), seen in 79% of patients. Other associations include VSD, PS or pulmonary atresia, PDA, and CoA. Of Ebstein anomaly patients, 20% will have an accessory pathway (Wolff-Parkinson-White) or other types of arrhythmias.

- Physiology: Depends on the severity of the malformation, degree of TR or RVOT obstruction, and size of the RV cavity.

Clinical Findings, Diagnosis, and Management

- Clinical presentation: Adults can present at any age and most commonly present with arrhythmia, exercise intolerance, or right heart failure. Sudden death can occur and has been attributed to atrial fibrillation with conduction through an accessory pathway or from ventricular arrhythmias. Paradoxical embolism may also occur, which suggests the presence of a concomitant ASD.

- Examination findings: A systolic murmur of TR may be heard; classically holosystolic at the left lower sternal border that increases with inspiration.

- Electrocardiogram: RA enlargement as evidenced by tall Himalayan P waves, QR in V1 up to lead V4, RBBB, splintered QRS complex. Accessory pathway is present in one-third of patients (Figure 17-44).

- Chest x-ray: May show cardiomegaly.

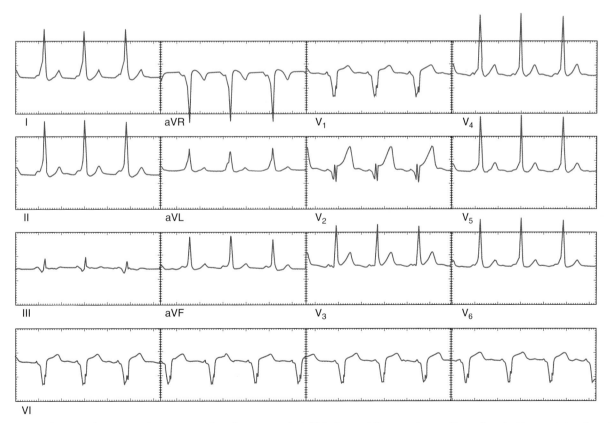

FIGURE 17-44 Electrocardiogram in Ebstein anomaly with associated Wolff-Parkinson-White syndrome. (Reproduced with permission from Crawford MH. *Current Diagnosis & Treatment: Cardiology.* 4th ed. New York, NY: McGraw-Hill Education; 2014. Figure 31-17.)

- Echocardiogram: This diagnosis is typically made with echo (apical displacement of septal tricuspid leaflet >8 mm/m^2 and the presence of redundant, elongated anterior leaflet and a septal leaflet tethered to the ventricular septum), which is also used to determine the degree of right atrial enlargement, TR, and presence of associated defects (Figure 17-45).

- Advanced imaging: Advanced imaging is not usually required unless there is a question about ventricular size/function.

- Catheterization: Not typically required.

- Management:
  - *Medical therapies:*
    - Anticoagulation with warfarin is recommended if there is history of paradoxical embolus or atrial fibrillation (class I indication).
  - *Class I indications for surgery:*
    - Repair or replace TV:
      - Symptoms or deteriorating exercise capacity
      - Paradoxical embolism
      - Progressive cardiomegaly on chest x-ray
      - Progressive RV dilation or reduction of RV systolic function
      - Cyanosis
    - Repeat repair/replacement:
      - Symptoms, deteriorating exercise capacity, or New York Heart Association functional class II or IV.
      - Severe TR after repair with progressive RV dilation, reduction RV systolic function, appearance/progression of atrial or ventricular arrhythmias.
      - If prosthetic valve is present, with evidence of significant prosthetic valve dysfunction.

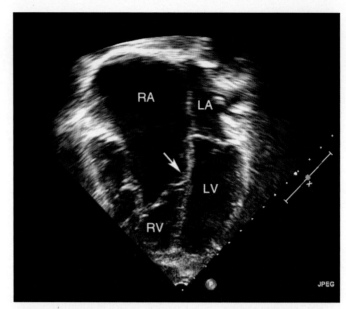

FIGURE 17-45 Ebstein anomaly of the tricuspid valve. Apical 4-chamber echocardiogram in a patient with Ebstein anomaly demonstrates severe apical displacement of the septal leaflet of the tricuspid valve (*arrow*), with resulting atrialization of a large portion of the right ventricular sinus. The anterior leaflet of the tricuspid valve is large (often described as sail-like) and has multiple attachments to the apex and anterior right ventricular wall (RV). Abbreviations: LA, left atrium; LV, left ventricle, RA, right atrium. (Reproduced with permission from Fuster V, Walsh RA, Harrington RA. *Hurst's the Heart*. 13th ed. New York, NY: McGraw-Hill Education; 2011. Figure 83-29.)

SINGLE VENTRICLE ANATOMY

Overview

Functional single ventricle anatomy results from a variety of congenital cardiac malformations. In the 21st century, the most common lesion leading to a Fontan palliation (Figure 17-46) is hypoplastic left heart syndrome (HLHS). Other anatomical lesions resulting in single ventricle anatomy are tricuspid atresia (TA) and double inlet left ventricle (DILV). A double outlet right ventricle (DORV) anatomy is highly variable and can result in either single or biventricular physiology after surgical correction.

The end result of single ventricle palliation is typically a Fontan circulation (Figure 17-46). The initial surgical palliation will vary depending on the underlying anatomy. For example, HLHS requires intervention to establish systemic blood flow, whereas TA requires intervention to establish pulmonary blood flow. Table 17-1 outlines the congenital heart lesions that lead to single ventricular repair, as well as surgical palliations.

Clinical Findings, Diagnosis, and Management

- Examination findings: Patients can have a variable physical examination depending on their underlying lesion and complications. Patients with Fontan circulation should exhibit a single S$_2$, given their single ventricular outflow track.

Lateral tunnel
Fontan

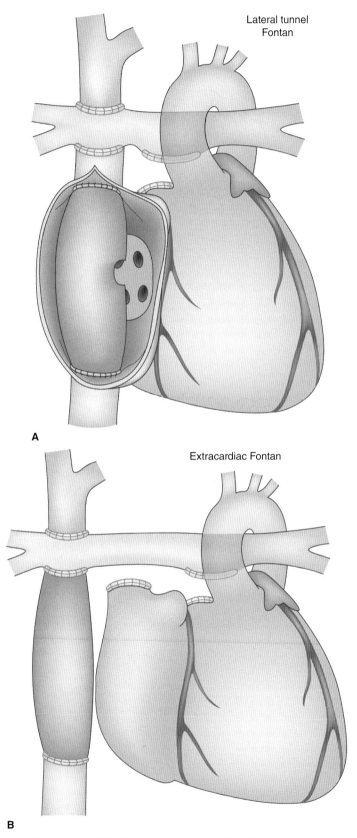

A

Extracardiac Fontan

B

FIGURE 17-46 **A.** Lateral tunnel Fontan with an interatrial baffle routes blood from the inferior vena cava along the lateral wall of the right atrium to the pulmonary artery, resulting in passive flow of systemic venous return from the lower body through the lung vascular bed. Note the fenestration in the baffle, often created to act as a pressure relief valve in the early postoperative period. **B.** Extracardiac Fontan with an interposition conduit outside the heart results in the same circulation, shown here without a fenestration. (Reproduced with permission of Springer Science and Business Media from Valente AM, Landzberg MJ, Powell AJ. Adult congenital heart disease. In: Libby P, ed. *Essential Atlas of Cardiovascular Disease.* Philadelphia, PA: Current Medicine Group; 2009.)

Table 17-1 Common Congenital Heart Disease Resulting in Single Ventricle Physiology

Type of Single Ventricle Lesion	Congenital Anatomy	Surgical Repair/Palliation
Hypoplastic left heart syndrome (HLHS) Hypoplasia or absence of the LV and severe hypoplasia of the ascending aorta. Variations include combinations of aortic and mitral valve stenosis and atresia. At birth, the descending aorta is essentially a continuation of the ductus arteriosus, with the ascending aorta and aortic arch a small branch off this vessel (Figure 17-47).	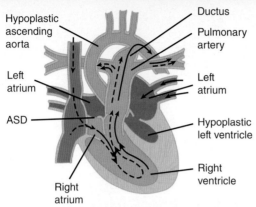 **FIGURE 17-47** Hypoplastic left heart syndrome. (Reproduced with permission from Schafermeyer R, Tenenbein M, Macias CG, Sharieff GQ, Yamamoto LG. *Strange and Schafermeyer's Pediatric Emergency Medicine.* 4th ed. New York, NY: McGraw-Hill Education; 2015. Figure 39-9.)	**Stage I:** Can be accomplished by either Norwood or hybrid Norwood 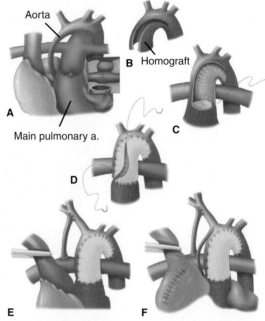 **FIGURE 17-48** Current techniques for first-stage palliation of the hypoplastic left-heart syndrome. **A.** Incisions used for the procedure, incorporating a cuff of arterial wall allograft. The distal divided main pulmonary artery may be closed by direct suture or with a patch. **B.** Dimensions of the cuff of the arterial wall allograft. **C.** The arterial wall allograft is used to supplement the anastomosis between the proximal divided main pulmonary artery and the ascending aorta, aortic arch, and proximal descending aorta. **D.** and **E.** The procedure is completed by atrial septectomy and a 3- to 5-mm modified right Blalock shunt. **F.** When the ascending aorta is particularly small, an alternative procedure involves placement of a complete tube of arterial allograft. The tiny ascending aorta may be left in situ, as indicated, or implanted into the side of the neoaorta. a. = artery. (From Castaneda AR, Jonas RA, Mayer JE, et al. *Cardiac Surgery of the Neonate and Infant.* Philadelphia: W.B. Saunders; 1994:371, with permission. Copyright Elsevier.)

(Continued)

Table 17-1 Common Congenital Heart Disease Resulting in Single Ventricle Physiology (Continued)

Type of Single Ventricle Lesion	Congenital Anatomy	Surgical Repair/Palliation

Hybrid

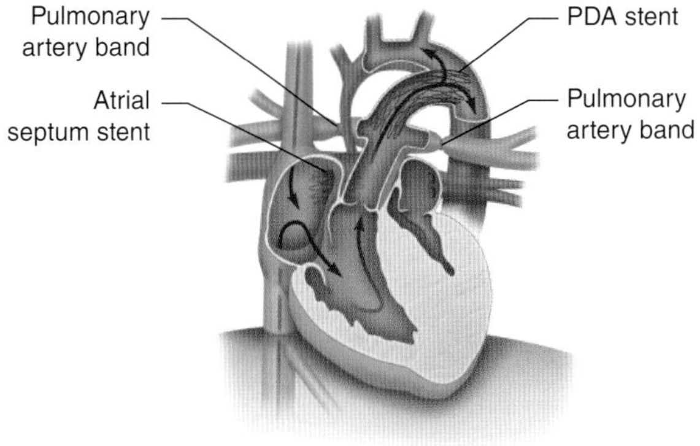

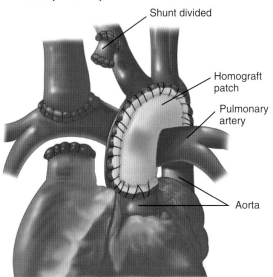

FIGURE 17-49 The hybrid stage 1 palliation. Note pulmonary artery (PA) bands on the left and right PAs, proximal to the upper lobe branches. Stents span the length of the patent ductus arteriosus and atrial septum. (Reproduced with permission from *Pediatric Cardiology*. 2005;26[2].)

Stage II: Bidirectional Cavopulmonary Anastomosis (BDCPA)

FIGURE 17-50 Technique of a bidirectional Glenn shunt. The divided right superior vena cava has been anastomosed at the previous site of the distal anastomosis of the modified right Blalock shunt. The cardiac end of the divided superior vena cava may also be anastomosed to the right pulmonary artery, with the internal orifice being closed with a Gore-Tex patch. (From Castaneda AR, Jonas RA, Mayer JE, et al. *Cardiac Surgery of the Neonate and Infant*. Philadelphia: W.B. Saunders; 1994:376, with permission. Copyright Elsevier.)

(Continued)

Table 17-1 Common Congenital Heart Disease Resulting in Single Ventricle Physiology (Continued)

Type of Single Ventricle Lesion	Congenital Anatomy	Surgical Repair/Palliation

Tricuspid atresia

Single ventricle heart with no communication between the RA and RV. Blood flows from the RA to LA via an ASD. The RV is primitive and connects to the LV through a VSD. Subclassified by the relationship of the great arteries and the degree of pulmonary blood flow obstruction (Figures 17-50, 17-51).

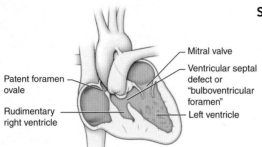

FIGURE 17-51 Tricuspid atresia. (Reproduced with permission from Crawford MH. *Current Diagnosis & Treatment: Cardiology.* 4th ed. New York, NY: McGraw-Hill Education; 2014. Figure 31-38.)

Stage III: Fontan

See Figure 17-46.

Stage I: Systemic to pulmonary shunt for pulmonary blood flow (eg, Blalock-Taussig-Thomas shunt)

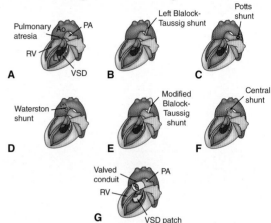

FIGURE 17-53 A. Unrepaired tetralogy of Fallot with pulmonary atresia. There is no anterograde flow from the right ventricle (RV) to the pulmonary artery (PA). A large nonrestrictive ventricular septal defect (VSD) allows communication between the left ventricle (LV) and the RV. There is an overriding aorta (Ao). **B.** Classic left Blalock-Taussig shunt consisting of direct connection of the divided left subclavian artery to the left pulmonary artery. **C.** Potts shunt consisting of a direct connection between the anterior wall of the descending Ao and left PA. **D.** Waterston shunt consisting of a direct connection of the posterior wall of the ascending Ao and the right PA. **E.** Modified Blalock-Taussig shunt consisting of a synthetic (Gore-Tex) tube connection from the left subclavian artery to the PA. **F.** Central shunt consisting of a synthetic tubular connection from the ascending Ao to the PA. **G.** Intracardiac repair consisting of VSD patch closure and placement of a valved conduit from the RV to the PA. (Reproduced with permission from Fuster V, Walsh RA, Harrington RA. *Hurst's the Heart.* 13th ed. New York, NY: McGraw-Hill Education; 2011. Figure 84-1.)

Stage II: Bidirectional cavopulmonary anastomosis (BDCPA)

See Figure 17-50.

Stage III: Fontan

See Figure 17-46.

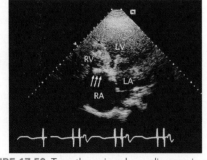

FIGURE 17-52 Transthoracic echocardiogram in a 30-year-old woman with tricuspid atresia. This 4-chamber view demonstrates the plate-like imperforate tricuspid annulus (*3 white arrows*). The right atrium (RA) is markedly dilated, and the right ventricle (RV) is hypoplastic. A ventricular septal defect (*black arrow*) is noted. Abbreviations: LA, left atrium; LV, left ventricle. (Reproduced with permission from Crawford MH. *Current Diagnosis & Treatment: Cardiology.* 4th ed. New York, NY: McGraw-Hill Education; 2014. Figure 31-29.)

(Continued)

Table 17-1 Common Congenital Heart Disease Resulting in Single Ventricle Physiology (Continued)

Type of Single Ventricle Lesion	Congenital Anatomy	Surgical Repair/Palliation
Double inlet left ventricle (DILV) Both the mitral and tricuspid valves enter a dominant left ventricle. There is variation in size of the right ventricle, typically with a VSD. The morphologic left ventricle is rightward and posterior, with the small right ventricle displaced leftward. In most cases, the aorta is leftward and anterior to the pulmonary artery. The aorta and pulmonary artery generally arise from the left ventricle and right ventricle, respectively (Figure 17-54).	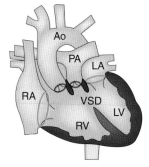 DILV **FIGURE 17-54** Double-inlet left ventricle (DILV). (Reproduced with permission from Rudolph CD, Rudolph AM, Lister GE, First LR, Gershon AA. *Rudolph's Pediatrics.* 22nd ed. New York, NY: McGraw-Hill Education; 2011. Figure 480-3F.)	May be able to undergo a 2-ventricle repair. If the right ventricle is small, this condition would generally lead to single ventricle repair as is outlined above (Fontan circulation).
Double outlet right ventricle (DORV) Both of the great arteries arise entirely or predominantly from the right ventricle. There is variation in size of left ventricle, typically with a VSD (Figure 17-55).	DORV **FIGURE 17-55** Double-outlet right ventricle (DORV). (Reproduced with permission from Rudolph CD, Rudolph AM, Lister GE, First LR, Gershon AA. *Rudolph's Pediatrics.* 22nd ed. New York, NY: McGraw-Hill Education; 2011. Figure 480-3E.)	May be able to undergo a 2-ventricle repair if there is reasonably good biventricular size. If the left ventricle is small, this would typically result in a single ventricle repair (Fontan).

Abbreviations: ASD, atrial septal defect; BDCPA, bidirectional cavopulmonary anastomosis; DORV, double outlet right ventricle; HLHS, hypoplastic left heart syndrome; LA, left atrium; LV, left ventricle; RA, right atrium; RV, right ventricle; VSD, ventricular septal defect.

- Electrocardiogram: ECG findings will vary, but providers need to have a high index of suspicion for atrial tachyarrhythmias.

- Echocardiogram: Echocardiography is important for evaluation of single ventricular function. TEE is often needed to image the entire Fontan pathway, evaluate for atrial thrombi, and measure the gradient if a fenestrated Fontan is present.

- Advanced Imaging: Cardiac CT or MRI is almost always required to fully characterize the Fontan anatomy as well as single ventricle anatomy, size, and function.

- Catheterization: Symptoms in the Fontan patient can be vague, and frequently may relate to late problems with the Fontan circuit (leaks, stenosis, and collaterals). Cardiac catheterization is used to evaluate for the cause of these symptoms and can be used to intervene on late sequelae that develop, such as arteriovenous malformations and systemic to pulmonary collaterals.

- Management: Overall patients with single ventricle physiology should be treated as if they have a chronic disease, which requires management to preserve ventricular function for as long as possible and prevent further disability. They should have at least yearly evaluation by an adult congenital cardiologist.

- Complications: Long-term complications related to the Fontan circulation include atrial arrhythmias, right atrial thrombus, systemic ventricular dysfunction, hepatic congestion leading to hepatic dysfunction (fibrosis and cirrhosis), and protein-losing enteropathy, to name a few. It is important to remember that late problems are unique to each patient given the heterogeneity in original anatomy and in surgical palliation.

REFERENCES

1. Williams RG, Person GD, Barst RJ, et al. Report of the National Heart Blood Lung Institute working group on research in adult congenital heart disease. *J Am Coll Cardiol.* 2006;47:701-707.

2. Marelli AJ, Ionescu-Ittu R, Mackie AS, Guo L, Dendukuri N, Kaouach M. The prevalence of congenital heart disease in the general population from 2000 to 2010. *Circulation.* 2014:130:749-756.

3. Marelli AJ, Mackie AS, Ionescu-Ittu R, Rahme E, Pilote L. Congenital heart disease in the general population: changing prevalence and age distribution. *Circulation.* 2007;115:163-172.

4. Mylotte D, Pilote L, Ionescu-Ittu R, et al. Specialized adult congenital heart disease care: the impact of policy on mortality. *Circulation.* 2014;129:1804-1812.

5. Bhatt AB, Foster E, Kuehl K, et al. Congenital heart disease in the older adult: a scientific statement from the American Heart Association. *Circulation.* 2015;131:1884-1931.

6. Baumgartner H, Hung J, Bermejo J, et al. Echocardiographic assessment of valve stenosis: EAE/ASE recommendations for clinical practice. *J Am Soc Echocardiogr.* 2009;22:1-23.

7. Khairy P, Van Hare G, Balaji S, et al. PACES/HRS expert consensus statement of the recognition and management of arrhythmias in adult congenital heart disease. *Heart Rhythm.* 2014;11:e102-e165.

8. Maron BJ, Zipes DP, et al. 36th Bethesda conference: eligibility recommendations for competitive athletes with cardiovascular abnormalities. *J Am Coll Cardiol.* 2005;45:1313-1375.

9. Nishimura RA, Otto C, Sorajja P, et al. 2014 AHA/ACC guidelines for the management of patients with valvular heart disease. *J Am Coll Cardiol.* 2014;63:e57-e185.

10. Warnes, CA, Williams RG, Bashore TM, et al. ACC/AHA 2008 guidelines for the management of adults with congenital heart disease: executive summary. *J Am Coll Cardiol.* 2008;52:1890-1947.

11. Zoghbi WA, Enriquez-Sarano M, Foster E, et al. Recommendations for evaluation of the severity of native valvular regurgitation with two-dimensional and Doppler echocardiography. *J Am Soc Echocardiogr.* 2003;16:777-802.

12. Schievink WI, Raissi SS, Maya MM, Velebir A. Screening for intracranial aneurysms in patients with bicuspid aortic valve. *Neurology.* 2010;74(18):1430-1433.

13. Khairy P, Aboulhosn J, Gurvitz MZ, et al. Arrhythmia burden in adults with surgically repaired tetralogy of Fallot. *Circulation.* 2010;122:868-875.

18 VENOUS THROMBOEMBOLIC DISEASE IN HEART FAILURE

Steven M. Dean, DO, FSVM, RPVI

PATIENT CASE

A 67-year-old man with a history of relapsing heart failure (left ventricular ejection fraction 25%-30%), hypertension, and dyslipidemia presents to the emergency department with a 1-week history of spontaneous pain and swelling within the left calf. His chronic dyspnea on exertion is unchanged and he denies pleuritic chest pain or cough.

On physical examination the patient is alert and in no acute distress with normal vital signs. Pulse oximetry obtained on room air is 95%. On physical examination the patient appears euvolemic with a murmur of aortic sclerosis, an S_4 gallop, and no adventitial lung sounds. His left calf is swollen, tender, and slightly warmer than the right calf. The muscle compartments are soft and distal pulses are intact bilaterally.

Duplex ultrasonography of the left leg documents an acute deep venous thrombosis within the gastrocnemius and popliteal veins (Figure 18-1). A complete blood count, chemistry profile, as well as prothrombin time/international normalized ratio (INR) and partial thromboplastin times are within normal limits. Anticoagulation is begun with therapeutic doses of apixaban and he is discharged to home with instructions to see his primary care provider in 1 week.

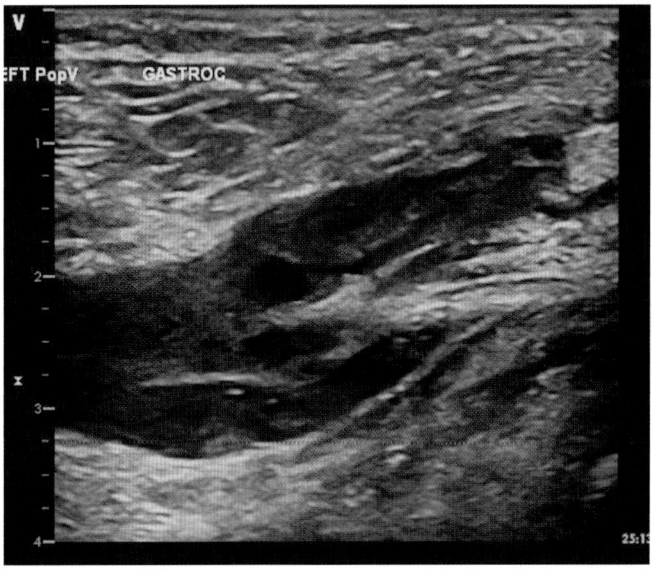

FIGURE 18-1 Venous duplex ultrasonography of the popliteal fossa demonstrating acute occlusive deep venous thrombosis within a dilated left gastrocnemius vein that has propagated into the juxtaposed popliteal vein.

EPIDEMIOLOGY

Heart failure (HF) is a major risk factor for venous thromboembolism (VTE) that is independent of concurrent coronary events or atrial fibrillation.

Although classically listed as a risk factor for decompensated hospitalized patients, HF increases the risk of VTE in stable outpatients as well.

In the absence of thromboprophylaxis, the prevalence of deep venous thrombosis (DVT) in patients hospitalized with HF traditionally ranges from 4% to 26%.[1] However, in a more contemporary 2014 prospective study of Japanese patients hospitalized for HF, DVT was remarkably detected in 34% despite the use of mechanical prophylaxis and/or antiplatelet therapy.[2]

In the Worcester Venous thromboembolism study of 1822 patients, the concurrence of HF in subjects with VTE yielded a 3-fold higher risk of in-hospital death and approximately 2.5-fold increased risk of dying within 30 days of the thrombotic diagnosis.[3]

In the U.S. National Hospital Discharge Survey (NHDS), a patient with HF was 2.2 times more likely to incur a pulmonary embolism (PE) when compared to patients without HF.[4] PE was documented in 9% of patients with decompensated HF admitted to an intensive care unit,[5] and 10% of the symptomatic PE patients enrolled in the RIETE registry had underlying HF.[6]

HF is a potent risk factor for VTE in young patients. For instance, in the NHDS the relative risk (RR) for PE in octogenarian congestive heart failure (CHF) patients was only 1.3; however, in patients younger than 40 years of age, the RR considerably escalated to 11.7. Similarly, the RR for DVT in patients <40 years was significantly increased at 5.5.[4]

Gender-based and racial differences may influence the risk of VTE in HF patients. For instance, HF appears to be a more potent risk factor for PE in women (RR, 2.45; 95% CI, 2.44-2.46) than in men (RR, 180;95% CI, 1.79-1.80). Additionally, black patients are at greater risk for PE (RR, 2.82; 95% CI, 2.79-2.84) than white patients (RR, 2.10; 95% CI, 2.09-2.11).[4]

A meta-analysis of 32 trials of angiotensin-converting enzyme (ACE) inhibitors in HF patients identified PE as 1 of the 5 primary causes of death.[7]

Postmortem studies of patients with HF have documented PE incidence rates ranging from 0.4% to 50%. However, it can be difficult to ascertain if PE is directly responsible for immediate mortality. Prospective analysis suggests that PE is the predominant cause of mortality in 3% to 10% of patients with HF.

ETIOLOGY AND PATHOPHYSIOLOGY

The prothrombotic tendency of HF is partially explained by Virchow classic triad. Stasis occurs due to depressed cardiac output as well as immobility. Endothelial dysfunction results from inhibition of endothelium-derived nitric oxide release as well as elevations in von Willebrand factor (vWF), thrombomodulin, and soluble E-selectin. Lastly, the thrombophilic component is reflected by elevated plasma viscosity, D-dimer, fibrinopeptide A, and fibrinogen levels in HF patients.

The link between thrombophilia and HF is also potentially related to an associated multifactorial chronic inflammatory state as proposed by Chong and Lip.[8] Figure 18-2 displays the intricate relationship between a variety of HF-elaborated inflammatory proteins, molecules, and cells that can ultimately culminate in VTE.

A striking inverse relationship exists between ejection fraction and risk of VTE (Table 18-1).[9]

HF severity is proportional to VTE risk. In the placebo arm of the MEDENOX trial, VTE was documented in 12.3% of the patients with New York Heart Association (NYHA) class III HF. However, VTE occurred in 21.7% of the patients with class IV HF.[10]

Elevated biomarkers have been increasingly linked to VTE risk in HF. In a subanalysis of the MAGELLAN trial, multivariable analysis documented that the N-terminal probrain natriuretic peptide (NT-proBNP) level independently predicted short-term (up to 10 days) VTE risk whereas elevated D-dimer concentrations predicted both short- and mid-term (up to 35 days) VTE susceptibilty.[11]

In both the Atherosclerosis Risk in Communities Study and Cardiovascular Health Study, a high sensitivity troponin (TnT) concentration was directly linked with the incidence of total and provoked VTE, but not with spontaneous VTE.[12]

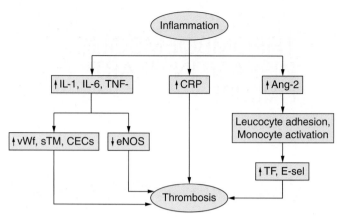

FIGURE 18-2 Relationship between the prothrombotic state and inflammation in heart failure. Abbreviations: Ang-2, angiopoietin-2; CEC, circulating endothelial cells; CRP, C-reactive protein; eNOS, endothelial nitrous oxide synthase; E-sel, E-selectin; IL-1, interleukin-1; IL-6, interleukin-6; sTM, soluble thrombomodulin; TF, tissue factor; TNF, tumor necrosis factor α; vWf, von Willebrand factor. (Reproduced with permission from Chong AY, Lip GY. Viewpoint: the prothrombotic state in heart failure: a maladaptive inflammatory response? *Eur J Heart Fail.* 2007;9:124-128.)

Table 18-1 Logistic Regression Model Evaluating LVEF and Risk of VTE

LVEF	Odd Ratio (95% Confidence Interval)
<20%	38.3 (9.6-152.5)
20%-44%	2.8 (1.4-5.7)
≥45%	1.7 (1.03-2.9)

Abbreviations: LVEF, left ventricular ejection fraction; VTE, venous thromboembolism. Adapted from Howell et al.[9]

DIAGNOSIS

CLINICAL FEATURES

Deep Venous Thrombosis

At least 50% of patients with an acute DVT are asymptomatic. Classic signs and symptoms include limb pain, tenderness, swelling, increased warmth, and/or increased venous collaterals (Figure 18-3). Unfortunately, these clinical manifestations (including Homan sign) are neither sensitive nor specific for the diagnosis of DVT.

The physical examination *is* relatively specific in 2 venous thromboembolic conditions: (1) Acute superficial venous thrombosis with a palpable tender, warm, erythematous cord (Figure 18-4), (2) Phlegmasia cerulea dolens manifested by a markedly turgid, blue, painful extremity (Figure 18-5), which can be both limb- and life-threatening.

Pulmonary Emboli

Acute PE frequently mimics other cardiopulmonary conditions (eg, HF) on account of its protean, nonspecific clinical manifestations. Consequently, it is imperative that a clinician maintains a high level of suspicion for PE, especially in the at-risk patient with HF.

Dyspnea is the most frequent symptom and tachypnea the most frequent sign. Other manifestations include pleuritic chest pain, cough, crackles, low-grade temperature, and/or an increased second heart sound.

Acute pulmonary infarction is associated with pleuritic chest pain, dyspnea, and hemoptysis. Physical findings include a pleural friction rub and possible decreased breath sounds due to a pleural effusion.

The presence of syncope, cyanosis, and/or cardiogenic shock suggests a massive PE.

LABORATORY

D-dimer

An elevated D-dimer via ELISA assay is highly sensitive for VTE; yet, the test is not specific. For example, various nonthrombotic disorders such as trauma, cancer, myocardial infarction, disseminated intravascular coagulation (DIC), pregnancy, and infection can increase D-dimer levels.

Consequently, elevated levels of D-dimer do not accurately predict the diagnosis of DVT/PE, yet normal or low levels have a very high negative predictive value (approaching 100%).

Arterial Blood Gas

Arterial blood gas (ABG) abnormalities in decreasing order of frequency include hypoxemia, widened alveolar-arterial gradient, and a respiratory alkalosis. None of these abnormalities are sensitive or specific for the PE, especially in the setting of coexistent HF.

The combination of cryptic hypoxemia and a normal chest x-ray should always raise the suspicion for PE. A pulse oximetry is extremely insensitive as it is normal in the majority of patients with PE.

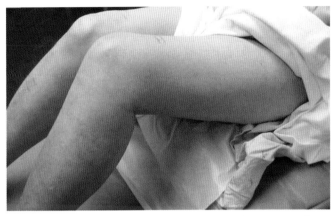

FIGURE 18-3 Although the clinical examination is often nonspecific and insensitive, this photograph demonstrates classic clinical manifestations of an acute left iliofemoral deep venous thrombosis including marked swelling, diffuse erythema, and a few dilated superficial collateral veins.

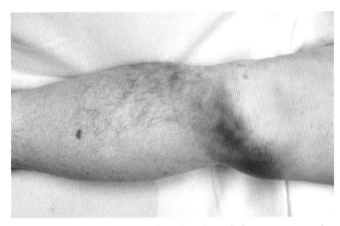

FIGURE 18-4 A tender inflamed cord on the right leg consistent with acute superficial venous thrombosis. (Reproduced with permission from Steven M. Dean, DO. As published in Dean SM, Satiani B, Abraham WT. *Color Atlas and Synopsis of Vascular Disease.* New York, NY: McGraw-Hill Education; 2014. Figure 51-1.)

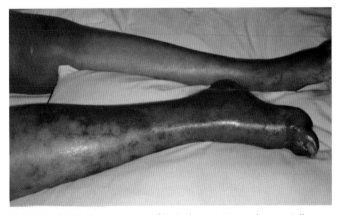

FIGURE 18-5 A dramatic case of limb-threatening and potentially life-threatening phlegmasia cerulea dolens of the right limb. Note the diffuse livedoid and purpuric ischemic mottling secondary to profound venous hypertension in association with multisegmental superficial and deep venous thrombosis. (Image used with permission from Dr. John R. Bartholomew.)

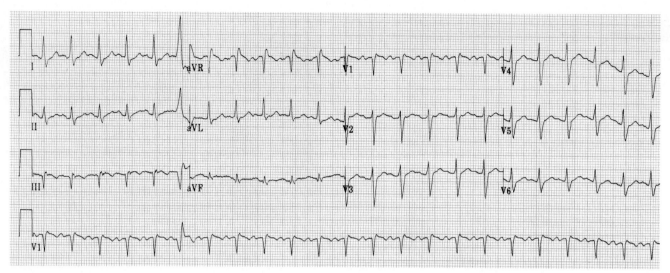

FIGURE 18-6 The rare but often-referenced S1Q3T3 electrocardiographic abnormality of acute pulmonary embolism. This pattern has been linked to a poor prognosis and usually connotes a large pulmonary embolic burden. (Image used with permission from James V. Ritchie, MD.)

Cardiac Biomarkers

Increased levels of brain natriuretic peptide (BNP) and high-sensitivity troponin T (TnT) can occur in response to significant right ventricular stretching and microinfarction, respectively.

BNP and TnT are both increased in the setting of moderate to large PE. Elevated levels of BNP and TnT are neither sensitive nor specific for diagnosing PE. These are best utilized for risk stratification and prognostication in patients with acute PE.

NONINVASIVE CARDIAC TESTING

Electrocardiography

Electrocardiographic (ECG) abnormalites are common in acute PE yet they lack sensitivity and specificity. The most common findings are tachycardia and nonspecific ST-segment and T-wave changes. In <10% of cases, ECG abnormalities frequently referenced in acute PE include the S1Q3T3 pattern (Figure 18-6), right ventricular strain, and/or a new incomplete right bundle branch block. Such abnormalities have been linked to a poor prognosis.

Additional ECG irregularities that predict a poor prognosis in acute PE include atrial arrhythmias (eg, atrial fibrillation), bradycardia or tachycardia, Q waves within the inferior leads (II, III, and aVF), and anterior ST-segment changes with T-wave inversion. An abnormal ECG is more likely to occur with a moderate to large PE.

Echocardiography

Echocardiography should not be routinely obtained when evaluating hemodynamically stable patients suspected of having a PE.

Echocardiographic findings are neither sensitive or specific for acute PE. Echo does yield valuable prognostic information by assessing the right ventricle in patients with acute PE. Approximately 30% to 40% of PE patients display echocardiographic abnormalities indicative of RV strain or overload, including increased RV diameter, impaired RV function, and/or acute tricuspid regurgitation. These findings are more common in large PE.

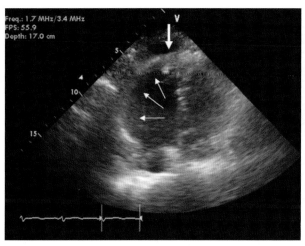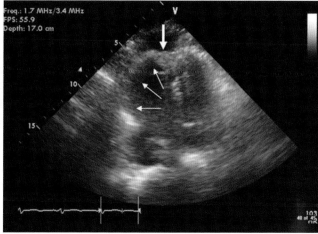

FIGURE 18-7 McConnell sign. Severe right ventricular (RV) hypokinesis with right apical sparing occurs in the setting of acute pressure overload from large pulmonary emboli. Tethering of the RV apex to a contracting and frequently hyperdynamic LV may account for the right apical sparing. The free wall of the RV, lacking the apical interventricular continuity (no LV tethering) is more notably dysfunctional. (Reproduced with permission from Pahlm O, Wagner GS. *Multimodal Cardiovascular Imaging: Principles and Clinical Applications*. New York, NY: McGraw-Hill Education; 2011. Figure 19-18A.)

Rare yet highly morbid echocardiographic defects in the setting of PE include thrombus within the RV, thrombus within the pulmonary artery and its main branches, and/or regional wall hypokinesis that spares the right ventricular apex (ie, McConnell sign, Figure 18-7).

RADIOLOGICAL IMAGING

Chest Radiography

The chest x-ray is often abnormal yet nondiagnostic, with abnormalities including parenchymal abnormalities, cardiomegaly, diaphragmatic elevation, platelike atelectasis, and pleural effusion.

A chest x-ray can be useful in evaluating other conditions that can mimic PE, including HF. Classically described, yet rare and nonspecific radiographic findings include Hampton hump (pleural-based, wedge-shaped abnormality) and Westermark sign (focal decreased pulmonary vascularity, Figure 18-8).

Chest x-ray can be deferred if a chest CT scan is intended.

Computed Tomographic Pulmonary Angiography

On account of its high sensitivity (>90%) and specificity (>90%), computed tomographic pulmonary angiography (CTPA) is the imaging modaility of choice for most patients with suspected PE.

In patients at intermediate to high risk of pulmonary embolism, the positive predictive value of CTPA is 92% to 96%. CTPA cannot dependably exclude PE when the clinical probability is high. In this setting the negative predictive value is only 60%. CTPA is most accurate in detecting PE within the main, lobar, and segmental pulmonary arteries and less effective in detecting small subsegmental emboli (Figure 18-9).

CTPA is useful in detecting alternative etiologies for pulmonary symptomatology. Potential contraindications include pregnancy, advanced chronic kidney disease, and contrast hypersensitivity.

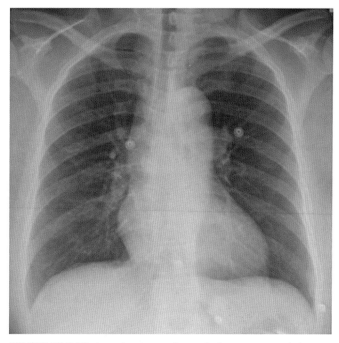

FIGURE 18-8 PA view of a chest radiograph demonstrates subtle decrease in vascular markings in the left lung as compared to the right consistent with a Westermark sign. (Reproduced with permission from Elsayes KM, Oldham SA. *Introduction to Diagnostic Radiology*. New York, NY: McGraw-Hill Education; 2014. Figure C6.8A.)

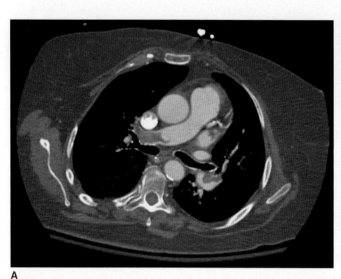 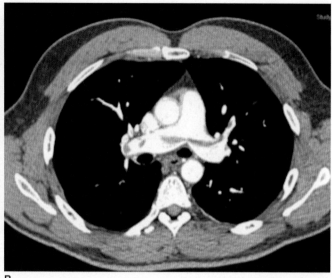

FIGURE 18-9 A. Computed tomographic pulmonary angiography (CTPA) illustrating large pulmonary emboli obstructing the right and left pulmonary arteries. No peripheral perfusion can be demonstrated in the bilateral lobar or segmental arteries. **B.** CTPA evidence of a life-threatening saddle embolus that straddles the main pulmonary arterial trunk at its bifurcation. (Image used with permission from Dr. Mitch Silver.)

Ventilation-Perfusion (V/Q) Lung Scan

A ventilation-perfusion (V/Q) lung scan can be useful in patients with CTPA contraindications, including renal disease, contrast hypersensitivity, and pregnancy.

The V/Q lung scan is most accurate in the absence of underlying cardiopulmonary disease. A normal V/Q lung scan essentially excludes acute PE. A high-probability scan is typically diagnostic of acute PE unless a history of a prior embolic event within the same segment exists (Figure 18-10).

The majority of V/Q lung scans are nondiagnostic (low or intermediate probability).

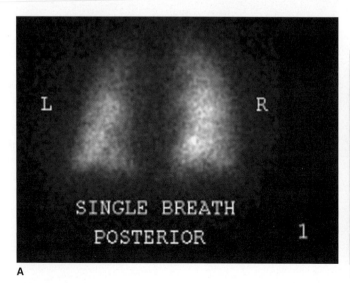 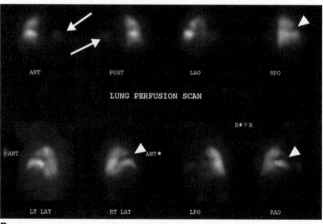

FIGURE 18-10 High-probability ventilation-perfusion lung scan in a patient with an acute pulmonary embolism. The ventilation scan is normal **(A)** but the perfusion scan demonstrates globally reduced perfusion to the left lung (*white arrows*) and a moderate sized segmental defect involving the anterior segment of the right upper lobe (*white arrowhead*) **(B)**. (Reproduced with permission from Elsayes KM, Oldham SA. *Introduction to Diagnostic Radiology.* New York, NY: McGraw-Hill Education; 2014. Figure C6.8BC.)

Magnetic Resonance Pulmonary Angiography

The magnetic resonance pulmonary angiography remains a second-line imaging test for the diagnosis of PE due to its higher cost, technical limitations (motion artifact, complicated blood flow patterns), and lower sensitivity when compared to CTPA or V/Q scanning.

Its sensitivity for detecting subsegmental PE is as low as 40%. Advantages of the magnetic resonance pulmonary angiography include the lack of associated ionizing radiation and iodinated contrast.

Contrast Pulmonary Arteriography

Contrast pulmonary arteriography is useful when the CTPA or V/Q scan is inconclusive or if negative studies conflict with a high clinical probability.

Additional advantages of pulmonary arteriography include (1) direct measurement of pulmonary artery pressure, and (2) ability to combine the procedure with catheter-directed thrombolysis and/or embolectomy (Figure 18-11).

With the emergence of CTPA, pulmonary arteriography is no longer considered the gold standard for detecting PE.

Venous Duplex Ultrasonography

Venous duplex ultrasonography (VDU) is the initial and primary modality for the diagnosis and exclusion of acute DVT.

The sensitivity and specificity of VDU for diagnosing symptomatic proximal DVT exceeds 90%. The accuracy of VDU decreases in the setting of asymptomatic proximal DVT, calf DVT, and pelvic (iliocaval) vein thrombosis.

The demonstration of venous incompressibility is the key ultrasonographic diagnostic criterion for acute DVT (Figure 18-12).

Alternative Deep Venous Thrombosis Imaging Modalities

When VDU is incomplete, unattainable, and/or inconclusive, contrast venography remains a useful diagnostic tool.

Magnetic resonance and CT venography are increasingly useful and accurate in the diagnosis of iliocaval pathology (Figure 18-13).

CLINICAL PREDICTION RULES

Deep Venous Thrombosis

Due to limitations of the clinical examination, validated clinical prediction rules such as the modified Wells criteria can be used to estimate the pretest probability of DVT.[13] In appropriately selected patients deemed unlikely to have a DVT (score <2), a normal high-sensitivity D-dimer essentially excludes the diagnosis and obviates ordering a VDU. In patients with a likely probability of lower-extremity DVT (score ≥2), ultrasonography is recommended (Table 18-2).

The Wells score performs better in younger patients without comorbidities or a history of VTE.

Pulmonary Embolism

Similar to DVT, the clinical probability of PE should be determined before proceeding with testing.

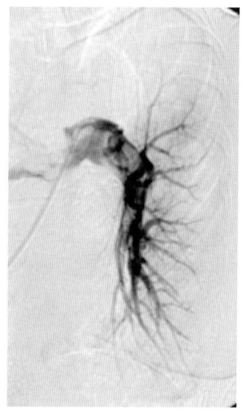

FIGURE 18-11 Contrast pulmonary arteriography demonstrating diffuse intraluminal filling defects throughout the left pulmonary artery, lobar, and segmental arteries consistent with a large embolic burden. (Image used with permission from Dr. Mitch Silver.)

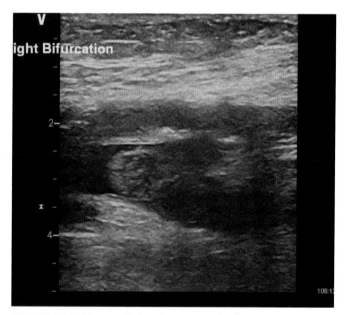

FIGURE 18-12 Venous duplex ultrasonography illustrating incompressible echogenic thrombus within dilated right proximal femoral and profunda femoral veins extending into the common femoral vein.

A 2011 prospective validation study evaluated the performance of 4 clinical decision rules in addition to D-dimer testing to exclude acute PE. All 4 rules (Wells rule, simplified Wells rule, revised Geneva score, and simplified revised Geneva score) displayed similar performance for excluding acute PE when combined with a normal D-dimer assay.[14]

The Clinical Guidelines Committee of American College of Physicians 2015 recommendations for evaluating patients with suspected acute PE are listed in Table 18-3.[15]

DIFFERENTIAL DIAGNOSIS

PULMONARY EMBOLUS

- Acute pericarditis
- Angina pectoris
- Atrial fibrillation
- Acute respiratory distress syndrome
- Anxiety
- Emphysema
- Fat embolism
- Mitral stenosis
- Myocardial infarction
- Pneumothorax
- Pneumonia
- Primary pulmonary hypertension
- Restrictive cardiomyopathy

DEEP VENOUS THROMBOSIS

- Abscess
- Cellulitis
- Chronic venous insufficiency
- Compartment syndrome
- Disuse/dependency
- Factitial
- Gastrocnemius muscle rupture
- Hematoma
- Lymphedema
- Osteomyelitis
- Popliteal cyst
- Popliteal artery aneurysm
- Superficial venous thrombosis
- Tumor
- Vascular malformation

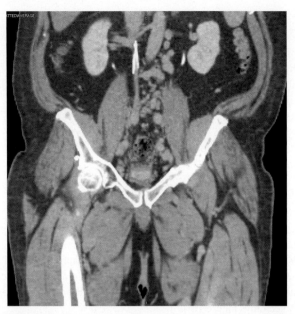

FIGURE 18-13 CT venography demonstrating a diffusely occluded post thrombotic iliocaval system inferior to a remotely placed inferior vena cava filter. (Image used with permission from Dr. Mitch Silver.)

Table 18-2 Modified Wells Criteria for Predicting the Pretest Probability of DVT[13]

Clinical Characteristic	Score
Active cancer (patient receiving treatment for cancer within the previous 6 mo or currently receiving palliative therapy)	+1
Paralysis, paresis, or recent plaster immobilization of the lower extremities	+1
Recently bedridden for 3 d or more, or major surgery within the previous 12 wk requiring general or regional anesthesia	+1
Localized tenderness along the distribution of the deep venous system	+1
Entire leg swollen	+1
Calf swelling at least 3 cm larger than on the asymptomatic side (measured 10 cm below the tibial tuberosity)	+1
Pitting edema confined to the symptomatic leg	+1
Collateral superficial veins (nonvaricose)	+1
Previously documented DVT	+1
Alternative diagnosis at least as likely as DVT	−2
Clinical Probability of DVT	
Likely	≥2
Unlikely	<2
In patients with symptoms in both legs, the more symptomatic leg is used.	

Abbreviation: DVT, deep venous thrombosis.

MANAGEMENT

The recently released 10th edition of the CHEST Guideline and Expert Panel Report on Antithrombotic Therapy for VTE Disease provided the following treatment guidelines for DVT and PE:[16]

- In patients with acute DVT of the lower extremity or acute PE and no cancer, a direct-acting oral anticoagulant (dabigatran, rivaroxaban, apixaban, or edoxaban) is now preferred over vitamin K antagonist (VKA) therapy (grade 2B).

- Initial parenteral anticoagulation (5-10 days) is required before initiating dabigatran and edoxaban, yet is not required when using rivaroxaban and apixaban.

- In patients with acute DVT of the lower extremity or acute PE and cancer, low molecular weight heparin (LMWH) remains the preferred therapy over VKA and direct-acting oral anticoagulants (grade 2C).

- In patients with distal (calf) or proximal DVT of the leg or PE provoked by either surgery or a nonsurgical risk factor, 3 months of anticoagulation is recommended over extended therapy (grade 1B).

- In patients with a first-time unprovoked proximal DVT of the leg or PE and who have a low or moderate bleeding risk, extended anticoagulant therapy (no scheduled stop date) is preferred over 3 months of therapy (grade 2B). When a high bleeding risk exists, 3 months of anticoagulant therapy is recommended over extended therapy (grade 1B).

- In patients with a second unprovoked VTE and low bleeding risk, extended anticoagulant therapy (no scheduled stop date) is recommended over 3 months (grade 1B). With a moderate bleeding risk, extended anticoagulant therapy is again recommended (grade 2B). However, when a high bleeding risk exists, 3 months of anticoagulant therapy is preferred over extended therapy (grade 2B).

- In patients with VTE and active cancer, extended anticoagulation therapy is recommended over 3 months of therapy, regardless of the bleeding risk.

- In patients with an unprovoked proximal DVT or PE who stop anticoagulation, aspirin is recommended over no aspirin to prevent recurrent VTE (grade 2B).

- In patients with acute proximal DVT of the leg, anticoagulation is suggested over catheter-directed thrombolysis (CDT) according to the recent CHEST Guidelines (grade 2C). However, the National Institute for Health and Care Excellence (NICE) guidelines recommend considering CDT therapy for patients with symptomatic *iliofemoral* DVT who have symptoms less than 14 days, good functional status, and a life expectancy of 1 year or more in the setting of a low risk of bleeding (Figure 18-14).[17] The American Heart Association (AHA) also recommends CDT for iliofemoral DVT when affected patients have phlegmasia, rapid thrombus extension, and/or clinical deterioration despite anticoagulation. The AHA additionally endorses CDT as a reasonable first-line treatment modality to prevent post-thrombotic syndrome in selected patients with iliofemoral DVT when the bleeding risk is low.[18]

Table 18-3 Evaluation of Patients with Suspected Acute Pulmonary Embolism

Best Practice Advice From the Clinical Guidelines Committee of the American College of Physicians[15]

*Best practice advise 1: Clinicians should use validated clinical prediction rules to estimate pretest probability in patients in whom acute PE is being considered.

*Best practice advise 2: Clinicians should not obtain D-dimer measurements or imaging studies in patients with a low pretest probability of PE and who meet all Pulmonary Embolism Rule-Out Criteria.

*Best practice advise 3: Clinicians should obtain a high-sensitivity D-dimer measurement as the initial diagnostic test in patients who have an intermediate pretest probability of PE or in patients with low pretest probability of PE who do not meet all Pulmonary Embolism Rule-Out Criteria. Clinicians should not use imaging studies as the initial test in patients who have a low or intermediate pretest probability of PE.

*Best practice advise 4: Clinicians should use age-adjusted D-dimer thresholds (age × 10 ng/mL rather than a generic value of 500 ng/mL) in patients older than 50 years to determine whether imaging is warranted.

*Best practice advise 5: Clinicians should not obtain any imaging studies in patients with a D-dimer level below the age-adjusted cutoff.

*Best practice advise 6: Clinicians should obtain imaging with CT pulmonary angiography (CTPA) in patients with high pretest probability of PE. Clinicians should reserve ventilation-perfusion scans for patients who have a contraindication to CTPA or if CTPA is not available. Clinicians should not obtain a D-dimer measurement in patients with a high pretest probability of PE.

Abbreviations: CTPA, computed tomography pulmonary angiography; PE, pulmonary embolism.

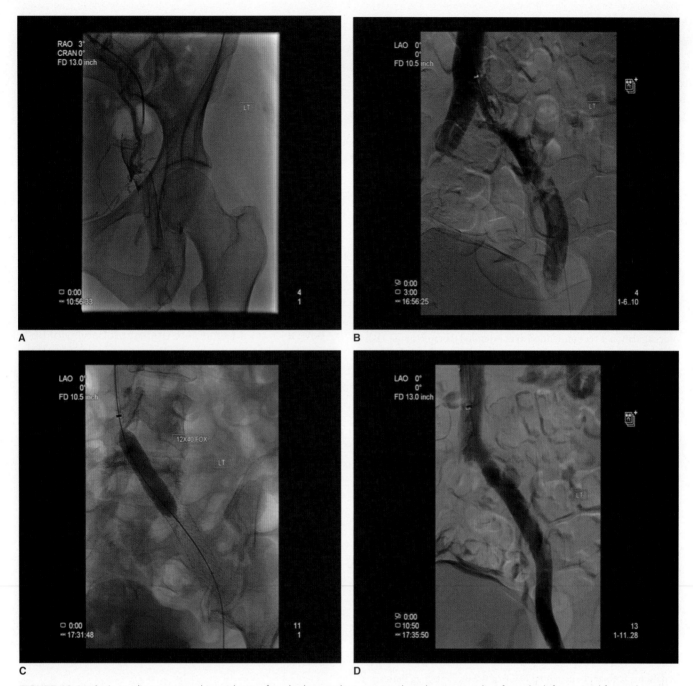

FIGURE 18-14 A. Ascending venographic evidence of marked acute deep venous thrombosis extending from the left proximal femoral vein to the proximal common iliac vein. Several collateral veins exist. **B.** Although the majority of the iliofemoral venous thrombosis has been successfully treated with catheter-directed thrombolysis (CDT), residual narrowing within the left proximal common iliac vein remains consistent with left iliac vein compression syndrome. **C.** Balloon venoplasty with stenting of the stenotic left common iliac vein. **D.** Ascending venographic evidence of successful restoration of left iliac venous flow after a combination of CDT and adjunctive venoplasty with stenting. (Image used with permission from Dr. Mitch Silver.)

In patients with acute DVT or PE who are treated with anticoagulants, insertion of an inferior vena cava (IVC) filter is not recommended (grade 1B).

In patients with subsegmental PE (no involvement of more proximal pulmonary arteries) and no proximal lower extremity DVT who are at low risk for recurrent VTE, clinical surveillance is suggested over anticoagulation; conversely, patients at high risk for recurrent VTE should receive anticoagulation (grade 2C).

PULMONARY EMBOLISM RISK STRATIFICATION

All patients presenting with an acute PE should quickly undergo risk stratification into 1 of 3 categories: low, intermediate, or high risk. The clinical assessment via the simplified Pulmonary Embolism Severity Index (sPESI) should be calculated where 1 point is scored for each of the items listed in Table 18-4.[19]

If sPESI is 0, the patient is considered low risk (30-day mortality risk: 1.1%) and can typically be treated with standard anticoagulation, often in an outpatient setting. A sPESI score of 1 or greater in a normotensive subject is at intermediate risk (30-day mortality 10.9%) and additional testing should be undertaken including a transthoracic echocardiography and cardiac biomarkers. Figure 18-15 documents how the combination of the sPESI and imaging/biomarker determination can be used to stratify and subsequently treat patients presenting with an acute PE.[20]

A 2014 meta-analysis of 16 randomized studies comparing thrombolytic therapy with anticoagulation therapy for acute PE (including intermediate-risk, hemodynamically stable patients with right ventricular dysfunction) identified that thrombolytic therapy was superior to standard anticoagulant therapy in reducing mortality by 47%. However, a 2.7-fold increase in major bleeding occurred in patients who received thrombolytic therapy.[21]

The risk of major bleeding (including up to 3% intracranial hemorrhage rate) associated with systemic thrombolytic therapy can be obviated by the use of contemporary CDT techniques (Figure 18-16). In the 2015 prospective SEATTLE II trial utilizing ultrasound-facilitated CDT for both massive and submassive PE, none of the 150 patients suffered an intracranial hemorrhage.[22]

Table 18-4 Simplified Pulmonary Embolism Severity Index[19]

The following clinical variables are worth 1 point:

Age >80 years

History of cancer

History of cardiopulmonary disease (heart failure and/or chronic lung disease)

Pulse >110 beats/min

Systolic blood pressure <100 mm Hg

Arterial saturation <90%

A total point score for a given patient is calculated by adding the points.

A score of 0 is low risk; 1 or more is high risk.

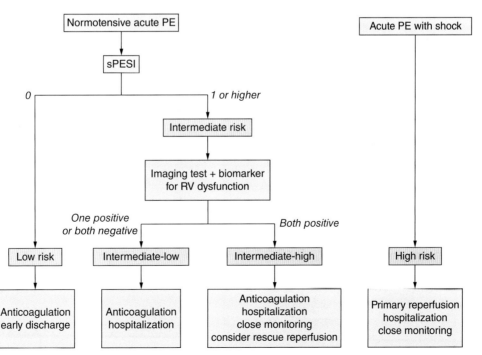

FIGURE 18-15 European Society of Cardiology Algorithm for Risk Stratification and Management of the patient with acute normotensive pulmonary embolism. (Reproduced from Handoko ML, de Man FS. Risk-stratification in normotensive acute pulmonary embolism. *Neth Heart J.* 2015;23:52-54).

PREVENTION

The ACCF/AHA 2013 HF guidelines class I recommend that a patient admitted to the hospital with decompensated HF should receive venous thromboembolism prophylaxis with an anticoagulant medication if the risk-benefit ratio is favorable (level of evidence: B).[23] For patients admitted specifically for decompensated HF and with adequate renal function (serum creatinine <2.0 mg/dL), either enoxaparin 40 mg subcutaneously once daily or unfractionated heparin 5000 units subcutaneously every 8 hours is recommended.

Although not a guideline-based recommendation, a direct oral anticoagulant could be effectively utilized for venous thromboprophylaxis in the hospitalized HF patient. In the MAGELLAN trial, rivaroxaban 10 mg once daily was noninferior to enoxaparin 40 mg once daily in preventing VTE in hospitalized acutely ill medical patients (1 in 3 patients had HF).[24]

PROGNOSIS

DEEP VENOUS THROMBOSIS

The dominant long-term morbidity from DVT is related to the post-thrombotic syndrome (PTS), which occurs in 20% to 50% of patients (Figure 18-17). PTS is less frequent after a distal (calf) DVT and more likely to complicate a larger proximal DVT.

PTS typically occurs within 2 years of the initial DVT. Nearly 1 in 5 cases have manifested by 1 year. Well-established risk factors for PTS include recurrent ipsilateral DVT (6- to 10-fold increase), proximal DVT (especially iliofemoral), obesity, and the presence of varicose veins *prior* to thrombosis.

PULMONARY EMBOLISM

The prognosis of patients with PE is dependent on a timely diagnosis and therapy as well as comorbid disease.

Approximately 10% of patients with acute PE die within 1 hour of symptom onset. Early PE mortality is directly related to thromboembolic burden upon presentation. Mortality rates for patients depending on PE size are nonmassive <1%, submassive 3% to 15%, and massive 20% to 60%.

Chronic thromboembolic pulmonary HTN develops in 0.5% to 3%.

VENOUS THROMBOEMBOLISM MORTALITY

Patients with PE have significantly higher in-hospital mortality than patients with DVT, but roughly the same mortality after the first month of therapy.

In an Italian cohort (n = 355) of patients followed after a first episode of symptomatic DVT, 90 (25%) died during follow-up. The majority of patients died from cancer (n = 52). Less frequent causes of mortality included cardiovascular disease (n = 12) and PE (n = 9). Survival was 83.3% after 1 year of follow-up and decreased to 74.6% at 5 years.[25]

In a 2011 study of 1023 patients with PE, the 5-year mortality was a remarkable 32% where approximately one-half of the patients died from underlying cardiovascular disease. Other causes for

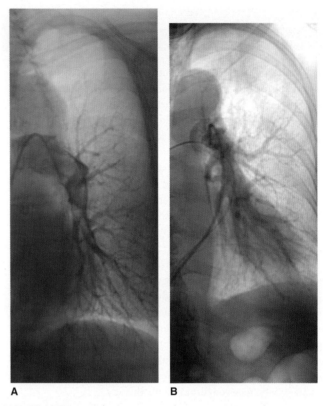

A   **B**

FIGURE 18-16 A. Prelytic contrast pulmonary arteriographic representation of a large embolus within the left pulmonary artery and associated branches; **B.** Resolution of the large left pulmonary artery embolus after catheter directed thrombolytic therapy. Note improved perfusion within the peripheral left segmental and subsegmental arteries.

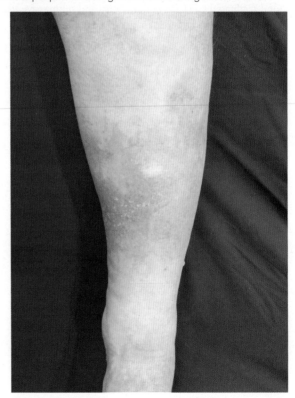

FIGURE 18-17 Post-thrombotic syndrome in the left calf with associated swelling, hyperpigmentation, and dermatitis. Lipodermatosclerosis of the distal medial calf is exemplified by sclerotic atrophy with increased concavity.

mortality included malignancy, chronic kidney disease, and neuro-degenerative disease.[26]

VENOUS THROMBOEMBOLISM RECURRENCE

In a prospective cohort study of 1626 patients with either a provoked or unprovoked proximal DVT and/or PE, the cumulative incidence of recurrent VTE after anticoagulation discontinuance was 11.0% after 1 year, 19.6% after 3 years, 29.1% after 5 years, and 39.9% after 10 years.[27] Patients with unprovoked VTE were nearly 2.5 times more likely to suffer a recurrence when compared to the provoked subset.

FOLLOW-UP

Patients should be monitored on a regular basis for signs of recurrent venous thromboembolic disease, especially if anticoagulation has been terminated.

Consider indefinite anticoagulation after a first unprovoked VTE event in the setting of HF, especially if 1 or more of the following high-risk factors for recurrence exists: male gender, severely depressed left ventricular ejection fraction (<20%), New York Heart Association class III or IV, elevated D-dimer, or concurrent traditional VTE risk factors (eg, thrombophilia, cancer, prior VTE).

Monitor patients with a prior DVT for manifestations of the post-thrombotic syndrome.

PATIENT EDUCATION

Health Media Network: https://www.acponline.org/system/files/documents/patients_families/products/facts/deep_vein_thrombosis.pdf; https://www.acponline.org/system/files/documents/patients_families/products/facts/pulmonary_embolism.pdf

UpToDate: http://www.uptodate.com/contents/pulmonary-embolism-beyond-the-basics

UpToDate: http://www.uptodate.com/contents/deep-vein-thrombosis-dvt-beyond-the-basics

Circulation: http://circ.ahajournals.org/content/129/17/e477.full

PATIENT RESOURCES

National Blood Clot Alliance: https://www.stoptheclot.org

Clot Connect: http://www.clotconnect.org/healthcare-professionals/patient-handouts

PROVIDER RESOURCES

UpToDate: http://www.uptodate.com/contents/overview-of-the-treatment-of-lower-extremity-deep-vein-thrombosis-dvt

Clot Connect: http://www.clotconnect.org/healthcare-professionals

Medscape: http://emedicine.medscape.com/article/1911303-overview

REFERENCES

1. Alikhan R, Spyropoulos AC. Epidemiology of venous thromboembolism in cardiorespiratory and infectious disease. *Am J Med.* 2008;121:935-942.

2. Matsuo H, Matsumura M, Nakajima Y, et al. Frequency of deep vein thrombosis among hospitalized non-surgical Japanese patients with congestive heart failure. *J Cardiol.* 2014;64:430-434.

3. Piazza G, Goldhaber SZ, Lessard DM, et al. Venous thromboembolism in heart failure: preventable deaths during and after hospitalization. *Am J Med.* 2011;124(3):252-259.

4. Beemath A, Stein PD, Skaf E, et al. Risk of venous thromboembolism in patients hospitalized with heart failure. *Am J Cardiol.* 2006;98:793-795.

5. Darze ES, Latado AL, Guimaraes AG, et al. Incidence and clinical predictors of pulmonary embolism in severe heart failure patients admitted to a coronary care unit. *Chest.* 2005;128:2576-2580.

6. Monreal M, Munoz-Torrero JF, Naraine VS, et al. Pulmonary embolism in patients with chronic obstructive pulmonary disease or congestive heart failure. *Am J Med.* 2006;119:851-858.

7. Garg R, Yusuf S. Overview of randomized trials of angiotensin-converting enzyme inhibitors on mortality and morbidity in patients with heart failure. Collaborative Group on ACE Inhibitor Trials. *JAMA.* 1995;273:1450-1456.

8. Chong AY, Lip GY. Viewpoint: the prothrombotic state in heart failure: a maladaptive inflammatory response? *Eur J Heart Fail.* 2007;9:124-128.

9. Howell MD, Geraci JM, Knowlton AA. Congestive heart failure and outpatient risk of venous thromboembolism: a retrospective, case-control study. *J Clin Epidemiol.* 2001;54:810-816.

10. Alikhan R, Cohen AT, Combe S, et al. Prevention of venous thromboembolism in medical patients with enoxaparin: a subgroup analysis of the MEDENOX study. *Blood Coagul Fibrinolysis.* 2003;14:341-346.

11. Mebazaa A, Spiro TE, Buller HR, et al. Predicting the risk of venous thromboembolism in patients hospitalized with heart failure. *Circ.* 2014;130:410-418.

12. Folsom AR, Lutsey PL, Nambi V, et al. Troponin T, NT-proBNP and venous thromboembolism: the Longitudinal Investigation of Thromboembolism Etiology (LITE). *Vasc Med.* 2014;19(1):33-41.

13. Well PS, Anderson DR, Rodger M, et al. Evaluation of d-Dimer in the diagnosis of suspected deep-vein thrombosis. *N Engl J Med.* 2003;349:1227-1235.

14. Douma RA, Mos IC, Erkens PM, et al. Performance of 4 clinical decision rules in the diagnostic management of acute pulmonary embolism: a prospective cohort study. *Ann Intern Med.* 2011;154(11):709-718.

15. Raja AS, Greenberg JO, Qaseem A, Denberg TD, et al. Evaluation of patients with suspected acute pulmonary embolism: best practice advice from the clinical guidelines committee

of the American College of Physicians. *Ann Intern Med.* 2015;163(9):701-711.

16. Kearon C, Aki EA, Ornelas J, et al. Antithrombotic therapy for VTE disease. CHEST guideline and expert panel report. *CHEST.* 2016;149(2):315-352.

17. Venous Thromboembolic Diseases: the Management of Venous Thromboembolic Diseases and the Role of Thrombophilia Testing. National Institute for Health and Clinical Excellence. website. Updated November 2015. http://guidance.nice.org.uk/CG144.

18. Jaff MR, McMurtry S, Archer SL, et al. Management of massive and submassive pulmonary embolism, iliofemoral deep vein thrombosis and chronic thromboembolic pulmonary hypertension: a scientific statement form the American Heart Association. *Circulation.* 2011;123:1788-1830.

19. Jiménez D, Aujesky D, Moores L, et al. Simplification of the pulmonary embolism severity index for prognostication in patients with acute symptomatic pulmonary embolism. *Arch Intern Med.* 2010;170:1383-1389.

20. Handoko ML, de Man FS. Risk-stratification in normotensive acute pulmonary embolism. *Neth Heart J.* 2015;23:52-54.

21. Chatterjee S, Chakraborty A, Weinberg I, et al. Thrombolysis for pulmonary embolism and risk of all-cause mortality, major bleeding, and intracranial hemorrhage: a meta-analysis. *JAMA.* 2014 Jun 18;311(23):2414-2421.

22. Piazza G, Hohlfelder B, Jaff MR. A prospective, single-Arm, multicenter trial of ultrasound-facilitated, catheter-directed, low-dose fibrinolysis for acute massive and submassive pulmonary embolism. The SEATTLE II Study. *J Am Coll Cardiol Intv.* 2015;8(10):1382-1392.

23. Yancy CW, Jessup M, Bozkurt B, et al. 2013 ACCF/AHA Guideline for the Management of Heart Failure. *J Am Coll Cardiol.* 2013;62(16):e147-e239.

24. Cohen AT, Spiro TE, Büller HR, et al. Rivaroxaban for thromboprophylaxis in acutely ill medical patients. *N Engl J Med.* 2013;368:513-523.

25. Prandoni P, Lensing A, Cogo A, et al. The long-term clinical course of acute deep venous thrombosis. *Ann Intern Med.* 1996;125(1):1-7.

26. Ng AC, Chung T, Yong AS, et al. Long-term cardiovascular and noncardiovascular mortality of 1023 patients with confirmed acute pulmonary embolism. *Circ Cardiovasc Qual Outcomes.* 2011;4:122-128.

27. Prandoni P, Noventa F, Ghirarduzzi A, et al. The risk of recurrent venous thromboembolism after discontinuing anticoagulation in patients with acute proximal deep vein thrombosis or pulmonary embolism: a prospective cohort study in 1,626 patients. *Haematologica.* February 2007;92:199-205.

19 ASSESSMENT OF VOLUME OVERLOAD IN ACUTE DECOMPENSATED HEART FAILURE

Heba R. Gaber, MD
Abeer Almasary, MD
W. Frank Peacock, MD, FACEP, FACC

PATIENT CASE

A 74-year-old man had been in his usual health and able to perform activities of daily living (including walking 1 block) until about 3 weeks ago, when he started to suffer shortness of breath that impaired his daily activity. He also found the need to sleep on 3 pillows. When asked, he complained of cough, but denied fever, and reported that his legs had become swollen. The patient's past medical history included hypertension (HTN), atrial fibrillation, chronic obstructive pulmonary disease, and ischemic heart disease (IHD). His medications were nifedipine, warfarin, amiodarone, and aspirin. Physical examination found an afebrile patient with an irregular heart rate (HR) at 110 beats per minute (Figure 19-1). His respiratory rate (RR) was 26 breaths per minute, blood pressure (BP) 160/92 mm Hg, and the oxygen saturation by pulse oximetry (SpO_2) was 92% on room air. His neck examination revealed jugular venous distention (Figure 19-2), he had an S_3 and rales on auscultation, as well as an enlarged liver and 3+ pretibial edema (Figure 19-3).

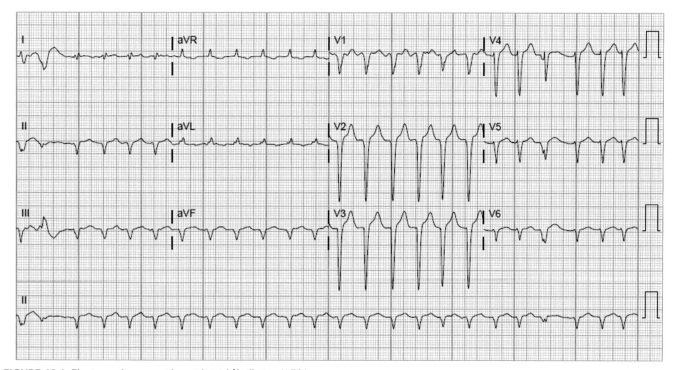

FIGURE 19-1 Electrocardiogram with rapid atrial fibrillation (AFib).

WHY IS VOLUME ASSESSMENT IMPORTANT?

When patients present acutely, one of the first challenges is to assess volume. The importance of an accurate volume assessment cannot be overstated. This is demonstrated by the results of a prehospital study of 493 patients transferred by ambulance with a chief complaint of dyspnea and suffering from suspected acute heart failure (AHF).[1] When patients with AHF received drugs targeting HF (furosemide, nitroglycerin, and morphine) their odds ratio for survival improved by 251%, thus demonstrating that correct volume assessment and early treatment has significant benefit. However, this compared to patients that did not have HF but mistakenly received HF treatment. The wrongly treated patients ultimately suffered a 13.6% mortality, which was even higher than that of the patients who received no treatment (8.2%). Thus, not only is it important to treat patients presenting with acute volume overload, it is important to not erroneously treat those who do not have excess volume. Getting it right is critical.

While the differential diagnosis of dyspnea is long and complicated, in the introductory Patient Case, the patient's volume overload is one of the predominant considerations. To accomplish an accurate diagnosis, a number of parameters must be weighed. The clinician must be careful in gathering a history from the patient and other sources to arrive at the correct diagnosis. Incorporating family members can be helpful in determining how compliant the patient is with medications and diet, and aid in a more rapid realization of what precipitated the episode of HF.

Several studies have examined the accuracy and reliability of the history and physical examination findings associated with excessive volume. Our patient complained of shortness of breath, orthopnea, and peripheral edema. In the ADHERE Registry (Acute Decompensated Heart Failure National Registry), which enrolled more than 190,000 episodes of patients hospitalized with HF, dyspnea was reported in about 89% of all patients presenting with HF.[2] As a predictor of volume overload, dyspnea on exertion has the highest sensitivity for circulatory congestion, and edema is also useful. The most specific symptoms consistent with volume overload are paroxysmal nocturnal dyspnea, orthopnea, and edema. Any of these increase the probability of an accurate HF diagnosis.[3,4] Edema may vary from being mild (Figure 19-4) or severe pitting edema (Figures 19-5 and 19-6). In most cases it is more prominent at the level of the ankles (Figures 19-7 through 19-10), but it may progress to the level of the knees (Figures 19-11 and 19-12).

Ultimately while paroxysmal nocturnal dyspnea is the most specific (positive likelihood ratio 2.6, 95% CI 1.5-4.5) of the historical symptoms, dyspnea on exertion is the most sensitive (negative likelihood ratio 0.45, 95% CI 0.35-0.67).[5] All of the historical and physical data are commonly synthesized into the physician's clinical impression, with variable accuracy. While Wang et al found the overall clinical gestalt of the emergency physician was associated with high sensitivity and specificity for the presence of volume overload from HF,[4] others have found that an initial impression, based only on history and physical is accurate only half the time.[6]

The possibility that low volume status is present must also be considered in patients with a history of HF, especially in the setting

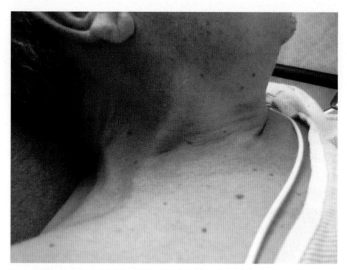

FIGURE 19-2 From introductory Patient Case, jugular venous distention (JVD).

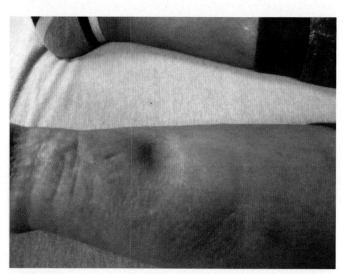

FIGURE 19-3 From introductory Patient Case, severe pitting edema +3 pretibial.

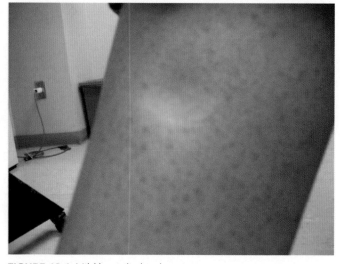

FIGURE 19-4 Mild lower limb edema.

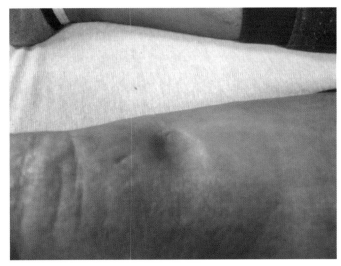

FIGURE 19-5 Severe pitting edema +3 above the level of the knee.

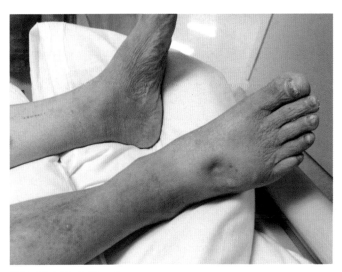

FIGURE 19-8 Ankle edema.

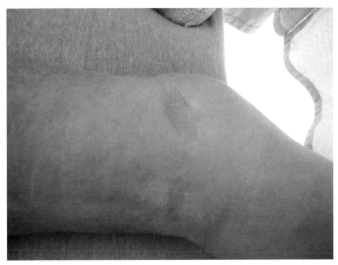

FIGURE 19-6 Pitting edema knee level.

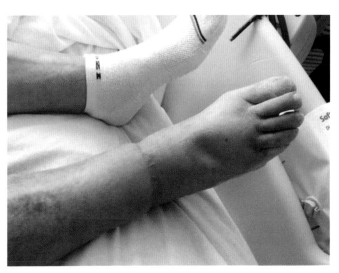

FIGURE 19-9 Ankle and leg edema.

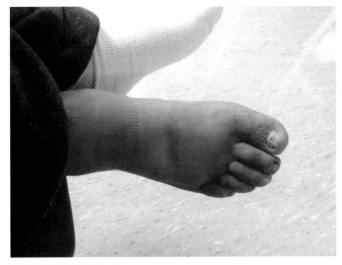

FIGURE 19-7 Ankle edema.

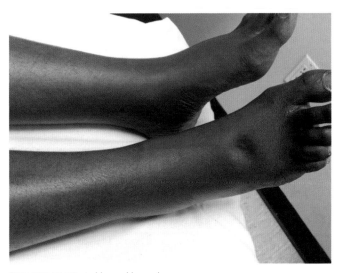

FIGURE 19-10 Ankle and leg edema.

of a low blood pressure. In a study examining 38 clinical indicators of dehydration in elderly patients,[7] the findings best correlated with the severity of volume deficit, and unrelated to the patient's age, included tongue dryness, longitudinal tongue furrows, dryness of the mouth mucous membranes, upper body muscle weakness, confusion, speech difficulty, and sunken eyes. Other indicators of low volume status had only weak associations with dehydration severity or were related to the patient's age. Unfortunately, the presence of thirst was not related to dehydration severity.[8]

ORTHOSTATIC VITAL SIGNS

Orthostatic hypotension, defined as a drop in systolic blood pressure (SBP) of >20 mm Hg or a drop in diastolic blood pressure >10 mm Hg, has been evaluated. A prospective study by Koziol-McLain et al[13] showed that out of 132 euvolemic patients, 43% were classified as hypovolemic, despite having orthostatic changes within 2 standard deviations of one another.[15] An orthostatic change in pulse of >30 bpm was also fraught with potential misclassification, having a sensitivity of 43% and specificity of 75%. Only in the setting of acute blood loss exceeding 1 L did the sensitivity and specificity improve to 97% and 98%, respectively.[9] Unfortunately, orthostatic vitals are not reliably sensitive to volume losses <1000 mL in adult patients.[10]

To add to the confusion, the procedure for measurement of orthostatic vital signs is not standardized as evidenced by a review of the literature reflecting significant variations in practice. The duration of position change differs between research studies, as do the position changes (lying to standing, lying to sitting to standing). There is even some debate as to which findings are the most important indicators of orthostatic hypotension and what are the best cutpoints for vital sign changes reflective of volume deficits.[11]

Levitt et al evaluated the degree of volume loss and orthostatic vital sign changes in emergency department (ED) patients. They found wide variation in orthostatic vital sign changes for healthy and ill individuals and poor correlation of vital signs for the severity of dehydration.[11] Heart rate (p = 0.0165) and age (p = 0.0047) had a small correlation (r2 = 0.098) with level of dehydration. While SBP did not demonstrate a statistically significant association with the degree of dehydration (r2 = 0.032, p = 0.56), a SBP change of −10.7 was the only vital sign to distinguish between patients with blood loss and healthy volunteers.[10,11]

PHYSICAL EXAMINATION

Of the physical examination, jugular venous distention (JVD) (Figure 19-13) may be the single best indicator of volume overload secondary to acute decompensated heart failure (ADHF) (positive likelihood ratio 5.1, 95% CI, 3.2-7.9; negative likelihood ratio 0.66, 95% CI, 0.57-0.77).[3] In one study a JVD exceeding 10 cm (Figure 19-14) was found to correspond to a pulmonary capillary wedge pressure (PCWP) of above 22 mm Hg, with an accuracy of 80%.[12] Another study (defining volume overload as a PCWP >18 mm Hg) reported that JVD and hepatojugular reflux had a predictive accuracy of only 81%. In this same analysis, the presence of rales had a positive predictive value of 100% for volume overload,

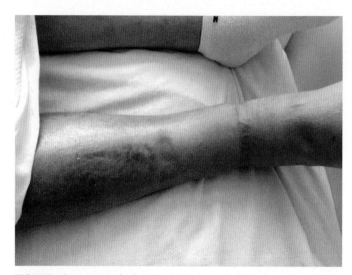

FIGURE 19-11 Lower limb edema below level of knees.

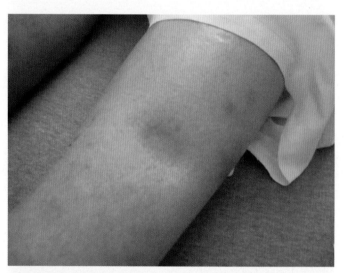

FIGURE 19-12 Pretibial edema.

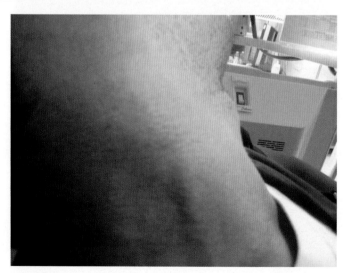

FIGURE 19-13 Jugular venous distention.

but their absence had a negative predictive value of only 35%. An alternative to passive observation of JVD is to evaluate volume status by determining if palpation of the liver results in JVD. Termed hepatojugular reflux (HJR), its presence is reported to be poorly sensitive (only 24%), but to have excellent specificity of 94%.[13] Finally, in severe chronic CHF, ascites may occur. Ascites may vary in its degree, from mild to severe. Tense ascites is shown in Figures 19-15 and 19-16; moderate to severe tense ascites is shown in Figures 19-17 through 19-19.

It must be considered that pathologies other than AHF may manifest as JVD. These include those conditions that result in marked increase in intrathoracic pressure and thus serve as an impediment to venous return. Thus while tension pneumothorax, hemothorax, chylothorax, and severe asthma or chronic obstructive pulmonary disease may all demonstrate findings of JVD, their presentations can be easily differentiated from that of AHF and thus are rarely clinically confused. Lastly, pericardial tamponade must be considered when JVD is found, but similar to elevated intrathoracic pressure, its presentation is usually easily discerned from that of AHF.

Other physical findings that may predict the presence of volume overload include extra cardiac sounds. Both the third and fourth heart sounds have been described as far back as the late 1800s.[14] Also known as a ventricular gallop, the third heart sound (S_3), occurs 0.12 to 0.16 seconds after the second heart sound in early diastole[15] and is indicative of an unfavorable prognosis in HF. The most likely explanation for the presence of the S_3 is when excessively rapid filling of a stiff ventricle is suddenly halted, causing vibrations audible as the third heart sound.[16] While accurate auscultation is challenging, especially in a noisy clinical environment, or when noise resulting from tachypnea obscures the heart sounds, when detected, the presence of an S_3 gallop has excellent specificity for the diagnosis of AHF.[17] Finally, it is important to recognize that the presence of an S_3 may be a normal finding in adolescents and young adults, but after the age of 40 years it is usually considered abnormal and indicative of left ventricular dysfunction.[18-20]

The fourth heart sound (S_4), also known as an atrial gallop, occurs just before the first heart sound in the cardiac cycle. It is the result of atrial contraction causing vibrations of the left ventricular muscle, mitral valve apparatus, and left ventricular blood mass.[21] The reported prevalence of an S_4 in healthy individuals is variable, ranging from 11% to 75%.[22-28]

Although history and physical are the easiest diagnostic tools, both have significant limitations in accuracy. Further challenges exist when patients present with multiple potential comorbidities, eg, simultaneous HF and sepsis. In these difficult cases, rapid objective measurement of volume status is needed. Several tests may be performed to determine the etiology and support the evaluation of volume status in suspected ADH.

INVESTIGATIONS

While an electrocardiogram (ECG) is helpful to detect acute myocardial infarction, ischemia, left ventricular (LV) hypertrophy (Figure 19-20), and arrhythmias, it is not particularly useful to

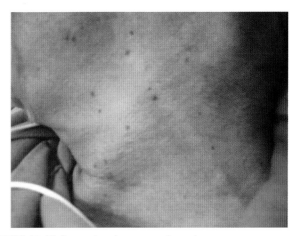
FIGURE 19-14 Severe jugular venous distention.

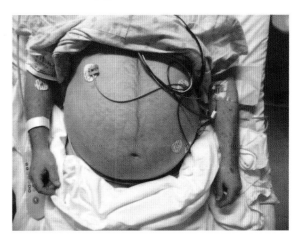
FIGURE 19-15 Tense ascites.

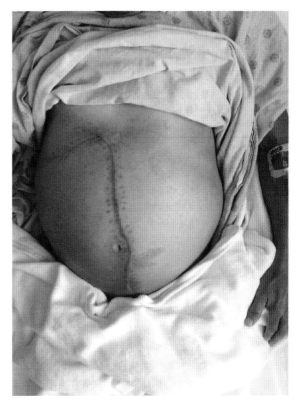
FIGURE 19-16 Tense ascites.

assess the presence of volume overload. Atrial fibrillation (Figure 19-21), which is present in about 31% of patients presenting with ADHF or heart block, also can contribute to HF symptoms and has little relation to volume status.[29]

The chest radiograph has been one of the earliest obtainable tests to estimate volume status. While its value in the setting of hypovolemia is limited to the exclusion of coexistent pathology (eg, coexistent pneumonia), it is of value in the setting of hypervolemia. When faced with an acutely dyspneic patient, the chest x-ray may exclude other significant confounding diagnoses, such as pneumothorax, infiltrative processes, and so on, from the differential diagnosis. Chest x-ray findings that suggest the diagnosis of HF with volume overload include Kerley lines (Figures 19-19 through 19-22), increased pulmonary vascularity, and pleural effusions. Cardiomegaly, which may be detectable by chest x-ray (Figures 19-23 and 19-24), is not a useful predictor of volume status, as it is as likely to be the consequence of chronic ventricular remodeling rather than represent an effect of acute volume overload. The chest x-ray may also reveal also underlying cardiac conditions such as the implanted cardiac device (ICD) shown in Figures 19-25 and 19-26. Figure 19-27 shows a chest x-ray with both an ICD and pulmonary congestion. Importantly, because the abnormal findings of chest radiographs may lag the clinical appearance by several hours, therapy should not be withheld while attempting to obtain the chest x-ray.

How the chest x-ray is obtained will have a critical impact on the ability of the clinician to accurately interpret the results. When obtained portably, the sensitivity of a chest x-ray for findings of volume overload is poor (Figure 19-28). In one study of mild HF, only dilated upper lobe vessels were found in >60% of acutely decompensated HF patients, thus failing to identify nearly half of the volume overloaded patients. It should be noted that the frequency of volume overload findings increases with the severity of presentation. Conversely, in one report of severe HF, x-ray findings of volume overload occurred in at least two-thirds of all patients, except for Kerley lines (occurring in only 11%) and a prominent vena cava (found in only 44%).[34] This suggests that the greater the volume overload, the more likely the chest radiograph is to demonstrate findings consistent with excess fluid. Finally, pleural effusion (Figure 19-29) can be missed by portable technique chest x-rays, especially if the patient is intubated, as in this scenario the film is performed supine. It may also show pleural effusion and interstitial congestion (Figures 19-30 and 19-31). In patients with pleural effusions, the sensitivity, specificity, and accuracy of the supine chest x-ray was reported to be 67%, 70%, and 67%, respectively.[30] Ultimately, acute pulmonary edema represents the greatest volume overload (Figures 19-32 and 19-33).

The gold standard for the quantification for thoracic fluid volumes is currently unclear, although computed tomography (CT) has been proposed. It has been promoted as being able to detect pleural fluid not noted on routine CT scanning; however, a small effusion is sometimes hard to differentiate from pleural thickening. Contrast enhancement is helpful in separating an effusion from an adjacent lung process (airspace disease or atelectasis). Unlike pleural fluid, lung tissue enhances with the administration of contrast material. CT scanning is superior to plain radiography in evaluating

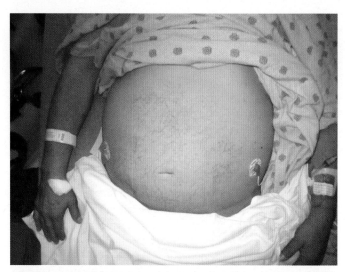

FIGURE 19-17 Moderate to severe ascites.

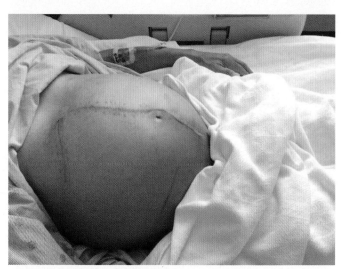

FIGURE 19-18 Severe ascites.

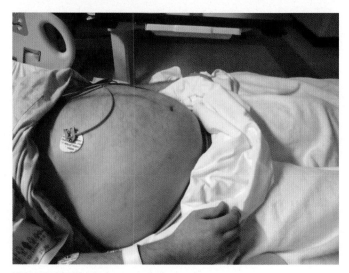

FIGURE 19-19 Moderate ascites.

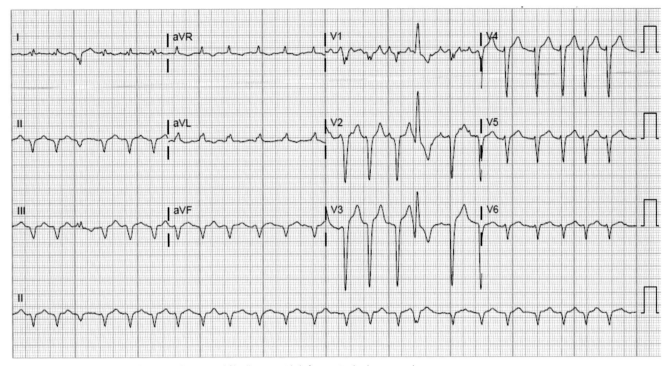

FIGURE 19-20 An electrocardiogram show atrial fibrillation with left ventricular hypertrophy.

the presence of loculated effusion or effusions with associated lung disease; this modality is also more helpful than plain radiography in evaluating the underlying etiology of effusion While CT may offer a diagnostic alternative, it is difficult in the unstable patient and cannot be recommended routinely.[31]

Chest x-rays were performed in evaluating our patient's case (Figure 19-34). They are consistent with a diagnosis of volume

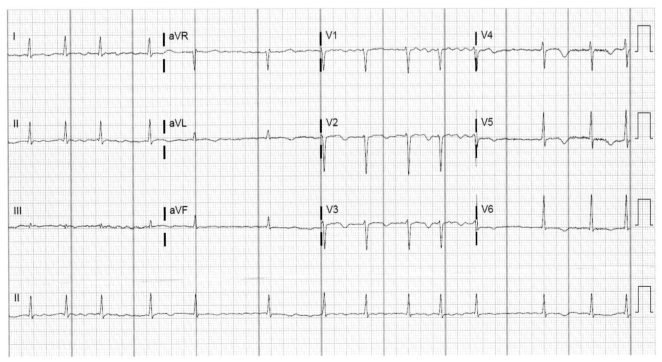

FIGURE 19-21 An electrocardiogram shows atrial fibrillation.

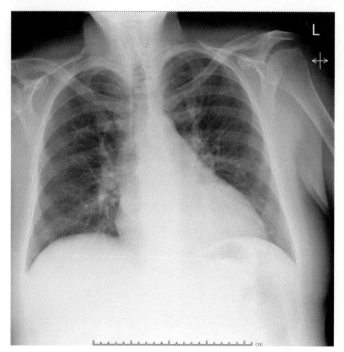

FIGURE 19-22 Chest x-ray posterior anterior view shows pulmonary congestion.

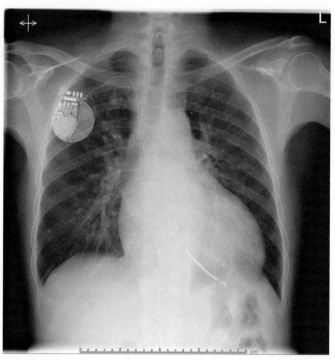

FIGURE 19-24 Chest x-ray shows implantable cardiac device (ICD) and cardiomegaly.

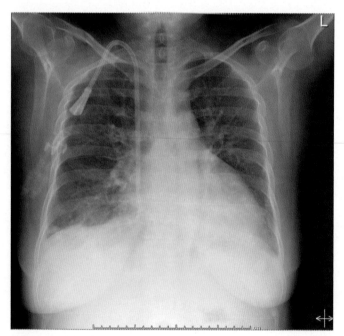

FIGURE 19-23 Chest x-ray shows pulmonary congestion and interstitial edema.

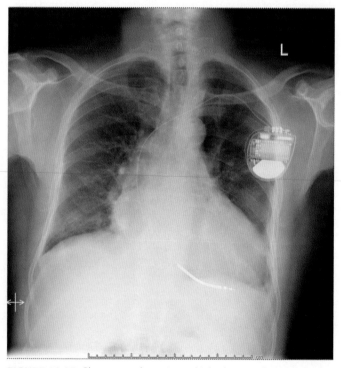

FIGURE 19-25 Chest x-ray shows interstitial edema, pulmonary venous congestion, and bilateral pleural effusion.

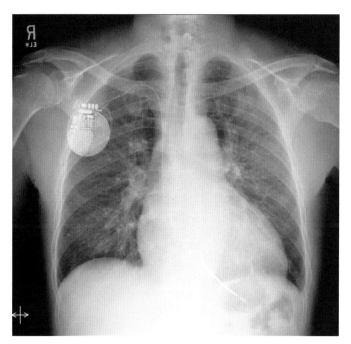

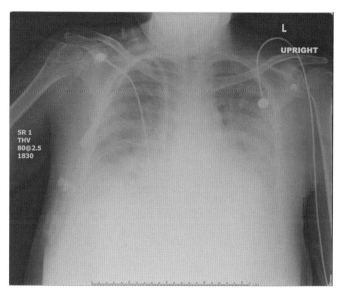

FIGURE 19-28 Chest x-ray shows pulmonary venous congestion and bilateral pleural effusions.

FIGURE 19-26 Chest x-ray shows implantable cardiac device (ICD), cardiomegaly, and pulmonary venous congestion.

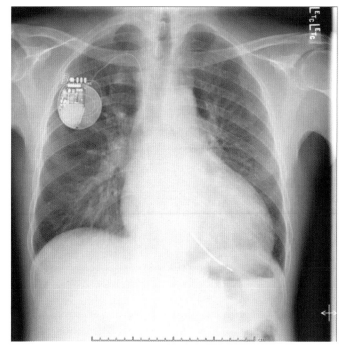

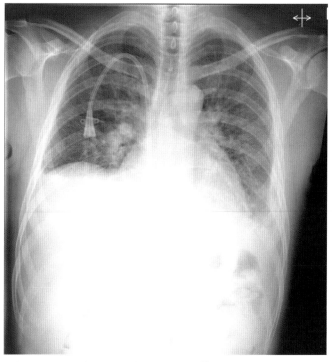

FIGURE 19-27 Chest x-ray shows implantable cardiac device (ICD), cardiomegaly, and pulmonary venous congestion.

FIGURE 19-29 Chest x-ray shows pleural effusion.

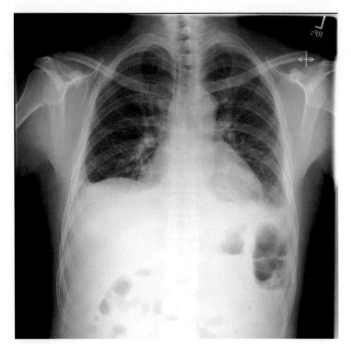

FIGURE 19-30 Chest x-ray shows congestion effusion and cardiomegaly.

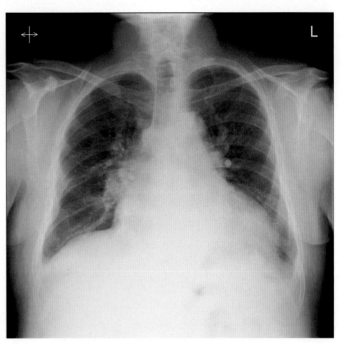

FIGURE 19-32 CXR pleural effusion cardiomegaly and congestion.

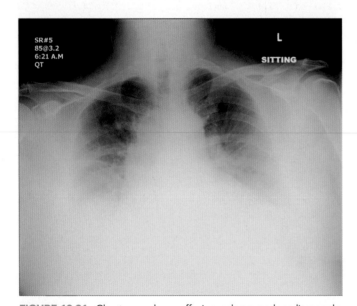

FIGURE 19-31 Chest x-ray shows effusion, edema, and cardiomegaly.

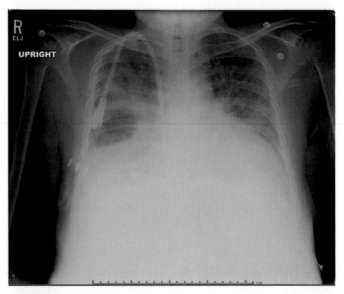

FIGURE 19-33 Chest x-ray shows pulmonary congestion with bilateral pleural effusion.

overload as they reveal an increase in the caliber of pulmonary vessels that have lost their definition because they are surrounded by edema. Kerley-B lines are also seen as peripheral short 1 cm to 2 cm horizontal lines near the costophrenic angles.

LABORATORY TESTING

A number of laboratory tests are recommended to be obtained in suspected AHF, and while they may suggest a contributing etiology to the presentation, few are actually helpful in volume assessment. Contrary to the general futility of laboratory testing providing insight into volume assessment, natriuretic peptides have demonstrated utility. The natriuretic peptides (NPs), termed B-type natriuretic peptide (BNP), its synthetic by-product N-terminal pro BNP (NT-proBNP), and the midregional prohormone of atrial natriuretic peptide (MR-proANP) are all elevated in the setting of myocardial stress. Consequently, levels of these molecules may be increased in the setting of volume overload. However, as there are many causes of myocardial stress unrelated to volume status (eg, myocardial infarction, pulmonary embolus), the NP level must be considered within the context of the clinical presentation. When NP levels are found to be low (<100 pg/mL for BNP, or <300 pg/mL for NT-proBNP), they have excellent negative predictive value, exceeding 95%, for the absence HF with volume overload. However, because of the long list of entities associated with increased myocardial stress, NP levels must be significantly elevated (>500 pg/mL for BNP, 900 pg/mL for NT-proBNP) before the positive predictive value for the presence of HF with volume overload exceeds 90%.

Finally, 3 important confounders can affect the clinical prediction of volume overload based on NP interpretation: obesity, renal failure, and drug effects. Because BNP is metabolized by endothelial C-receptors, and each pound of fat adds a significant volume of endothelial surface that is capable of metabolizing BNP, there is a marked negative correlation between obesity and NP levels such that it is generally recommended to double the BNP level if the body mass index (BMI) exceeds 35. Conversely, as a significant proportion of BNP and NT-proBNP metabolism is a function of renal integrity, decreases in estimated glomerular filtration rate (eGFR) are associated with a proportional increase in NP levels such that it is recommend if the eGFR is below 60 mL/min, that the NP level should be halved.

Lastly, several drugs may affect the measures of BNP. If nesiritide is administered to the HF patient, because it is recombinant DNA-synthesized BNP, levels of BNP are markedly increased so that no interpretation of clinical status based on BNP measurement is possible. Most recently the combination drug sacubitril/valsartan became available, the first part of which is a neprilysin antagonist. As neprilysin is the endogenous enzyme responsible for BNP metabolism, its inhibition results in higher endogenous BNP levels, although it does not appear to affect NT-proBNP in the same fashion. In what manner sacubitril/valsartan should affect treatment algorithms is unclear; however, its diagnostic impact should be considered when attempting to ascertain volume status in a patient currently taking this drug.

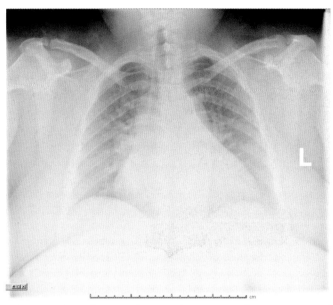

FIGURE 19-34 Volume resulting in pulmonary vascular congestion and interstitial edema.

It is important to recognize that some patients will have chronically elevated NP levels. When this occurs, knowledge of their dry weight NP is critical for accurate interpretation. If the baseline levels are known, then increases exceeding 50% suggest clinically relevant changes, where smaller fluctuations may simply reflect biologic variation. Ultimately, while NPs can be performed rapidly as a bedside test and thus satisfy the need for objective assessment in critically ill presentations, in patients in whom knowledge of prior NP test results are unknown, their greatest utility is in the absence of elevation.

ULTRASOUND

Bedside ultrasound can provide timely data sufficient to support or refute the diagnosis of volume overload. It also allows treating physicians to begin therapy, even in the most unstable patients with ADHF, before the traditional diagnostic tests are available. The ability to perform bedside ultrasound has rapidly become part of the emergency physician's armamentarium, such to the point that a basic skill is now a requisite part of all emergency medicine training programs.

INFERIOR VENA CAVA ULTRASOUND

As recently as 2008 the American College of Emergency Physicians issued a policy statement for emergency ultrasound. This includes the evaluation of intravascular volume status and the estimation of central venous pressure (CVP) based on sonographic examination of the inferior vena cava (IVC). The IVC is a thin-walled compliant vessel that adjusts to the body's volume status by changing its diameter depending on the total body fluid volume. The IVC also contracts and expands with each respiration. This is a function of blood flow into the thoracic cavity as a result of the negative intrathoracic pressure created by the inspiration, which results in briefly collapsing the IVC. Conversely, with exhalation intrathoracic pressure increases, which is associated with decreased venous return and expansion of the IVC to its baseline diameter as blood backs up in the IVC. Changes in volume status will be reflected in the sonographic evaluation of the IVC, where increased or decreased collapsibility of the vessel will help guide clinical management of the patient. The combination of the absolute diameter of the IVC and the degree of collapse with respiration may give an estimate of central venous pressure and substitute for more invasive measurements.

In states of low intravascular volume, the percentage collapse of the vessel will be proportionally higher than in intravascular volume overload states Figure 19-35. This is quantified by the calculation of the caval index, which is defined as the IVC expiratory diameter minus IVC inspiratory diameter, divided by IVC expiratory diameter × 100. The caval index is written as a percentage, where a number close to 100% is indicative of almost complete collapse (and therefore severe volume depletion), whereas a number close to 0% suggests minimal collapse (ie, likely volume overload, or restriction to blood flow). A caval index >50% predicts a central venous pressure <8 with a sensitivity of 91% and a specificity of 94%. The corresponding positive and negative predictive values were 87%

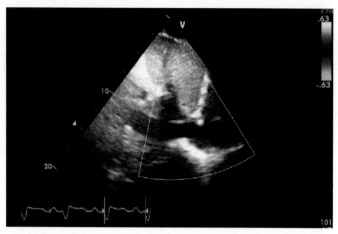

FIGURE 19-35 Ultrasound of the heart shows IVC where it should be measured 2 cm from the right atrium.

and 96%, respectively.[32] The diameter of the IVC for calculation of the caval index should be measured 2 cm from where it enters the right atrium. An alternative way to visualize respiratory variation is to use M-mode, with the beam overlying the IVC 2 cm from the right atrium. The inspiratory and expiratory diameter can then be measured on the M-mode image, at the smallest and largest locations, respectively.

In the setting of volume depletion, the diameter of the IVC will be decreased and the percentage collapse will be greater than 50%. With complete collapse, the IVC may become difficult to visualize (Figure 19-36). Conversely, with volume overload, patients will have a large IVC diameter and minimal collapse on inspiration and in severe cases, there may not be any notable respiratory variation seen in M-mode (Figure 19-37).

PULMONARY ULTRASOUND

The utility of lung ultrasound is based upon an acoustic artifact known as the B-line. Ziskin et al first described this artifact in 1982.[33] B-lines constitute a significant lung ultrasound finding. Lichtenstein et al first used the presence of at least 3 B-lines per field of scan seen longitudinally between 2 ribs, with a distance between 2 B-lines <7 ± 1 mm, as criteria for abnormality. Most authors have followed this convention.[34-37] These criteria have been used irrespective of scan technique, whether transverse in the intercostal space or longitudinal across ribs. Usually, a microconvex or phased array probe with a narrow footprint is used. Some operators choose to use a linear or curvilinear probe with a broad footprint. These probes allow views across several rib spaces, or a longer view of the pleural line. A positive scan with these probes should be similar to the general convention of at least 3 B-lines less than 7 mm apart.

As to what scan technique is optimal, several approaches have been used. One simple approach is to divide the chest wall into anterior and lateral areas. Another approach divides the chest wall into anterior and lateral portions, upper and lower halves, for 4 zones per hemithorax. Irrespective of the scan technique, a positive test is defined as multiple bilateral B-lines in an anterolateral or lateral location. A positive lung ultrasound has a sensitivity and specificity of 100% and 92%, respectively, for the diagnosis of cardiogenic pulmonary edema.[36]

BIOIMPEDANCE TECHNOLOGIES

Bioimpedance involves the injection of a small amount of electrical current into the thorax with simultaneous measurement of the voltage drop using electrodes placed on the chest or extremities (Figure 19-38). The basic principle of measurement is based on Ohm's law, which states that impedance to an alternating current (Z) is equal to the voltage drop[38] between 2 ends of a circuit divided by the flow of electrical current (I). Bioimpedance analysis (BIA) is an objective quantitative method of volume assessment based on the principle that the human body acts as a circuit BIVA device (Figure 19-39). As total body water increases, the resistance (Rz) and reactance (Xc) of the body decrease. Bioimpedance has excellent correlation with the radioactive isotope dilution studies

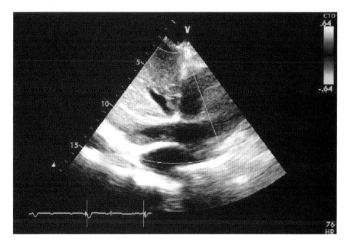

FIGURE 19-36 Subxiphoid view of the heart with difficult-to-estimate IVC diameter.

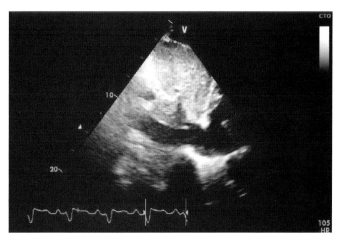

FIGURE 19-37 Ultrasound of the heart shows plethoric IVC.

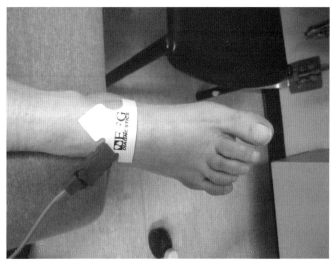

FIGURE 19-38 BIVA trodes foot.

(r = 0.996), the gold standard method for volume assessment.[39] Unfortunately, isotopic dilution is not feasible in the acute-care environment because of the lengthy time and high costs required for its performance.[40]

Bioimpedance vector analysis (BIVA) represents an improvement of BIA. BIVA, which calculates bioimpedance from the measured height-corrected reactance (Xc/Hh) and resistance (Rz/Hh), is not affected by weight. Bioimpedance (Z/h) is the calculated vector sum of the height-corrected resistance and reactance.[41] Low bioimpedance values are associated with fluid retention. BIVA is rapid (can be determined within 1 minute), noninvasive, and requires minimal training to perform. For accurate results, BIVA requires adequate cutaneous contact and patients who are able to lie supine. Limitations to the use of impedance measurements include skin-related conditions (crusting skin, ulcers, wounds, eshcars, excessive sweating, inadequate cleaning, and excessive hair that would interfere with electrode placement), misplacement of the electrodes, severe obesity, if the patient cannot maintain body position (eg, in cases of severe psychiatric disease), and contact with an electrical ground (as metal bed frame) or electrical interference. With these few limitations, BIVA has been used to manage hemodialysis,[42] investigate the progression of liver disease,[43] predict mortality in cancer patients,[44] as well as diagnose and manage AHF.[45,46] BIA techniques are safe, portable, relatively inexpensive, objective, and require very little training to assess body fluid status. A BIVA reading is shown in Figure 19-40.

It has been reported that the impedance and hydration scores derived from BIVA measurements objectively correlate with volume overload, and can be presented as BIVA hydration status (Figure 19-41). In addition, they are also associated with an increased need for volume reduction and hospitalization rates. Patients who present to the ED with a higher degree of fluid overload may have a more serious or longstanding pathology than patients who are more euvolemic, and their early identification may be clinically valuable. Importantly, hydration scores and bioimpedance had similar or better predictive abilities for volume overload, the need for volume reduction, and the requirement for hospitalization when compared with either BNP or chest x-ray. Because measurements from the BIVA device are readily determined, objective, inexpensive, and noninvasive, its use may aid in clinical management.

Another monitoring device for HF is CardioMEMS (St. Jude Medical, St. Paul, MN). It consists of 3 parts: a small permanent sensor implanted in the pulmonary artery, a catheter-based delivery system, and a system that acquires and processes PA pressure measurements from the implanted monitor and transfers the data to a secure database. The small implantable device provides daily pulmonary artery pressure measurements to guide physicians in their treatment of NYHA class III HF patients who have been hospitalized for HF in the previous year. The FDA's Circulatory System Devices Panel has agreed that the device was safe but that it had not been shown to be effective or that the benefits of the device outweighed the risks. Future studies are warranted.

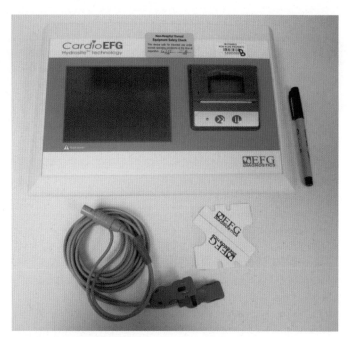

FIGURE 19-39 BIVA device.

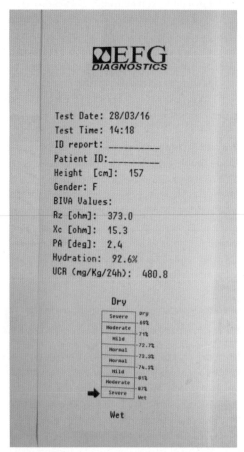

FIGURE 19-40 BIVA reading.

THERAPEUTIC CHALLENGE

Some investigators have reported that a diuretic challenge may be of utility in the evaluation of volume status. While this does have some theoretical support, when evaluated objectively its utility is limited. This is because those patients who are diuretic naïve may have the most robust response, and conversely the most resistant patients to the effect of intravenous loop diuretic may simply be those with the most advanced disease, most prior exposure, or suffering coexistent renal insufficiency. While a diuretic trial may result in clinical improvement, as a diagnostic adjunct for volume overload, its utility cannot be recommended.

SUMMARY

Assessment of volume status of patients who present acutely can be challenging. While it is important to rapidly treat patients presenting with acute volume overload, it is equally important to not erroneously diagnose those who do not have excess volume. The differential diagnosis of dyspnea is long and complicated. Reliability of the history and physical examination findings associated with volume overload are debatable and still suffer from significant limitations in accuracy. Rapid objective measurement is needed to determine the etiology and support the evaluation of volume status in ADHF. Chest x-rays have been one of the earliest noninvasive tests to estimate volume status, but their sensitivity for identifying volume overload is poor. While CT may offer diagnostic alternatives, it is difficult in unstable patients and cannot be routinely recommended. NPs can be performed rapidly as a bedside test and thus satisfy the need for objective assessment in critically ill presentations; however, in patients in whom knowledge of prior NP test results is unknown, their greatest utility may be in the absence of elevation. Bedside ultrasound can provide timely data sufficient to support or refute the diagnosis of volume overload. In the setting of volume depletion, the diameter of the IVC will be decreased and the percentage collapse will exceed 50%. Conversely, with volume overload, patients will have a large IVC diameter and minimal collapse on inspiration. Additionally, IVC scan lung ultrasound with optimal technique has sensitivity and specificity of 100% and 92%, respectively, for the diagnosis of cardiogenic pulmonary edema. Lastly, BIA techniques are safe, portable, relatively inexpensive, objective, and require very little training to assess body fluid status. Ultimately the clinician must consider the patient's history and physical, with the corroboration by the various data sources, to construct an accurate assessment and interventional plan.

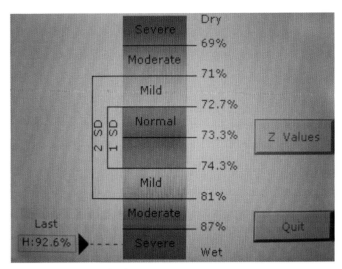

FIGURE 19-41 BIVA hydration 1.

REFERENCES

1. Wuerz RC, Meador SA. Effects of prehospital medications on mortality and length of stay in congestive heart failure. *Ann Emerg Med.* 1992;21(6):669-667.

2. Fonarow GC. The Acute Decompensated Heart Failure National Registry (ADHERE): opportunities to improve care of patients hospitalized with acute decompensated heart failure. *Rev Cardiovasc Med.* 2003;(4 Suppl 7):S21-S30.

3. Wang CS, Fitzgerald JM, Schulzer M, et al. Does this dyspneic patient in the emergency department have congestive heart failure? *J Am Med Assoc.* 2005;294:1944-1956.

4. Wong GC, Ayas NT. Clinical approaches to the diagnosis of acute heart failure. *Curr Opin Cardiol.* 2007;22:207-213.

5. Allen LA, O'Connor CM. Management of acute decompensated heart failure. *CMAJ.* 2007;176(6):797-805.

6. Remes J, Miettinen H, Reunanen A, et al. Validity of clinical diagnosis of heart failure in primary health care. *Eur Heart J.* 1991;12(3):315-321.

7. Gross CR, Lindquist RD, Woolley AC, Granieri R, Allard K, Webster B. Clinical indicators of dehydration severity in elderly patients. *J Emerg Med.* 1992 May-Jun;10(3):267-274.

8. Peacock WF, Soto KM. Current techniques of fluid status assessment. *Contrib Nephrol.* 2010;164:128-142. doi: 10.1159/000313726. Epub 2010 Apr 20.

9. Koziol-McLain J, Lowenstein SR, Fuller B. Orthostatic vital signs in emergency department patients. *Ann Emerg Med.* 1991;20(6):606-610.

10. Barraf LJ, Schriger DL. Orthostatic vital signs: variation with age, specificity, and sensitivity in detecting a 450-mL blood loss. *Am J Emerg Med.* 1992;10(2):99-103.

11. Levitt MA, Lopez B, Lieberman ME, Sutton M. Evaluation of the tilt test in an adult emergency medicine population. *Ann Emerg Med.* 1992;21(6):713-718.

12. Stevenson LW, Perloff JK. The limited reliability of physical signs for estimating hemodynamics in chronic heart failure. *JAMA.* 1989;261(6):884-888.

13. Marantz PR, Kaplan MC, Alderman MH. Clinical diagnosis of congestive heart failure in patients with acute dyspnea. *Chest.* 1990;97(4):776-781.

14. Potain C. Du bruit de galop. *Gaz D Hop.* 1880;53:529-531.

15. Sokolow M. Physical examination. In: Sokolow M, McIlroy MB, eds. *Clinical Cardiology.* 5th ed. Norwalk, CT: Appleton & Lange.

16. Joshi N. The third heart sound. *South Med J.* 1999;92:756-761.

17. Dao Q, et al. Utility of B-type natriuretic peptide in the diagnoses of congestive heart failure in an urgent care setting. *J Am Coll Cardiol.* 2001;37(2):379-385.

18. Reddy PS. The third heart sound. *Int J Cardiol.* 1985;7(3):213-221.

19. Sloan A. Cardiac gallop rhythm. *Medicine (Baltimore).* 1958;37:197-215.

20. Evans W. The use of phonocardiography in clinical medicine. *Lancet.* 1951;1:1083-1085.

21. Abrams J. Current concepts of the genesis of heart sounds. II. Third and fourth sounds. *JAMA.* 1978;239(26):2790-2791.

22. Benchimol A, Desser KB. The fourth heart sound in patients without demonstrable heart disease. *Am Heart J.* 1977;93(3):298-301.

23. Erikssen J, Rasmussen K. Prevalence and significance of the fourth heart sound (S4) in presumably healthy middle-aged men, with particular relation to latent coronary heart disease. *Eur J Cardiol.* 1979;9(1):63-75.

24. Spodick DH, Quarry VM. Prevalence of the fourth heart sound by phonocardiography in the absence of cardiac disease. *Am Heart J.* 1974;87(1):11-14.

25. Jordan MD, Taylor CR, Nyhuis AW, et al. Audibility of the fourth heart sound. Relationship to presence of disease and examiner experience. *Arch Intern Med.* 1987;147(4):721-726.

26. Prakash R, Aytan N, Dhingra R, et al. Variability in the detection of a fourth heart sound—its clinical significance in elderly subjects. *Cardiology.* 1974;59(1):49-56.

27. Swistak M, Mushlin H, Spodick DH. Comparative prevalence of the fourth heart sound in hypertensive and matched normal persons. *Am J Cardiol.* 1974;33(5):614-616.

28. Aronow WS, Uyeyama RR, Cassidy J, et al. Resting and postexercise phonocardiogram and electrocardiogram in patients with angina pectoris and in normal subjects. *Circulation.* 1971;43(2):273-277.

29. Fonarow GC, et al. Risk stratification for in-hospital mortality in acutely decompensated heart failure: classification and regression tree analysis. *JAMA.* 2005;293(5):572-580.

30. Ruskin JA, Gurney JW, Thorsen MK, Goodman LR. Detection of pleural effusions on supine chest radiographs. *AJR.* 1987;148:681-683.

31. Çullu N, Kalemci S, Karakaş Ö, Eser İ, Yalçin F, Boyacı FN, Karakaş E. Efficacy of CT in diagnosis of transudates and exudates in patients with pleural effusion. *Diagn Interv Radiol.* 2014 Mar-Apr;20(2):116-120. doi: 10.5152/dir.2013.13066.

32. Stawicki SPA, Bahner DP. Evidence tables: inferior vena cava collapsibility index (IVC-CI). OPUS 12. *Scientist.* 2012;6(1):3-5.

33. ACEP Policy Statement on Emergency Ultrasound Guidelines. *Ann Emerg Med.* 2009;53:550-570.

34. Blehar DJ, Dickman E, Gaspari R. Identification of congestive heart failure via respiratory variation of inferior vena cava diameter. *Am J Emerg Med.* 2009;27:71-75.

35. Ziskin MC, Thickman DI, Goldenberg NJ, Lapayowker MS, Becker JM. The comet tail artifact. *J Ultrasound Med.* 1982;1(1):1-7.

36. Lichtenstein D, Mézière G, Biderman P, Gepner A, Barré O. The comet-tail artifact: an ultrasound sign of alveolar-interstitial syndrome. *Am J Respir Crit Care Med.* 1997;156(5):1640-1646.

37. Soldati G, Copetti R, Sher S. Sonographic interstitial syndrome: the sound of lung water. *J Ultrasound Med.* 2009 Feb;28(2):163-174.

38. Voroneanu L, Cusai C, Hogas S, et al. The relationship between chronic volume overload and elevated blood pressure in hemodialysis patients: use of bioimpedance provides a different perspective from echocardiography and biomarker methodologies. *Int Urol Nephrol.* 2010;42(3):789-797.

39. Kushner R, Schoeller D, Fjeld C, Danford L. Is the impedance index (ht2/R) significant in predicting total body water? *Am J Clin Nutr.* 1992;56(5):835-839.

40. Piccoli A. Whole body—single frequency bioimpedance. *Contrib Nephrol.* 2005;149:150-161.

41. Piccoli A, Nigrelli S, Caberlotto A, et al. Bivariate normal values of the bioelectrical impedance vector in adult and elderly populations. *Am J Clin Nutr.* 1995;61(2):269-270.

42. Piccoli A, Rossi B, Pillon L, et al. A new method for monitoring body fluid variation by bioimpedance analysis: the RXc graph. *Kidney Int.* 1994;46(2):534-539.

43. Panella C, Guglielmi FW, Mastronuzzi T, et al. Whole-body and segmental bioelectrical parameters in chronic liver disease: effect of gender and disease stages. *Hepatology.* 1995;21(2):352-358.

44. Paiva SI, Borges LR, Halpern-Silveira D, et al. Standardized phase angle from bioelectrical impedance analysis as prognostic factor for survival in patients with cancer. *Support Care Cancer.* 2010;19(2):187-192.

45. Parrinello G, Paterna S, Di Pasquale P, et al. The usefulness of bioelectrical impedance analysis in differentiating dyspnea due to decompensated heart failure. J Card Fail. 2008;14(8):676-686.

46. Valle R, Aspromonte N, Milani L, et al. Optimizing fluid management in patients with acute decompensated heart failure (ADHF): the emerging role of combined measurement of body hydration status and brain natriuretic peptide (BNP) levels. *Heart Fail Rev.* 2011;16(6):519-529.

20 BIOMARKERS IN HEART FAILURE

Sutton Fox, MPH
Cecilia Berardi, MD
Ha Mieu Ho, BS
Alan S. Maisel, MD

PATIENT CASE

A 35-year-old man arrives by ambulance to the emergency department (ED) with chief complaints of chest pain, shortness of breath, nausea, and dizziness. Physician interviews reveal no relevant risk factors for cardiovascular disease and no family history of cardiovascular events. Because his electrocardiogram (ECG) does not show any alterations, and the chest x-ray is normal, he is promptly discharged with possible diagnoses of influenza or stress. A few days later, he returns to the ED for severe chest pain accompanied again by shortness of breath and dizziness. Both ECG and chest x-ray do not show relevant alterations, so he is again discharged. Less than 30 hours later, he is found on his kitchen floor, unresponsive. First responders declare him dead at 3:30 that morning. The following day, his autopsy reveals the cause of death: aortic dissection.

Biomarkers have risen to popularity for their ability to promote timely diagnoses, reveal prognostic information, monitor disease progression, and predict therapeutic response. In the context of emergency medicine, biomarkers can serve as rule-in or rule-out diagnostic tools to supplement the emergency physician's knowledge and judgment. In the Patient Case above, laboratory tests may have served both secondary and tertiary prevention roles in the optimal course of treatment. In the context of the continuous management of a chronic disease, such as heart failure (HF), biomarkers can help evaluate whether therapies are effective, guide management, and predict adverse outcomes.[1,2]

DIFFERENTIAL DIAGNOSIS

In the ED, the most common and concerning symptoms are nontraumatic chest pain and shortness of breath, especially among older populations; they represent, respectively, 9% to 10% of ED complaints, followed by abdominal pain and general weakness. This equates to more than 1.5 million visits out of a total of more than 5.0 million visits a year in the United States alone, and this figure has steadily grown over the past decade. Often, patients experience concomitant chest pain and shortness of breath, but dizziness, nausea, and diaphoresis can commonly present as well.[1]

Cases with these symptoms share a wide variety of etiologies; the most concerning, ie, those that must be most promptly included or excluded, can either have cardiac or respiratory etiologies. Acute myocardial infarction (AMI), acute heart failure (AHF), aortic dissection, and pulmonary embolism (PE) are the most common

diagnoses, but pneumothorax, asthma, or a panic attack can present with these symptoms. For this reason, accurate and specific diagnostic techniques are crucial for timely treatment. The patient's history, clinical evaluation with an accurate physical examination, biomarkers, and some diagnostic tools—such as ECG, x-ray, and other imaging techniques—are fundamental in identifying the disease.[2] The efficacy depends on biomarker predictive accuracy; based on the etiology of biomarker release, the marker may have high sensitivity, specificity, positive predictive value, or negative predictive value (Figure 20-1).

Recent advances in biomarker detection have given the emergency medicine community cause to diagnose and treat persons with acute coronary syndrome (ACS) much more quickly, methodically, and quantitatively. The world of cardiac symptoms has become increasingly biochemical with the goal of improving diagnosis and prognosis, from the emergency setting to the chronic management of the patient.[2] In this chapter, we outline the most common uses of cardiac biomarkers in the clinical setting and alert the reader to recent advances, particularly with regards to prognosis.

There is a strong association between the type of damage or alteration that characterizes a pathological condition and the mechanism of biomarker release. In this review, we outline the utility of several biomarkers in relation to both their biochemistry and associated dynamics in pathophysiology and their practical utility in the clinical setting.

Several biomarkers, the most important of which are cardiac peptides, show vastly increased sensitivity and specificity over canonical ECG changes and chest x-ray techniques.[2-4] Hundreds of novel cardiac biomarkers, such as microRNAs (miRNAs), in conjunction with well-known biomarkers of more generalized necrosis, fibrosis, and systemic stress have also been proposed as biomarkers for both rule-in and rule-out for potential cardiac pathologies presenting with the traditional symptoms described above.

Essentially, a constellation of biomarkers must be considered in conjunction with the physician's best judgment to differentially diagnose the etiologic pathology of these symptoms, especially as new markers are discovered for specific cellular and biochemical processes.[2] Figure 20-2 shows just some of the signals that may or may not manifest clinically in cardiac pathophysiology. It behooves the physician to consider the multidimensionality of biomarker elevation; compartmentalization, pharmacological history, biochemistry, and metabolism of such markers all play a role when considering the clinical picture of the patient, particularly in differential diagnosis.

BIOMARKERS DESCRIBED: BRIEF BIOCHEMISTRY

To lend insight into the impetus behind the use of biomarkers in differential diagnosis of common cardiac diseases, we outline briefly some biochemical features of the most commonly used markers in clinical practice. Also we will mention some of the emerging biomarkers that are still under study but are promising as both diagnostic and emerging prognostic tools (Table 20-1).

Myoglobin

Myoglobin (Mb) is a carrier of oxygen, ubiquitously present in both cardiac and skeletal muscle types. It serves as a reserve of aerobic fuel when hemoglobin reserves deplete or when myocytes undergo necrotic damage. Because it infiltrates the bloodstream in both skeletal and cardiac muscle damage, its specificity is low in the clinical setting for acute cardiac distress. Normal levels rest between 0 and 85 ng/mL.[5]

Creatine Kinase-MB

Creatine kinase-MB (CK-MB) is a heterodimer in a family of molecules that catalyzes the phosphorylation of creatine, a ubiquitous byproduct of amino acid catabolism. It is highly linked to transmitochondrial energy pathways and serves as a key regulator of ATP inside the mitochondrial lumen and in the cytosol. The MB isoform is present in myocytes' cytosol, so it is strongly related to this type of cell damage. However, this marker has still proven less sensitive than other acute cardiac biomarkers. Normal levels rest between 5 and 25 IU/L, though it can also be reported as a ratio of isoforms. In this case, a 3% to 5% ratio of CK-MB to total CK blood content is typical in a healthy patient.[6]

	Disease	No Disease
Test (+)	a	b
Test (−)	c	d

1. Sensitivity $= \dfrac{a}{a+c}$

2. Specificity $= \dfrac{d}{b+d}$

3. Positive predictive value $= \dfrac{a}{a+b}$

4. Negative predictive value $= \dfrac{d}{b+d}$

FIGURE 20-1 The 4 main accuracy values associated with a quantitative biomarker. Sensitivity and specificity evaluate the probability of correct testing status given disease state, while predictive values assess the patient's likelihood of disease in the context of the associated positive or negative test result. While sensitivity and specificity are often the chief focus of biomarker evaluation and utility, positive—but mostly negative—predictive value presents a particular proclivity for clinical rule-out in the differential diagnosis, management, and prognosis of cardiac diseases.

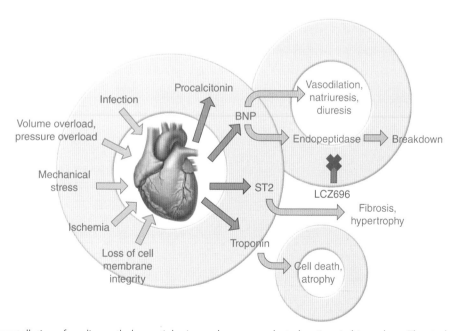

FIGURE 20-2 Clinical constellation of cardiac pathology etiologies and correspondent elevations in biomarkers. Elevated or suppressed biomarkers (*red*) must be clinically considered together with other disease inputs (*green*), and metabolic or pharmacologic clearance (*purple*) to arrive at an accurate clinical diagnosis, especially in the context of multiple comorbidities. Though certain markers will point positively to certain disease state etiologies (eg, procalcitonin and infection), negative predictive value should also be considered to rule out other etiologies, a valuable tool in the context of differential diagnosis.

Table 20-1 Summary Information for Biomarkers of Current and Future Utility in Differential Diagnosis of Common Cardiac Pathologies

Molecule	Characteristics	Normal Levels	Altered In
Myoglobin (Mb)	• Ubiquitously present in cardiac and skeletal muscle. • Released precociously into the bloodstream during muscular necrosis. • If rise is sustained for more than 24 h the cardiac ischemic event is likely still going on.	0-85 ng/mL	AMI Timeline of detectability after the ischemic event • Rise <2 h • Peak 8-12 h • Decrease within 24 h
Creatine kinase-MB (CK-MB)	• 2 genes, dimeric structure: multiple and ubiquitary distributed isoforms (MM1-3, MB1, MB2, BB). • MB isoform is present in myocytes' cytosol, so it is strongly related to these cells' damage.	5-25 IU/L 3%-5% (ratio CKMB/total CK)	AMI Timeline of detectability after the ischemic event • Rise 6-10 h • Peak 24 h • Decrease/normalization in 72 h
Lactate dehydrogenase (LDH)	• 5 types of isoenzymes: LDH-1 (HHHH) and LDH-2 (HHHM) are typically in myocytes. • Produced in response to increased metabolic stress in cardiomyocytes.	105-333 IU/L	AMI Timeline of detectability after the ischemic event • Rise between 8-12 h • Peak 28-48 h • Normalization in 10 d
Troponin I (TnI)	• Normally resides in the cytosol of cardiac myocytes.	99th percentile	AMI Timeline of detectability after the ischemic event • Rise 2-3 h • Peak 24 h • Normalization within 2 wk
High-sensitivity troponin I (hsTnI)	• High-sensitivity assays have increased ability to detect cardiac troponin isoforms even in healthy patient plasma. • Reduced specificity compared to less modern assays.	Assay dependent	As above
MicroRNA (miRNA/miR)	• Small transcripts of noncoding RNA. • Dynamically upregulated in cardiac distress as initial markers of cardiac hypertrophy. • Several subtypes are under study, including miR-1, -33, -21, -18b, -26a, -191, -197, -208b, and -233.	Under investigation	AMI and HF

(Continued)

Table 20-1 Summary Information for Biomarkers of Current and Future Utility in Differential Diagnosis of Common Cardiac Pathologies (Continued)

Molecule	Characteristics	Normal Levels	Altered In
Copeptin	• C-terminal part of pro-AVP and is released together with AVP during processing of the precursor peptide. • Secreted from the neurohypophysis upon hemodynamic or osmotic stimuli. • Appears to be superior to cortisol in determination of the stress level; cortisol is further downstream in the stress response, has a strong circadian rhythm, and is also challenging to measure as a free hormone.	Under investigation	AMI and HF
Soluble ST2 (sST2)	• Family of interleukin I (IL-1), binds to ligand IL-33. Another isoform, ST2L, is membrane-bound. • IL-33 exerts protective effects in myocardial cells when bound to ST2L. • sST2 competitively inhibits these effects when released in response to cardiac distress.	Under investigation	AMI and HF
Pro-N-terminus brain natriuretic peptide (NT-proBNP)	• Released in equimolar amounts to BNP, this is an inactive fragment of the lysis of pre-proBNP bended by neprolysin. • Synthesized and released when ventricular wall stress is increased.	<300 pg/mL	HF (see Figure 20-3)

Brain natriuretic peptide (BNP)	• Active part of the lysis of pre-proBNP.
	• Exerts hormonal effects on the heart and kidneys:
	  ◦ Decreases sympathetic tone;
	  ◦ Reduces afterload by inducing the secretion of sodium and water into the urine;
	  ◦ Inhibits RAAS mechanisms.
		<100 pg/mL	HF (see Figure 20-3)

D-dimer	• Thrombus degradation by-product: fibrin-derived homodimer. • Circulates in the blood in response to any thrombotic event. • Notably increased in major inflammatory events such as aortic dissection, though it is not specific to these conditions.	<500 ng/mL	PE and aortic dissection

Lactate Dehydrogenase

Lactate dehydrogenase (LDH) is produced in response to increased metabolic stress in cardiomyocytes. Anaerobic metabolism produces lactate in the cytosol of diseased cardiomyocytes, necessitating the production of increased LDH. The enzyme is released from the cytosol when cardiomyocytes undergo necrosis, particularly in AMI. Normal levels of LDH fall between 105 and 133 IU/L, though this can vary slightly and should always be adjusted relative to a cohort of healthy controls for individual assay kits.[7]

Troponin I and High-Sensitivity Troponin I

Troponin I (TnI) is 1 of the 3 troponin isoforms, and it inhibits the ATPase activity of myosin complexes. The peptide binds to actin in thin myofilaments to hold the troponin-tropomyosin complex in place. Primarily residing in the cytosol of cardiac myocytes, TnI comprises 1 of the most localized detectable known cardiac biomarkers, yielding high sensitivity and specificity. Because assays vary, typical TnI levels are determined based on individual assay comparison to a cohort of healthy control patients. A TnI reading above the 99th percentile in a control cohort of healthy patients indicates significant cardiac myocyte necrosis.

More sensitive assays have recently emerged to detect extremely low levels of circulating TnI even in healthy patients. In these so-called hsTnI assays, levels below 0.01 ng/mL are considered normal (a typical cutoff for normal TnI assays is 0.07 ng/mL).[8]

ST2

ST2 is a member of the family of interleukin 1, and its ligand is interleukin 33 (IL33). It has 2 isoforms: 1 soluble (sST2), detectable in serum; and 1 membrane-bound (ST2L). Both have different roles related to cardiac pathology. In the case of cardiac injury, ST2L binds IL33, and it exerts a preservative effect on heart function. In fact, IL33 has antihypertrophic and antifibrotic effects on myocardium, in part due to reduction in proapoptotic pathways. However, because IL33 also binds to sST2, when higher serum levels of sST2 are present, there is increased competition between the 2 ST2 isoforms; thus, the cardioprotective effect is decreased by increased sST2 plasma levels.[9]

Brain Natriuretic Peptide and N-Terminal Pro-Brain Natriuretic Peptide

The prohormone pre-proBNP is secreted from the myocardium, whereupon it is processed into the active hormone BNP-32 and the inactive amino-terminal fragment NT-proBNP-76. The active part of this lysis, BNP, exerts hormonal effects on the heart and kidneys, decreasing sympathetic tone, reducing afterload by inducing the secretion of sodium and water into the urine, and inhibiting RAAS mechanisms. It is released into the bloodstream in response to increased ventricular load, and is broken down into inactive fragments by the enzyme neprilysin. Normal levels in healthy patients vary, but cutoff schemes pivoting about 100 pg/mL are usually employed (see the upcoming section, Diagnosis: "Heart Failure").

Released in equimolar amounts to BNP, NT-proBNP is an inactive fragment byproduct of pre-proBNP lysis that is not broken down by neprilysin. Increased ventricular wall stress promotes the synthesis of BNP, releasing NT-proBNP into the bloodstream as a result. The sensitivity of this marker has been debated and is still under investigation with respect to diagnostic ability.[10]

D-Dimer

D-dimer is a thrombus degradation byproduct that circulates in the blood in response to thrombotic events such as emboli. It is notably increased in events such as aortic dissection, though it is not specific to these conditions; any thrombotic event will result in increased levels of this fibrin-derived homodimer, so it can be considered highly sensitive, but not specific. A normal D-dimer value is typically under 500 ng/dL in healthy populations.[11]

DIAGNOSES

HEART FAILURE

The insufficiency in the heart's ability to pump blood in response to the body's needs is a serious condition with high mortality, morbidity, and frequent visits to the ED and/or multiple rehospitalizations. This condition represents a major cause of hospitalization in people >65 years old, and the incidence of new cases has been predicted at >550,000 cases/year, adding to some 5.8 million prevalent cases in the United States alone.[1,12] HF usually has a typical presentation: dyspnea, low extremities edema, fatigue, orthopnea and paroxysmal nocturnal dyspnea or episodes of obstructive sleep apnea, and weight gain not related to diet. Detectable signs can be distinguished in these typical of left- or right-sided HF, but usually there is the copresence of both dysfunctions.[2-4,12] When one suspects HF, BNP and NT-proBNP levels are usually examined.

In the Breathing Not Properly trials, BNP levels were shown to vary in diagnostic power with age but not sex or race. Now a standard for cardiac health care, BNP and NT-proBNP tests bring both high sensitivity and negative predictive value to the differential diagnosis of HF in the acute setting.[13] One proposed scheme includes a stratification structure for likelihood of HF in the context of symptoms of acute cardiac decompensation. We particularly highlight the gray zone of 100 to 400 pg/mL (Figure 20-3). In the presence of chest pain or shortness of breath, we stress the importance of clinical judgment including patient history, risk factors, and physical examination in diagnosing HF when natriuretic peptides fall in this range.[14]

In contrast, the predictive accuracy of NT-proBNP has been shown to interact with age, likely due to naturally progressive decreases in left ventricular compliance and glomerular filtration rate (GFR). Figure 20-3 highlights the lower cutoff of 300 ng/mL for likelihood of HF diagnosis in the appropriate clinical presence. After age 50 years, the likelihood of HF increases with age at the rate of about 2 times the lower NT-proBNP cutoff per 25 years thereafter. NT-proBNP is not as widely utilized as BNP in the clinical setting, but studies continue to emerge with the promise of increasing its predictive power.

Particular attention has to be given to patients with elevated body mass index (BMI). In fact, an inverse relationship between BNP and NT-proBNP levels and BMI has been found. Obesity is a risk factor for systemic hypertension, hyperlipidemia, diabetes mellitus, and left ventricular hypertrophy. These conditions, in turn, are associated with an increased prevalence of chronic heart failure (CHF) and an increased mortality rate of about half of the patient population within 5 years of diagnosis. Obese patients can present with common symptoms and signs of HF, such as low extremities edema, dyspnea, and orthopnea; also, diagnostic tools such as chest x-rays and cardiac echocardiograms can be difficult to perform or to interpret due to body habitus.

Biomarkers can significantly aid in the management of HF patients in the emergency setting. As already mentioned, higher levels of natriuretic peptides in the bloodstream in patients with dyspnea are likely related to HF, but obese patients unfortunately could possibly not present with elevated natriuretic peptides. In 2004, Wang et al were the first to describe the inverse relationship between obesity and BNP levels and none of the subjects had HF. The mean plasma BNP levels were 21.4, 15.5, and 12.7 pg/mL in patients who were lean (BMI <25), overweight (BMI of 25-29.9), and obese (BMI ≥ 30), respectively. Subsequently, the Dallas Heart Study confirmed the report of Wang et al and demonstrated the inverse relationship among BMI, BNP, and NT-proBNP levels, both in stable and acute CHF patients.

According to these results, several studies had been completed in order to establish a punctual cutoff; lower thresholds were considered for diagnoses of the CHF patient population. In one study, based on the established clinical threshold of 100 pg/mL, BNP testing yielded false-negative results in 20% of obese HF patients, so, to rule out CHF, the cutoff point should be BNP ≤54 pg/mL in severely obese patients (BMI ≥35).[15]

It is also suggested that a higher BNP cutoff point of ≥170 pg/mL in lean patients increases specificity. In contrast to BNP cutoff points, relatively lower concentrations of NT-proBNP in overweight and obese patients with acute dyspnea retain their diagnostic and prognostic capacity. A cutoff point of 300 ng/L NT-proBNP had highly significant negative likelihood ratio of 0.02, 0.03, and 0.08 for BMI of <25.0, 25.0 to 29.9, and ≥30.0, respectively, ruling out acute HF. Also, a NT-proBNP cutoff point of >986 ng/L remained strongly prognostic across all 3 BMI groups.[16]

CARDIORENAL SYNDROME

Cardiorenal syndrome (CRS) describes any type of alteration in the heart and/or kidneys, as acute or chronic dysfunction in 1 organ may induce acute or chronic dysfunction of the other.[17] Ronco et al classified 5 types of CRS and their different pathophysiology in 2010. Type 1, or acute CRS, is linked to HF and is caused by an abrupt worsening of cardiac function leading to kidney injury and dysfunction (ie, acute cardiogenic shock or acute decompensated HF). Type 2, or chronic CRS, is characterized by chronic abnormalities in heart function leading to kidney injury or dysfunction (ie, CHF). Acute kidney injury (AKI) in patients with cardiac dysfunction has been recognized as an independent risk factor for morbidity and mortality and in fact impaired renal function has been found as an independent risk factor for 1-year mortality in patients with AHF. Also, approximately 25% of patients with CHF have renal dysfunction.[18]

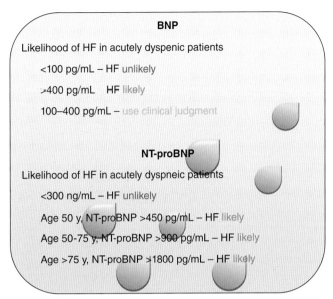

FIGURE 20-3 BNP and NT-proBNP stratification schemes in the context of heart failure differential diagnosis. While these figures are often used in conjunction with imaging data to diagnose heart failure, these ranges may change with age and weight, as discussed in the text. Despite the range of values, both BNP and NT-proBNP have high sensitivity and specificity for heart failure in the context of volume overload, and larger increases should correlate with likelihood of heart failure in the appropriate age ranges.

Early recognition of patients at risk of CRS allows a better assessment of the patients and their therapies. Thus, CRS has come to the forefront of biomarker research since its delineation within the past decade.[18] Though increases in the serum creatinine (sCr) renal marker are used to track kidney health during treatment of CRS2, sCr is a marker of tertiary utility; that is, by the time a creatinine increase is detected in the blood, kidney injury has most likely already occurred. As a consequence, other markers have been examined in concert with sCr to differentially diagnose cardiorenal comorbidity.

A hotly contested marker in the differential diagnosis of CRS, neutrophil gelatinase-associated lipocalin (NGAL) may or may not be diagnostically conclusive alone due to its low specificity; it is secreted by organs other than the kidney.[18] However, NGAL has been shown to have diagnostic use in combination with sCr, reinforcing that biomarkers must be considered within the context of the suspected organs at risk to diagnose complicated, potentially multisystemic pathologies involving HF.[19,20]

Another promising marker is cystatin C (CysC). This molecule is a functional marker of GFR, as opposed to NGAL, which is a structural marker of cell damage. CysC is freely filtered by the glomerulus and not secreted from the tubules, although it can be reabsorbed and catabolized.[20]

Unlike sCr, CysC is not influenced by gender, muscle mass, or race, so it is increasingly considered as a useful and trustable marker of glomerular function, especially in elderly, cachectic patients, or those with multiple comorbidities.[21] In a study conducted in 85 intensive care units (ICUs), both the analysis of baseline sCr and CysC were performed. CysC was able to detect AKI 1 to 2 days earlier than sCr with 82% of sensitivity and 95% of specificity, showing a good prognostic value.[19] In fact, in patients with HF, CysC >1.30 mg/L had been related to their highest adjusted hazards ratio of 3.2 (95% CI:2.0-5.3; P <0.0001) for all-cause mortality at 12 months. Combining tertiles of CysC with NT-proBNP, the prognostic value is even stronger.[22]

In the FINN-AKVA study group study of inpatients admitted for acute decompensated heart failure (ADHF), CysC was measured on admission and at 48 hours. When an increase >0.3 mg/L in CysC was present, a longer hospitalization was revealed, associated to an increased patient mortality and also recognized as an independent predictor of 90-day mortality.[23] In any case, as with NGAL, CysC has been shown to have some limitations. For example, CysC was not found to be a better estimator of GFR than sCr in a cohort of middle-aged patients from the general population, excluding coronary or kidney disease.[24] In conclusion, even though many potential biomarkers were pointed out as useful in detecting CRS and AKI, they all have weaknesses that make further analysis and studies necessary in order to find the best diagnostic tool for both these pathological conditions.

ACUTE MYOCARDIAL INFARCTION

Rapidly diagnosing or ruling out acute ischemic cardiac events pivots on several diagnostic decisions. In the example of our introductory Patient Case, a highly negatively predictive cardiac biomarker panel with TnI could have confirmed the negative ECG findings, while inflammatory biomarkers may have urged the physician to consider other pathologies. We emphasize that an ECG is absolutely necessary in the acute presentation described to assess ST elevation and other canonical changes while consulting blood biomarkers, pursuant to AHA guidelines.[2] Furthermore, the thorough physician utilizes both biomarkers of necrosis and biomarkers of inflammation to differentially diagnose time-sensitive cases of MI and ensure the smallest amount of time between pain onset and vascular treatment.[2]

TnI and hsTnI currently represent the gold standard for diagnosing AMI in several regards. Inexpensive and rapid, the assay is currently used as a standard of diagnostic decision for AMI across the globe. In practice, serial hsTnI—preferred over serial TnI—lab values predict AMI to high sensitivity if the marker value crosses above the 99th percentile of a control cohort of healthy patients. The initial rise occurs within 2 to 3 hours after onset of the ischemic event, peaks within 24 hours, then remains elevated for up to 2 weeks after the event has subsided. The corresponding absolute values for the 99th percentile in healthy controls, discussed previously, strictly depend on the assay used, though one can generally trust a negative result (<99th percentile) due to this molecule's high degree of compartmentalization in cardiomyocytes. TnI tests of increasing sensitivity continue to push the lower limit of detection, so this paradigm of relativity may change as typical values and ranges of absolute plasma levels are better characterized and assays become more uniform.

Markers of cytolysis still have prevalence in the differential diagnosis of AMI despite their low specificity. LDH and CK-MB laboratory tests are still carried out in concert with other traditional "cardiac enzyme" panels because of their low cost, availability, and efficacy within the context of other newer markers. Early seminal sources indicate that the ratio of 2 LDH isoforms, LDH-1 to LDH-2, is usually examined. A value exceeding 0.76 has been found to indicate inflammatory/necrotic pathology such as AMI, and a ratio exceeding unity is highly sensitive to a diagnosis of AMI. This increase in plasma levels occurs from 8 to 12 hours after the ischemic event, peaks at 28 to 48 hours, and usually normalizes by day 10.[25]

A somewhat historical cardiac enzyme, CK-MB has imprinted itself in the diagnostic realm as a classic, though nonspecific, marker for AMI. An increased ratio of CK-MB to total CK rests between 3% and 5%, as mentioned previously. In AMI, this kinase rises as a percentage between 6 and 10 hours after the initiation of the ischemic event, reaching its peak at 24 hours. The enzyme should decrease back to proportions of 3% to 5% 36 to 72 hours after the event terminates. It is well established that levels of CK-MB may also spike in cases of skeletal muscle degeneration, so this cytolysis marker should be used in conjunction with other markers to diagnose AMI.[26]

Myoglobin (Mb) too hearkens back to the early days of AMI biomarkers, and its clinical utility mirrors that of CK-MB in several ways. Particularly in suspected AMI, Mb is measured as a percentage with time in certain cases of acute dyspnea. Traditionally known as the fastest biomarker to respond to ischemic events, Mb can be detected in the plasma just 2 hours after ischemia onset, generally reaching a peak from 8 to 12 hours thereafter. Clinicians should suspect AMI when increases fall between (or above) 25% to 40% of the baseline value. Importantly, return to normal values should occur after the ischemic episode has subsided; that is, elongated periods (beyond 24 hours) of above-threshold Mb lab values strongly indicate that the ischemic episode has not terminated and should strongly encourage follow-up for prolonged ischemia. Like other mentioned markers of cytosolic release, Mb is released in pathologies other than AMI, so clinicians would also expect to see increased levels in pathologies of skeletal muscle and also nonischemic cardiac injury in addition to AMI.[27]

To summarize, these standard markers are of particular value during distinct periods of chest pain and clinical examination (Figure 20-4). While the aforementioned biomarkers constitute the vast majority of the physician's biochemical toolbox, several new

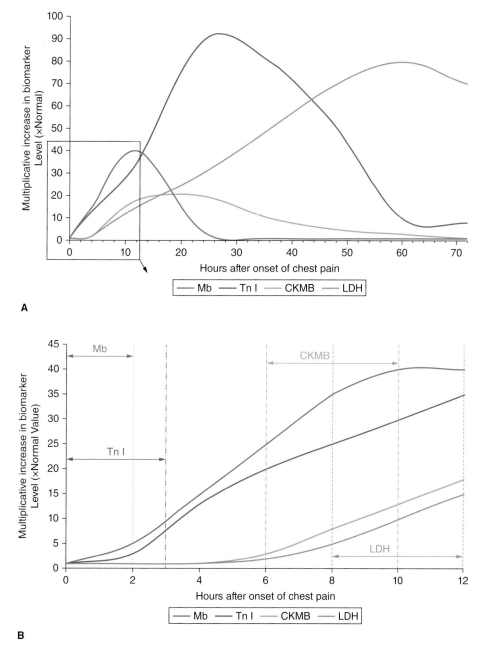

FIGURE 20-4 A. Timeline of biomarker increase and decrease over the course of typically presenting acute myocardial infarction, including presentation and recovery, and assuming survival over the shown time course. We draw the reader's attention particularly to the time scales on which changes are observed, as fold-changes in individual biomarkers may vary from what is shown. Note that several biomarker characteristics affect time of observed increase; nonspecific markers like Mb or LDH increase and decrease on drastically different time periods due to differential metabolism and clearance from serum. **B.** Common biomarker changes over acute phases succeeding chest pain in acute myocardial infarction. We highlight intervals over which biomarkers typically show elevation in the first hours of admission (*dotted lines*). Laboratory testing should optimally occur at baseline presentation and within the time intervals of maximum increase shown, post onset, according to available patient history.

molecules have come under scrutiny to detect MI faster and with more predictive power. We discuss these below.

Small transcripts of noncoding RNA, microRNAs (miRNAs) are propeptides that bind to complementary coding sections of other single-stranded RNA to block translation into several proteins implicated in cardiac hypertrophy. These molecules are on the order of 22 nucleotides long and are dynamically upregulated in cardiac distress as initial markers of cardiac hypertrophy, though the timeline of upregulation versus pathology currently presents an investigational opportunity in the face of modern epigenomic characterization methods and bioinformatics. Several subtypes are under study, including miRNA-1, -33, -21, -18b, -26a, -191, -197, -208b, and -233. For example, some studies revealed that miRNA-26a and -191 are significantly increased in early stages of AMI, whereas miRNA-208b levels increase in those patients with STEMI.[28] These studies are in their infancy, and further defining which and when miRNAs rule in or rule out AMI on rapid time scales could potentially improve both sensitivity in the face of traditional indicators of STEMI and specificity in cases like our introductory Patient Case, where ECG and chest x-ray changes are not apparent.

We mention copeptin as a final novel marker of potential diagnostic value for AMI. Produced as a cotranscript byproduct with arginine vasopressin, or antidiuretic hormone (ADH), this 39-amino acid peptide is an indicator of increased endocrine activity, secreted in excess by the anterior pituitary in times of cardiac distress.[29] One multicenter study of 1386 patients with suspected ACS revealed that, when combined with troponin T (TnT, another troponin isoform generally associated with cardiac necrosis when detected in the plasma), copeptin had a negative predictive value of 92.4% with respect to AMI, a significant improvement over traditional, nonsensitive troponin assays.[30] A potentially multifaceted marker for both acute and chronic use in both AMI and HF, this novel marker has great potential for prognosis as well, and we detail additional studies in that section.

One can easily comprehend the seriousness of rapid and accurate diagnosis of AMI, and, while biomarkers old and new aid in making this determination in ED presentations of acute dyspnea and/or chest pain, several other clinical judgments must be made to arrive at the correct diagnosis. To illustrate this, we elaborate on the introductory Patient Case with an example flowchart (Figure 20-5). As faster, more sensitive, and more specific biomarkers emerge, this workflow will no doubt become obsolete in the management of ACS, replaced by more complete biochemical pictures of AMI; thus, we encourage healthcare professionals to stay in touch with the most current research in the biomarkers described here.

PULMONARY EMBOLISM

Pulmonary embolism (PE) can have a wide variety of causes. In fact, the occlusion of pulmonary arteries can be related to genetic or acquired coagulation disorders that can increase the risk of formation of clots, prolonged immobility due to surgical interventions (especially orthopedic), recent traumas or compromised health conditions that force the patient in the lying-flat position, estrogenic therapies or pregnancy—common in young women, obesity, smoking, and cancer. Usual presentation of a patient with PE consists of shortness of breath, SpO$_2$ <95%, tachycardia, unilateral leg swelling, and deep venous thrombosis (DVT), when this condition is the thromboembolic source. Also, patients could complain of atypical chest pain characterized by sudden onset and increase of intensity during deep breathing (pleuritic chest pain). In any case, sometimes the only symptom of presentation can be the shortness of breath with no other significant signs suggestive of this clinical entity. Misunderstanding the correct diagnostic orientation can lead to a delayed identification of the PE, and this can be lethal—not casually, it is also known as the silent killer. For this reason, it is very important to collect the patient's past medical history and identify the risk factors mentioned above.

The so-called Wells score can be used to predict the likelihood of PE based on clinical criteria. Chest x-rays are not sensitive for differential diagnosis of PE, but these are usually performed as first-step imaging exams to rule out other causes of shortness of breath (eg, acute pulmonary edema in HF, rib fractures). In normal cases, chest x-rays are not diriment for PE diagnosis.

D-dimer is a biomarker that is highly sensitive in the exclusion of PE if its levels are within the normal range (<500 μg/L). An elevation of D-dimer levels over 500 μg/L is not specific for PE (present also in other conditions such as aortic dissection) but it rules in those patients who need further investigation to diagnose PE. It is also very important to consider that the baseline values of D-dimer increase with age after the age of 50 years; the cutoff value should be adjusted to the person's age multiplied by 10 μg/L. This adjustment increases specificity without modifying sensitivity, thereby improving the clinical utility of D-dimer testing in patients aged 50 years or more with a seemingly low clinical probability.[31] Upon identifying the patients at highest risk for PE according to the D-dimer testing, the gold standard for the evaluation is computed tomography pulmonary angiography (CTPA). An alternative for patients who have a contraindication to CTPA (or if CTPA is not available) are ventilation-perfusion scans.

AORTIC DISSECTION

This condition might not be identified until sudden, sharp stabbing or tearing onset of chest or abdominal migrant pain, usually accompanied by dizziness and nausea. In aortic dissection, the detachment of the aortic tunica allows the progressive flow of blood to tear the layers apart. Usually the characteristics of the pain and the absence of coronary artery disease (CAD) risk factors can hint toward this emergency condition. In fact, according to the position of the involved tract, different organs may be involved and lead to insufficiencies. For example, when the aortic root is engaged, the dissection can spread forward in the direction of flow and tear the coronary arteries. In this case, the resulting chest pain would have both characteristics of AMI and dissection, and cardiac biomarkers such as TnI/hsTnI would rise due to the cardiac ischemia.

Because of aortic dissection's lethality, a quick diagnosis is necessary. Usually an ECG will not show any significant changes, if coronary arteries are not involved. A chest x-ray may show some alterations, such as widening of the mediastinum or other alteration of the aortic knob's normal shape; this is more likely in DeBakey types I and II (Stanford type A). In any case, chest x-ray analysis has low specificity, considering that about 12% to 20% of individuals presenting with an aortic dissection could have a normal imaging.[32]

To rule out aortic dissection, D-dimer levels are the most important tool. In fact, patients with levels <500 ng/mL are less likely to

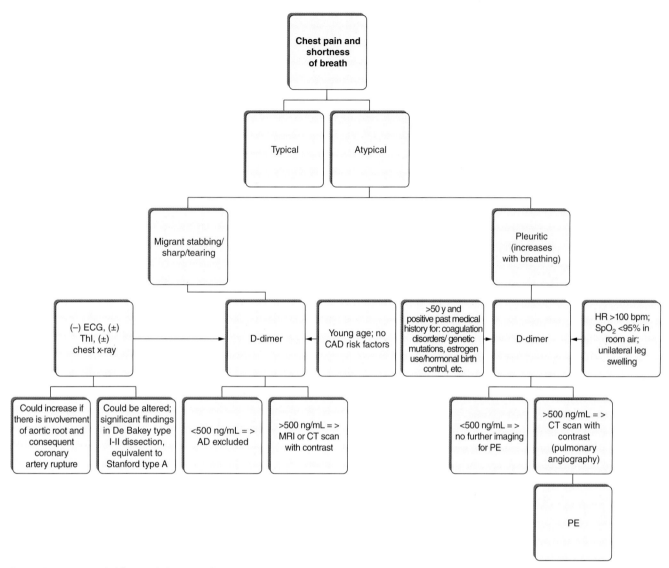

FIGURE 20-5 Potential differential diagnosis flowchart that a physician may have alternatively applied to the Patient Case at the beginning of the chapter. Note the supplemental role of biomarkers at key clinical presentations and findings in concordance with each marker's predictive value for necrotic, inflammatory, or thrombotic damage, and observe how results are used to indicate further imaging and/or alternative physiological biomarker testing.

have an aortic dissection, especially if the patients are classified at low risk and if the test is performed within 24 hours from the onset of the pain.[33,34] Conversely, D-dimer levels >500 ng/mL should guide physicians' decisions to pursue the gold standard (imaging) for aortic dissection diagnosis. MRI is the gold standard for detection and assessment (with a sensitivity and specificity of 98%), but the performance is highly time consuming and often not suitable for an emergency setting as a result. For this reason, a very valid alternative is the CT scan with iodate contrast, which has both sensitivity and specificity from 96% to 100%.

MANAGEMENT

HEART FAILURE

Several options are available to the physician in the management of HF, and biomarker-guided therapy has been rigorously shown to improve prognosis. The bread and butter of HF treatment is medication; administration of diuretics, beta blockers, vasodilators (nitrates), antiarrhythmics, angiotensin receptor blockers (ARBs), aldosterone inhibitors, and calcium channel blockers has been extensively described and tested for treating patients with HF, of varied etiological pathways, especially in the context of volume overload and ventricular wall stress. Essentially, natriuretic peptide levels should decrease over the course of successful treatment, and much evidence has warranted increased frequency of biomarker—and in particular, natriuretic peptide—monitoring to guide intensity of treatment.

As mentioned previously, the physician should be aware that changes in BNP level appear to vary less in elderly and obese individuals. In 2013, Januzzi and Troughton argued, based on evidence gathered from the TIME-CHF trial, that though BNP-guided therapy was particularly robust in younger patients, there were significant benefits to modeling treatment based on natriuretic peptides across both severity of disease and age. The authors cite the significance level of a successful treatment relative to a given previous measurement rests at 40% for BNP and 25% for NT-proBNP. Changes such as these should guide dose titration for the drug classes mentioned above. Diuretics in particular reduce ventricular stress and remodeling and have been shown to lead to better prognoses.[35]

However, caveats exist, especially with regard to kidney function in the administration of diuretics. Along with the natriuretic peptides, sCr should be monitored regularly to determine presence of AKI, and increases in this biomarker often point the physician toward a reduction in diuretic administration, all other factors equal. Because sCr often only increases after postdiuretic kidney injury has occurred, there is much room in the field of clinical research to discover a more prompt biomarker of kidney function in the management of HF.[19] The optimal increase for a novel biomarker with respect to kidney injury is illustrated in Figure 20-6.

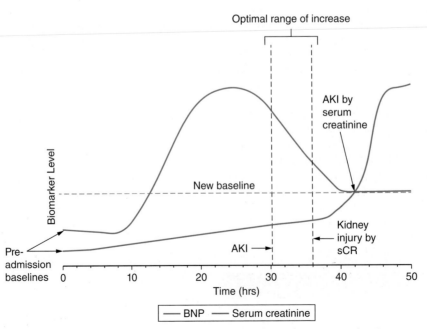

FIGURE 20-6 Model for a novel biomarker of renal function indication along the cardiorenal axis. Currently, sCr is a post hoc marker of acute kidney injury and increases only after renal damage; optimally, a new biomarker would predict kidney injury as it occurs (*AKI*) rather than after (*AKI by serum creatinine*). This would more precisely guide management and may improve prognosis in patients with heart failure.

PROGNOSIS

A fascinating cross between the worlds of biochemistry, medicine, and epidemiology, the use of biomarkers as predictors of health outcomes rather than determinants of differential diagnosis has revealed a paradigm shift for research in recent years. Here, we again examine the most prevalent cardiac pathologies—HF and AMI—with respect to recent studies, delineating the predictive values of known and recently discovered and/or re-adapted biomarkers with respect to clinical outcomes on chronic time periods, generally defined here as 30 days postdischarge.

HEART FAILURE: BNP, ST2, AND sCR

We first examine current studies aimed at using BNP as a predictor for adverse HF events beyond diagnosis and admission. The Rapid Emergency Department (RED) prospective cohort, conducted at the Sant'Andrea Hospital in Rome from 2006-2007, examined the BNP levels of 180 patients presenting with ADHF at 30, 90, and 180 days postdischarge.[36] All patients were over 70 years of age, and exclusion criteria included patients with ACS, diagnosis of AMI, obesity defined by BMI greater than 30 kg/m^2, renal failure necessitating dialysis, and noncardiac-related dyspnea. Postdischarge, patients' BNP levels were measured, and they were simultaneously examined for any adverse events related to their cardiac diagnosis including dyspnea, respiratory rate above 30 breaths/minute, oxygen saturation below 90%, appreciated rales on exam, or lower extremity edema.

The investigators used a BNP cutoff point of 400 pg/mL to evaluate predictive metrics and investigated optimal predictive relative BNP increase (Δ%BNP). Ultimately, a significant predictive value (P <0.05) for adverse events with cutoffs of 400 pg/mL and 4% BNP increases was noted (1) at 30 days postdischarge, and (2) between 30 and 90 days postdischarge. At 30 days, receiving characteristic (ROC) area-under-the-curve (AUC) values were 0.842 and 0.851 for the absolute and relative cutoffs, respectively, while sensitivities were 83% and 78%, and specificities came in at 69% and 82%.[36] Thus, early serial BNP values taken in elderly ADHF patients at 30 days, and levels above 400 pg/mL or 4Δ%BNP might serve as a reasonably sensitive prognosticative alert for rehospitalization, exacerbation, or death in time spans of approximately half a year. As a result, treatment plans for CHF might be better tailored according to prognostic BNP profiles given sufficient attention and measurement on time scales shortly following discharge.

A study from the Multinational Observational Cohort on Acute heart failure (MOCA) examined the added clinical prognostic value of the plasma interleukin sST2 in determining outcomes at 30 days and 1 year in patients hospitalized for ADHF.[37] A retrospective cohort study, this investigation examined sST2 levels in 576 patients whose data were obtained from 12 centers across the globe (Austria, Czech Republic, Finland, France, Italy, Japan, Netherlands, Spain, Switzerland, Tunisia, and the United States; n unknown for patients in which sST2 was collected). The investigators devised a multivariate "clinical" regression model for predicting likelihood of mortality at 30 days and 1 year, which included

adjustments for age, gender, both systolic and diastolic blood pressure, heart rate, renal function estimated by the MDRD equation (<60 mL/min/1.73 m^2), sodium level, hemoglobin level, and place of data collection. Clinical mortality was modeled first with these variables alone and subsequently with the biomarker of interest added. In a similar fashion, both models were also run according to a risk stratification scheme, where low-, medium-, and high-risk were defined disparately for 30-day mortality and 1-year mortality. They found that positive sST2 levels, defined as >35 ng/mL, had significantly better prognostic ability than the clinical model alone in both 30-day (ΔAUC = 0.05, P = 0.03) and 1-year mortality (ΔAUC = 0.04, P = 0.02), and had a reclassification index of 25.5% (P <0.001) at 30 days and 10.2% (P <0.001) at 1 year. Furthermore, combining C-reactive protein (CRP) and ST2 in the model together resulted in a risk reclassification of 30.8% at 30 days and 20.3% at 1 year (both P <0.001) compared to the clinical model alone. sST2, as a marker of remodeling in HF, certainly shows promise as a potential prognostic biomarker on longitudinal time scales, especially when used in conjunction with relatively nonspecific markers of inflammation such as CRP.[37]

In another analysis of patients who participated in the STRATIFY study, sST2 predicted adverse events at 30 days in patients presenting to 3 ED centers with probable acute heart failure syndromes (AHFS) as judged by an expert panel of cardiologists. However, this only occurred in unadjusted models, which did not take into account inpatient medications. Clearly, more data on specific HF events with similar covariate adjustments and at more granular time points are needed to reconcile the results between this study and the MOCA subanalysis mentioned previously.[38]

Estimates of cardiorenal function based on creatinine levels have also been shown to predict worse outcomes in patients with ADHF and congestion. One recent review highlights the sensitive interaction between the preservation of renal function; typically, one attempts to estimate clearance from the kidney via a calculated estimated glomerular filtration rate (eGFR), using tested equations such as the Cockcroft-Gault model or the MDRD equation. Several extensive studies have shown an eGFR cutoff of 60 mL/min/1.73 m^2 to be prognostic as it relates to multiple cardiorenally derived pathologies, including albuminuria and anemia.

Both the MDRD and Cockcroft-Gault models rely on measurements of sCr; thus, one could argue that this basic laboratory measurement is the key factor in monitoring renal function during the course of HF and thus prognosis, even in complex interactions with commonly administered pharmaceuticals. For example, it has been shown that the loop diuretic furosemide is consistently associated with dose-responsive mortality and renal dysfunction hazard ratios greater than 1.5 over 5 years, especially at doses over 120 mg/day during hospitalization. On the other hand, angiotensin converting enzyme (ACE) inhibitors and ARBs were shown to be preservative of renal function at up to a 30% increase in sCr levels from baseline during the first 2 months of drug administration.[39]

Several studies have correlated worsening renal function (WRF) with adverse outcomes. In one study, a daily measured sCr in 599 patients showed that WRF, defined as an increase greater than or equal to 0.3 mg/dL in sCr at admission, demonstrated higher mortality or readmission for acute HF at 1 year, but, interestingly, only in the presence of congestion.[40] A large meta-analysis of 39,372 HF patients showed sCr to be the fourth most significant predictor of mortality at a median follow-up of 2.5 years, behind age, lower ejection fraction, and New York Heart Association HF class (rate ratio: 1.039, 95% CI: [1.035, 1.042]). Authors consistently cite the added prognostic value of elevated, frequently measured sCr and derived eGFR values with respect to treatment and management of HF.[41]

ACUTE MYOCARDIAL INFARCTION: hsTnI, sST2, AND COPEPTIN

Most modern clinical diagnostic techniques surrounding AMI focus on differential diagnosis, as hinted previously. However, significant current research has examined traditional biomarkers of cellular necrosis in a new light, ie, predicting adverse outcomes on chronic timelines. Results are fascinating and merit further investigation, especially with respect to traditional markers of acute necrosis such as TnI in the context of high-sensitivity testing.

Added prognostic value of hsTnI versus traditional TnI assays appears to have an impact up to 4 years postdischarge. A study was conducted in Deutsches Herzzentrum from 2005 to 2006 involving 1578 patients who presented with symptomatic CAD and underwent revascularization (including percutaneous coronary intervention or aortocoronary bypass surgery). Enrollees did not have detectable TnI in a traditional assay, and the investigators found that, in the 103 patients who were followed for 4 years postprocedure, a cutoff value of preoperative hsTnI equal to 0.016 μg/L resulted in an AUC of 0.742 (P <0.001) for all-cause mortality at 4 years. A dose-response trend in observed hsTnI increases was also significant. Other variables such as age, smoking, left ventricular ejection fraction, diabetic status, and HF class were taken into account in this model. Though these patients were not diagnosed with AMI according to traditional assay TnI cutoffs, this study clearly shows that detecting low values of circulating troponin may predict mortality on time scales of years, even after controlling for standard clinical predictors of cardiovascular death in the face of myocytic ischemia. Additional studies should focus on the variation of this marker with postdischarge lifestyle modification and/or treatment upon rehospitalization to guide therapy and assess the use of the hsTnI assay as a long-term health indicator.[42]

Some concerns that have arisen with respect to prognosis post-AMI are whether the cutoff for diagnosing AMI in high-sensitivity assays reduces specificity, forces excess AMI intervention, and results in a higher rate of recurrent AMI. A study conducted at the Royal Infirmary, Edinburgh, United Kingdom, examined the outcome implications of a diagnostic hsTnI cutoff of 0.05 μg/L for AMI, stratifying risk between 0.012 μg/L and this value.[43] At a median of 446 days postdischarge, an adjusted odds ratio of 2.5 (95% CI: 1.5-4.3) delineated a greater chance of death or recurrent myocardial infarction at 1 year in those patients with hsTnI values between 0.012 and 0.049 μg/L. Similar risk was observed for values above 0.05 μg/L, and, in fact, negative predictive value improved by 3% (94%-97%) when the cutoff was lowered to 0.012 μg/L (though this was accompanied by a concomitant decrease in positive predictive value).[43] Lowering the cutoff of certain hsTnI assays beyond the current diagnostic guidelines at requisite assay precision levels may have value in predicting the course of future acute ischemic events, and individual assays should be investigated for prognostic value post-AMI.

We have previously discussed the role of sST2 in the diagnosis of acute HF. However, this novel biomarker role has also been analyzed in ACS patients. A substudy of the MERLIN-TIMI 36 trial clearly demonstrated how patients with higher serum levels of sST2 at ED presentation are strongly susceptible to adverse outcomes at 30 days and at 1 year. In this particular study, at 30 days, patients with sST2 >35 μg/L had a higher risk of cardiovascular disease (CVD)/HF, including significant relationships individually with CVD, HF, sudden cardiac death, and all-cause death. These relationships remained significant at 1 year.[44] This study, in conjunction with those discussed previously, shows that biomarkers of cardiac necrosis and subsequent remodeling not only have value in acute clinical decision-making alone but also that, taken together and at different clinical thresholds, these markers signal long-term cardiac response to such acute events. In particular, studies of new hsTnI assays and markers of cardiac remodeling in the context of prognosis should be viewed less as reassessments of their current diagnostic utility and more as extensions of and transitions in the heart's response to traumatic pathological conditions.

We have previously discussed copeptin as a novel biomarker of diagnosis in HF, but it too has come under scrutiny as a predictor of mortality, usually in concert with TnI or hsTnI to boost the negative predictive value in a prognostic setting. Here, we briefly mention a study conducted in 2700 patients undergoing catheterization due to ischemic AMI or stable angina pectoris: copeptin alone predicted mortality, rehospitalization secondary to cardiovascular events, and stroke at 3 months postdischarge (AUC = 0.703) using a cutoff of 21.6 pmol/L; this value in fact exceeded that of TnI (P <0.0001) and also better reclassified patients into risk categories on this time scale, presenting significant value as a marker of prognosis, even when considered separately from TnI.[45] The role of copeptin not solely as a tandem biomarker to troponins and natriuretic peptides should continue to present a hot-button topic in both diagnosis and prognosis.

miRNAs: AT THE FRONTIER OF PROGNOSIS

A review was recently published on works investigating highly ribonuclease-resistant miRNAs with respect to both diagnosis and prognosis of cardiac diseases.[46] The variety of these molecules clearly presents a new universe of epigenetic biomarker monitoring for cardiac processes. Having been proven to correlate with cardiac health in the context of both solidarity and in conjunction with previously mentioned markers of prognosis, it is clear that there is still much to learn about both the clinical utility and the biochemical origin of release in these short nucleotide sequences; their demonstrated stability under physiological conditions certainly makes miRNAs attractive in the view of long-term outcomes on time scales of pathologically induced genetic regulation. Surely, as assay technology becomes more and more sensitive and specific to small circulating epigenetic silencers, so will clinical utility and marketability for these new assays increase in the setting of both rapid testing in acute conditions and follow-up testing for prognostic monitoring.

FOLLOW-UP

HEART FAILURE

We have discussed at length the role of natriuretic peptides in the prognosis of HF. It has been recognized by several sources that in the follow-up period shortly following discharge, providers should remain in contact with patients via in-home and clinic visits, telemonitoring, and/or telephone communication to titrate fluid-altering medications. To this end, resources recommend frequent measurements of natriuretic peptides and renal markers such as sCr to assess treatment efficacy and prognosis, particularly in the short term. Increases in either of these sets of markers beyond normal limits (see "Prognosis") should warrant a change in the course of management according to the needs of the patient, including adjustment of diuretics, antihypertensive medications, and electrolyte-sparing medications. While these measures are recommended on a general scale, there is a call for the standardization of the use of biomarkers in the follow-up of HF.[47]

One novel technology that may spur this standardization is the home-use BNP finger-stick. In the HABIT trial, a double-blinded prospective clinical trial, it was shown that 163 patients trained in the use of a novel BNP sandwich immunoassay device underwent a median of 65 days of follow-up, with clinic visits at 30 and 60 days postconsent. Forty patients had adverse events, revealing a hazard ratio per unit increase in $\ln(\text{BNP})$ of 1.8 (95% CI: [1.4, 2.4]) and a hazard ratio of 3.6 (95% CI: [1.8-7.2]) on days of weight gain. Thus, daily home measurement of natriuretic peptides may present a novel opportunity for high-frequency, highly predictive follow-up for HF patients.[48]

ACUTE MYOCARDIAL INFARCTION

The 2013 AHA Guidelines for the Management of ST-elevation myocardial infarction mention that, following treatment of AMI, basic proatherosclerotic and prothrombotic markers should be measured during subsequent clinic visits, especially low-density lipoproteins (LDL). Statin therapy is recommended even in patients with <70 mg/dL LDL cholesterol; thus, close monitoring is crucial to maintaining healthy lipid balance and reducing the advancement of atherosclerosis. In addition, high triglyceride measurements (>150 mg/dL) and detection of low high-density lipoprotein (HDL) cholesterol (<40 mg/dL in men and 50 mg/dL in women) have been cited as recommended follow-up measures, especially in patients with metabolic dysregulation such as metabolic syndrome.[49,50]

PATIENT EDUCATION

For now, biomarkers chiefly prove the most useful in clinical decision-making. Patients should be counseled on known risk factors for cardiovascular disease such as smoking, diet, physical activity, and sedentary lifestyle. However, physicians should keep a close

eye on the horizon for novel patient-initiated biomarker testing. As discussed in the follow-up of HF, home measurement of natriuretic peptides may soon come onto the scene as a patient-utilizable tool of prognosis for cardiac health.[48]

PROVIDER RESOURCES

AHA/ACC Guidelines: http://circ.ahajournals.org/content/130/25/e344.full.pdf

European Society of Cardiology: https://www.escardio.org

REFERENCES

1. Pines JM, Mullins PM, Cooper JK, Feng LB, Roth KE. National trends in emergency department use, care patterns, and quality of care of older adults in the United States. *J Am Geriatr Soc.* 2013;61(1):12-17.

2. Mann DL, Zipes DP, Libby P, Bonow RO, Braunwald E. *Braunwald's Heart Disease: A Textbook of Cardiovascular Medicine.* Philadelphia, PA: Elsevier/Saunders; 2015.

3. Amsterdam EA, Wenger NK, Brindis RG, et al. 2014 AHA/ACC guideline for the management of patients with non-ST-elevation acute coronary syndromes: a report of the American College of Cardiology/American Heart Association Task Force on practice guidelines. *J Am Coll Cardiol.* 2014;64(24):e139-e228.

4. McMurray JJV, Adamopoulos S, et al. ESC guidelines for the diagnosis and treatment of acute and chronic heart failure 2012. *Eur J Heart Fail.* 2012;14(8):803-869.

5. Winter RJ de, Koster RW, Sturk A, Sanders GT. Value of myoglobin, troponin T, and CK-MB mass in ruling out an acute myocardial infarction in the emergency room. *Circulation.* 1995;92(12):3401-3407.

6. Wallimann T, Tokarska-Schlattner M, Schlattner U. The creatine kinase system and pleiotropic effects of creatine. *Amino Acids.* 2011;40(5):1271-1296.

7. Armstrong AJ, George DJ, Halabi S. Serum lactate dehydrogenase predicts for overall survival benefit in patients with metastatic renal cell carcinoma treated with inhibition of mammalian target of rapamycin. *J Clin Oncol.* 2012;30(27):3402-3407.

8. Patil H, Vaidya O, Bogart D. A review of causes and systemic approach to cardiac troponin elevation. *Clin Cardiol.* 2011;34(12):723-728.

9. Friões F, Lourenço P, Laszczynska O, et al. Prognostic value of sST2 added to BNP in acute heart failure with preserved or reduced ejection fraction. *Clin Res Cardiol.* 2015;104(6):491-499.

10. Nishikimi T, Kuwahara K, Nakao K. Current biochemistry, molecular biology, and clinical relevance of natriuretic peptides. *J Cardiol.* 2011;57(2):131-140.

11. Perrier A, Bounameaux H, Morabia A, et al. Diagnosis of pulmonary embolism by a decision analysis-based strategy including clinical probability, d-dimer levels, and ultrasonography: a management study. *Arch Intern Med.* 1996;156(5):531-536.

12. Roger VL. Epidemiology of heart failure. *Circ Res.* 2013;113(6):646-659.

13. Maisel AS, Daniels LB. Breathing not properly 10 years later: what we have learned and what we still need to learn. *J Am Coll Cardiol.* 2012;60(4):277-282.

14. Maisel A, Mueller C, Adams K Jr, et al. State of the art: using natriuretic peptide levels in clinical practice. *Eur J Heart Fail.* 2008;10(9):824-839.

15. Wang TJ, Larson MG, Levy D, et al. Impact of obesity on plasma natriuretic peptide levels. *Circulation.* 2004;109(5):594-600.

16. Madamanchi C, Alhosaini H, Sumida A, Runge MS. Obesity and natriuretic peptides, BNP and NT-proBNP: mechanisms and diagnostic implications for heart failure. *Int J Cardiol.* 2014;176(3):611-617.

17. Ronco C, McCullough P, Anker SD, et al. Cardio-renal syndromes: report from the consensus conference of the Acute Dialysis Quality Initiative. *Eur Heart J.* 2010;31(6):703-711.

18. Ronco C, Haapio M, House AA, Anavekar N, Bellomo R. Cardiorenal syndrome. *J Am Coll Cardiol.* 2008;52(19):1527-1539.

19. Taub PR, Borden KC, Fard A, Maisel A. Role of biomarkers in the diagnosis and prognosis of acute kidney injury in patients with cardiorenal syndrome. *Expert Rev Cardiovasc Ther.* 2012;10(5):657-667.

20. Haase M, Devarajan P, Haase-Fielitz A, et al. The outcome of neutrophil gelatinase-associated lipocalin-positive subclinical acute kidney injury: a multicenter pooled analysis of prospective studies. *J Am Coll Cardiol.* 2011;57(17):1752-1761.

21. Lassus J, Harjola V-P. Cystatin C: a step forward in assessing kidney function and cardiovascular risk. *Heart Fail Rev.* 2011;17(2):251-61.

22. Lassus J, Harjola VP, Sund R, et al. Prognostic value of cystatin C in acute heart failure in relation to other markers of renal function and NT-proBNP. *Eur Heart J.* 2007;28(15):1841-1847.

23. Lassus JPE, Nieminen MS, Peuhkurinen K, et al. Markers of renal function and acute kidney injury in acute heart failure: definitions and impact on outcomes of the cardiorenal syndrome. *Eur Heart J.* 2010;31(22):2791-2798.

24. Eriksen BO, Mathisen UD, Melsom T, et al. Cystatin C is not a better estimator of GFR than plasma creatinine in the general population. *Kidney Int.* 2010;78(12):1305-1311.

25. Marshall T, Williams J, Williams KM. Electrophoresis of serum isoenzymes and proteins following acute myocardial infarction. *J Chromatogr.* 1991;569(1):323-345.

26. Sobel BE, Shell WE. Serum enzyme determinations in the diagnosis and assessment of myocardial infarction. *Circulation.* 1972;45(2):471-482.

27. Stone MJ, Willerson JT, Gomez-Sanchez CE, Waterman MR. Radioimmunoassay of myoglobin in human serum. Results in patients with acute myocardial infarction. *J Clin Invest.* 1975;56(5):1334-1339.

28. Li C, Chen X, Huang J, Sun Q, Wang L. Clinical impact of circulating miR-26a, miR-191, and miR-208b in plasma of patients with acute myocardial infarction. *Eur J Med Res.* 2015;20(1)58.

29. Nickel CH, Bingisser R, Morgenthaler NG. The role of copeptin as a diagnostic and prognostic biomarker for risk stratification in the emergency department. *BMC Medicine.* 2012;10:7.

30. Keller T, Tzikas S, Zeller T, et al. Copeptin improves early diagnosis of acute myocardial infarction. *J Am Coll Cardiol.* 2010;55(19):2096-2106.

31. Schouten HJ, Geersing GJ, Koek HL, et al. Diagnostic accuracy of conventional or age adjusted D-dimer cut-off values in older patients with suspected venous thromboembolism: systematic review and meta-analysis. *BMJ.* 2013;346:f2492.

32. Strayer RJ, Shearer PL, Hermann LK. Screening, evaluation, and early management of acute aortic dissection in the ED. *Curr Cardiol Rev.* 2012;8(2):152-157.

33. Asha SE, Miers JW. A systematic review and meta-analysis of D-dimer as a rule-out test for suspected acute aortic dissection. *Ann Emerg Med.* 2015;66(4):368-378.

34. Bossone E, Suzuki T, Eagle KA, Weinsaft JW. Diagnosis of acute aortic syndromes: imaging and beyond. *Herz.* 2013;38(3):269-276.

35. Januzzi JL, Troughton R. Are serial BNP measurements useful in heart failure management? Serial natriuretic peptide measurements are useful in heart failure management. *Circulation.* 2013;127(4):500-508.

36. Di Somma S, Marino R, Zampini G, et al. Predictive value for death and rehospitalization of 30-day postdischarge B-type natriuretic peptide (BNP) in elderly patients with heart failure. Sub-analysis of Italian RED Study. *Clin Chem Lab Med.* 2014;53(3):507-513.

37. Lassus J, Gayat E, Mueller C, et al. Incremental value of biomarkers to clinical variables for mortality prediction in acutely decompensated heart failure: the Multinational Observational Cohort on Acute Heart Failure (MOCA) study. *Int J Cardiol.* 2013;168(3):2186-2194.

38. Henry-Okafor Q, Collins SP, Jenkins CA, et al. Soluble ST2 as a diagnostic and prognostic marker for acute heart failure syndromes. *Open Biomark J.* 2012;2012(5):1-8.

39. Abdel-Qadir HM, Chugh S, Lee DS, Abdel-Qadir HM, Chugh S, Lee DS. Improving prognosis estimation in patients with heart failure and the cardiorenal syndrome. *Int J Nephrol.* 2011;2011:e351672.

40. Metra M, Davison B, Bettari L, et al. Is worsening renal function an ominous prognostic sign in patients with acute heart failure? The role of congestion and its interaction with renal function. *Circ Heart Fail.* 2012;5(1):54-62.

41. Pocock SJ, Ariti CA, McMurray JJV, et al. Predicting survival in heart failure: a risk score based on 39372 patients from 30 studies. *Eur Heart J.* 2012. doi: 10.1093/eurheartj/ehs337.

42. Ndrepepa G, Braun S, Mehilli J, et al. Prognostic value of sensitive troponin T in patients with stable and unstable angina and undetectable conventional troponin. *Am Heart J.* 2011;161(1):68-75.

43. Mills NL, Lee KK, McAllister DA, et al. Implications of lowering threshold of plasma troponin concentration in diagnosis of myocardial infarction: cohort study. *BMJ.* 2012;344:e1533.

44. Kohli P, Bonaca MP, Kakkar R, et al. Role of ST2 in non–ST-elevation acute coronary syndrome in the MERLIN-TIMI 36 trial. *Clin Chem.* 2012;58(1):257-266.

45. von Haehling S, Papassotiriou J, Morgenthaler NG, et al. Copeptin as a prognostic factor for major adverse cardiovascular events in patients with coronary artery disease. *Int J Cardiol.* 2012;162(1):27-32.

46. Sayed ASM, Xia K, Salma U, Yang T, Peng J. Diagnosis, prognosis and therapeutic role of circulating miRNAs in cardiovascular diseases. *Heart Lung Circ.* 2014;23(6):503-510.

47. Gheorghiade M, Vaduganathan M, Fonarow GC, Bonow RO. Rehospitalization for heart failure problems and perspectives. *J Am Coll Cardiol.* 2013;61(4):391-403.

48. Maisel A, Barnard D, Jaski B, et al. Primary results of the HABIT trial (Heart Failure Assessment With BNP in the Home). *J Am Coll Cardiol.* 2013;61(16):1726-1735.

49. O'Gara PT, Kushner FG, Ascheim DD, et al. 2013 ACCF/AHA guideline for the management of ST-Elevation myocardial infarction: a report of the American College of Cardiology Foundation/American Heart Association Task Force on practice guidelines. *J Am Coll Cardiol.* 2013;61(4):e78-e140.

50. Novo S, Peritore A, Guarneri FP, et al. Metabolic syndrome (MetS) predicts cardio and cerebrovascular events in a twenty years follow-up. A prospective study. *Atherosclerosis.* 2012;223(2):468-472.

21 ECHOCARDIOGRAPHY IN CONGESTIVE HEART FAILURE

Gbemiga G. Sofowora, MBChB, FACC
Abiodun Ishola, MD

INTRODUCTION

Congestive heart failure has been defined as a clinical syndrome that occurs when the heart is unable to meet the demands of actively metabolizing tissue without increasing filling pressures. Myocardial causes of heart failure (HF) may be systolic and/or diastolic. The versatile, noninvasive nature of echocardiography means that it plays a part in the diagnosis, determining the etiology, and noninvasive evaluation of HF guide management. This chapter will highlight the role of echo in evaluating a few cases of systolic dysfunction and diastolic dysfunction.

PATIENT CASE: ISCHEMIC CARDIOMYOPATHY

Mrs. LH is a 66-year-old woman who uses a wheelchair. She has a past history of recent myocardial infarction s/p percutaneous coronary intervention (PCI) to a large left anterior descending artery (LAD) (Video 21-1*, Figure 21-1, Video 21-2, Video 21-3) and left circumflex artery (LCX), and history of congestive heart failure (CHF) with medical noncompliance, hypertension (HTN), and hyperlipidemia. Mrs. LH was seen in clinic with worsening pedal swelling and decreased ability to lie down flat at night. She had a history of dietary and medical noncompliance and was brought in by her husband who complained that his wife was getting worse. She denied new onset of chest pain but admitted that she had not been compliant with her carvedilol medication out of concerns that it may precipitate an undue drop in blood pressure.

On examination, Mrs. LH's jugular venous pressure was elevated with a prominent V wave and she had a soft systolic murmur over her tricuspid area, which got louder with inspiration. Also present was a soft S_1 with a prominent third heart sound. She also had bilateral crackles over her lung bases, bilateral pedal edema, and chronic stasis dermatitis. Her electrocardiogram (ECG) was unchanged from her previous ECGs and 3 sets of troponins were negative. Echocardiography revealed an ejection fraction (EF) of 32% with anterior wall motion abnormalities and a prominent left ventricular thrombus at the apex (Video 21-1, Video 21-4, Video 21-5). She was then admitted and maintained on oral lisinopril daily, intravenous (IV) frusemide, and IV heparin with warfarin. She was eventually discharged after achieving euvolemic status on the same medicines with aspirin 81 mg daily, atorvastatin 40 mg daily, carvedilol 12.5 mg twice daily and spironolactone 25 mg daily. Her

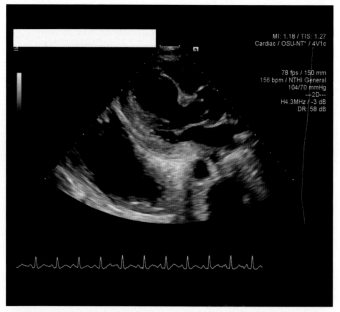

FIGURE 21-1 Parasternal long-axis view of another patient with thinned anteroseptal wall. Three-chamber view of patient with ischemic cardiomyopathy showing severely hypokinetic anterior wall and apex.

*Videos available on www.BaligaHeartFailureCh21.com.

discharge INR was 2.6 and she was asked to follow up with her cardiologist for consideration of stress testing and implantable cardioverter defibrillator (ICD) placement.

CLINICAL FEATURES

The signs and symptoms are at first predominantly that of coronary artery disease (CAD) but also include signs and symptoms of CHF.

- May present with classic signs of chest pain radiating to the left arm, jaw, or neck.
- Women tend to have atypical symptoms.
- Pain is usually described as crushing.
- Associated nausea or vomiting may be present.
- May be asymptomatic. This is more common in:
  - The elderly
  - Patients with diabetes mellitus
  - Women
- Lightheadedness and dizziness may be a feature.
- Shortness of breath
- Leg swelling
- Dyspnea on exertion
- Orthopnea
- Paroxysmal nocturnal dyspnea
   Signs include:
- Pedal edema
- Raised jugular venous pulse (JVP)
- Displaced apex beat
- A third heart sound that may be due to ischemic mitral regurgitation or systolic dysfunction.

ETIOLOGY AND EPIDEMIOLOGY

According to the NHANES study, 13,643 men and women were followed up for 19 years and 1382 developed congestive cardiac failure. Of these, CAD was associated with a RR of 8.1 and a population-attributable risk of 62%.[1] The resulting cardiomyopathy after a coronary insult may be due to:

- Irreversible loss of myocardium after an ischemic insult.
- Stunned or hibernating myocardium.
  - Stunned myocardium refers to transient post ischemic dysfunction, whereas hibernating myocardium refers to contractile dysfunction that improves after revascularization.

PATHOPHYSIOLOGY

Multiple factors contribute to the development of the atherosclerotic plaque from formation of fatty streaks in childhood to eventual development of a fibrous plaque and neovascularization as well as inflammation. An acute obstruction may be due to rupture of vulnerable plaque with eventual platelet activation, adhesion, and aggregation leading to occlusion of the vessel wall. Plaque erosion may also lead to platelet aggregation.

Major risk factors for atherosclerosis include:

- HTN
- Diabetes mellitus
- Cigarette smoking
- Hyperlipidemia
- Family history of premature CAD

DIAGNOSIS

This usually involves some form of ischemic evaluation. These include:

- Stress testing
- Computed tomography (CT) angiography
- Coronary angiography
- Echocardiogram may demonstrate wall motion abnormalities suggesting ischemia. The presence and location of wall motion abnormalities also give clues about the location of the coronary insult. Due to its noninvasive nature and lack of need for radioactive contrast, echocardiography is widely used to determine the EF and can also give useful information about myocardial viability. The presence of end-diastolic wall thickness <0.6 cm (Video 21-6 and Figure 21-2) excluded the potential for functional recovery with a sensitivity of 94% and a specificity of 49%,[2] while a deceleration time >150 ms predicted an increase in EF after coronary artery bypass grafting (CABG) with sensitivity and specificity of 80%.[3] Echocardiography may also show complications of a myocardial infarction such as:
  - Ventricular septal defect (VSD)
  - Pericardial effusion (Figure 21-2)
  - Ruptured papillary muscle and severe mitral regurgitation
  - Cardiac rupture
- Other findings would include a B bump to suggest an elevated Left ventricular end diastolic pressure (LVEDP),[4] increased E-point septal separation (EPSS) suggesting decreased stroke volume, and/or a dilated left ventricle and increased E/e' ratio with bulging of the interatrial septum to the right suggesting increased left atrial pressure.[5]
- ECG may show evidence of ischemia or Q waves correlating with a coronary artery distribution.

MANAGEMENT

This involves treatment of the CHF as well as the underlying CAD with coronary artery revascularization either percutaneously or by surgery. Patients need to be on

- Aspirin
- Beta blocker
- Angiotensin-converting enzyme (ACE) inhibitor, angiotensin receptor blocker (ARB) or sacubitril/valsartan.
- Statin: For secondary prevention of myocardial infarction. The high-intensity statins are preferred.
- Spironolactone: For patients with NYHA class II-IV symptoms and EF <35% who have normal renal function and normal potassium concentration.
- Loop diuretic: This provides a symptomatic benefit.
- ICD or cardiac resynchronization therapy.

PATIENT CASE: DILATED CARDIOMYOPATHY

Mr. BB is a 43-year-old man who presented to the hospital with shortness of breath and leg swelling. He had a flu-like illness 3 weeks prior. He said the "flu" never got better, but was now associated with worsening shortness of breath on exertion and he had been unable to sleep for 3 days. He also described progressive leg swelling and early satiety. On examination, he had a jugular venous pulse which was raised all the way to the jaw, a displaced apex beat, and a soft systolic murmur over his tricuspid and mitral areas, which increased with inspiration and radiated to his axilla respectively. Abdominal examination demonstrated a fluid thrill by examination and he had 1+ pedal edema. Echocardiography showed a dilated left ventricle measuring 6.5 cm with a reduced EF of 30% (Figure 21-3, Figure 21-4, Video 21-7, Figure 21-5, Figure 21-6, Video 21-8, Figure 21-7), a B bump and increased EPSS on M mode (Figure 21-8) with an E/e' of 18. M mode through the base of the heart at the level of the aorta also demonstrated minimal movement of the aortic root (Figure 21-9). Spectral Doppler showed mild pulmonic and tricuspid regurgitation with elevated right ventricular (RV) systolic pressures (Figures 21-10 and 21-11). His atria were mildly dilated and his inferior vena cava (IVC) was dilated with minimal compressibility with sniff (Video 21-9). His hepatic veins showed diastolic predominance of hepatic flow. A left and right heart catheterization was performed. These showed luminal irregularities in his coronaries and right atrial (RA) pressure of 19 mm Hg, RV pressure of 50/19 mm Hg, pulmonary artery (PA) pressures of 50/23 mm Hg, and a wedge pressure of 21 mm Hg. His cardiac index (CI) was 2.0 L/min/m². He was subsequently started on IV doses of a loop diuretic and an oral ACE inhibitor. He was net negative 8.0 L over the course of his admission and was discharged on furosemide, lisinopril, carvedilol and spironolactone, to follow up with his outpatient cardiologist for consideration of ICD placement if his EF failed to improve (Figure 21-12).

CLINICAL FEATURES

Symptoms

- Shortness of breath
- Leg swelling
- Orthopnea
- Paroxysmal nocturnal dyspnea
- Early satiety

Signs

- Pedal edema
- Raised JVP
- Displaced apex beat
- Third heart sound
- Systolic murmur loudest at the apex and radiating to the axilla

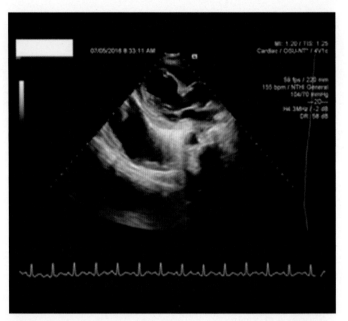

FIGURE 21-2 Same patient with akinetic and thinned anteroseptal wall with pericardial and pleural effusions.

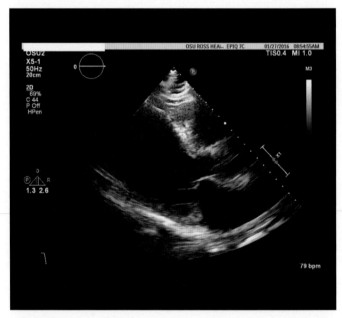

FIGURE 21-3 Parasternal long-axis view of patient with dilated cardiomyopathy. Notice dilated left ventricle.

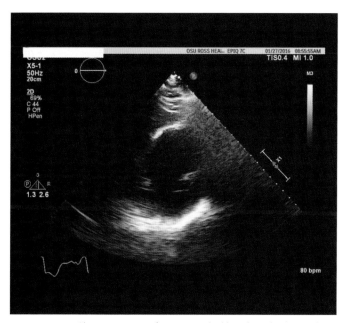

FIGURE 21-4 Short-axis view of patient with dilated cardiomyopathy.

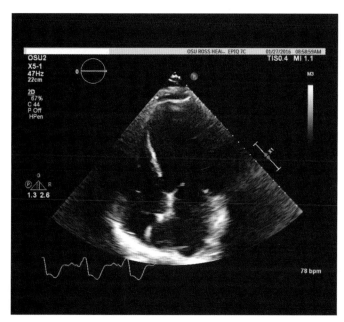

FIGURE 21-5 Four-chamber view of patient with dilated cardiomyopathy. Notice bulging of interatrial septum to the right, suggestive of increased left atrial pressure.

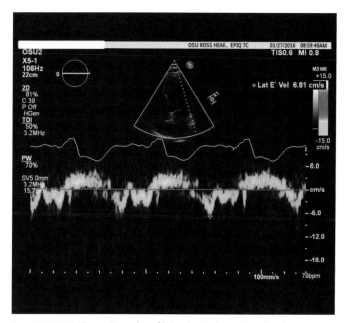

FIGURE 21-6 Tissue Doppler of lateral mitral annulus showing reduced e' velocity.

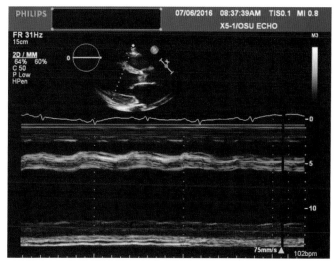

FIGURE 21-7 M mode of the left ventricle showing significant dilation.

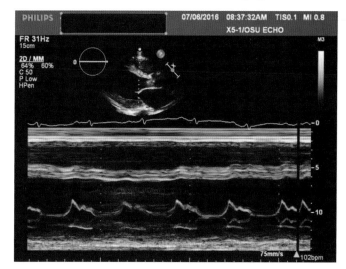

FIGURE 21-8 M mode of the left ventricle showing increased E-point septal separation (EPSS) and B bump.

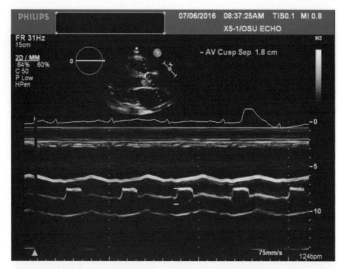

FIGURE 21-9 M mode through the aortic root showing relatively minimal movement of the aortic root in severe cardiomyopathy.

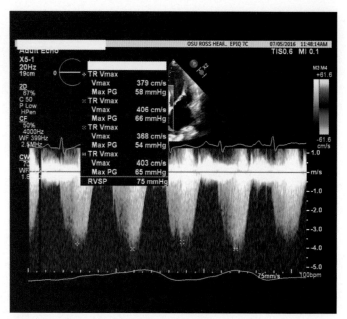

FIGURE 21-11 Continuous-wave Doppler through a jet of tricuspid regurgitation showing a wide pressure gradient between the right atrium and right ventricle. The estimated right atrial pressure was 15 mm Hg.

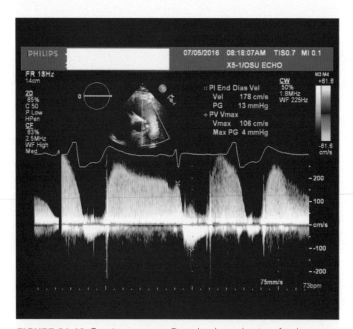

FIGURE 21-10 Continuous-wave Doppler through a jet of pulmonary regurgitation showing increased pulmonary regurgitation end diastolic gradients. The estimated RA pressure was 15 mm Hg.

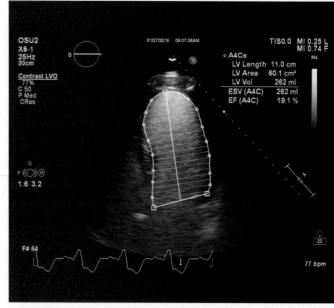

FIGURE 21-12 Estimated ejection fraction using Simpson's rule of discs.

DIAGNOSIS

Echocardiography: Findings on echocardiography in decompensated nonischemic cardiomyopathy include:

- Decreased EF (Video 21-9)
- B bump and increased EPSS on M mode of the mitral valve (Figure 21-8)
- Gradual aortic valve closure and decreased movement of the aortic root on M mode of the aortic valve (Figure 21-9)
- Decreased left ventricular outflow tract (LVOT) velocity time integral (VTI) reflecting the decreased stroke volume and cardiac output
- Decreased mitral annular planar systolic excursion (MAPSE) and mitral annular S' (Figure 21-6)
- Dilated atria reflecting chronically increased filling pressures
- Dilated IVC (Video 21-9)
- D wave predominance with hepatic vein Doppler
- E/e' >15
- Associated features of diastolic dysfunction

Some form of ischemic evaluation is appropriate to exclude ischemic cardiomyopathy. Cardiac magnetic resonance (MRI) has utility, not only in demonstrating the reduced systolic function, but in determining possible etiology based on the distribution pattern of fibrosis.

MANAGEMENT

- Beta blocker
- ACE inhibitor or ARB
- Spironolactone: For patients with NYHA class II-IV symptoms and EF <35% who have normal renal function and normal potassium concentration
- Loop diuretic: This provides a symptomatic benefit.
- Digoxin: May help reduce hospitalizations
- ICD or cardiac resynchronization therapy
- Ivabradine
- Valsartan/Sacubitril in place of an ACE inhibitor

PATIENT CASE: LEFT VENTRICULAR NONCOMPACTION

Mr. AA is a 53-year-old man with a family history of sudden cardiac death who presented to the clinic with gradual onset shortness of breath. He was a previously healthy man who used to be able to walk with his dog in the evenings but noticed that he was becoming increasingly short of breath. On further questioning he admitted to waking up at night short of breath twice in the previous week but assumed it was because his bedroom was stuffy.

Examination revealed a mildly anxious man with visible neck veins midway up his neck, tachycardia, and a displaced apex beat with a soft systolic murmur radiation to the axilla and a third heart sound. Echocardiography revealed a dilated left ventricle with prominent trabeculations (Figures 21-13 through 21-18, Video 21-10) in the left

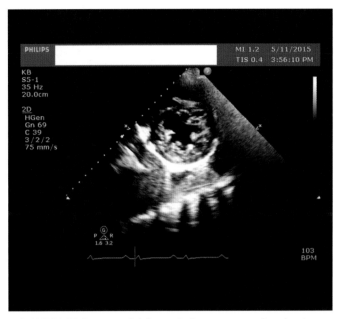

FIGURE 21-13 Patient with left ventricular noncompaction showing trabeculations involving the inferior and lateral walls in end diastole.

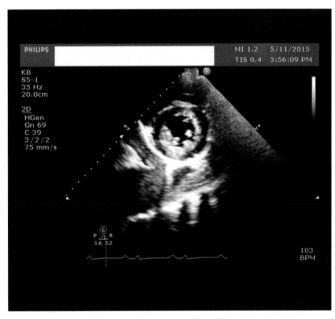

FIGURE 21-14 Same patient showing trabeculations involving the inferior and lateral walls at end systole.

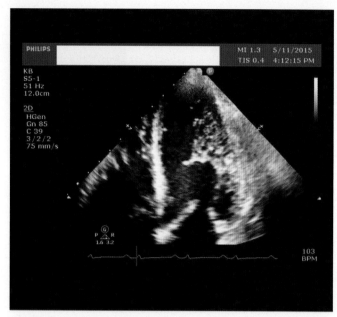

FIGURE 21-15 Four-chamber view of patient with left ventricular non-compaction showing trabeculations involving the lateral wall.

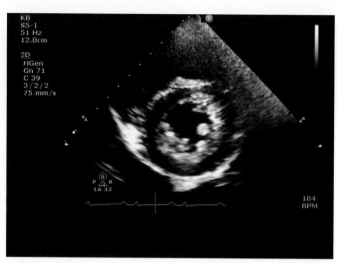

FIGURE 21-17 A short-axis view of another patient with left ventricular noncompaction illustrating the spongy myocardium at end systole.

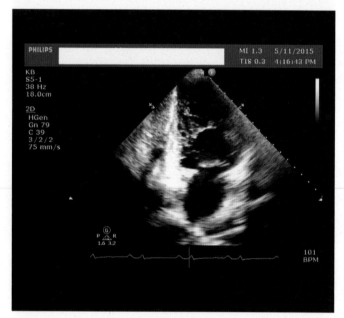

FIGURE 21-16 Two-chamber view of same patient showing trabeculations involving the inferior wall.

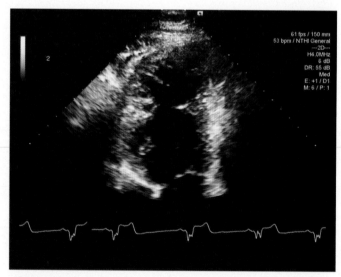

FIGURE 21-18 Three-chamber view of patient with left ventricular noncompaction showing prominent trabeculae in the inferolateral wall.

ventricle just distal to the papillary muscles, multiple intraventricular recesses, and an EF of 35% to 40%. His left atrium was mildly dilated. He was promptly admitted and diuresed with furosemide and eventually discharged home on carvedilol 25 mg bid, lisinopril 5 mg daily, and spironolactone 25 mg daily as well as oral warfarin.

CLINICAL FEATURES

- May be asymptomatic
- May present with signs and symptoms of CHF
- Nonsustained and sustained ventricular tachycardias (VT) are found in up to 27%[6] of patients.
- Thromboembolism is a feature and occurs in 5-38% of cases[7] and is high in the presence of atrial fibrillation and LV systolic dysfunction.
- Mortality varies greatly from 48% death or transplantation rate in 44 months[8] to a mean survival rate of 97% in 46 months.[9] This discrepancy may reflect differences in patient phenotype. In the former group the patients were symptomatic.

EPIDEMIOLOGY

- Prevalence is uncertain but has been reported to be as high as 1:500.[10]

ETIOLOGY AND PATHOPHYSIOLOGY

Mutations in cardiac sarcomeric proteins are associated with left ventricular noncompaction cardiomyopathy (LVNC) including genes encoding β-myosin heavy chain, α-dystrobrevin, and Cypher/ZASP.

During fetal cardiac development, trabeculations emerge by the fifth week of development and typically involute or compact by the 70th day. This process of compaction starts at the base and progresses toward the apex. Noncompaction is due to failure of compaction during embryogenesis leaving persistent trabeculations and intertrabecular recesses.

DIAGNOSIS

Several echocardiographic criteria exist:
Chin et al[11]

- The ratio of the compacted layer to the sum of the noncompacted and compacted layers is <0.5 at end diastole (Figure 21-13).
Jenni et al[12]
- Ratio of the noncompacted to the compacted layer at end systole >2 (Figures 21-14 and 21-17).
- Prominent trabeculations affecting the lateral and inferior walls from apex to mid ventricle.
- Evidence of intertrabecular recesses filled with blood from the LV cavity.
Stollberger and Finsterer[13]
- Four or more trabeculations protruding from the LV wall in end diastole (Figure 21-18 and Video 21-10)
- MRI criteria also exist and they include:

  ○ Ratio of the noncompacted to compacted layer at end diastole >2.3
  ○ Noncompacted mass >20% of LV global mass

Differential Diagnosis

- Normal variants: Pregnancy, highly trained athletes, sickle cell disease
- Hypertrophic cardiomyopathy: Apical
- Endomyocardial fibrosis affecting the left ventricle
- False tendons
- Eosinophilic heart disease

MANAGEMENT

This depends on the phenotype.

- CHF is managed according to the current HF guidelines.
- ICD therapy may be used for secondary prevention after VT or primary prevention after cardiomyopathy.
- The use of anticoagulation has been debated but is appropriate in the presence of atrial fibrillation or demonstrated LV or atrial thrombi.

PATIENT CASE: HYPERTENSIVE HEART DISEASE

Mr. EY is a 50-year immigrant from West Africa who was diagnosed with HTN for the first time in the United States 10 years ago. He was being treated with furosemide, metolazone, clonidine, and minoxidil but claimed that the "medicines did not work." He had noticed progressive shortness of breath, abdominal swelling, and leg swelling and had been to several hospitals for paracentesis. He claimed that after each tap he tended to reaccumulate fluids quickly. His weight had increased from 155 pounds to 175 pounds and he had noticed progressive shortness of breath and leg swelling but denied waking up at night short of breath. The morning of admission, he woke up in the morning short of breath but was asked by his wife to help move some furniture. He promptly passed out and the squad was called.

Examination revealed an asthenic man, with a JVP that extended all the way up to his earlobes. His chest was clear to auscultation but auscultation of his heart revealed an apex beat displaced to the sixth intercostal space midaxillary line with a palpable left parasternal heave. He had a systolic murmur located over the tricuspid area, which increased in intensity with inspiration and he had an S_4 gallop rhythm. His abdomen was grossly distended with a palpable fluid thrill and he had a liver palpable up to 11 cm below the right costal margin and slightly tender. He had bilateral pitting pedal edema.

An echocardiogram revealed severe left ventricular hypertrophy (LVH) (Video 21-11, Figure 21-19, Video 21-12, Figure 21-20, Video 21-14, Figure 21-21) with an EF of >70% and a small LV cavity. He had grade II diastolic dysfunction and moderate to severe tricuspid regurgitation. A subsequent MRI done to rule out hypertrophic cardiomyopathy was negative but raised a concern for amyloid heart disease. A subsequent myocardial biopsy was negative for amyloid heart disease. He was subsequently diuresed and had a paracentesis done that drained 2.5 L of fluid. He had a brief episode of sustained VT and his abdominal girth decreased from 49 cm at the umbilicus to 33 cm. He was eventually sent home on furosemide 20 mg daily, lisinopril 40 mg daily, carvedilol 25 mg bid, and amlodipine 10 mg daily.

CLINICAL FEATURES

Symptoms

- Shortness of breath
- Leg swelling
- Orthopnea
- Paroxysmal nocturnal dyspnea
- Early satiety

Signs

- Pedal edema
- Raised JVP
- Displaced apex beat
- Fourth heart sound (if not in atrial fibrillation)
- Third heart sound
- Mitral or tricuspid regurgitation murmurs may be heard due to chamber dilation.

EPIDEMIOLOGY

- In 2011-2012, the age-adjusted prevalence of HTN was 29.1%.[14]
- HTN prevalence is greatest among non-Hispanic black adults.
- Men and women had similar prevalence of HTN.

DIAGNOSIS

The diagnosis is made by a clinical history of HTN, symptoms and signs of heart failure, characteristic features of LVH, and left atrial enlargement (LAE) on ECG and echocardiography.

Echocardiography

- LVH or concentric remodeling
- M mode may show increased LV thickness and impaired relaxation of the LV wall (Figure 21-22).
- Diastolic dysfunction with reduced medial and lateral e' (Figure 21-23)
- Dilated left atrium (Video 21-13, Figure 21-24)
- ± impaired systolic function

Differential Diagnosis

- Hypertrophic cardiomyopathy
- Amyloid heart disease
- Aortic stenosis with LVH
- Fabry disease

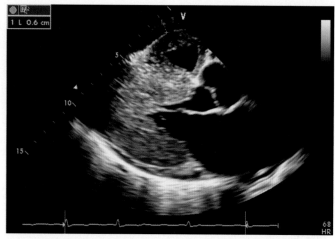

FIGURE 21-19 Parasternal long-axis view of patient with severe left ventricular hypertrophy secondary to hypertension—still image.

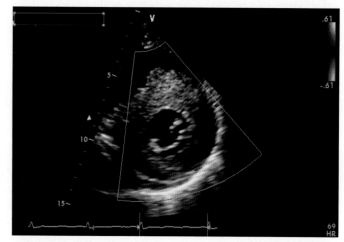

FIGURE 21-20 Parasternal short-axis view of patient with severe left ventricular hypertrophy secondary to hypertension—still image.

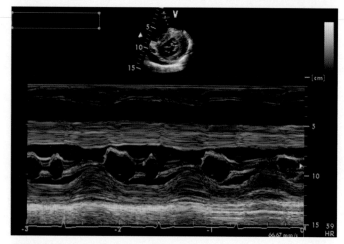

FIGURE 21-21 M mode of patient with severe left ventricular hypertrophy secondary to hypertension.

MANAGEMENT

This involves blood pressure control and HF management. Blood pressure control involves:

- Salt restriction
- Weight reduction
- The DASH diet, which is a diet rich in fruits, vegetables, nuts, low-fat dairy, skinless poultry, fish, and nontropical vegetable oils
- Regular exercise
- Limited alcohol intake
- Antihypertensive drugs

    HF is managed using current guideline-directed medical therapy.

PATIENT CASE: ARRHYTHMOGENIC RIGHT VENTRICULAR CARDIOMYOPATHY

Mr. CB is a 45-year-old man with a known history of dilated cardiomyopathy thought to be secondary to mitochondrial myopathy, though this was never confirmed on biopsy, who came to the emergency department with chest "burning." He described his discomfort as a burn not consistently brought on by exertion nor relieved by rest but that tended to last several seconds at a time. His ECG showed Q waves and T-wave inversions in leads II, III, and AVF as well as T-wave inversions in V1 to V6 and his troponins peaked at 0.07. He underwent a CT angiogram in the ED, which showed no significant atherosclerotic narrowing but showed a possible LV thrombus and evidence of RV dysplasia. An echocardiogram done showed an EF of 40% and reduced RV systolic function. A subsequent MRI showed a dilated right ventricle with severe RV systolic dysfunction and multiple areas of RV aneurysmal dilation and dyskinesis. This met criteria for arrhythmogenic right ventricular cardiomyopathy (ARVC). A thrombus was also noted at the apex. Late-gadolinium enhancement imaging also demonstrated transmural scar of the LV lateral wall and apex. Septal midwall and RV myocardial enhancement were also present. He was maintained on goal-directed therapy for systolic HF with Toprol XL 150 mg daily, lisinopril 5 mg daily, and spironolactone 25 mg daily, and warfarin for his LV thrombus. The electrophysiology team placed a primary prevention ICD on him prior to discharge.

CLINICAL FEATURES

- May be asymptomatic
- Palpitations
- Syncope
- Ventricular arrhythmias ranging from isolated premature ventricular contractions to VT/VF
- Isolated RV failure
- Biventricular failure
- Sudden cardiac death

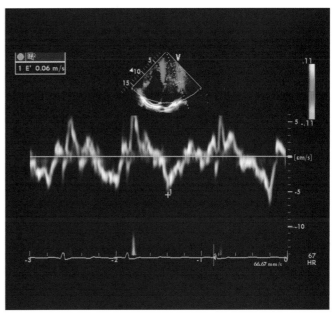

FIGURE 21-22 Tissue Doppler of lateral mitral annulus showing reduced e' velocity due to impaired relaxation.

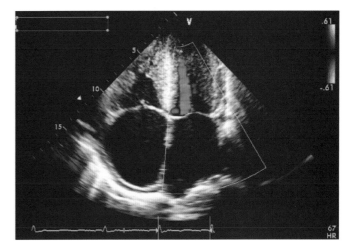

FIGURE 21-23 Four-chamber view of patient with severe left ventricular hypertrophy due to hypertension showing biatrial enlargement due to diastolic dysfunction—still image.

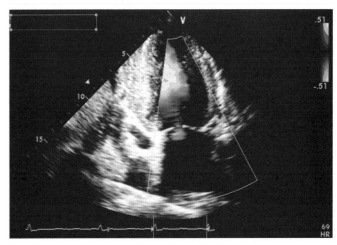

FIGURE 21-24 Two-chamber view of patient with severe left ventricular hypertrophy—still image.

EPIDEMIOLOGY

- The estimated prevalence of ARVC ranges from 1:1000 to 1:5000 although the condition appears to be more common in the Veneto region of Italy.[15,16]
- ARVC is inherited in an autosomal-dominant trait with variable penetrance although recessive forms exist: Naxos disease and Carvajal disease.

DIAGNOSIS

This is according to the Modified Task Force criteria for the diagnosis of arrhythmogenic right ventricular cardiomyopathy/dysplasia.[17]

Revised Task Force Criteria

1. Global or regional dysfunction and structural alterations
   Major   By 2D echo

   - Regional RV akinesia, dyskinesia, or aneurysm
   - And 1 of the following at end diastole
     - PLAX RVOT ≥32 mm (or PLAX/BSA ≥19 mm/m^2)
     - PSAX RVOT ≥36 mm (or PSAX/BSA ≥21 mm/m^2)
     - Or fractional area change ≤33%

   By MRI

   - Regional RV akinesia or dyskinesia or dyssynchronous RV contraction
   - And 1 of the following
     - Ratio of RV end-diastolic volume to BSA ≥110 mL/m^2 (male) or ≥100 mL/m^2 (female)
     - Or RV EF ≤40%

   By RV angiography
   - Regional RV akinesia, dyskinesia, or aneurysm

   Minor   By 2D echo

   - Regional RV akinesia, or dyskinesia
   - And 1 of the following at end diastole
     - PLAX RVOT ≥29 to <32 mm (or PLAX/BSA ≥16 to <19 mm/m^2)
     - PSAX RVOT ≥32 to <36 mm (or PSAX/BSA ≥18 to <21 mm/m^2)
     - Or fractional area change >33% to ≤40%

   By MRI
   - Regional RV akinesia or dyskinesia or dyssynchronous RV contraction
   - And 1 of the following
     - Ratio of RV end-diastolic volume to BSA ≥100 to <110 mL/m^2 (male) or ≥90 to <100 mL/m^2 (female)
     - Or RV EF >40% to ≤45%

2. Tissue characteristics of wall
   Major   Residual myocytes <60% by morphometric analysis (or <50% if estimated), with fibrous replacement of the RV free wall myocardium in ≥ sample, with or without fatty replacement of tissue on endomyocardial biopsy

   Minor   Residual myocytes 60% to 75% by morphometric analysis (or 50%-65% if estimated) with fibrous replacement of the RV free wall myocardium in ≥1 sample, with or without fatty replacement of tissue on endomyocardial biopsy

3. Repolarization abnormalities
   Major   Inverted T waves in the right precordial leads (V1, V2, V3) or beyond in individuals >14 years of age (in the absence of complete right bundle branch block QRS ≥120 ms)

   Minor   Inverted T waves in leads V1 and V2 in individuals >14 years of age (in the absence of complete right bundle branch block) or in V4, V5 or V6
   Inverted T waves in V1, V2, V3, and V4 in individuals >14 years of age in the presence of complete right bundle branch block

4. Depolarization/conduction abnormalities
   Major   Epsilon wave (reproducible low-amplitude signals between end of QRS complex to onset of the T wave) in the right precordial leads V1 to V3

   Minor   Late potentials by SAECG in ≥1 of 3 parameters in the absence of a QRS duration of ≥110 ms on the standard ECG
   Filtered QRS duration ≥114 ms
   Duration of terminal QRS <40 µV (low-amplitude signal duration) ≥38 ms
   Root mean square voltage of terminal 40 ms ≤20 µV
   Terminal activation duration of QRS ≥55 ms measured from the nadir of the S wave to the end of the QRS, including R' in V1, V2, or V3 in the absence of complete right bundle branch block

5. Arrhythmias
   Major   Nonsustained or sustained ventricular tachycardia of left bundle branch morphology with superior axis (negative or indeterminate QRS in leads II, III, and AVF and positive in lead AVL)

   Minor   Nonsustained or sustained ventricular tachycardia of RV outflow configuration, left bundle branch morphology with inferior axis (positive QRS in leads II, III, and AVF and negative in AVL) or unknown axis
   500 ventricular extrasystoles per 24 hours Holter monitoring

6. Family history
   Major   ARVC/D confirmed in a first-degree relative who meets task force criteria
   ARVC/D confirmed pathologically at autopsy or surgery in a first-degree relative
   Identification of a pathogenic mutation categorized as associated or probably associated with ARVC/D in the patient under evaluation

| Minor | History of ARVC/D in a first-degree relative in whom it is not possible or practical to determine whether the family member meets current Task Force criteria |
| | Premature sudden death (<35 years of age) due to suspected ARVC/D in a first-degree relative ARVC/D confirmed pathologically or by current Task Force criteria in a second-degree relative |

Two major, 1 major and 2 minor, or 4 minor criteria are required for diagnosis.

Echo findings[18]

- RV function may be mildly or severely reduced although normal function does not exclude ARVC/D[18] as up to 38% of patients meeting Task Force criteria for ARVC/D had normal RV function.
- Regional wall motion abnormalities affecting the RV
  - Hyper-reflective moderator band
  - Excessive abnormal trabeculations
  - Sacculations
  - An RVOT long-axis dimension of >30 mm had the greatest sensitivity (89%) and specificity (86%) for the diagnosis of ARVD.[18]

Differential Diagnosis

RVOT tachycardia

MANAGEMENT[19]

- Restriction from competitive and endurance sports
- Beta blockers and ACE inhibitors/ARBs for HF
- Anticoagulation for intracardiac thrombi
- Antiarrhythmic drugs and catheter ablation for arrhythmias
- ICD for high-risk subjects

REFERENCES

1. He J, Ogden LG, Bazzano LA, Vupputuri S, Loria C, Whelton PK. Risk factors for congestive heart failure in US men and women: NHANES I epidemiologic follow-up study. *Arch Intern Med*. 2001;161(7):996-1002.

2. Cwajg JM, Cwajg E, Nagueh SF, et al. End-diastolic wall thickness as a predictor of recovery of function in myocardial hibernation: relation to rest-redistribution T1-201 tomography and dobutamine stress echocardiography. *J Am Coll Cardiol*. 2000;35(5):1152-1161.

3. Yong Y, Nagueh SF, Shimoni S, et al. Deceleration time in ischemic cardiomyopathy: relation to echocardiographic and scintigraphic indices of myocardial viability and functional recovery after revascularization. *Circulation*. 2001;103(9):1232-1237.

4. Feigenbaum H. Role of M-mode technique in today's echocardiography. *J Am Soc Echocardiogr*. 2010;23(3):240-257;335-337.

5. Ommen SR, Nishimura RA, Appleton CP, et al. Clinical utility of Doppler echocardiography and tissue Doppler imaging in the estimation of left ventricular filling pressures: a comparative simultaneous Doppler-catheterization study. *Circulation*. 2000;102(15):1788-1794.

6. Stanton C, Bruce C, Connolly H, et al. Isolated left ventricular noncompaction syndrome. *Am J Cardiol*. 2009;104(8):1135-1138.

7. Paterick TE, Umland MM, Jan MF, et al. Left ventricular noncompaction: a 25-year odyssey. *J Am Soc Echocardiogr*. 2012;25(4):363-375.

8. Oechslin EN, Attenhofer Jost CH, Rojas JR, Kaufmann PA, Jenni R. Long-term follow-up of 34 adults with isolated left ventricular noncompaction: a distinct cardiomyopathy with poor prognosis. *J Am Coll Cardiol*. 2000;36(2):493-500.

9. Murphy RT, Thaman R, Blanes JG, et al. Natural history and familial characteristics of isolated left ventricular non-compaction. *Eur Heart J*. 2005;26(2):187-192.

10. Sandhu R, Finkelhor RS, Gunawardena DR, Bahler RC. Prevalence and characteristics of left ventricular noncompaction in a community hospital cohort of patients with systolic dysfunction. *Echocardiography*. 2008;25(1):8-12.

11. Chin TK, Perloff JK, Williams RG, Jue K, Mohrmann R. Isolated noncompaction of left ventricular myocardium. A study of eight cases. *Circulation*. 1990;82(2):507-513.

12. Jenni R, Oechslin E, Schneider J, Attenhofer Jost C, Kaufmann PA. Echocardiographic and pathoanatomical characteristics of isolated left ventricular non-compaction: a step towards classification as a distinct cardiomyopathy. *Heart*. 2001;86(6):666-671.

13. Stollberger C, Finsterer J. Left ventricular hypertrabeculation/noncompaction. *J Am Soc Echocardiogr*. 2004;17(1):91-100.

14. Nwankwo T, Yoon SS, Burt V, Gu Q. Hypertension among adults in the United States: National Health and Nutrition Examination Survey, 2011-2012. *NCHS Data Brief*. Oct 2013;(133):1-8.

15. Basso C, Corrado D, Marcus FI, Nava A, Thiene G. Arrhythmogenic right ventricular cardiomyopathy. *Lancet*. 2009;373(9671):1289-1300.

16. Peters S, Trummel M, Meyners W. Prevalence of right ventricular dysplasia-cardiomyopathy in a non-referral hospital. *Int J Cardiol*. 2004;97(3):499-501.

17. Marcus FI, McKenna WJ, Sherrill D, et al. Diagnosis of arrhythmogenic right ventricular cardiomyopathy/dysplasia: proposed modification of the task force criteria. *Circulation*. 2010;121(13):1533-1541.

18. Yoerger DM, Marcus F, Sherrill D, et al. Echocardiographic findings in patients meeting task force criteria for arrhythmogenic right ventricular dysplasia: new insights from the multidisciplinary study of right ventricular dysplasia. *J Am Coll Cardiol.* 2005;45(6):860-865.

19. Corrado D, Wichter T, Link MS, et al. Treatment of arrhythmogenic right ventricular cardiomyopathy/dysplasia: an international task force consensus statement. *Circulation.* 2015;132(5):441-453.

22 CARDIOPULMONARY STRESS TESTING IN HEART FAILURE

Eugene E. Wolfel, MD

PATIENT CASE

A 46-year-old man with a dilated cardiomyopathy and known chronic HFrEF for the last two years now presents with a recent history of worsening shortness of breath and fatigue with physical activity. His LVEF is 25% and he has enlargement of all four chambers of his heart on echocardiography. He was last hospitalized two months ago with fluid retention that responded to high dose intravenous diuretic therapy. He did not need an intravenous inotropic or vasodilator drug. He is taking maximally tolerated doses of carvedilol, sacubitril/valsartan, spironolactone, and bumetanide. He remains in sinus rhythm and has an ICD for primary prevention of sudden cardiac death. His QRS duration on his ECG is only 100 msec; therefore, he is not a candidate for chronic resynchronization therapy. Because of his worsening exercise tolerance, he is referred for a cardiopulmonary exercise test to evaluate his functional limitation and to assess his prognosis and candidacy for advanced heart failure therapies. He walked for 4 minutes on a treadmill following a modified Naughton protocol and stopped due to dyspnea and fatigue. He only attained 70% of his predicted maximal heart rate as he was taking a beta-blocker. There were occasional premature ventricular beats during exercise but no sustained arrhythmia. His oxygen saturation by pulse oximetry remained greater than 90% throughout exercise. He had a 10 mmHg decrease in systolic blood pressure at peak exercise. His heart rate recovery was abnormal with only a 5 bpm decrease at one minute of recovery during a slow walking cool-down period. His peak VO$_2$ was 10.5 mL/kg/min which is 29% predicted for his age and gender. His peak respiratory exchange ratio (RER) was 1.20, indicating a near maximal effort. His VE/VCO$_2$ slope was 48 and his oxygen uptake efficiency slope (OUES) was 1.1. He had evidence of oscillatory ventilation during exercise. His end-tidal CO2 (PETCO$_2$) at rest was 28 mmHg and it decreased during exercise to 22 mmHg. The results of this test confirmed his severe exercise limitation and were consistent with diminished cardiac output and the development of pulmonary hypertension during exercise. In addition, the low peak VO$_2$, elevated VE/VCO$_2$ slope, decreased OUES, abnormal PETCO$_2$ response, oscillatory ventilation, exertional hypotension, and abnormal heart rate recovery all indicated that this patient had a poor prognosis with his HFrEF over the next year. A subsequent right heart catheterization confirmed the presence of a low resting cardiac index and pulmonary hypertension due to an elevated pulmonary capillary wedge pressure of 34 mmHg. His transpulmonary gradient was elevated at 15 mmHg but he had a favorable response to intravenous nitroprusside with a resulting pulmonary vascular resistance (PVR) of 2.1 Wood units. Based on these studies he was listed for cardiac transplantation. He subsequently required several hospitalizations for volume overload in the next few months and required

inotropic therapy. He was unable to be weaned from milrinone and a left ventricular assist device was implanted as a bridge to transplantation as he had type O blood and his waiting time on the transplant list was expected to be prolonged.

INTRODUCTION

Exercise intolerance is a hallmark of both chronic heart failure with reduced ejection fraction (HFrEF) and chronic heart failure with preserved ejection fraction (HFpEF). Patients complain of exertional dyspnea and fatigue and these symptoms relate to both elevated cardiac filling pressures and reduced cardiac output. In addition, there are abnormalities in the peripheral extraction of oxygen that limit exercise performance. It is plausible that patients with more severe heart failure (HF), both HFrEF and HFpEF, would have more functional limitation due to worsening of both cardiac and peripheral maladaptations. Thus, determination of exercise capacity becomes an important aspect of the care of these patients. It is important to realize that the syndrome of HF affects more than the cardiovascular system. There are abnormalities in the respiratory, skeletal muscle, and nervous system that play important roles in the regulation of cardiac and respiratory responses during exercise. Testing that incorporates an analysis of the interplay between these systems would be the ideal way to evaluate disease severity, categorize the degree of disability, and potentially assess prognosis in patients with HF. Routine treadmill testing has been used to evaluate exercise capacity in HF patients with some limited success in estimating functional capacity and assessing prognosis. This type of testing has limited value due to concerns about reproducibility and limited data about mechanisms responsible for the observed reduction in exercise capacity. In addition, exercise capacity as determined by an estimated metabolic equivalent (MET) level is often overestimated on these tests in HF and other cardiac patients. Cardiopulmonary exercise (CPX) testing has been recognized as a noninvasive tool to assess the interactions of the cardiovascular system with gas exchange physiology during exercise in normal subjects and patients with a variety of cardiovascular disorders. The American Heart Association and the European Association of Cardiovascular Prevention and Rehabilitation have both produced scientific statements describing the use and interpretation of these tests in a variety of clinical conditions, including HF.[1,2] CPX testing in HF patients has several important benefits including determining whether exertional dyspnea is caused by HF, determining the severity of disease, providing important prognostic information that may lead to advanced HF therapy in HFrEF patients, determining the efficacy of new pharmacologic or device therapies, and creating an exercise prescription for cardiac rehabilitation.

The conduct of a CPX test is similar to a regular exercise test with the addition of expired gas (O$_2$ and CO$_2$) analysis and quantification of ventilation. Heart rate (HR), blood pressure (BP), electrocardiogram

(ECG) recordings, and usually O_2 saturation by pulse oximetry are obtained at rest, during exercise, and in early recovery. The patient also breathes through a mouthpiece or face mask in a closed system with a 1-way valve that allows room air for inspiration and the capture of all expired air for analysis. The expired air is analyzed with a metabolic cart. The basic components of the equipment contained in a metabolic cart in CPX testing are illustrated in Figure 22-1. Analyzers are used for the determination of expired O_2 and CO_2 and usually a pneumotachometer is used to determine ventilation. These data are used to determine oxygen consumption (VO_2), carbon dioxide production (VCO_2), and minute ventilation (VE). The VO_2 and VCO_2 are reported as both mL/min and mL/kg/min and VE is reported as L/min. From these directly measured factors a variety of derived (calculated) parameters can be obtained including the respiratory exchange ratio (RER), which is the ratio of VCO_2 to VO_2, oxygen pulse (VO_2/HR), work rate (VO_2/watts), and ventilatory parameters including the VE/VCO_2 slope, the oxygen uptake efficiency slope (OUES), and end-tidal CO_2 ($PETCO_2$). Normal values are available to interpret these data in individual patients.[3] Patients can exercise on either a treadmill or cycle ergometer but in nontrained individuals, there is a 10% to 20% lower peak VO_2 on a cycle compared to a treadmill. Exercise testing protocols are usually less aggressive in HF patients with more gradual increases in workloads. Low-level protocols with 1-MET increments in workload, such as the Naughton protocol, are often used. Ramp testing with gradual increases in speed and grade on a treadmill or progressive increases in resistance on a cycle ergometer are becoming the standard and are replacing the step-wise increases in workload seen in various protocols such as modifications of the Bruce protocol and Balke protocol.

One may ask how respiratory measurements, such as VO_2, relate to the cardiovascular system. In Figure 22-2, the Fick equation is presented. VO_2 is the product of cardiac output (oxygen transport) and the arteriovenous (a-v) O_2 content difference (oxygen extraction). Thus, the measurement of VO_2 reflects both cardiovascular function (cardiac output and muscle blood flow) and the peripheral utilization of O_2. Because cardiac output is the product of HR and stroke volume, the Fick equation can be modified to represent the relationship of VO_2/HR (oxygen pulse) to both stroke volume and the a-v O_2 content difference. During heavy and near maximal exercise, the O_2 extraction is maximal and the O_2 pulse serves as a good surrogate of the stroke volume response. Patients with chronic HF, both HFrEF and HFpEF, have both reduced cardiac output and altered O_2 extraction during exercise. In one of the first clinical experiments using both CPX testing and invasive hemodynamic monitoring, Weber and colleagues demonstrated that the peak exercise VO_2 was more closely related to the cardiac output response to exercise.[4] Thus, in most patients with chronic HF the VO_2 at peak exercise is a good surrogate for the cardiac output response. Similar studies performed in patients with HFpEF also show a strong relationship between VO_2 and cardiac output, although there is more of a role for altered a-v O_2 content difference in the determination of peak exercise VO_2.

PHYSIOLOGIC RESPONSES DURING CARDIOPULMONARY EXERCISE TESTING

During progressive exercise there is a similar increase in both HR and VO_2 up to maximally tolerated exercise (Figure 22-3). Thus,

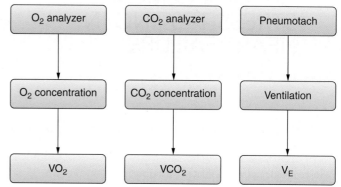

Components of metabolic chart

FIGURE 22-1 Components of equipment for cardiopulmonary exercise testing.

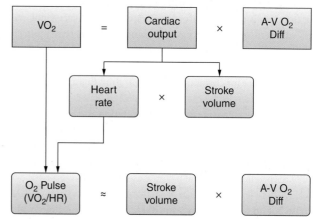

Correlates with the Fick equation

FIGURE 22-2 Relationship between VO_2 and cardiovascular components of the Fick equation during exercise. Abbreviations: HR, heart rate; VO_2, oxygen consumption.

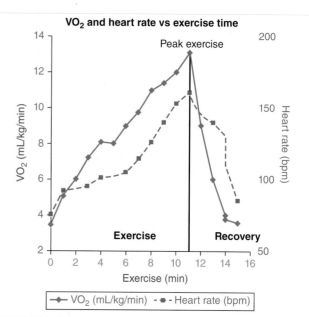

FIGURE 22-3 Oxygen consumption (VO_2) and heart rate responses during exercise and early recovery.

there is a direct relationship between HR and VO_2 even in the presence of cardiac disease or pharmacologic therapy. However, the magnitude of the relationship can be altered. In patients with HF there is a reduction in the VO_2 at a given workload and this will influence both the O_2 pulse (VO_2/HR) and the work rate (VO_2/watt). The VO_2 at maximally tolerated work is the gold standard for the description of aerobic exercise performance. If the VO_2 value reaches a plateau despite an increase in workload, this is termed "VO_2 max" (Figure 22-4). However, patients with cardiac disease are unable to attain such a high level of exertion; the VO_2 attained in the last 15 seconds of exercise is termed the "peak VO_2," and this value has been shown to be reproducible in HF patients. The peak RER is often used to determine if the patient has reached near maximal exercise capacity. A RER of 1.20 is considered near maximal capacity and a CPX test in a HF patient has good test-retest reproducibility if the RER is >1.05.[5] The maximal or peak VO_2 is influenced by age, gender, genetic disposition, training or deconditioning, environment, disease, and medications. In recovery there is a rapid decrease in both HR and VO_2 and the rate of recovery is influenced by both parasympathetic activation and the rate of recovery of the oxygen deficit incurred during exercise. These responses are usually abnormal in HF patients with more prolonged rates of recovery. Heart rate recovery has been shown to have important clinical and prognostic value in HF patients. To date, evaluation of VO_2 recovery has limited clinical utility in HF patients. The determination of VO_2 during submaximal exercise also has important physiologic and clinical significance. The ventilatory threshold (VT) is the highest attained VO_2 where there is still no significant accumulation of lactic acid in skeletal muscle and no switch to anaerobic metabolism. This threshold was formerly termed the anaerobic threshold, but anaerobic metabolism is not always present. At the VT there is an increase in ventilation to accommodate the increase in CO_2 produced by the conversion of lactic acid to lactate. Thus, there is a change in the relationship between VO_2 and ventilation but not between VCO_2 and ventilation as ventilation increases to eliminate the excess CO_2 produced in higher-intensity exercise. Physical activity above the VT will never reach a physiologic steady state and there will be progressive increases in HR, BP, sympathetic stimulation, and eventual cessation of exercise. The VT can be determined by various methods (Figures 22-5 and 22-6). The most reliable method is the V-slope method (Figure 22-5) where the relationship changes between VCO_2 and VO_2. The other represented method uses the ventilatory equivalents for VO_2 and VCO_2 (Figure 22-6). In this method the relationship between VE and VCO_2 remains unchanged due to the increase in ventilation required to eliminate excessive CO_2 while there is an increase in the VE and VO_2 relationship. A third method (not shown) uses the end-tidal O_2 and CO_2 responses during exercise. The VT is reported as the VO_2 at the threshold and is normalized as the percent of peak VO_2. In healthy, untrained subjects, the VO_2 at VT occurs at 45% to 65%. This measurement can be difficult to validate in HF patients due to a greater likelihood of a submaximal effort and ventilatory fluctuations that impede its determination. Patients with HF have been shown to have lower VO_2 values at VT related to the severity of their illness and there has been some limited data indicating a worse prognosis with a lower VT.

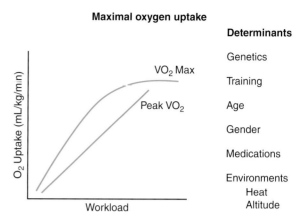

FIGURE 22-4 Description of maximal and peak exercise oxygen consumption (VO_2) and influencing factors.

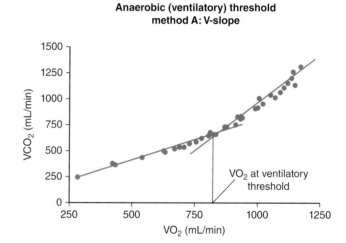

FIGURE 22-5 Determination of the ventilatory (anaerobic) threshold using the carbon dioxide production (VCO_2) vs oxygen consumption (VO_2) (V-slope) method.

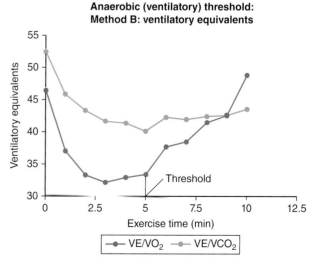

FIGURE 22-6 Determination of the ventilatory (anaerobic) threshold using the ventilatory equivalents method.

Minute ventilation (VE) also increases progressively during exercise (Figure 22-7). In HF patients, VE at any given submaximal exercise workload is usually greater than in a normal subject while the peak exercise VE is lower due to a lower attainable workload. RER initially decreases early in exercise but then gradually increases through peak exercise (Figure 22-7). The RER is usually ≥1.10 at peak exercise and continues to increase due to the increase in VCO_2 related to the respiratory removal of CO_2. RER can be used as a determination of near maximal exercise capacity and is more reliable than the percent predicted maximal HR. However, a RER ≥1.1 should not be used as the determination for stopping a CPX test.

VENTILATORY RELATIONSHIPS DURING EXERCISE

As noted earlier, patients with HF have a higher VE at submaximal exercise and a lower VE at peak exercise when compared to a healthy person (Figure 22-8). The decrease in peak exercise VE is related to a lower workload and subsequently lower peak VO_2 than in a healthy subject. However, the higher VE during submaximal exercise represents excessive ventilation during exercise that is commonly seen in HF, both HFrEF and HFpEF. This increase in ventilation is a result of several mechanisms that influence ventilatory drive (Figure 22-9). With progressive HF there is an increase in cardiac filling pressures (LV end-diastolic pressure and pulmonary capillary wedge pressure) and a decrease in cardiac output/index. These hemodynamic alterations result in an increase in ventilation/perfusion mismatch in the lungs with adequate ventilation but poor perfusion. In addition, there is an increase in chemoreceptor and ergoreceptor sensitivity and activation that results in an increase in the rate and depth of breathing. Thus, there is excessive ventilation for any given VCO_2 during exercise. This relationship has been described throughout exercise, at the VT, and at peak exercise. The most common description of this relationship is the linear relationship between VE and VCO_2 throughout exercise, described as the VE/VCO_2 slope. This slope is not influenced by the mode of exercise or the aggressiveness of the exercise protocol and does not require near-maximal exercise. It can be obtained during submaximal exercise in most patients and is highly reproducible with repeated testing in a given subject. This relationship was reported to be elevated with prognostic significance in systolic HF patients.[6] A normal VE/VCO_2 slope is shown in Figure 22-10. In Figure 22-11, a HF patient has an abnormally elevated VE/VCO_2 slope of 42.5. In both examples it is clear that there is a very statistically significant linear relationship between VE and VCO_2, with the HF patient having a much steeper slope, indicating excessive or inefficient ventilation during exercise. A normal VE/VCO_2 is <30. Patients with both HFrEF and HFpEF can have mild (30.0-35.9), moderate (36.0-44.8), and severe (≥45) excessive ventilation as represented by VE/VCO_2. Values greater than 34 to 36 have been associated with worse prognosis in HFrEF patients.[6] Patients with HFpEF can also have elevated VE/VCO_2 slopes but the values are usually less than in patients with HFrEF. It is important to note that patients with pulmonary hypertension (HTN) and chronic

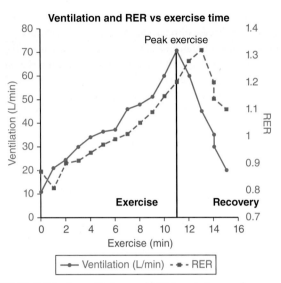

FIGURE 22-7 Minute ventilation and RER (respiratory exchange ratio) during exercise and early recovery.

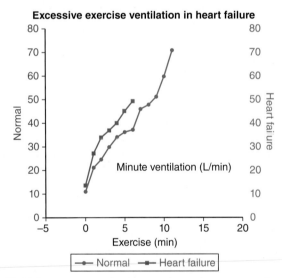

FIGURE 22-8 Comparison of minute ventilation during exercise between a normal subject and a patient with systolic heart failure (HFrEF).

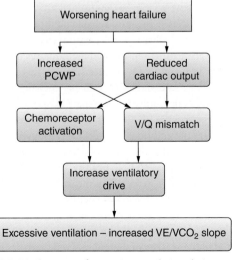

FIGURE 22-9 Mechanisms of excessive ventilation during exercise, resulting in an increased VE/VCO_2 slope.

lung disease can also have elevated VE/VCO_2 slopes and by itself, an elevated VE/VCO_2 slope during exercise is not diagnostic for HF. In patients with very elevated VE/VCO_2 slopes >50, pulmonary disease alone or a mixed picture of HF and pulmonary disease should be considered.

The relationship between VO_2 and VE during exercise is more complex. Because ventilation progresses at a more rapid rate than VO_2 during exercise, the relationship is logarithmic (Figure 22-12). However, this relationship becomes linear when the log transformation of VE is related to VO_2 (Figure 22-13). This relationship has been designated as the oxygen uptake efficiency slope (OUES). It represents the rate of increase in VO_2 in response to a given VE during incremental exercise. Similar to the VE/VCO_2 slope, this parameter can be obtained during submaximal exercise and a near-maximal exercise effort is not required. The OUES has been reported to be a measurement of the efficiency of O_2 extraction and uptake. It is influenced by muscle mass, oxygen extraction and utilization, the level of $PaCO_2$ set point during exercise, physiologic dead space in the lung with ventilation/perfusion mismatch, and the onset of lactic acidosis. More than VE/VCO_2, the OUES incorporates cardiovascular, musculoskeletal, and respiratory function in a single index. As opposed to VE/VCO_2, a lower OUES is more abnormal as it indicates more ventilation being required to consume the same amount of VO_2. The OUES declines with age and is affected by lean body mass. In a study of normal subjects and patients with cardiac disease, the normal values for OUES were determined to be as follows: $1,175 - (15.8 \times age) + (841 \times body$ surface area) in women and $1,320 - (26.7 \times age) + (1,394 \times body$ surface area) in men.[7] OUES has also been shown to have additional prognostic value when compared to peak VO_2 and VE/VCO_2 slope in chronic HF patients with a value <1.47.[8] In Figure 22-14, there is a comparison between the OUES in a healthy subject and a patient with chronic HFrEF. The nonlogarithmic relationships are shown. The slope of the HF patient is substantially lower (23%) compared to that in the normal subject and it falls in the poor prognostic category. This patient went on to have a heart transplant. Despite its physiologic and potential clinical relevance, the OUES is rarely used alone to determine prognosis and therapy. Its use is limited by a few studies with limited numbers of patients, the lack of standardization of units, an unclear understanding of the most important physiologic mechanism explaining the relationship, the influence of body weight on the measurement, and the questionable additional prognostic value to other CPX variables. In addition, the OUES can also be abnormal in patients with pulmonary disease; however, there is less of an abnormality in pulmonary disease and a severely low OUES may discriminate between HF and lung disease.

The behavior of $PETCO_2$ during exercise can provide important information on pulmonary blood flow (cardiac output) and pulmonary artery pressure (PAP) and resistance (PVR). $PETCO_2$ represents the pressure of CO_2 at the end of every breath. CO_2 is carried to the lungs by pulmonary blood flow and the amount of measured $PETCO_2$ in the expired air is directly related to pulmonary blood flow and the resistance to flow in the pulmonary circulation. The $PETCO_2$ is ≥34 mm Hg at rest in healthy subjects. During moderate exercise up until the VT, the $PETCO_2$ increases relative to the increase in pulmonary blood flow (cardiac output). In healthy

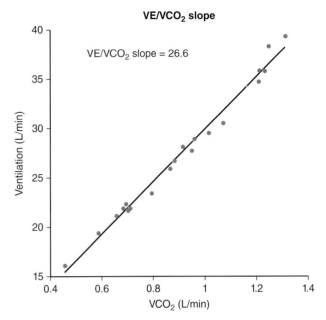

FIGURE 22-10 Normal VE/VCO_2 slope.

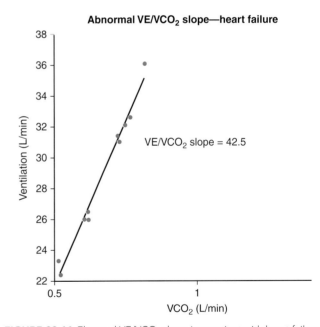

FIGURE 22-11 Elevated VE/VCO_2 slope in a patient with heart failure (either HFrEF or HFpEF).

subjects this represents an increase of 3 to 8 mm Hg. During more intense exercise above the VT, there is a rise in lactic acid with an associated heightened ventilatory response. This results in a decrease in the PETCO$_2$ to levels below that at the VT but greater than at rest. Patients with HF and pulmonary HTN have a different response related to decreases in pulmonary blood flow and increases in PVR. These changes in PETCO$_2$ at rest and during exercise in HF and pulmonary HTN patients compared to healthy subjects are illustrated in Figure 22-15. Resting PETCO$_2$ is usually lower in patients with significant HFrEF and even lower in patients with pulmonary HTN. This finding can be related to lower resting cardiac output and increased PVR secondary to pulmonary HTN. However, a low resting PETCO$_2$ could also be related to hyperventilation in patients who are naive to CPX testing and the use of a mouthpiece or face mask. Therefore, resting PETCO$_2$ has decreased specificity in determining a low resting cardiac output or pulmonary HTN. However, the response during submaximal exercise is clearly abnormal. In HF patients there is a blunted to no increase in PETCO$_2$ up to the VT. An increase ≤1.8 mm Hg has been associated with a worse clinical outcome.[9] In patients with pulmonary HTN, there is a paradoxical decrease in PETCO$_2$ between rest and exercise up to the VT. This abnormal response occurs in both precapillary (normal PCWP) and postcapillary (PCWP >15 mm Hg) pulmonary HTN but patients with precapillary pulmonary HTN usually have a more dramatic decrease. Thus the PETCO$_2$ response during exercise can indicate if there are abnormal cardiac hemodynamic responses in HF patients, with or without pulmonary HTN. Most of the data on PETCO$_2$ responses to exercise have been obtained in patients with HFrEF with limited information in HFpEF patients.

The pattern of ventilation during exercise can be important in determining the severity of HF with implications about prognosis. In Figure 22-16, there are regular oscillations of minute ventilation, VO$_2$, and VCO$_2$, all ventilatory-derived parameters. This regular waxing and waning of breathing is associated with fluctuation in O$_2$ and CO$_2$ tension. This variation in the pattern of ventilation during exercise is termed exercise oscillatory ventilation (EOV) and is associated with other forms of abnormal respiratory drive such as Cheyne-Stokes respiration and central sleep apnea. This pattern

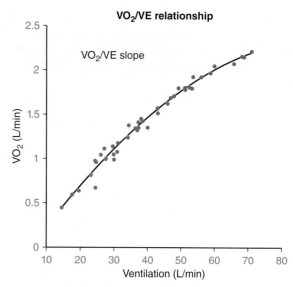

FIGURE 22-12 VE/VO$_2$ relationship during exercise.

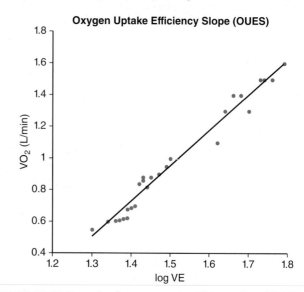

FIGURE 22-13 Example of oxygen uptake efficiency slope (OUES). Note that the log VE is used to get a linear regression line.

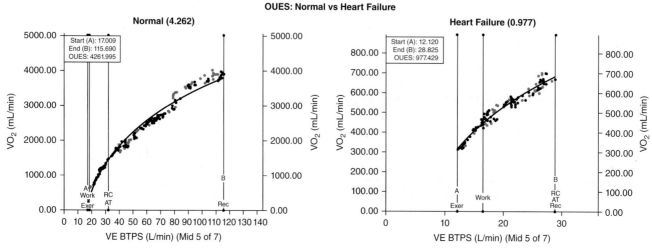

FIGURE 22-14 Comparison of the oxygen uptake efficiency slope (OUES) curves in a normal subject and a patient with systolic heart failure (HFrEF). A lower value for the OUES is indicative of excessive ventilation.

can occur at levels of exercise below the VT as demonstrated in Figure 22-17. Here the patient has not reached a RER of 1.0, indicating submaximal exercise, but he clearly has EOV. The probable mechanism for his pattern of breathing during exercise is illustrated in Figure 22-18. The driving factor appears to be a decreased cardiac output as demonstrated in invasive hemodynamic exercise studies in HF patients.[10] A decrease in cardiac output during exercise leads to circulatory delay and hypersensitivity of chemoreceptors results in both central and peripheral chemoreceptor activation. There is an increase in ventilatory drive alternating with periods of hypopnea related to frequent fluctuations in PaO_2 and $PaCO_2$. The exact mechanism has yet to be determined but the current data suggest a deregulation of the mechanisms involved in the neural and mechanical control of the circulatory system and respiration during exercise. Patients with EOV often have central sleep apnea and they should be screened for this disorder. The definition of EOV is related to the duration of the oscillations as well as the depth and duration of the VE curve. The current definition is the presence of oscillations in at least 60% of exercise with amplitudes that are at least 15% of the average resting values. In Figure 22-19, the Quantitation of a case of severe EOV is illustrated. Commercially available programs, such as the example MedGraphics instrument, can provide rapid analysis of the ventilatory pattern during exercise. This form of periodic breathing during exercise can limit the analysis of various ventilatory components during CPX testing such as VT, VE/VCO$_2$ slope, and OUES, due to the variability of the data. The prevalence of this finding has been reported to be between 12% and 30% in HF patients and EOV has been reported in both HFrEF

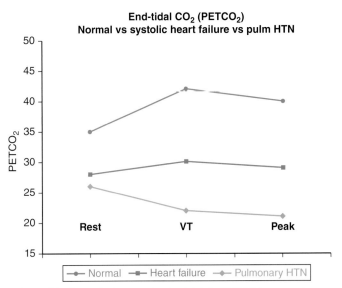

FIGURE 22-15 The behavior of end-tidal CO$_2$ (PETCO$_2$) at rest, the ventilatory threshold (VT), and peak exercise in a normal subject, a patient with HFrEF, and a patient who develops pulmonary hypertension during exercise.

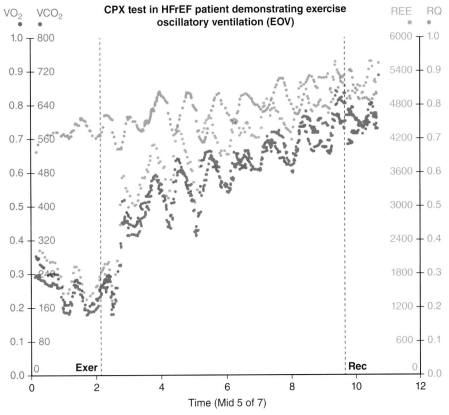

FIGURE 22-16 Minute ventilation, oxygen consumption (VO$_2$), carbon dioxide production (VCO$_2$), and respiratory exchange ratio (RER) responses during exercise in a heart failure patient with exercise oscillatory ventilation.

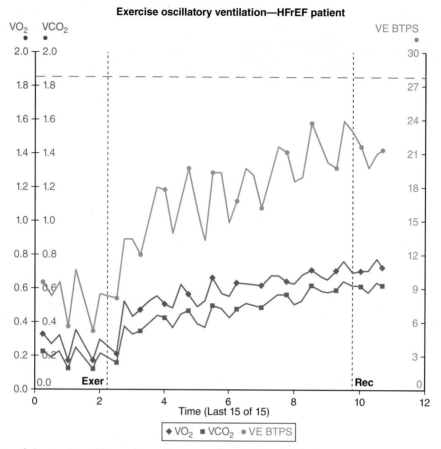

FIGURE 22-17 Another heart failure patient with exercise oscillatory ventilation. Note that the VCO$_2$ never exceeds the VO$_2$ during exercise, indicating a peak exercise RER <1.0. Despite not achieving near-maximal exercise, this patient displays very abnormal ventilatory behavior during exercise that suggests severe heart failure and a poor prognosis.

and HFpEF patients. Patients with EOV, especially early during exercise, have more severe HF with a poorer prognosis reported in HFrEF patients. In one study, systolic HF patients with EOV had a higher incidence of sudden death.[11] There is minimal information on the response of EOV to pharmacologic therapy but one study demonstrated an improvement related to an increase in cardiac index with sildenafil therapy.[10]

ASSIMILATION OF CARDIAC AND VENTILATORY DATA DURING A CARDIOPULMONARY EXERCISE TEST

Many of the described ventilatory responses to exercise during a CPX test require detailed analysis with the construction of specific graphs to complete the analysis. Although tabular data of VO$_2$, VCO$_2$, VE, RER, PETCO$_2$, PETO$_2$, VE/CO$_2$, and VE/O$_2$ are provided, it is difficult to determine the interrelationships of these physiologic parameters. Fortunately, the various measured and derived ventilatory and noninvasive cardiovascular data can be evaluated by analyzing the Wasserman 9-plot graph obtained with most commercial instruments (Figure 22-20). An analysis of the graphs from left to right and top to bottom can provide an overview of the findings in a CPX test and allow a noninvasive determination of the cardiovascular and ventilatory systems during exercise.

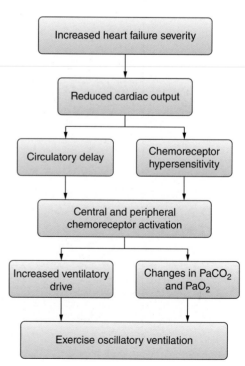

FIGURE 22-18 Potential mechanisms of the development of exercise oscillatory ventilation in heart failure.

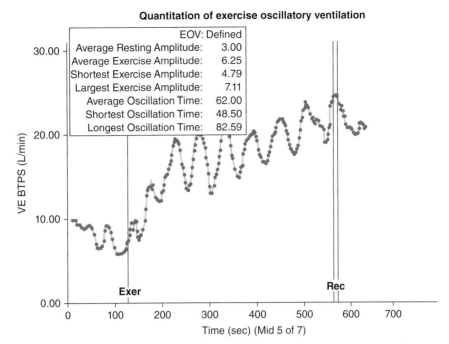

FIGURE 22-19 Quantitation of the amplitude and duration of ventilatory oscillations during exercise in a heart failure patient. This patient has ventilatory oscillations throughout exercise.

Information can be readily obtained about the uniformity of matching of ventilation to blood flow. Panels 2, 3, and 5 demonstrate the cardiovascular responses to exercise. Panel 2 demonstrates the HR and O_2 pulse responses to progressive exercise. Panel 3 indicates VO_2 and VCO_2 versus time and the work rate (WR). This allows an analysis of the $\Delta VO_2/\Delta WR$ relationship that is often abnormal in cardiac patients. Plot 5 indicates the HR versus VO_2 and the VCO_2 versus VO_2. An approximation of the VT can also be made from the data on this plot. Panels 1, 4, and 7 describe the ventilatory responses to exercise including VE versus time and work rate in panel 1, the VE/VCO_2 slope in panel 4, and the tidal volume versus VE in panel 7. Panels 5, 6, and 9 demonstrate the 3 methods than can be used to determine VT. In panel 9, O_2 saturation data from a pulse oximeter can also be evaluated. Panel 8 indicates the RER pattern during exercise.

ROLE OF PEAK EXERCISE VO₂ IN THE ASSESSMENT OF SEVERITY OF HEART FAILURE

Early studies using CPX testing in HF patients demonstrated that patients with higher New York Heart Association functional class had lower peak exercise VO_2 values. These patients often had elevated cardiac filling pressures and lower cardiac outputs. The use of resting LV ejection alone did not discriminate between patients with clinically stable and very symptomatic HF. The landmark study that demonstrated the clinical relevance of measuring peak VO_2 during exercise in patients with systolic HF was performed by Dr. Michael Weber at the University of Pennsylvania. Using CPX testing with invasive hemodynamic measurements, he demonstrated that patients with lower exercise cardiac indices had lower peak VO_2 values.[4] The systolic HF patients in his study were

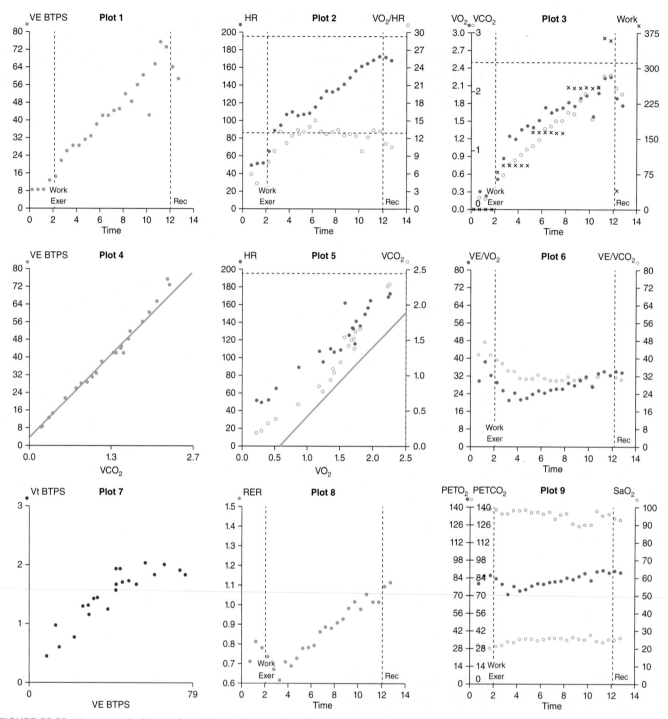

FIGURE 22-20 Wasserman 9-plot graph used to evaluate cardiac (plots 2, 3, 5), ventilation (plots 1, 4, 7), and ventilatory threshold (plots 5, 6, 9) during cardiopulmonary exercise testing. (Graph Plots Courtesy of MGC Diagnostics Corporation.)

divided into 4 groups, based on the severity of HF as determined by peak VO_2. The Weber classification was developed and categorized patients based on their exercise performance and not resting measurements of cardiac dysfunction (Figure 22-21). Patients in class D and E had lower cardiac indices at rest and during submaximal and peak exercise. The rate of increase in cardiac index with progressive exercise was also blunted. Although patients in class D and E had great O_2 extraction to compensate for the decrease in O_2 delivery, the Weber classes were defined more by the differences

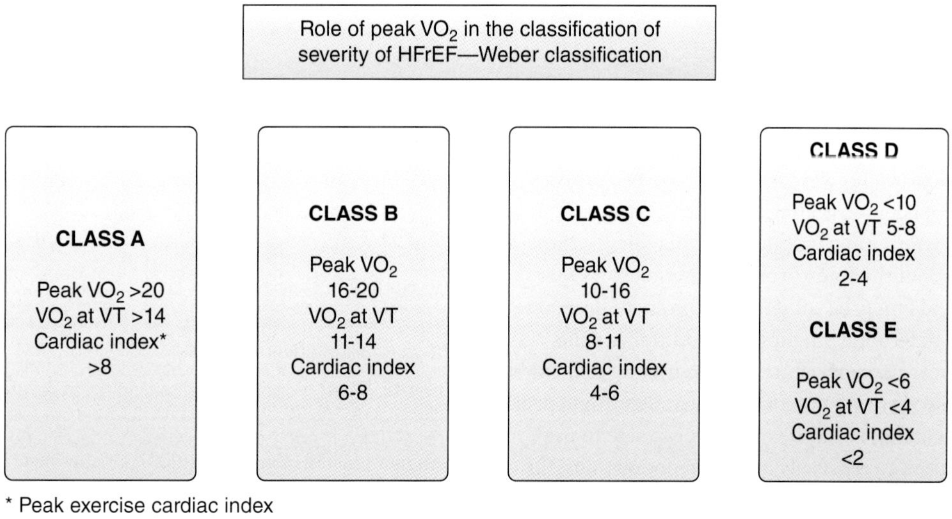

Role of peak VO$_2$ in the classification of
severity of HFrEF—Weber classification

CLASS A

Peak VO$_2$ >20
VO$_2$ at VT >14
Cardiac index*
>8

CLASS B

Peak VO$_2$
16-20
VO$_2$ at VT
11-14
Cardiac index
6-8

CLASS C

Peak VO$_2$
10-16
VO$_2$ at VT
8-11
Cardiac index
4-6

CLASS D

Peak VO$_2$ <10
VO$_2$ at VT 5-8
Cardiac index
2-4

CLASS E

Peak VO$_2$ <6
VO$_2$ at VT <4
Cardiac index
<2

* Peak exercise cardiac index

FIGURE 22-21 Weber classification of peak exercise VO$_2$ related to severity of systolic heart failure as indicated by progressive reduction in peak exercise cardiac index. (Data from Weber KT, Kinasewitz GT, Janicki JS, Fishman AP. Oxygen utilization and ventilation during exercise in patients with chronic cardiac failure. *Circulation.* 1982;65:1213-1223.)

in the cardiac index responses to exercise. These data validated the link between a ventilatory measurement, VO$_2$, and cardiovascular function as predicted by the Fick equation. In more recent studies, patients with HFpEF have also been found to have lower peak VO$_2$ values that correspond with greater severity of HF symptoms.

ROLE OF CPX TESTING IN ASSESSING PROGNOSIS IN SYSTOLIC HEART FAILURE

Because peak VO$_2$ is an indicator of severity in systolic HF, studies were performed to determine if a certain peak VO$_2$ value would indicate a poorer prognosis and determine the need for cardiac transplantation. Mancini and colleagues demonstrated that patients with a low left ventricular ejection fraction (LVEF) but a peak VO$_2$ >18 mL/kg/min had a good 1-year survival without transplantation.[12] Conversely, patients with a peak VO$_2$ <14 mL/kg/min and especially those with a peak VO$_2$ <10 mL/kg/min had a higher mortality without transplantation. Peak VO$_2$ was subsequently included in the Heart Failure Survival Score that included other clinical and hemodynamic variables that improved the determination of prognosis in systolic HF patients.[13] Other studies were also performed that demonstrated the prognostic value of a percent predicted peak VO$_2$ <50% and a peak VO$_2$ corrected for lean body mass (LBM) of <19 mL/kg. These studies were performed prior to the use of beta blockers in the treatment of HF. Patients taking beta blockers may not improve their peak VO$_2$ substantially but generally have a greater survival than patients with comparable peak VO$_2$ values without beta blockade. More recent studies in systolic HF patients taking beta blockers have confirmed the value of peak exercise VO$_2$ in determining prognosis. However, the peak VO$_2$ values are lower than those obtained in the earlier studies. A peak exercise VO$_2$ <12 mL/kg/min has been accepted as the new prognostic threshold in systolic HF. The addition of peak VO$_2$ to the Seattle Heart Failure Model was also shown to have added prognostic value. In 2 large CPX testing cohorts, the HF-ACTION trial and the Henry Ford Hospital Cardiopulmonary Exercise Test-ing (FIT-CPX) Project, peak VO_2, percent predicted peak VO_2, and exercise duration retained their prognostic values in systolic HF patients after multivariable analyses.[14,15] In a small retrospective study of patients with HFpEF in the FIT-CPX Project, peak VO_2 and percent predicted peak VO_2 were shown to have prognostic value. Despite these data demonstrating the potential value of peak exercise VO_2 in determining prognosis in HF patients, there are several concerns about the sole use of this parameter. VO_2 is a continuous variable and it may be somewhat arbitrary to designate a certain threshold to determine prognosis. In addition, a valid peak VO_2 requires a near-maximal effort and this may be difficult in many HF patients. Also there are other factors that determine peak VO_2, such as age and gender; it may be more appropriate to use percent predicted peak VO_2, especially in certain populations. Of course, this method assumes that the prediction equation is valid for a given population. Because of these concerns about the use of peak VO_2 in assessing prognosis in chronic systolic HF, other CPX parameters have also been evaluated. The most consistent finding is the validation of the VE/VCO_2 slope as an important predictor of survival in patients with chronic systolic HF. Values >34 have been associated with a poorer clinical outcome[4] and a ventilatory classification schema has been developed to assess severity and risk of adverse cardiac events at 2 years after evalua-tion.[16] This schema is presented in Figure 22-22. Patients with a very high VE/VCO_2 slope have the worse outcome. It should be noted that patients with a relatively good peak exercise VO_2 but a significantly elevated VE/VCO_2 slope still had a higher rate of adverse events. In addition to an elevated VE/VCO_2 slope, other CPX variables have been shown to have prognostic value in HF patients. These include a VO_2 <11 mL/kg/min at the VT, OUES <1.47, $\Delta PETCO_2$ ≤1.8 mm Hg, $PETCO_2$ during exercise <33 mm Hg, presence of EOV, abnormal HR recovery ≤6 bpm at 1 min, and a peak systolic BP <120 mm Hg. A meta-analysis of 30 studies that reported the prognostic value of CPX variables indicated that peak VO_2, VE/VCO_2 slope, and EOV were all highly significant prognostic indicators.[17] OUES was also found to be a potentially valuable prognostic indicator but there were only 2 studies that supported its use. Because these variables may have different prog-nostic values, attempts have been made to consolidate these various factors into a unified concept. A CPX test score has been evaluated and validated in HF patients.[18] CPX test variables were assigned numerical values based on their statistical strength in determining prognosis. VE/VCO_2 slope ≥34 received 7 points, abnormal HR recovery ≤6 bpm at 1 min received 5 points, OUES ≤1.4 received 3 points, $PETCO_2$ <33 mm Hg received 3 points, and peak VO_2 ≤14 mL/kg/min received 1 point. Patients with a score >15 had the worse outcome (death, transplantation, or LV assist device) at 2 years with event-free survival <50%. In contrast, a score of 0 to 5 indicated an event-free survival of >90% at 2 years. A recent position paper by the European Society of Cardiology also recom-mends the use of multiple CPX parameters to assess prognosis in HFrEF patients.[19] In a recent review of cardiopulmonary test-ing in HF, an integrated assessment of CPX variable for cardiac risk stratification was presented.[20] This schema is represented in Figure 22-23. Systolic HF patients at low risk of a cardiac event had

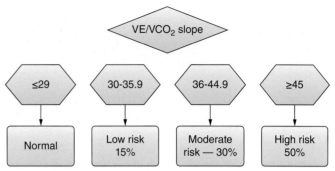

FIGURE 22-22 Ventilatory classification of severity of systolic heart failure using VE/VCO_2 slope data. (Data from Arena R, Myers J, Abella J, et al. Development of a ventilatory classification system in patients with heart failure. *Circulation.* 2007;115:2410-2417.)

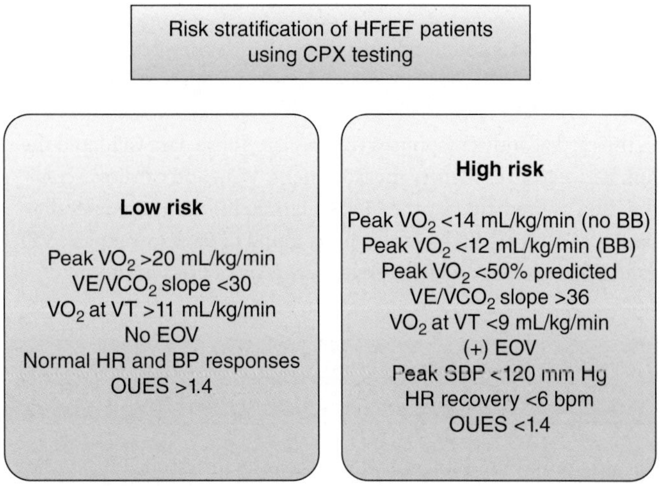

Risk stratification of HFrEF patients using CPX testing

Low risk

Peak VO_2 >20 mL/kg/min
VE/VCO_2 slope <30
VO_2 at VT >11 mL/kg/min
No EOV
Normal HR and BP responses
OUES >1.4

High risk

Peak VO_2 <14 mL/kg/min (no BB)
Peak VO_2 <12 mL/kg/min (BB)
Peak VO_2 <50% predicted
VE/VCO_2 slope >36
VO_2 at VT <9 mL/kg/min
(+) EOV
Peak SBP <120 mm Hg
HR recovery <6 bpm
OUES <1.4

FIGURE 22-23 Integrated approach of using multiple ventilatory and noninvasive hemodynamic variables in the assessment of risk of mor-tality in patients with chronic systolic heart failure. (Data from Malhotra R, Bakken K, D'Elia E, Lewis GD. Cardiopulmonary exercise testing in heart failure. *J Am Coll Cardiol HF.* 2016;4:607-616.)

a higher peak VO_2, lower VE/VCO_2 and OUES, normal systolic BP and HR recovery responses, and no EOV. Patients at high risk (>20% 1-year mortality) have a combination of abnormal findings including a low peak VO_2 significantly elevated VE/VCO^2 and OUES, EOV, a blunted or decrease in systolic blood pressure at peak exercise, and delayed HR recovery. These patients should be considered for advanced HF therapy including heart transplantation and mechanical circulatory support.

USING CARDIOPULMONARY EXERCISE TESTING TO ASSESS FOR PULMONARY HYPERTENSION

Pulmonary HTN is commonly seen in patients with both HFrEF and HFpEF and this finding is usually associated with worsening symptoms and outcomes. Severe mitral regurgitation is frequently observed in patients with progressive systolic HF, leading to high PCWP and PA pressures. In addition, patients with precapillary pulmonary HTN can present with exertional dyspnea and signs and symptoms of RV dysfunction that mimic left-sided HF. Some patients, especially those with HFpEF, may have normal pulmonary artery pressures at rest but they become significantly elevated during exercise. CPX testing may help detect some of these patients by the analysis of several ventilatory parameters (Figure 22-24). Several studies have shown the predictive value of elevated VE/VCO_2 slopes, the lack of decrease in VE/VCO_2 from rest to a fixed submaximal workload, a minimal increase or decrease in $PETCO_2$ with exercise, a peak $PETCO_2$ of ≤34 mm Hg during exercise, and the presence of EOV.[21,22] The sensitivity and specificity of CPX testing for detecting pulmonary HTN is significantly increased when abnormalities in VE/VCO_2 slope, $PETCO_2$, and EOV are all present. In addition, the more abnormal the findings, the more likely there is precapillary or irreversible pulmonary HTN. The pathophysiology of these findings includes abnormalities in perfusion and cardiac filling pressures. The blunting or prevention of an increase in $PETCO_2$ during exercise can be explained by increased PVR and possibly low cardiac output. With high cardiac filling pressures and altered perfusion of the lung, there is V/Q mismatch, leading to enhanced ventilatory drive and an increase in the VE/VCO_2 slope. Finally, with hypoperfusion of the lung from decreased pulmonary blood flow, there is circulatory delay and deregulation of the mechanical and neural control mechanisms of breathing and circulation leading to EOV. These CPX parameters will be more abnormal with more severe pulmonary HTN. These findings have important clinical implications in the management of these HF patients.

THE ROLE OF CARDIOPULMONAR EXERCISE TESTING IN THE ASSESSMENT OF EXERTIONAL DYSPNEA

Although dyspnea on exertion is a common symptom of HF, this symptom is also frequently seen in patients with chronic lung disease. Most studies performed to evaluate structure and function in HF patients occur at rest. CPX testing in combination with resting spirometry can be useful to differentiate between a cardiac and pulmonary cause of dyspnea. Many CPX findings are similar in HF

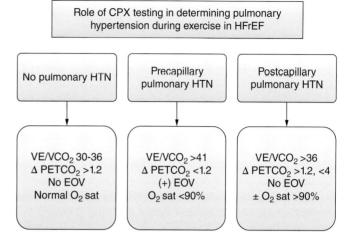

FIGURE 22-24 Use of CPX data to evaluate the presence of precapillary and postcapillary pulmonary hypertension in patients with systolic heart failure. (Data from Woods PR, Frantz RP, Taylor BJ, et al. The usefulness of submaximal gas exchange to define pulmonary arterial hypertension. *J Heart Lung Transplant.* 2011;30:1133-1142 and Guazzi M, Cahalin LP, Arena R. Cardiopulmonary exercise testing as a diagnostic tool for the detection of left-sided pulmonary hypertension in heart failure. *J Card Fail.* 2013;19:461-467.)

and pulmonary patients including a low peak VO_2, an increased VE/VCO_2 slope, and a reduced VO_2 at the VT. In some cases, patients with lung disease will not be able to exercise sufficiently to obtain a valid VT but the discriminating value of this finding is low. Patients with HF usually do not breathe at a high percent of their breathing reserve, which is defined as (1-peak exercise VE – maximal voluntary ventilation). Maximal voluntary ventilation (MVV) can be accurately estimated as $41 \times FEV_1$ from spirometry testing. A breathing reserve <20% means that a patient is breathing at >80% of his or her MVV and this finding is usually seen in patients with chronic lung disease. OUES is also less dependent on lung function and is often normal in patients with lung disease. In contrast, HF patients often have a low OUES and it is a marker of severity and predictor of poorer clinical outcomes. A recent study evaluating many CPX testing parameters in HF and chronic obstructive pulmonary disease (COPD) patients determined that breathing reserve and OUES were the most reliable factors to differentiate between the 2 disease states.[23] A flow diagram describing the evaluation of patients with exertional dyspnea is presented in Figure 22-25. The evaluation of the relationship between mixed-expired CO_2 ($PECO_2$) and $PETCO_2$ can also be used to determine if the primary disease state is COPD or HF.[24] $PECO_2$ can be estimated by dividing 863 by the VE/VCO_2 ratio. $PETCO_2$ is directly measured in the expired air. $PECO_2$ is always lower than $PETCO_2$. These measurements relate to both the dead space/tidal volume relationship in the lung and pulmonary blood flow (V/Q mismatch). The ratio of $PECO_2/PETCO_2$ is an indicator of alterations in ventilation and perfusion. Even in the absence of disease there is some physiologic dead space in the lung, represented as VD/VT. In normal subjects this ratio is approximately 0.75. In the patient with HF, dead space increases but perfusion decreases to nearly the same extent. The same physiology occurs in pulmonary HTN. The $PECO_2$ pressure does not decrease out of proportion to the decrease in $PETCO_2$ and the ratio of both of these factors does not significantly change. It is mildly reduced in both HF at 0.7 and pulmonary HTN at 0.7 to 0.75. The behavior in $PETCO_2$ during exercise can help differentiate between the 2 disease states. In contrast, the $PECO_2/PETCO_2$ ratio is reduced to 0.6 in chronic obstructive pulmonary disease (COPD). Therefore, this ratio may help differentiate HF from COPD as a cause of dyspnea.

CPX FINDINGS WITH DEVELOPMENT OF MYOCARDIAL ISCHEMIA

Many patients with HFrEF have ischemic cardiomyopathy and coronary artery disease is common in patients with HFpEF. The development of myocardial ischemia could be the cause of exertional dyspnea or fatigue in some of these patients. CPX testing not only provides information on functional capacity but there are findings that suggest the development of myocardial ischemia during exercise. Oxygen pulse (VO_2/HR) is a surrogate for stroke volume during exercise and changes in the character of the VO_2/HR response to progressive exercise have been associated with the development of myocardial ischemia.[25] As shown in Figure 22-26, VO_2/HR increases during progressive exercise in a normal subject.

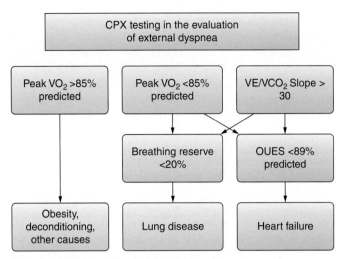

FIGURE 22-25 Use of CPX testing data to determine a pulmonary versus cardiac cause of dyspnea. This analysis is relevant in patients with both HFrEF and HFpEF. (Data from Barron A, Francis DP, Mayet J, et al. Oxygen uptake efficiency slope and breathing reserve, not anaerobic threshold, discriminate between patients with cardiovascular disease over chronic obstructive pulmonary disease. *J Am Coll Cardiol HF.* 2016;4:252-261.)

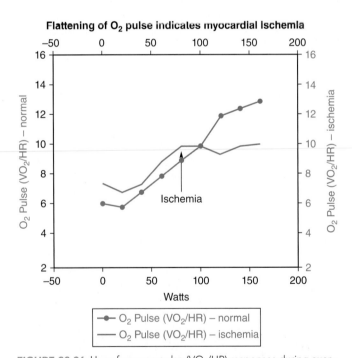

FIGURE 22-26 Use of oxygen pulse (VO_2/HR) responses during exercise to determine the onset and presence of myocardial ischemia. (Data from Belardinelli R, Lacalaprice F, Carle F, et al. Exercise-induced myocardial ischemia detected by cardiopulmonary exercise testing. *Eur Heart J.* 2003;24:1304-1313.)

However, in the patient with myocardial ischemia, there is a plateau in the VO_2/HR response throughout the remainder of exercise. A similar finding can be seen when evaluating the VO_2 response to progressive exercise. There is a flattening of the VO_2 response with ischemia as illustrated in Figure 22-27. Myocardial ischemia can also be suspected with an acceleration of the HR response during exercise.[26] In Figure 22-28, there is an abrupt increase in the slope of the HR/workload relationship at the onset of symptoms of ischemia. The mechanism responsible for this change has not been determined but could be related to a reduction in stroke volume or heightened sympathetic stimulation. Although these findings on CPX testing in the setting of myocardial ischemia are provocative, there are several unanswered questions including the effect of cardiac medications, the adaptability to treadmill testing as all these studies were performed with a cycle ergometer, and the effect of gender and exercise capacity. Although changes in VO_2/HR, VO_2/WR, and HR/WR have been observed on CPX testing in HF patients, there is usually no abrupt change in the pattern. Therefore, an abrupt change in 1 of these parameters could indicate myocardial ischemia.

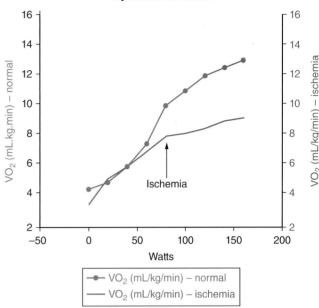

FIGURE 22-27 Use of VO_2 response to progressive exercise workload in determining the onset of myocardial ischemia during exercise. (Data from Belardinelli R, Lacalaprice F, Carle F, et al. Exercise-induced myocardial ischemia detected by cardiopulmonary exercise testing. *Eur Heart J.* 2003;24:1304 1313.)

SAFETY OF CARDIOPULMONARY EXERCISE TESTING IN SYSTOLIC HEART FAILURE PATIENTS

The safety of CPX testing in patients with chronic systolic HF and a LVEF <35% was evaluated in the HF-ACTION study.[27] In the study, 2331 patients with NYHA class II-IV systolic HF performed 4411 CPX tests using a standard protocol. There were no test-related exacerbations of HF, myocardial infarctions or acute coronary syndromes, transient ischemic attacks, strokes, or deaths. There was 1 episode of ventricular fibrillation and 1 sustained ventricular tachycardia that occurred within 24 hours of testing. Both were successfully treated. There were no ICD discharges during exercise testing in these subjects. There were 0 deaths and 0.45 nonfatal major cardiovascular events per 1000 exercise tests. It is important to note that >90% of the subjects were taking appropriate doses of evidence-based HF medications and they were clinically stable at the time of testing. Due to orthopedic/musculoskeletal complaints, 13% of the patients stopped the exercise test. These patients were older, less physically fit as determined by peak exercise VO_2, and were Caucasian. There were no other demographic differences from the patients who stopped exercise due to cardiorespiratory signs and symptoms. The results of this study indicate that symptom-limited CPX testing is safe in stable, chronic systolic HF patients on optimal medical therapy.

SUMMARY

CPX testing is an important part of the management schema in patients with both HFrEF and HFpEF. The results of this testing provide important information on the physiology of exercise, the degree of functional impairment, the severity of HF, and the

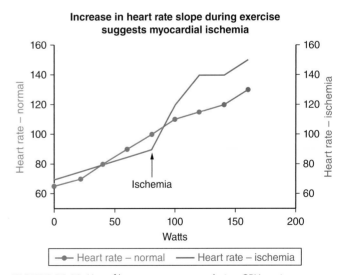

FIGURE 22-28 Use of heart rate response during CPX testing to determine the onset and presence of myocardial ischemia in a patient with nonobstructive coronary disease. (Data from Chaudhry S, Kumar N, Behbahani H, et al. Abnormal heart-rate response during cardiopulmonary exercise testing identifies cardiac dysfunction in symptomatic patients with non-obstructive coronary artery disease. *Int J Cardiol.* 2017;228:114-121.)

assessment of prognosis that will guide future therapeutic endeavors. There are both cardiovascular and ventilatory parameters obtained during CPX testing that provide a composite evaluation of the interaction between the cardiovascular, respiratory, musculoskeletal, and nervous systems during exercise in these patients. It is clearly superior to other forms of testing used to evaluate functional capacity due to its wealth of clinically and physiologically relevant data.

Recent studies have included other forms of cardiovascular testing performed in combination with CPX testing. These include the use of invasive hemodynamic testing and echocardiography to better define the pathophysiology of exercise in both HFrEF and HFpEF patients. There are also instruments available that will measure cardiac output by an inert gas rebreathing technique or impedance cardiography. This allows the generation of additional parameters such as cardiac output, stroke volume, cardiac power (mean arterial pressure × cardiac output/451) to aid in the evaluation and therapy of patients with chronic HF. It is too premature to determine if any of these additional parameters will improve the diagnostic capabilities of standard CPX testing but the application of noninvasive testing will have more general appeal to both clinicians and HF patients.

ACKNOWLEDGMENT

This chapter is dedicated to my parents, Edward and Helen Wolfel. They are responsible for providing me the opportunity to pursue a medical career and achieve success in life. They have also instilled in me the importance of caring for other people and this attitude has resulted in my desire to be involved in the management of patients with chronic heart failure.

REFERENCES

1. Balady GJ, Arena R, Sietsema K, et al. Clinician's guide to cardiopulmonary exercise testing in adults: a scientific statement from the American Heart Association. *Circulation.* 2010;122:1191-1225.

2. Mezzani A, Agostoni P, Cohen-Solal A, et al. Standards for the use of cardiopulmonary exercise testing for the functional evaluation of cardiac patients: a report from the Exercise Physiology Section of the European Association of Cardiovascular Prevention and Rehabilitation. *Eur J Cardiovasc Prev Rehabil.* 2009;16:249-267.

3. Wasserman K, Hansen JE, Sue DY, et al. Normal values. In: *Principles of Exercise Testing and Interpretation.* 5th ed. Philadelphia, PA: Lippincott Williams & Wilkins; 2012:154-180.

4. Weber KT, Kinasewitz GT, Janicki JS, Fishman AP. Oxygen utilization and ventilation during exercise in patients with chronic cardiac failure. *Circulation.* 1982;65:1213-1223.

5. Keteyian SJ, Brawner CA, Ehrman JK, et al. Reproducibility of peak oxygen uptake and other cardiopulmonary exercise parameters: implications for clinical trials and clinical practice. *Chest.* 2010;138:950-955.

6. Chua TP, Ponikowski P, Harrington D, et al. Clinical correlates and prognostic significance of the ventilatory response to exercise in chronic heart failure. *J Am Coll Cardiol.* 1997;29:1585-1590.

7. Hollenberg M, Tager IR. Oxygen uptake efficiency slope: an index of exercise performance and cardiopulmonary reserve requiring only submaximal exercise. *J Am Coll Cardiol.* 2000;36:194-201.

8. Davies LC, Wensel R, Georgiadou P, et al. Enhanced prognostic value from cardiopulmonary exercise testing in chronic heart failure by nonlinear analysis: oxygen uptake efficiency slope. *Eur Heart J.* 2006;27:684-690.

9. Arena R, Guazzi M, Myers J. Prognostic value of end-tidal carbon dioxide during exercise testing in heart failure. *Int J Cardiol.* 2007;117:103-108.

10. Murphy RM, Shah RV, Malhotra R, et al. Exercise oscillatory ventilation in systolic heart failure: an indicator of impaired hemodynamic response to exercise. *Circulation.* 2011;124:1442-1451.

11. Guazzi M, Raimondo R, Vicenzi M, et al. Exercise oscillatory ventilation may predict sudden cardiac death in heart failure patients. *J Am Coll Cardiol.* 2007;50:299-308.

12. Mancini DM, Eisen H, Kussmaul W, et al. Value of peak exercise oxygen consumption for optimal timing of cardiac transplantation in ambulatory patients with heart failure. *Circulation.* 1991;83:778-786.

13. Aaronson KD, Schwartz SJ, Chen JM, et al. Development and prospective validation of a clinical index to predict survival in ambulatory patients referred for cardiac transplant evaluation. *Circulation.* 1997;95:2660-2667.

14. Brawner CA, Shafiq A, Aldred HA, et al. Comprehensive analysis of cardiopulmonary exercise testing and mortality in patients with systolic heart failure: The Henry Ford Hospital Cardiopulmonary Exercise Testing (FIT-CPX) Project. *J Card Fail.* 2015;21:710-718.

15. Keteyian SJ, Patel M, Kraus WE, et al. Variables measured during cardiopulmonary exercise testing as predictors of mortality in chronic systolic heart failure. *J Am Coll Cardiol.* 2016;67:780-789.

16. Arena R, Myers J, Abella J, et al. Development of a ventilatory classification system in patients with heart failure. *Circulation.* 2007;115:2410-2417.

17. Cahalin LP, Chase P, Arena R, et al. A meta-analysis of the prognostic significance of cardiopulmonary exercise testing in patients with heart failure. *Heart Fail Rev.* 2013;18:79-84.

18. Myers J, Arena R, Dewey F. A CPX testing score for predicting outcome in patients with heart failure. *Am Heart J.* 2008;156:1177-1183.

19. Corra U, Piepolo MF, Adamopoulos S, et al. Cardiopulmonary exercise testing in systolic heart failure in 2014: the evolving prognostic role. A position paper from the committee on exercise physiology and training of the heart failure association of the ESC. *Eur Heart J.* 2014;16:929-941.

20. Malhotra R, Bakken K, D'Elia E, Lewis GD. Cardiopulmonary exercise testing in heart failure. *J Am Coll Cardiol HF.* 2016;4:607-616.

21. Woods PR, Frantz RP, Taylor BJ, et al. The usefulness of submaximal gas exchange to define pulmonary arterial hypertension. *J Heart Lung Transplant.* 2011;30:1133-1142.

22. Guazzi M, Cahalin LP, Arena R. Cardiopulmonary exercise testing as a diagnostic tool for the detection of left-sided pulmonary hypertension in heart failure. *J Card Fail.* 2013;19:461-467.

23. Barron A, Francis DP, Mayet J, et al. Oxygen uptake efficiency slope and breathing reserve, not anaerobic threshold, discriminate between patients with cardiovascular disease over chronic obstructive pulmonary disease. *J Am Coll Cardiol HF.* 2016;4:252-261.

24. Hansen JE, Ulubay G, Chow BF, et al. Mixed-expired and end-tidal CO_2 distinguish between ventilation and perfusion defects during exercise testing in patients with lung and heart diseases. *Chest.* 2007;132:977-983.

25. Belardinelli R, Lacalaprice F, Carle F, et al. Exercise-induced myocardial ischemia detected by cardiopulmonary exercise testing. *Eur Heart J.* 2003;24:1304-1313.

26. Chaudhry S, Kumar N, Behbahani H, et al. Abnormal heart-rate response during cardiopulmonary exercise testing identifies cardiac dysfunction in symptomatic patients with non-obstructive coronary artery disease. *Int J Cardiol.* 2017;228:114-121.

27. Keteyian SJ, Isaac D, Thadani U, et al. Safety of symptom-limited cardiopulmonary exercise testing in patients with chronic heart failure due to severe left ventricular systolic dysfunction. *Am Heart J.* 2009;158:S72-S77.

23 CARDIAC MAGNETIC RESONANCE IMAGING

Emily A. Ruden, MD
Karolina M. Zareba, MD

INTRODUCTION

Cardiac magnetic resonance (CMR) imaging has become a powerful diagnostic tool in the assessment of cardiomyopathy. CMR not only provides a comprehensive evaluation of structure and function, but also allows for tissue characterization. CMR is the gold standard for quantification of cardiac volumes and function; it allows 3-dimensional visualization of the heart, as well as detailed flow evaluation with velocity encoded cine imaging. Tissue characterization has become the most exciting aspect of CMR in the field of heart failure (HF). The use of late gadolinium enhancement (LGE) allows for direct visualization of focal ischemic and nonischemic scar. Advances in T1 mapping now enable quantification of diffuse myocardial fibrosis by measuring the extent of interstitial expansion via extracellular volume (ECV) fraction. Further tissue characterization is performed with T2 mapping allowing for visualization of myocardial edema, while T2 star mapping directly quantifies myocardial iron content. The comprehensive nature of CMR not only yields high-quality diagnostic data, but also significant prognostic information, especially in patients with HF. This chapter will highlight the critical role of CMR in the assessment of cardiomyopathies.

ISCHEMIC CARDIOMYOPATHY

PATIENT CASE 1: DETERMINING VIABILITY

A 50-year-old woman with a history of coronary artery disease (CAD) and coronary artery bypass grafting, prior myocardial infarction (MI), and ischemic cardiomyopathy presented with dyspnea and decompensated systolic HF. Her bypass grafts were

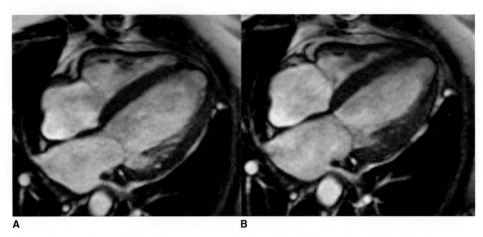

A   **B**

FIGURE 23-1 Horizontal long-axis steady-state free precession (SSFP) cine at end diastole (A) and end systole (B) in a patient with severe ischemic cardiomyopathy.

found to be occluded, including her left internal mammary artery, and she was being evaluated for possible repeat bypass surgery. CMR was ordered to assess myocardial viability.

Assessment of cardiac function with electrocardiogram (ECG)-gated steady-state free precession (SSFP) cine imaging, a key element of the standard CMR cardiomyopathy protocol, demonstrated multiple regional wall motion abnormalities (Figure 23-1) and moderate to severe left ventricular (LV) systolic dysfunction. LGE imaging showed near transmural MI of the basal to mid inferolateral wall and the entire apex (Figure 23-2), consistent with nonviable myocardium. Subendocardial infarction involving 50% of myocardial wall thickness was present in the anteroseptal, anterior, and anterolateral segments (Figure 23-3), suggesting partial viability. Given multiple segments with limited to no viability, high risk of redo sternotomy, and concern for medication noncompliance with dual antiplatelet therapy, the patient was managed with aggressive goal-directed medical therapy.

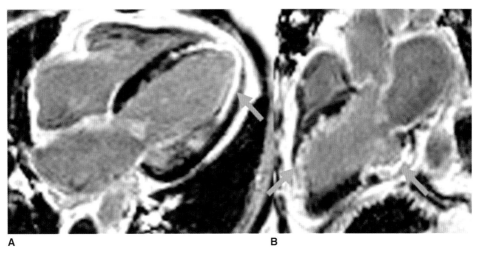

FIGURE 23-2 Subendocardial to transmural hyperenhancement (*blue arrows*) in horizontal long-axis (A) and 3-chamber (B) views on late gadolinium enhancement images represents infarcted myocardium.

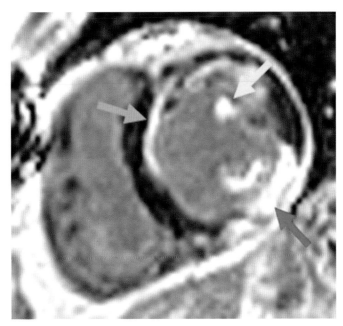

FIGURE 23-3 Subendocardial myocardial infarction (*blue arrow*), transmural myocardial infarction (*red arrow*), and papillary muscle infarction (*yellow arrow*) on late gadolinium enhancement short-axis image.

DISCUSSION

In acute MI, damaged myocyte membranes allow gadolinium to diffuse into the intracellular space, resulting in increased tissue concentration of gadolinium compared with normal myocardium. Likewise, in chronic infarction, as necrotic tissue is replaced by collagenous scar, the interstitial space expands, which leads to increased gadolinium tissue concentration. Higher tissue concentrations of gadolinium shorten the T1 relaxation time and thus appear bright, or hyperenhanced, whereas viable regions appear black, or nulled.[1] In patients with ischemic cardiomyopathy, the transmural extent of infarction predicts improvement in contractile function, with 51% to 75% transmural extent associated with limited viability and 76% to 100% associated with virtually no viability.[2,3] The high spatial resolution of CMR allows for a more accurate determination of the transmural extent of viability as opposed to other imaging methods. This distinction is critical because it has been repeatedly shown that revascularization of patients with viable myocardium leads to significant improvement in clinical outcome.[3]

PATIENT CASE 2: ANTERIOR MYOCARDIAL INFARCTION COMPLICATED BY LEFT VENTRICULAR THROMBUS

A 55-year-old man with a history of diabetes mellitus type 2 and hypertension (HTN) presented to the emergency department with 4 days of chest pain associated with nausea. His ECG showed anterior and lateral ST elevations, for which he was emergently taken to the cardiac catheterization laboratory. Angiographic imaging demonstrated 100% occlusion of his mid left anterior descending artery (LAD), at which time he received a bare metal stent with restoration of TIMI-3 flow (Figure 23-4). Subsequent echocardiogram showed moderate, segmental LV dysfunction with an ejection fraction (EF) of 35% to 40% (Figure 23-5) and an apical LV

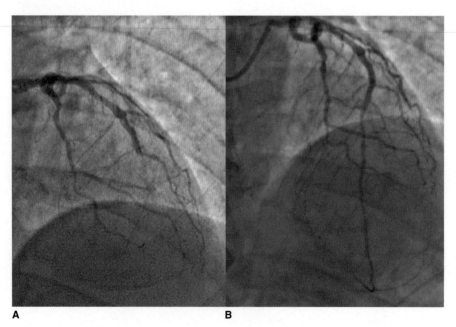

A   **B**

FIGURE 23-4 Angiography demonstrating 100% left anterior descending artery (LAD) occlusion before (A) and after (B) percutaneous intervention in a patient presenting with an anterior STEMI.

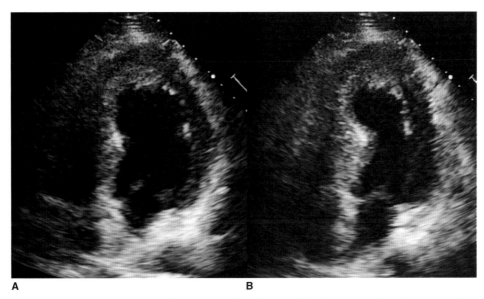

FIGURE 23-5 Apical 4-chamber echocardiogram at end diastole (A) and end systole (B) with apical wall motion abnormality after an anterior STEMI.

thrombus (Figure 23-6), for which he was placed on warfarin. Six months after his MI, he was enrolled in a research trial and received intracoronary stem cell therapy. He was referred for CMR imaging as part of the research protocol.

Cine SSFP imaging (Figure 23-7) demonstrated persistent anterior and anteroseptal akinesis with moderate LV systolic dysfunction. LGE imaging (Figure 23-8) demonstrated transmural scar of the apical anterior, septal, and inferior walls, and the true apex, along with near transmural extension of the infarct into the distal portion of the mid anteroseptum and inferoseptum, consistent with prior LAD-territory infarction. CMR confirmed a large residual thrombus in the LV apex (Figure 23-8).

DISCUSSION

In a large cohort of 738 ST elevation myocardial infarction (STEMI) patients, the prevalence of LV thrombus as assessed by CMR was 3.5% and increased to 7.1% for anterior STEMIs. The presence of an LV thrombus was associated with larger infarct size, lesser myocardial salvage, and a lower EF. Moreover, LV thrombus was independently associated with major adverse cardiac events at 1 year.[4] CMR is superior to transthoracic echocardiography for the detection of LV thrombus, with reported sensitivities of 88% and 33% to 40%, respectively.[5] On LGE imaging, thrombus appears as a low-signal-intensity mass surrounded by high-signal-intensity structures including the ventricular cavity and surrounding myocardium. The absence of contrast enhancement can be used to distinguish thrombus from other masses such as neoplasm, which typically demonstrate contrast uptake due to tumor-associated vascularity. LGE imaging can be further tailored for thrombus assessment by prolonging the inversion time, thus exploiting the avascular tissue properties of the thrombus. At prolonged inversion times, even severely damaged myocardium with microvascular obstruction exhibits some degree of contrast uptake, whereas the thrombus exhibits none and appears black.[6] Delayed enhancement

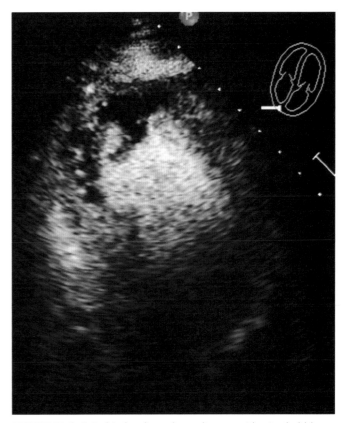

FIGURE 23-6 Apical 4-chamber echocardiogram with microbubble contrast demonstrating an apical filling defect.

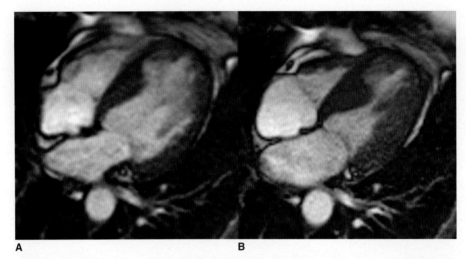

FIGURE 23-7 Horizontal long-axis steady-state free precession (SSFP) cine at end diastole (A) and end systole (B) demonstrating ischemic cardiomyopathy after an anterior STEMI.

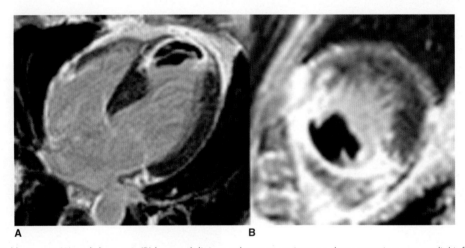

FIGURE 23-8 Horizontal long-axis (A) and short-axis (B) late gadolinium enhancement images demonstrating myocardial infarction (*white*) and a large apical left ventricular (LV) thrombus (*black*).

CMR is thus highly superior to anatomic cine imaging at identifying the presence of even small thrombi.

■ NONISCHEMIC CARDIOMYOPATHIES

PATIENT CASE 3: DILATED CARDIOMYOPATHY

A 42-year-old man with no prior medical history presented with 3 months of dyspnea, orthopnea, paroxysmal nocturnal dyspnea (PND), and lower extremity edema. He was initially treated with inhalers for an upper respiratory infection, but his symptoms did not improve. Chest radiography demonstrated cardiomegaly, for which he was referred to cardiology, and subsequent transthoracic echocardiography (TTE) revealed an EF of 5%. Resting nuclear perfusion images demonstrated an extensive area of decreased perfusion within the inferoposterior and inferolateral segments from base to apex but no evidence of ischemia. Cardiac catheterization showed normal coronary arteries. He was referred for CMR to evaluate his cardiomyopathy.

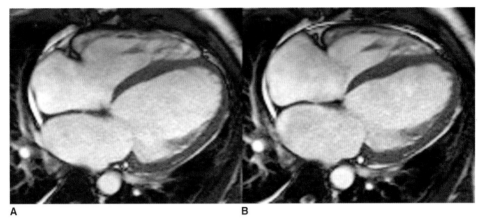

FIGURE 23-9 Horizontal long-axis steady-state free precession (SSFP) cine at end diastole (A) and end systole (B) in a patient with idiopathic, dilated cardiomyopathy.

Cine SSFP imaging confirmed severe biventricular dilatation and systolic dysfunction (Figure 23-9). LGE imaging demonstrated striking, linear midmyocardial fibrosis in the septum of nonischemic etiology (Figure 23-10). There was no CMR evidence of prior MI. The ECV fraction was significantly elevated at 35% (normal <29%) signifying diffuse interstitial expansion. With goal-directed medical therapy, his EF by echocardiography improved to 30%. He declined cardioverter defibrillator implantation at that time due to concern that it would interfere with his occupation as an arc welder. Following 6 months of medical therapy, his EF had improved to 48% by multigated acquisition (MUGA) scan (Figure 23-11).

DISCUSSION

CMR imaging allows the differentiation of ischemic and nonischemic cardiomyopathy based on the location and pattern of LGE; and further delineates nonischemic cardiomyopathies based on morphology, scar, and novel tissue characterization techniques (Figure 23-12).[7,8] Midmyocardial fibrosis as noted by LGE has been shown to be an independent and incremental predictor of ventricular arrhythmias, mortality, and morbidity in patients with nonischemic dilated cardiomyopathy.[9] This and numerous other studies have found that the presence of LGE was the best predictor of sudden cardiac death in dilated cardiomyopathy patients, and ultimately can aid in selecting ideal candidates for defibrillator implantation.

LGE imaging is an accurate method to measure focal myocardial replacement fibrosis; however, it cannot assess diffuse interstitial fibrosis as image contrast relies on the different signal intensities between fibrotic and normal myocardium.[10] In diffuse nonischemic processes these differences may not exist. Novel T1 mapping can now quantify diffuse myocardial fibrosis with measurement of ECV fraction, which has been shown to highly correlate with the histologic extent of collagen.[11] An elevated ECV is known to portend worse outcomes in multiple disease states, including the nonischemic patient population and has the ability to detect the ameliorating effects of renin angiotensin aldosterone system inhibition.[12] Specifically in patients with dilated cardiomyopathy, ECV measurements reflect myocardial collagen content, and can serve as a noninvasive tool for quantifying myocardial fibrosis to aid in risk stratification and to monitor response to therapy.[13]

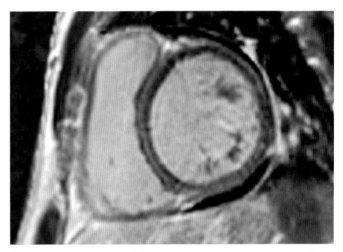

FIGURE 23-10 Short-axis late gadolinium enhancement image with linear midmyocardial hyperenhancement/fibrosis within the septum in a patient with idiopathic, dilated cardiomyopathy.

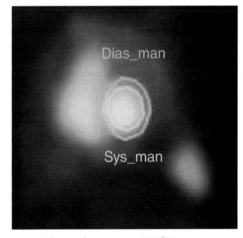

FIGURE 23-11 Multigated acquisition (MUGA) contours at end diastole and end systole in a patient with dilated cardiomyopathy.

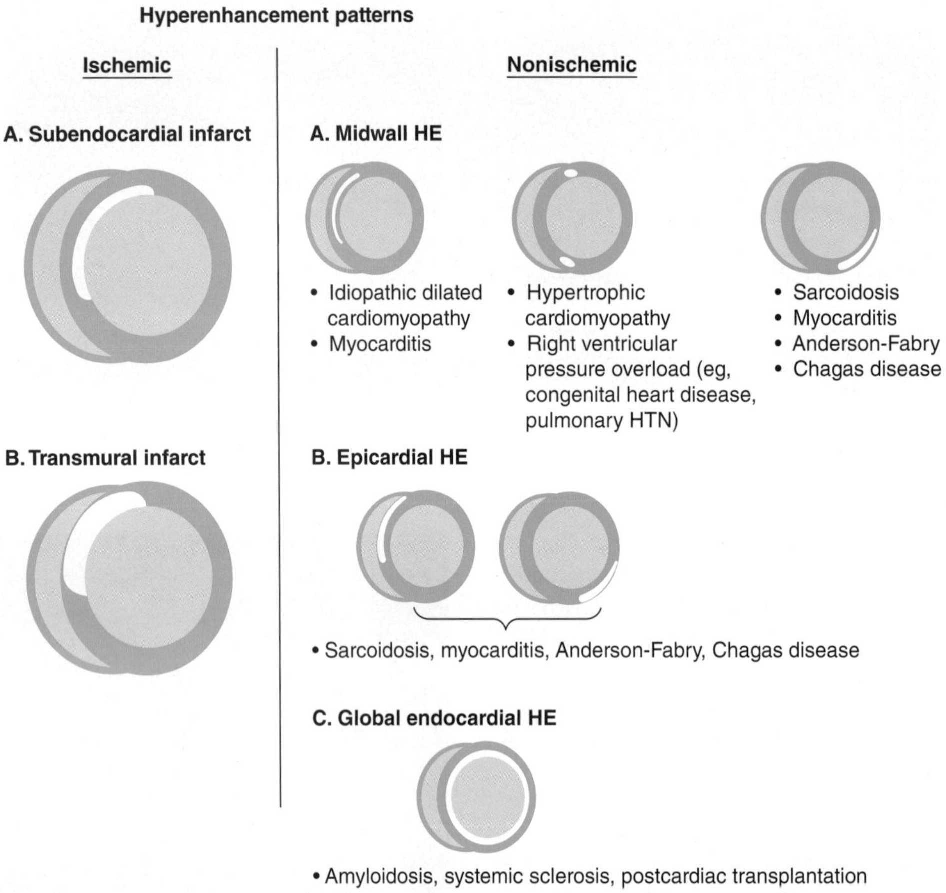

Hyperenhancement patterns

Ischemic	Nonischemic

A. Subendocardial infarct

A. Midwall HE

- Idiopathic dilated cardiomyopathy
- Myocarditis

- Hypertrophic cardiomyopathy
- Right ventricular pressure overload (eg, congenital heart disease, pulmonary HTN)

- Sarcoidosis
- Myocarditis
- Anderson-Fabry
- Chagas disease

B. Transmural infarct

B. Epicardial HE

- Sarcoidosis, myocarditis, Anderson-Fabry, Chagas disease

C. Global endocardial HE

- Amyloidosis, systemic sclerosis, postcardiac transplantation

FIGURE 23-12 Different hyperenhancement patterns in both ischemic and nonischemic cardiomyopathies.

PATIENT CASE 4: LEFT VENTRICULAR NONCOMPACTION

A 59-year-old woman with a history of Laing skeletal myopathy presented for cardiac evaluation. She began experiencing falls in her 30s, which led to genetic testing and demonstration of a myosin heavy chain mutation (MYH7). She was identified as the proband of a large autosomal-dominant family pedigree that was diagnosed with the MYH7 mutation. She experienced an episode of chest pain 8 years prior to her current presentation and reportedly had abnormal cardiac biomarkers at that time, but her workup was otherwise unremarkable. On presentation, she complained of chest pain with emotional stress and with exertion. She was referred for CMR to evaluate for myocardial involvement of her skeletal myopathy.

Cine imaging (Figures 23-13 and 23-14) demonstrated heavily trabeculated left and right ventricles, meeting diagnostic imaging criteria for noncompaction. Biventricular systolic function was normal. She had no fibrosis on LGE imaging and no evidence of LV thrombus at long inversion times. Her chest pain has improved with long-acting nitrate therapy.

DISCUSSION

Left ventricular noncompaction cardiomyopathy (LVNC) is a rare abnormality of the LV wall resulting from developmental arrest of the normal compaction process of the myocardium leading to the

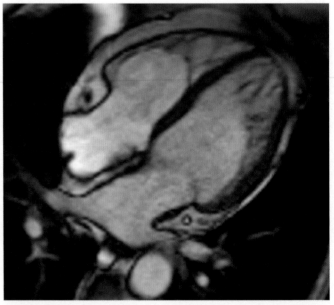

FIGURE 23-13 Horizontal long-axis SSFP cine at end diastole showing prominent trabeculae along the anterolateral and apical walls consistent with LV noncompaction.

formation of 2 layers of the myocardium: the compacted and the noncompacted layer. The spectrum of myocardial phenotypes is broad and can present as dilated, hypertrophy, mixed, restrictive, or arrhythmogenic cardiomyopathy.[14] Multiple genes have been implicated in LVNC, which can be familial or sporadic, isolated or associated with other cardiomyopathies, congenital heart disease, mitochondrial diseases, or complex multiorgan syndromes. The primary phenotype can result in progressive cardiac dysfunction and be associated with dysrhythmias or thromboembolic events.

CMR is uniquely suited for evaluating LVNC as it can easily identify the noncompacted layer predominantly located in the apical and lateral segments. A noncompacted to compacted layer ratio of >2.3 in diastole yields a high diagnostic accuracy for distinguishing pathologic LVNC.[15] Given the diverse phenotypic presentation in LVNC, numerous LGE patterns have been described including subendocardial, trabecular, midmyocardial, and transmural.[16] The presence of myocardial fibrosis itself has been shown to relate to clinical disease severity and LV systolic dysfunction. In addition, CMR can better visualize right ventricular (RV) involvement as well as identify apical thrombi.

PATIENT CASE 5: CHEMOTHERAPY-INDUCED CARDIOMYOPATHY

A 62-year-old woman with ER/PR+ metastatic breast cancer presented 16 years after her diagnosis with supraventricular tachycardia. Subsequent echocardiogram showed new biventricular systolic dysfunction with an LVEF of 25% to 30%. Her oncologic history was notable for full treatment with cyclophosphamide, doxorubicin, and 5-fluorouracil with subsequent tamoxifen therapy after her initial diagnosis. Her disease progressed 10 years after her diagnosis, and she was subsequently treated with letrozole followed by docetaxel and later fulvestrant with additional thoracic radiation. She developed leptomeningeal involvement, for which she received capecitabine and intrathecal cytarabine, and had recently been started on exemestane and everolimus at the time of her cardiac presentation. She was referred for CMR to evaluate her cardiomyopathy.

SSFP cine imaging demonstrated LV dilatation and severe LV systolic dysfunction (Figure 23-15). LGE imaging revealed the presence of midmyocardial fibrosis within the septum, consistent with an underlying nonischemic myopathic process (Figure 23-16). She had no evidence of myocardial inflammation, fatty infiltration, or iron overload. Her native T1 time was elevated at 1082 ms. Her cardiomyopathy was presumed to be secondary to her intensive and prolonged chemotherapy regimens. She was placed on goal-directed medical therapy with an improvement in her EF to 39%. She developed angioedema with lisinopril and did not tolerate long-acting nitrate therapy due to headaches; thus, she remains on beta blocker and hydralazine therapies and has demonstrated sustained improvement in LV systolic function.

DISCUSSION

Autopsy data have shown that myocardial fibrosis is a key feature of patients with late anthracycline-induced cardiomyopathy,[17] which CMR imaging is best suited to detect. CMR imaging also adds diagnostic value for its accurate assessment of LVEF, proving to be a

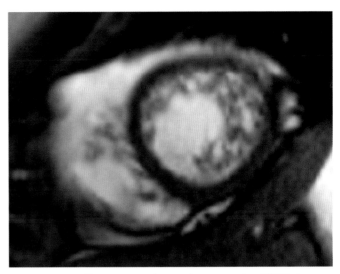

FIGURE 23-14 Short-axis steady-state free precession (SSFP) cine at end diastole with prominent trabeculae of left ventricular (LV) noncompaction.

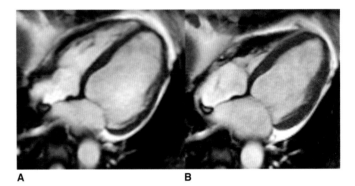

A   **B**

FIGURE 23-15 Horizontal long-axis steady-state free precession (SSFP) cine at end diastole (A) and end systole (B) in a patient with chemotherapy-induced cardiomyopathy.

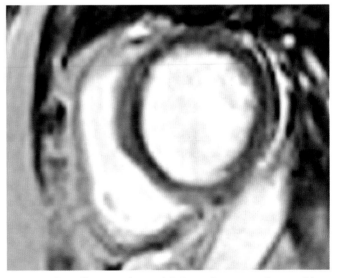

FIGURE 23-16 Short-axis late gadolinium enhancement image with patchy and linear midmyocardial hyperenhancement/fibrosis within the anteroseptum and inferolateral wall consistent with an underlying nonischemic myopathic process.

more precise tool than echocardiography for screening this at-risk population.[18]

However, early detection of chemotherapy-induced cardiotoxicity is also critically important. Current surveillance strategies rely on changes in LV systolic function to identify cardiotoxicity, a feature that is now thought to be a late finding.[19] Newer diagnostic techniques are emerging that may allow for earlier detection of cardiotoxicity secondary to chemotherapy. Research has shown that patients treated with anthracyclines have higher native T1 times and ECVs as calculated from T1 mapping than controls, even in the absence of LV dysfunction.[20,21] In a cohort of cancer patients, changes in T1 signal intensity correlated to small but significant decreases in LVEF just 3 months after the receipt of potentially cardiotoxic chemotherapy, suggesting that T1-weighted signal intensity may serve as an early marker of injury.[20] Further research in this area is ongoing. However, the ability of CMR to accurately assess LV systolic function with the added benefit of myocardial tissue characterization may lead to more accurate and more timely diagnosis of this form of cardiomyopathy.

■ INFILTRATIVE CARDIOMYOPATHIES

PATIENT CASE 6: CARDIAC AMYLOIDOSIS

A 58-year-old woman with atrial fibrillation, HTN, stroke, and gastroparesis was previously diagnosed with a nonischemic cardiomyopathy after an unremarkable workup, including negative fat pad, bone marrow, and gastric biopsies. Her mother died from a nonischemic cardiomyopathy at age 50 years. She presented acutely 4 years later with decompensated systolic HF, and a CMR examination was performed.

Breath-held SSFP cine imaging was obtained and demonstrated severe concentric left ventricular hypertrophy (LVH), right ventricular hypertrophy (RVH), biatrial enlargement with wall thickening, a moderate sized pericardial effusion, and bilateral pleural effusions (Figure 23-17). Biventricular systolic function was moderately to severely reduced. LGE imaging demonstrated diffuse hyperenhancement of the myocardium and atrial walls with the inability to null the myocardium (Figures 23-18 and 23-19). Calculated ECV fraction by T1 mapping (Figure 23-20) was 82% (normal <29%).[22] Together these findings were diagnostic for classic cardiac amyloidosis. Subsequent right heart catheterization showed elevated filling pressures and endomyocardial biopsy demonstrated positive Congo red staining, and immunohistochemical staining confirmed transthyretin-related amyloid (ATTR) deposition within the heart. No amino acid sequence abnormalities in the transthyretin protein were detected, making wild-type ATTR amyloidosis the most likely etiology. Of note, urine and serum protein electrophoreses were normal.

DISCUSSION

ATTR amyloidosis is a fatal disorder characterized primarily by progressive neuropathy and cardiomyopathy. Mutant (with autosomal-dominant inheritance) and wild-type (with predominant

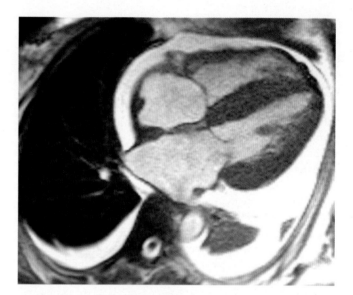

FIGURE 23-17 Horizontal long-axis steady-state free precession (SSFP) cine at end diastole showing left ventricular (LV), right ventricular (RV), and atrial wall hypertrophy, moderate pericardial effusion, and bilateral pleural effusions in a patient with cardiac amyloidosis.

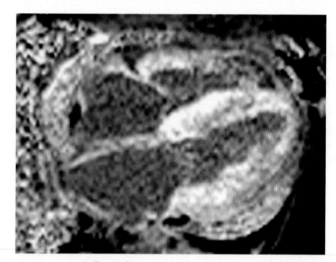

FIGURE 23-18 Diffuse left ventricular (LV), right ventricular (RV), and atrial wall hyperenhancement and characteristic dark blood pool in a horizontal long-axis late gadolinium enhancement image classic for cardiac amyloidosis.

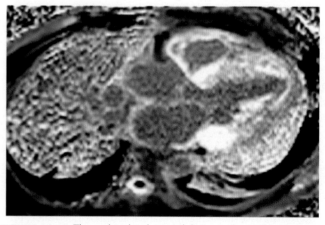

FIGURE 23-19 Three-chamber late gadolinium enhancement image with diffuse left ventricular (LV) hyperenhancement and dark blood pool characteristic of cardiac amyloidosis.

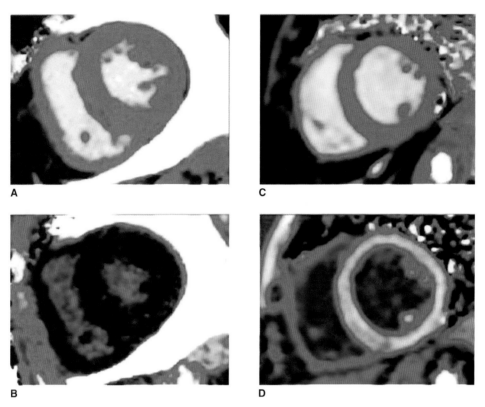

FIGURE 23-20 T1 mapping (MOLLI sequence) in a patient with cardiac amyloidosis before (A) and after (B) gadolinium contrast compared to T1 mapping in a normal patient before (C) and after (D) gadolinium contrast.

cardiac involvement) forms exist.[23] The prognosis of wild-type ATTR is better than other forms of amyloid cardiomyopathy, with median survival of 60 months from presentation with HF symptoms versus only 5.4 months in patients with cardiomyopathy from light chain (AL) amyloidosis.[24] In a large series of more than 100 patients with wild-type ATTR, median survival from onset of symptoms was 6.07 years.[25] Our patient survived 4 years after her initial presentation with HF.

CMR is uniquely suited for the diagnosis of cardiac amyloidosis. In this disease, insoluble fibrillar amyloid protein deposits within the myocardial interstitium. CMR T1 mapping allows for quantification of extracellular interstitial matrix expansion via the measurement of ECV fraction.[26,27] ECV is uniformly and uniquely elevated in cardiac amyloidosis[28] and provides significant prognostic value.[29] Figure 23-27 demonstrates the striking difference between precontrast and postcontrast T1 maps in a patient with cardiac amyloid (panel A and B) and a healthy individual (panel C and D). Additionally, amyloid infiltrative disease is associated with distinct patterns of LGE. Gadolinium-based contrast agents accumulate in extracellular spaces without crossing intact myocardial cell membranes and result in T1 shortening. In cardiac amyloid, there is increased gadolinium contrast in areas of amyloid deposition, resulting in substantial lowering of myocardial T1 and prominent hyperenhancement on LGE imaging. LGE patterns in amyloidosis may be patchy, transmural, or subendocardial.[30] Recent literature suggests that the LGE pattern may be able to distinguish between various subtypes of cardiac amyloidosis.[31]

PATIENT CASE 7: HEMOCHROMATOSIS WITH CARDIAC IRON OVERLOAD

A 51-year-old man with a known history of hereditary hemochromatosis (HH) was admitted with altered mental status due to severe diabetic ketoacidosis. Genetic testing 10 years earlier confirmed the presence of a C282Y mutation in the *HH* gene, but he had previously refused treatment. Abdominal imaging on presentation showed iron deposition within the liver, pancreas, and adrenal glands. His hospital course was complicated by paroxysmal atrial fibrillation and nonsustained ventricular tachycardia. He was referred for CMR to assess for cardiac involvement.

T2-star (T2*) imaging demonstrated severe cardiac and hepatic iron overload (Figure 23-21). Both myocardial and hepatic T2* values were <1.8 ms (shortest echo time) (normal >20 ms),[32] which precluded precise calculation of tissue iron content. LV systolic function was mildly reduced on cine imaging with no evident fibrosis on LGE imaging. The patient was subsequently started on goal-directed medical therapy and underwent phlebotomy for iron overload. His disease was felt to be too advanced to realize any significant benefit from chelation therapy.

DISCUSSION

In the early stages of disease, myocardial iron overload results in diastolic LV dysfunction but, if left untreated, will lead to progressive LV dilatation and systolic dysfunction. Myocardial iron uptake is much slower in comparison with hepatic uptake, and thus myocardial iron overload develops at a later stage in comparison with hepatic iron overload.[33]

CMR T2* imaging has transformed the diagnostic landscape for this condition. Validated against direct quantification of tissue iron content,[32] T2* relaxometry can reproducibly quantify myocardial iron deposition, unlike serum ferritin and liver iron measurements. T2* values <20 ms are inversely correlated with LVEF, and T2* values <10 ms (severe) are associated with an increased annual risk of the development of HF or arrhythmias.[34] Moreover, serial CMR T2* imaging can be useful in guiding and monitoring chelation therapy.[33]

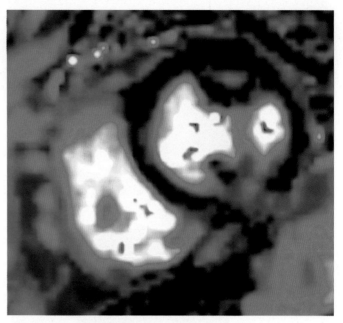

FIGURE 23-21 T2* map of a mid short-axis slice in a patient with hereditary hemochromatosis.

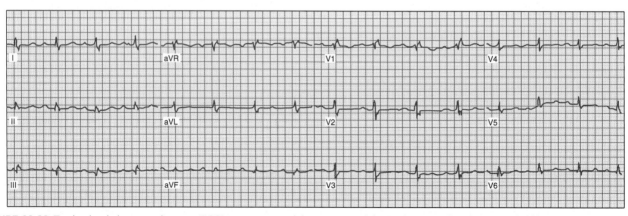

FIGURE 23-22 Twelve-lead electrocardiogram (ECG) in a patient with hypereosinophilic syndrome and endomyocardial fibrosis.

PATIENT CASE 8: HYPEREOSINOPHILIC SYNDROME WITH ENDOMYOCARDIAL FIBROSIS

A 65-year-old man from Somalia presented with 2 years of progressive HF. His ECG demonstrated first-degree atrioventricular block, right bundle branch block, and low voltage (Figure 23-22). Admission labs were notable for eosinophilia (13.9%; normal 0%-5%), and an echocardiogram that demonstrated an RV mass (Figure 23-23). CMR was ordered to characterize the mass.

Cine imaging revealed near-obliteration of the RV cavity and RV outflow tract by the suspected mass (Figure 23-24). The right atrium was severely dilated and hypokinetic, and flow through the right heart appeared swirling and sluggish on SSFP imaging. LGE imaging demonstrated diffuse hyperenhancement of the RV free wall that extended into the proximal RV outflow tract, along with nearly diffuse subendocardial LV hyperenhancement. The heterogeneous LGE characteristics of the material lining the RV and RV outflow tract suggested a mixture of fibrosis and thrombus (Figure 23-25). The diagnosis of hypereosinophilic syndrome with endomyocardial fibrosis was made.

DISCUSSION

Cardiac involvement in hypereosinophilic syndrome is a major cause of morbidity and mortality. In its earliest stage, eosinophils and lymphocytes infiltrate cardiac tissue and release toxic proteins, resulting in myocyte necrosis. At later stages, thrombi form along the marred endocardium with the potential for thromboembolism. In its most advanced form, fibrosis replaces these thrombi, leading to scarring of the myocardium and subsequent restrictive cardiomyopathy. CMR can detect ventricular thrombi with a higher degree of sensitivity and specificity than echocardiography, and contrast-enhanced CMR can identify inflammation and fibrosis, making it a particularly useful imaging modality for this scenario.[35]

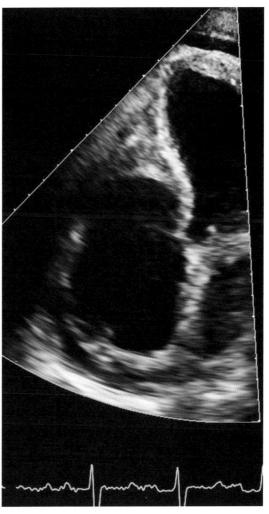

FIGURE 23-23 Apical 4-chamber echocardiogram demonstrating RV cavity obliteration by an echogenic material in a patient with endomyocardial fibrosis.

■ GENETIC CARDIOMYOPATHIES

PATIENT CASE 9: ANDERSON-FABRY CARDIOMYOPATHY

A 40-year-old man with a long-standing history of proteinuria and a lower extremity rash presented to a dermatologist for worsening rash. Additional symptoms included paresthesias and hypohydrosis. Skin biopsy demonstrated features of angiokeratoma, and subsequent testing revealed advanced kidney disease. Enzymatic testing confirmed alpha-galactosidase A deficiency, consistent with Anderson-Fabry disease (AFD). He subsequently developed dyspnea with exertion, lower extremity edema, and was noted to have LVH on his ECG, thus prompting CMR examination to evaluate for cardiac involvement.

Breath-held SSFP cine imaging demonstrated concentric LVH with preserved systolic function (Figure 23-26). T1 mapping revealed a native T1 time of 885 ms (Figure 23-27), highly suggestive of AFD in the setting of LVH. Due to advanced renal disease,

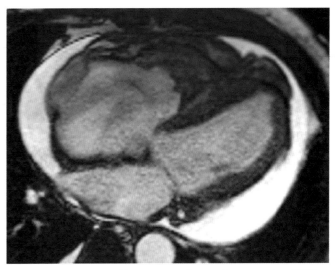

FIGURE 23-24 Horizontal long-axis steady-state free precession (SSFP) cine at end systole in a patient with endomyocardial fibrosis showing right ventricular (RV) cavity obliteration by thrombus and spontaneous contrast swirling through the right atrium due to stagnant blood flow.

gadolinium-based contrast could not be administered during his CMR examination.

DISCUSSION

AFD is an uncommon X-linked disorder caused by deficient activity of the lysosomal enzyme alpha-galactosidase A, resulting in intracellular accumulation of glycosphingolipids within various organ systems. Cardiac manifestations include progressive left ventricular hypertrophy (LVH), myocardial fibrosis, and systolic and diastolic dysfunction. AFD accounts for at least 3% of unexplained LVH in middle-aged men.[36] Treatment with recombinant enzyme has been shown to reverse or slow disease progression when initiated before reversible end-organ damage has occurred, underscoring the importance of early detection of this rare disease.[37,38]

T1 relaxation time is a fundamental property of tissue, with fat characterized by very low T1 relative to other tissue types. Intracellular accumulation of myocardial glycosphingolipid results in dramatic shortening of myocardial T1. Noncontrast T1 mapping has been shown to distinguish AFD from other causes of LVH (eg, hypertensive heart disease, hypertrophic cardiomyopathy, severe aortic stenosis, and cardiac amyloidosis)[39] with high reproducibility.

PATIENT CASE 10: ARRHYTHMOGENIC RIGHT VENTRICULAR CARDIOMYOPATHY/ DYSPLASIA

A 33-year-old man presented with near-syncope and monomorphic ventricular tachycardia. His ECG revealed abnormal T-wave inversions in leads V1 and V2 (Figure 23-28), and a signal-averaged ECG confirmed the presence of late potentials. He had no structural heart disease identified by echocardiography, and subsequent endomyocardial biopsy showed only mild endocardial thickening without interstitial deposition. He was referred for CMR.

CMR cine imaging confirmed the presence of RV dilatation, RV systolic dysfunction, and regional RV dyskinesis (Figure 23-29), consistent with major imaging criteria for arrhythmogenic right ventricular dysplasia (ARVD).[40] Indexed RV end-diastolic volume (RVEDVI) was 121 mL/m^2, and right ventricular ejection fraction (RVEF) was 29%. He was subsequently placed on sotalol with excellent control of his arrhythmia and continues to decline implantable cardioverter defibrillator (ICD) placement despite extensive counseling.

DISCUSSION

ARVC/D is an autosomal-dominant myocardial disease caused by mutations in desmosomal proteins resulting in progressive fibrofatty replacement of the myocardium with eventual wall thinning and aneurysm formation due to the loss of structural integrity of the myocardium. Fibrofatty replacement interferes with electrical impulse conduction, which is responsible for the characteristic ECG abnormalities, late potentials, and arrhythmias experienced by patients with this condition.[41]

CMR imaging is well-suited for the evaluation of ARVC/D, as evidenced by its inclusion in revised Task Force Criteria,[40] owing to its superior imaging of the right ventricle. Cine imaging is

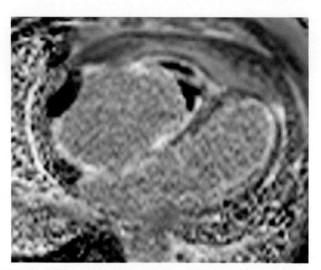

FIGURE 23-25 Horizontal long-axis late gadolinium enhancement image in a patient with endomyocardial fibrosis showing right ventricular (RV) free wall hyperenhancement and a hybrid pattern of fibrosis and thrombus filling the RV.

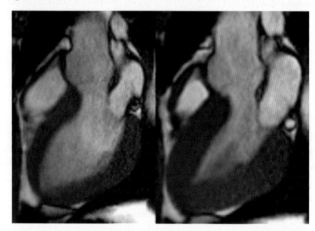

FIGURE 23-26 Three-chamber axis steady-state free precession (SSFP) cine at end diastole (A) and end systole (B) in a patient with Anderson-Fabry disease.

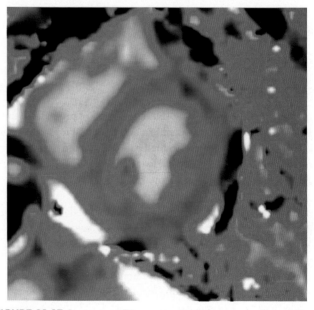

FIGURE 23-27 Precontrast T1 mapping (MOLLI sequence) in a patient with Anderson-Fabry disease. Native T1 time was 885 ms.

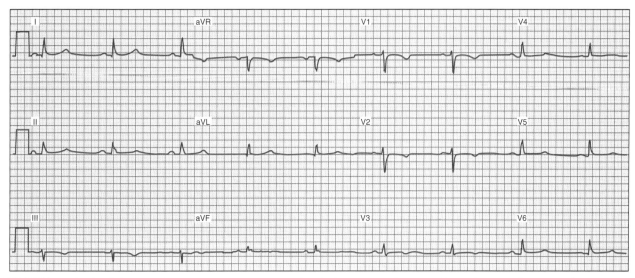

FIGURE 23-28 Twelve-lead electrocardiogram (ECG) in a patient with arrhythmogenic right ventricular cardiomyopathy (ARVC) showing T-wave inversions in precordial leads V1-V3.

particularly useful for the quantification of RV volumes and for the assessment of regional wall motion abnormalities so characteristic of ARVC/D.[42] When compared with prospective clinical diagnosis and gene-carrier status, CMR performed better than Task Force Criteria[43] in the diagnosis of ARVC/D, suggesting that CMR may allow for disease detection at an earlier stage.

PATIENT CASE 11: DUCHENNE MUSCULAR DYSTROPHY

A 13-year-old boy with Duchenne muscular dystrophy (DMD) presented to discuss enrollment in a research study. He had no cardiovascular symptoms or history of major adverse cardiovascular events. CMR was ordered as part of the research protocol.

Cine imaging demonstrated mild lateral wall hypokinesis with overall low-normal LV systolic function. LGE imaging revealed striking hyperenhancement of the lateral wall, most prominent at the base (Figures 23-30 and 23-31), consistent with cardiac involvement.

DISCUSSION

DMD is an X-linked recessive disorder caused by mutations in the dystrophin gene, which lead to destabilization of the sarcolemma. Death is usually due to cardiac disease, which may include ventricular dysfunction and/or malignant arrhythmias. Overt HF may be delayed or absent. Interestingly, female carriers may also manifest cardiac involvement.[44] CMR has proven to be a valuable tool in the diagnosis and prognosis of this select group. Fibrosis, as identified by late gadolinium enhancement, is progressive and increases with both age and decreasing LVEF.[45] Its presence has been linked to adverse cardiac events in DMD patients,[46] making CMR an imperative risk stratification tool and an opportunity to identify DMD patients who are most likely to benefit from aggressive medical therapy and/or ICD therapy.

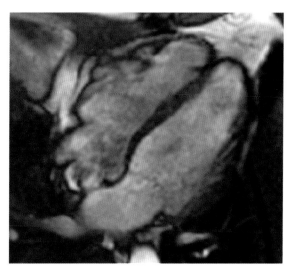

FIGURE 23-29 Horizontal long-axis steady-state free precession (SSFP) cine at end diastole in a patient with arrhythmogenic right ventricular cardiomyopathy (ARVC) showing right ventricular (RV) dilatation and multiple irregularities and aneurysms of the RV free wall.

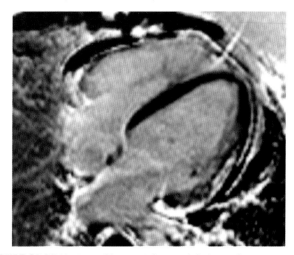

FIGURE 23-30 Horizontal long-axis late gadolinium enhancement image in a patient with Duchenne muscular dystrophy showing characteristic lateral wall hyperenhancement.

PATIENT CASE 12: HYPERTROPHIC CARDIOMYOPATHY

A 45-year-old man with a history of hypertrophic cardiomyopathy (HCM) presented to re-establish cardiology care. He was diagnosed with HCM at the age of 24 following an abnormal screening ECG performed by the U.S. Navy. Subsequent echocardiography confirmed the diagnosis. His family history was notable only for a paternal grandfather who died at the age of 41 years, though not all of his first-degree relatives agreed to testing. He had no history of syncope, ventricular arrhythmias on surveillance monitoring, or abnormal blood pressure response to exercise on prior treadmill stress testing. He reported occasional chest discomfort, and CMR was ordered.

SSFP cine imaging demonstrated severe, asymmetric septal and anterior wall hypertrophy with a maximum septal wall thickness of 2.5 cm (Figure 23-32). There was flow acceleration across the LV outflow tract and mild systolic anterior motion of the mitral valve resulting in mild late, eccentric mitral regurgitation. Single-shot SSFP LGE imaging was remarkable for striking, extensive fibrosis throughout the septum (Figures 23-33 and 23-34). The extent of LGE was calculated at 19% LGE/gram of LV mass. Given the magnitude of his fibrosis, he was referred to electrophysiology for consideration of ICD for primary prevention. However, he was admittedly resistant to the idea. Because the extent of CMR-detected fibrosis has not yet been incorporated into society guidelines, the patient and his electrophysiologist agreed to continue vigilant monitoring with ECG and stress testing.

DISCUSSION

Traditional risk factors for sudden cardiac death (SCD) in patients with HCM fail to adequately capture all patients at risk,[47] complicating the process of appropriate selection for primary prevention ICD. In fact, ICD implantation based on traditional risk factors has been shown to result in more inappropriate shocks and complications than appropriate shocks.[48]

CMR is a powerful diagnostic tool in HCM patients and has been recognized for its potential utility in improved risk stratification. The presence of LGE has been shown to be an independent risk factor for adverse outcomes, and a meta-analysis demonstrated significant relationships between LGE and cardiovascular mortality,

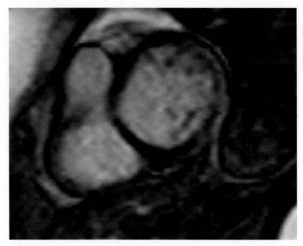

FIGURE 23-31 Short-axis late gadolinium enhancement image in a patient with Duchenne muscular dystrophy showing characteristic lateral wall hyperenhancement.

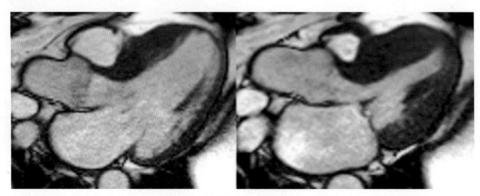

FIGURE 23-32 Three-chamber axis steady-state free precession (SSFP) cine at end diastole (A) and end systole (B) in a patient with hypertrophic cardiomyopathy.

HF death, and all-cause mortality in HCM patients.[49] In fact, LGE ≥15% of LV mass has been linked to a 2-fold increase in SCD risk in otherwise lower risk patients.[50] Currently, the first prospective international registry in HCM is actively enrolling patients in an effort to identify novel prognostic markers, including CMR markers of fibrosis, genetic markers, and biomarkers, that will in turn allow for better risk stratification of this population.[51]

■ INFLAMMATORY CARDIOMYOPATHIES

PATIENT CASE 13: MYOCARDITIS

A 20-year-old male college student with no significant past medical history experienced 5 days of sore throat, productive cough, fever, and chills followed by nausea, vomiting, and diarrhea. He subsequently developed sharp positional chest discomfort, which improved with upright position and ibuprofen, prompting a visit to the emergency department. His ECG demonstrated diffuse ST elevations (Figure 23-35), his C-reactive protein (CRP) was 98.9 mg/L (normal <10.00 mg/L), and his troponin peaked at 52 ng/mL (normal <0.11 ng/mL). He was referred to for CMR to evaluate for myopericarditis.

Initial evaluation with SSFP cine imaging demonstrated low normal systolic function with an EF of 52% and lack of regional wall motion abnormalities. However, T2 mapping (Figure 23-36) revealed markedly abnormal T2 signal (up to 73 ms), most prominent in the lateral and anterior walls, consistent with myocardial inflammation and edema. LGE imaging (Figures 23-37 and 23-38) demonstrated striking epicardial enhancement of the lateral wall as well as patchy areas of midmyocardial enhancement. These findings were classic for myocarditis. Viral testing did not elucidate an etiology for his myocarditis; however, he clinically improved with aspirin and colchicine therapy. Repeat CMR imaging to evaluate residual scar is scheduled at 6-month follow-up.

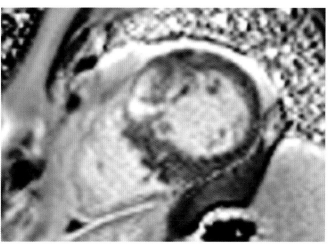

FIGURE 23-33 Short-axis late gadolinium enhancement image in a patient with hypertrophic cardiomyopathy illustrating prominent patchy midmyocardial fibrosis in a hypertrophied segment.

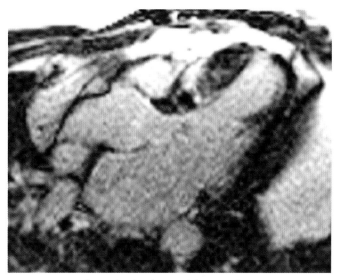

FIGURE 23-34 Three-chamber late gadolinium enhancement image in a patient with hypertrophic cardiomyopathy illustrating prominent patchy midmyocardial fibrosis in a hypertrophied segment.

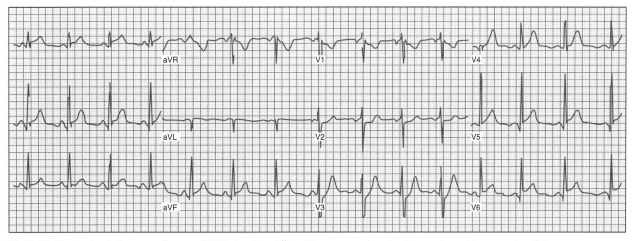

FIGURE 23-35 Twelve-lead electrocardiogram (ECG) showing diffuse ST segment elevation in a patient with myopericarditis.

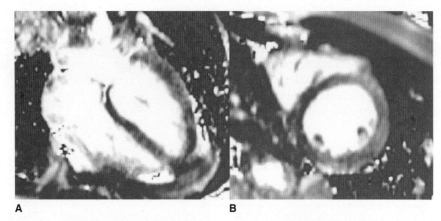

FIGURE 23-36 Horizontal long-axis (A) and short-axis (B) T2 maps in a patient with myocarditis demonstrating diffusely abnormal T2 signal, most prominent within the lateral wall.

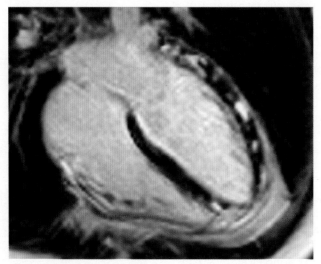

FIGURE 23-37 Horizontal long-axis late gadolinium enhancement image in a patient with myocarditis demonstrating patchy mid to epicardial hyperenhancement of the lateral wall.

DISCUSSION

CMR is an important diagnostic and prognostic tool in patients with acute myocarditis. Not only does CMR allow for differentiation between ischemic and nonischemic injury, but also provides key information on tissue characterization. Increased T2 signal is a reflection of increased water content, which accompanies tissue inflammation and/or tissue edema. T2 mapping offers a quantitative assessment of myocardial T2[52] and has been shown to reliably identify myocardial involvement in patients with myocarditis.[53] Moreover, in a cohort of patients with biopsy-proven myocarditis, LGE was shown to be the best independent predictor of all-cause and cardiac mortality, above and beyond initial LVEF. Interestingly, in the same cohort of patients, there were no SCD events in LGE-negative patients, despite LV dilation and severely reduced EF.[54]

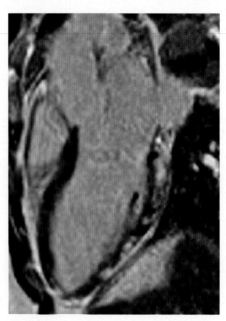

FIGURE 23-38 Three-chamber long-axis late gadolinium enhancement image in a patient with myocarditis demonstrating patchy mid to epicardial hyperenhancement of the lateral wall.

PATIENT CASE 14: STRESS (TAKOTSUBO) CARDIOMYOPATHY

A 54-year old woman with a history of fibromyalgia presented with chest discomfort radiating to her left arm. Her ECG showed frequent premature ventricular contractions (PVCs) and ST elevations prompting emergent cardiac catheterization. Angiographic imaging demonstrated normal coronary arteries, but left ventriculography demonstrated apical ballooning (Figure 23-39). Additional history from the patient identified significant stress from both personal and family health problems. Troponin peaked at 8.9 ng/mL (normal <0.11 ng/mL), and CMR was ordered.

Breath-held cine imaging revealed moderately depressed LV systolic function with mid and apical segmental hypokinesis and apical ballooning (Figure 23-40). T2 mapping confirmed regional elevation of T2 signal in the mid and apical segments (Figure 23-41), consistent with myocardial edema/inflammation. No evidence of hyperenhancement was noted on LGE imaging. Follow-up echocardiogram 2 months later showed normal LV systolic function with resolution of previously observed wall motion abnormalities.

DISCUSSION

CMR plays an important role in the diagnosis of stress cardiomyopathy due to its ability to noninvasively characterize the ventricular myocardium. Most of these patients present with symptoms and findings concerning for acute coronary syndrome despite lack of obstructive coronary disease. The ability to discriminate between ischemic injury, classic myocarditis, and stress cardiomyopathy has significant prognostic implications given the excellent survival and prognosis in patients with takotsubo cardiomyopathy. Important diagnostic CMR features include severe LV dysfunction in a noncoronary distribution, myocardial edema within affected LV segments, and minimal to no hyperenhancement on LGE imaging.[55] Similar to myocarditis, T2 mapping has emerged as an important tool for the detection of myocardial inflammation/edema in this patient population.[53]

PATIENT CASE 15: CARDIAC SARCOIDOSIS

A 41-year-old man with sarcoidosis involving the skin, lungs, and lymph nodes presented with left bundle branch block. He was referred for CMR to assess for cardiac sarcoid involvement.

Cine imaging demonstrated low normal LV systolic function. T2 mapping revealed areas of increased T2 signal most prominent in the inferior and inferolateral walls suggestive of myocardial edema/inflammation (Figure 23-42). Patchy fibrosis was noted in the basal anterolateral and inferolateral walls as well as mid inferoseptum on LGE imaging (Figures 23-43 and 23-44). Following initial CMR imaging, he was started on immunosuppressive therapy with prednisone and methotrexate. He did not qualify for defibrillator implantation given his EF. CMR performed 1 year later demonstrated normalization of T2 signal (Figure 23-45) after immunosuppressive therapy, and stable LGE findings.

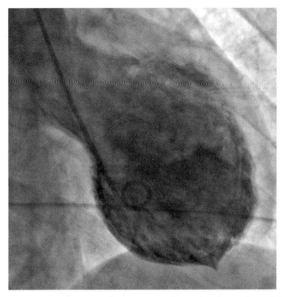

FIGURE 23-39 Left ventriculogram at end systole of a patient with takotsubo cardiomyopathy.

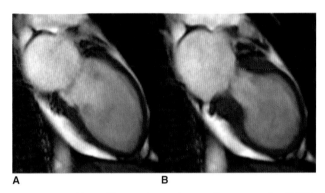

A   **B**

FIGURE 23-40 Vertical long-axis steady-state free precession (SSFP) cine at end diastole (A) and end systole (B) in a patient with takotsubo cardiomyopathy.

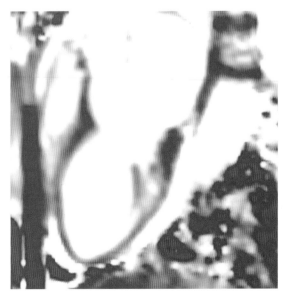

FIGURE 23-41 Three-chamber T2 map in a patient with takotsubo cardiomyopathy demonstrating diffusely abnormal T2 signal in mid and apical segments, corresponding to areas of abnormal wall motion on cine imaging.

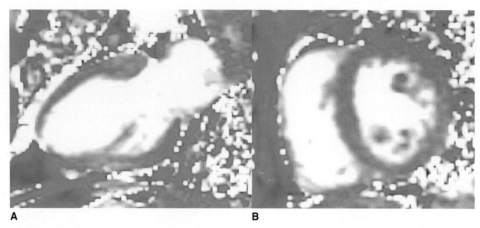

A   **B**

FIGURE 23-42 Vertical long-axis (A) and mid short-axis (B) T2 maps demonstrating patchy abnormal T2 signal in the inferior and inferolateral walls in a patient with active cardiac sarcoidosis before immunosuppressive therapy.

DISCUSSION

The primary clinical manifestations of cardiac sarcoidosis include conduction abnormalities and arrhythmias, congestive HF, and sudden death. The most important clinical predictor of mortality among patients with cardiac sarcoidosis has traditionally been LVEF.[56] However, recent data suggest that LGE may be equally as important in cardiac sarcoidosis with higher rates of death and ventricular arrhythmias in patients with LGE positivity as noted in multiple cohorts.[57,58] Additionally, T2 mapping is able to identify patients with active inflammation, which has been shown to correspond to ECG and arrhythmic abnormalities.[59] Increased T2 signal may represent early clinical disease and be a potentially reversible target. Collectively, CMR shows great promise in cardiac sarcoidosis due to its ability to identify reversible inflamed myocardium (T2) and irreversible scarred myocardium (LGE).

Conventional primary and secondary prevention indications for ICD implantation apply for patients with cardiac sarcoidosis. However, in light of emerging data, the recent Heart Rhythm Society (HRS) expert consensus statement suggests it may be appropriate to consider ICD placement in cardiac sarcoidosis patients with fibrosis or inflammation detected by advanced imaging.[60]

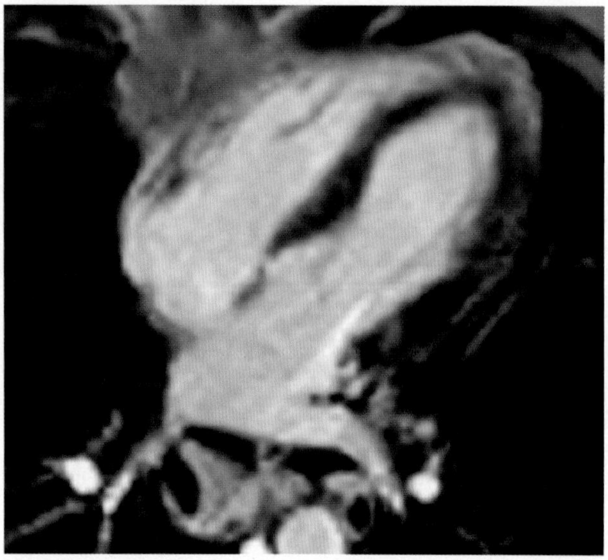

PATIENT CASE 16: CHAGAS CARDIOMYOPATHY

A 67-year-old Bolivian woman was diagnosed with Chagas disease via routine screening prior to volunteer blood donation. She presented with chronic, intermittent chest pressure and fatigue. Nuclear stress testing was negative for ischemia, and her echocardiogram showed normal LV systolic function. A Holter monitor demonstrated a wandering atrial pacemaker with frequent, multifocal supraventricular ectopic complexes and 2 runs of nonsustained ventricular tachycardia. Blood testing confirmed IgG positivity for trypanosoma cruzi without evidence of active parasitemia. She was referred for CMR to evaluate for cardiac involvement.

LGE imaging (Figures 23-46 and 23-47) demonstrated sharply delineated transmural hyperenhancement of the basal inferolateral wall with additional small areas of patchy hyperenhancement in the apical portion of the anterior septum and true apex. T2 mapping

FIGURE 23-43 Horizontal long-axis late gadolinium enhancement image showing patchy midmyocardial fibrosis of the basal and mid anterolateral segments in a patient with cardiac sarcoidosis.

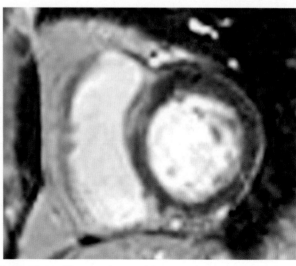

FIGURE 23-44 Short-axis late gadolinium enhancement image showing patchy midmyocardial fibrosis of the anteroseptum and inferolateral wall in a patient with cardiac sarcoidosis.

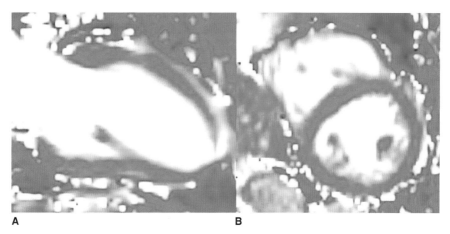

FIGURE 23-45 Vertical long-axis (A) and mid short-axis (B) T2 maps demonstrating normalization of T2 signal in a patient with cardiac sarcoidosis after immunosuppressive therapy.

revealed elevated T2 signal in the basal anterior, and basal to mid anteroseptal walls, suggesting myocardial inflammation and/or edema.

DISCUSSION

Cardiac involvement is the most serious complication of Chagas disease, affecting approximately one-third of seropositive individuals and serving as the leading cause of death from HF in Latin America. The asymptomatic phase can last for decades until unknown triggers initiate the development of arrhythmias and clinical HF. A low-intensity, slowly progressive but persistent myocarditis has been implicated, ultimately resulting in impairment of contractile function and dilatation of all 4 chambers.[61] In a cohort of patients with and without cardiac involvement, abnormal T2 signal and LGE were detected by CMR in all patients, even those without established cardiac involvement by ECG or echocardiography,[62] thus making CMR an important tool for early diagnosis and risk stratification in this population.

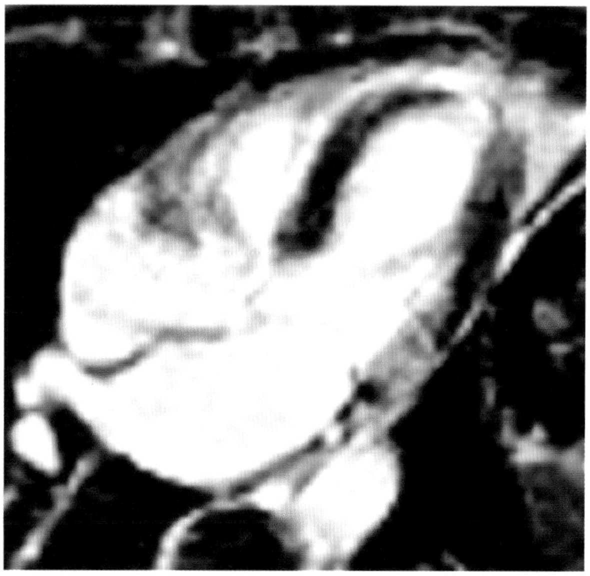

▨ MISCELLANEOUS

PATIENT CASE 17: PULMONARY ARTERIAL HYPERTENSION

A 55-year-old man presented to an outside hospital with lower extremity edema and an echocardiogram showing a dilated right ventricle with evidence of pulmonary arterial hypertension (PAH) (RV systolic pressure of 54 mm Hg). His edema improved with furosemide, but he developed progressive dyspnea with exertion. He underwent right and left heart catheterization, which demonstrated severely elevated right-and left -sided pressures—RA 20 mm Hg, RV 120/25 mm Hg, PA 123/58 mm Hg, PCWP 40 mm Hg—and reduced cardiac output and index (1.8 l/min; 1.0). He was admitted to the hospital for diuresis augmented by milrinone. Physical examination was remarkable for facial telangiectasias. Diagnostic workup was notable for an elevated ANA (1:1280) and rheumatoid factor (64; normal 0-14 IU/mL) as well as positive anti-SSa antibody. He was referred for CMR.

FIGURE 23-46 Three-chamber late gadolinium enhancement image showing dense fibrosis of the basal inferolateral wall in a patient with Chagas disease.

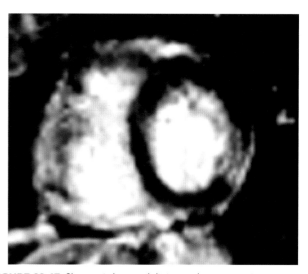

FIGURE 23-47 Short-axis late gadolinium enhancement image showing dense fibrosis of the basal inferolateral wall in a patient with Chagas disease.

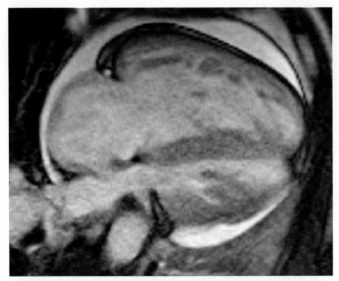

FIGURE 23-48 Horizontal long-axis steady-state free precession (SSFP) cine at end diastole in a patient with pulmonary hypertension showing right atrium (RA) and right ventricular (RV) dilatation, septal flattening, and a moderate-sized pericardial effusion.

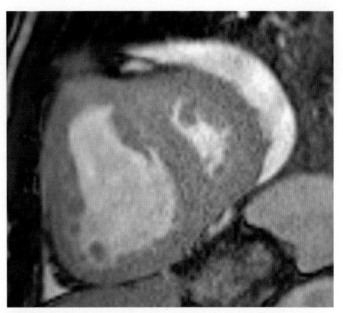

FIGURE 23-49 Short-axis steady-state free precession (SSFP) cine at end-inspiration in a patient with pulmonary hypertension showing marked septal flattening consistent with right ventricular (RV) overload.

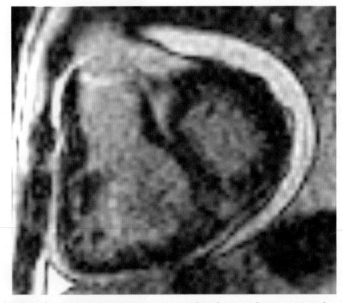

FIGURE 23-50 Short-axis late gadolinium enhancement image in a patient with pulmonary hypertension demonstrating prominent superior and inferior insertion point fibrosis.

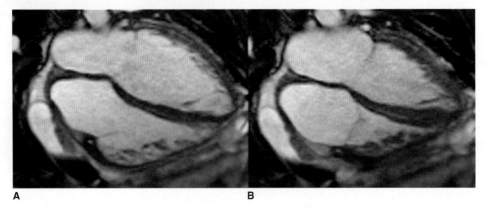

A   B

FIGURE 23-51 Horizontal long-axis steady-state free precession (SSFP) cine at end diastole (A) and end systole (B) in a patient with rejection status post orthotopic heart transplant.

Cine SSFP imaging demonstrated a dilated, apex-forming, hypertrophied RV with a D-shaped ventricular septum consistent with RV overload (Figures 23-48 and 23-49), along with a moderate-sized pericardial effusion. RV function was severely depressed with an RVEF of 12% and free wall akinesis. LGE imaging showed patchy fibrosis at the superior and inferior LV-RV insertion points, a pattern commonly observed in PAH (Figure 23-50). There was no imaging evidence of myocardial inflammation or infiltration.

Subsequent high-resolution chest CT showed basilar fibrosis and honeycombing as well as cystic and emphysematous changes. The patient's V/Q scan suggested a high probability for pulmonary embolism, and a subsequent pulmonary angiogram confirmed multiple bilateral filling defects consistent with acute and chronic thromboembolic disease. The final diagnosis was PAH associated with mixed collagen vascular disease confounded by CTEPH. He was considered a reasonable candidate for thromboendarterectomy but was clinically improving on a trial of PDE-5 inhibitors; thus surgery was deferred.

DISCUSSION

The RV plays a central role in the management of patients with PAH, and its structure and function serve as powerful indicators of prognosis.[63] CMR allows for improved right heart imaging compared to other imaging modalities, making it the optimal imaging test for patients with RV pathology/dysfunction.[64,65] Certain CMR features portend a worse prognosis in PAH patients. In a meta-analysis of longitudinal studies in PAH patients, RVEF was the strongest CMR predictor of mortality.[66] Additionally, the presence of RV insertion point (RVIP) fibrosis on LGE imaging is a marker of more advanced disease and poor prognosis.[67] Lastly, pericardial effusion is yet another indicator of poor outcome.[68]

PATIENT CASE 18: HEART TRANSPLANT

A 28-year-old man with a history of pre-B-cell acute lymphoblastic leukemia (ALL) status post chemotherapy complicated by severe nonischemic cardiomyopathy underwent orthotopic heart transplantation. Two months post transplant he was found to have reduced LV systolic function and grade 1A rejection, for which he received high-dose immunosuppression. Follow-up biopsy was negative, but LV systolic dysfunction persisted. He was referred for CMR to evaluate for myocardial inflammation and for assessment of LV systolic function.

CMR imaging confirmed moderately reduced LV systolic function (Figure 23-51). Markedly elevated myocardial T2 signal (>80 ms, normal <60 ms) (Figure 23-52) indicated diffuse myocardial edema/inflammation. Additionally, there was striking, diffuse midmyocardial hyperenhancement sparing only the mid to distal inferior wall and apex (Figures 23-53 and 23-54). ECV fraction was 37% (normal <29%), suggestive of significant interstitial expansion. His immunosuppression regimen was subsequently intensified.

DISCUSSION

Acute rejection remains a leading cause of morbidity and mortality in heart transplant recipients. Clinical features are unreliable, and

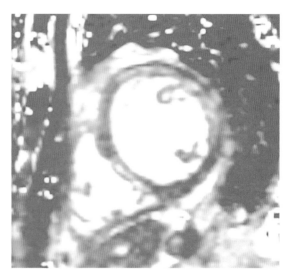

FIGURE 23-52 Short-axis T2 map in a patient with rejection status post orthotopic heart transplant showing markedly abnormal T2 signal throughout the myocardium.

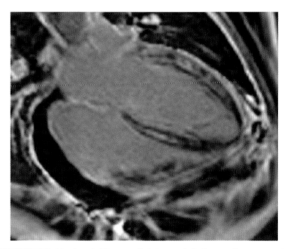

FIGURE 23-53 Horizontal long-axis late gadolinium enhancement image showing diffuse midmyocardial hyperenhancement in a patient with rejection status post orthotopic heart transplant.

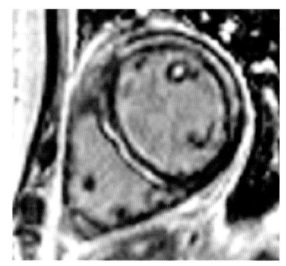

FIGURE 23-54 Short-axis late gadolinium enhancement image showing striking linear midmyocardial hyperenhancement in a patient with rejection status post orthotopic heart transplant.

current standard of care requires routine surveillance endomyocardial biopsies to detect rejection at an early stage. However, biopsy-negative rejection has been reported in up to 20% of patients.[69] Hence, there has been considerable interest in noninvasive screening to allow for more comprehensive monitoring.

T2 imaging has been proposed as a comprehensive, noninvasive tool for assessment of myocardial inflammation. In fact, higher T2 times have been linked to the presence of rejection on biopsy and to the risk of subsequent rejection.[70,71] Currently, a multicenter prospective diagnostic study (DRAGET) is enrolling patients to further characterize this relationship. Patients will undergo T2 quantification and endomyocardial biopsy within 24 hours of each other several times during the first year after transplantation to quantify CMR sensitivity and specificity for graft rejection.[72]

Even beyond the first year, CMR imaging has been shown to provide prognostic information in transplant recipients. An elevated T2 signal and the presence of myocardial fibrosis are both independently associated with adverse cardiovascular outcomes at 5 years of follow-up.[73,74]

REFERENCES

1. Rehwald WG, Fieno DS, Chen E-L, Kim RJ, Judd RM. Myocardial magnetic resonance imaging contrast agent concentrations after reversible and irreversible ischemic injury. *Circulation.* 2002;105(2):224-229.

2. Choi KM, Kim RJ, Gubernikoff G, Vargas JD, Parker M, Judd RM. Transmural extent of acute myocardial infarction predicts long-term improvement in contractile function. *Circulation.* 2001;104(10):1101-1107.

3. Kim RJ, Wu E, Rafael A, et al. The use of contrast-enhanced magnetic resonance imaging to identify reversible myocardial dysfunction. *N Engl J Med.* 2000;343:1445-1453.

4. Pöss J, Desch S, Eitel C, de Waha S, Thiele H, Eitel I. Left ventricular thrombus formation after ST-segment–elevation myocardial infarction: insights from a cardiac magnetic resonance multicenter study. *Circ Cardiovasc Imaging.* 2015;8(10): e003417.

5. Delewi R, Zijlstra F, Piek JJ. Left ventricular thrombus formation after acute myocardial infarction. *Heart.* 2012;98(23):1743-1749.

6. Kim J, Weinsaft JW. Thrombosis and prognosis following ST-elevation myocardial infarction: left ventricular thrombus assessment by cardiac magnetic resonance. *Circ Cardiovasc Imaging.* 2015;8(10):e004098.

7. Mahrholdt H, Wagner A, Judd RM, Sechtem U, Kim RJ. Delayed enhancement cardiovascular magnetic resonance assessment of non-ischaemic cardiomyopathies. *Eur Heart J.* 2005;26(15):1461-1474.

8. Almehmadi F, Joncas SX, Nevis I, et al. Prevalence of myocardial fibrosis patterns in patients with systolic dysfunction: prognostic significance for the prediction of sudden cardiac arrest or appropriate implantable cardiac defibrillator therapy. *Circ Cardiovasc Imaging.* 2014;7(4):593-600.

9. Gulati A, Jabbour A, Ismail TF, et al. Association of fibrosis with mortality and sudden cardiac death in patients with nonischemic dilated cardiomyopathy. *JAMA.* 2013;309(9):896-908.

10. Mewton N, Liu CY, Croisille P, Bluemke D, Lima JA. Assessment of myocardial fibrosis with cardiovascular magnetic resonance. *J Am Coll Cardiol.* 2011;57(8):891-903.

11. Miller CA, Naish JH, Bishop P, et al. Comprehensive validation of cardiovascular magnetic resonance techniques for the assessment of myocardial extracellular volume. *Circ Cardiovasc Imaging.* 2013;6(3):373-383.

12. Zareba K, Wong T, Kellman P, et al. Myocardial fibrosis quantified by CMR extracellular volume fraction predicts mortality in the non-ischemic patient population. *JACC.* 2013;61(10):E829.

13. aus dem Siepen F, Buss SJ, Messroghli D, et al. T1 mapping in dilated cardiomyopathy with cardiac magnetic resonance: quantification of diffuse myocardial fibrosis and comparison with endomyocardial biopsy. *Eur Heart J Cardiovasc Imaging.* 2015;16(2):210-216.

14. Towbin JA, Lorts A, Jefferies JL. Left ventricular non-compaction cardiomyopathy. *Lancet.* 2015;386(9995):813-825.

15. Petersen SE, Selvanayagam JB, Wiesmann F, et al. Left ventricular non-compaction: insights from cardiovascular magnetic resonance imaging. *J Am Coll Cardiol.* 2005;46(1):101-105.

16. Nucifora G, Aquaro GD, Pingitore A, Masci PG, Lombardi M. Myocardial fibrosis in isolated left ventricular non-compaction and its relation to disease severity. *Eur J Heart Fail.* 2011;13(2):170-176.

17. Bernaba BN, Chan JB, Lai CK, Fishbein MC. Pathology of late-onset anthracycline cardiomyopathy. *Cardiovasc Pathol.* 2010;19(5):308-311.

18. Armstrong GT, Plana JC, Zhang N, et al. Screening adult survivors of childhood cancer for cardiomyopathy: comparison of echocardiography and cardiac magnetic resonance imaging. *J Clin Oncol.* 2012;30(23):2876-2884.

19. Yeh ET, Bickford CL. Cardiovascular complications of cancer therapy: incidence, pathogenesis, diagnosis, and management. *J Am Coll Cardiol.* 2009;53(24):2231-2247.

20. Jordan JH, D'Agostino RB, Jr., Hamilton CA, et al. Longitudinal assessment of concurrent changes in left ventricular ejection fraction and left ventricular myocardial tissue characteristics after administration of cardiotoxic chemotherapies using T1-weighted and T2-weighted cardiovascular magnetic resonance. *Circ Cardiovasc Imaging.* 2014;7(6):872-879.

21. Neilan TG, Coelho-Filho OR, Shah RV, et al. Myocardial extracellular volume by cardiac magnetic resonance imaging in patients treated with anthracycline-based chemotherapy. *Am J Cardiol.* 2013;111(5):717-722.

22. Kellman P, Wilson JR, Xue H, et al. Extracellular volume fraction mapping in the myocardium, part 2: initial clinical experience. *J Cardiovasc Magn Reson.* 2012;14:64.

23. Gertz MA, Benson MD, Dyck PJ, et al. Diagnosis, prognosis, and therapy of transthyretin amyloidosis. *J Am Coll Cardiol.* 2015;66(21):2451-2466.

24. Kyle RA, Spittell PC, Gertz MA, et al. The premortem recognition of systemic senile amyloidosis with cardiac involvement. *Am J Med.* 1996;101(4):395-400.

25. Pinney JH, Whelan CJ, Petrie A, et al. Senile systemic amyloidosis: clinical features at presentation and outcome. *J Am Heart Assoc.* 2013;2(2):e000098.

26. Messroghli DR, Radjenovic A, Kozerke S, Higgins DM, Sivananthan MU, Ridgway JP. Modified Look-Locker inversion recovery (MOLLI) for high-resolution T1 mapping of the heart. *Magn Reson Med.* 2004;52(1):141-146.

27. Moon JC, Messroghli DR, Kellman P, et al. Myocardial T1 mapping and extracellular volume quantification: a Society for Cardiovascular Magnetic Resonance (SCMR) and CMR Working Group of the European Society of Cardiology consensus statement. *J Cardiovasc Magn Reson.* 2013;15:92.

28. Banypersad SM, Sado DM, Flett AS, et al. Quantification of myocardial extracellular volume fraction in systemic AL amyloidosis: an equilibrium contrast cardiovascular magnetic resonance study. *Circ Cardiovasc Imaging.* 2013;6(1):34-39.

29. Banypersad SM, Fontana M, Maestrini V, et al. T1 mapping and survival in systemic light-chain amyloidosis. *Eur Heart J.* 2015;36(4):244-251.

30. Syed IS, Glockner JF, Feng D, et al. Role of cardiac magnetic resonance imaging in the detection of cardiac amyloidosis. *JACC Cardiovasc Imaging.* 2010;3(2):155-164.

31. Dungu JN, Valencia O, Pinney JH, et al. CMR-based differentiation of AL and ATTR cardiac amyloidosis. *JACC Cardiovasc Imaging.* 2014;7(2):133-142.

32. Anderson LJ, Holden S, Davis B, et al. Cardiovascular T2-star (T2*) magnetic resonance for the early diagnosis of myocardial iron overload. *Eur Heart J.* 2001;22(23):2171-2179.

33. Kremastinos DT, Farmakis D. Iron overload cardiomyopathy in clinical practice. *Circulation.* 2011;124(20):2253-2263.

34. Kirk P, Roughton M, Porter JB, et al. Cardiac T2* magnetic resonance for prediction of cardiac complications in thalassemia major. *Circulation.* 2009;120(20):1961-1968.

35. Mankad R, Bonnichsen C, Mankad S. Hypereosinophilic syndrome: cardiac diagnosis and management. *Heart.* 2016;102(2):100-106.

36. Linhart A, Elliott PM. The heart in Anderson-Fabry disease and other lysosomal storage disorders. *Heart.* 2007;93(4):528-535.

37. Eng CM, Guffon N, Wilcox WR, et al. Safety and efficacy of recombinant human α-galactosidase a replacement therapy in Fabry's disease. *N Engl J Med.* 2001;345:9-16.

38. Hughes DA, Elliott PM, Shah J, et al. Effects of enzyme replacement therapy on the cardiomyopathy of Anderson–Fabry disease: a randomised, double-blind, placebo-controlled clinical trial of agalsidase alfa. *Heart.* 2008;94(2):153-158.

39. Sado DM, White SK, Piechnik SK, et al. Identification and assessment of Anderson-Fabry disease by cardiovascular magnetic resonance noncontrast myocardial T1 mapping. *Circ Cardiovasc Imaging.* 2013;6(3):392-398.

40. Marcus FI, McKenna WJ, Sherrill D, et al. Diagnosis of arrhythmogenic right ventricular cardiomyopathy/dysplasia: proposed modification of the task force criteria. *Circulation.* 2010;121(13):1533-1541.

41. Basso C, Corrado D, Marcus FI, Nava A, Thiene G. Arrhythmogenic right ventricular cardiomyopathy. *Lancet.* 2009;373(9671):1289-1300.

42. Tandri H, Macedo R, Calkins H, et al. Role of magnetic resonance imaging in arrhythmogenic right ventricular dysplasia: insights from the North American arrhythmogenic right ventricular dysplasia (ARVD/C) study. *Am Heart J.* 2008;155(1):147-153.

43. Sen-Chowdhry S, Prasad SK, Syrris P, et al. Cardiovascular magnetic resonance in arrhythmogenic right ventricular cardiomyopathy revisited: comparison with task force criteria and genotype. *J Am Coll Cardiol.* 2006;48(10):2132-2140.

44. Mavrogeni S, Markousis-Mavrogenis G, Papavasiliou A, Kolovou G. Cardiac involvement in Duchenne and Becker muscular dystrophy. *World J Cardiol.* 2015;7(7):410-414.

45. Hor KN, Taylor MD, Al-Khalidi HR, et al. Prevalence and distribution of late gadolinium enhancement in a large population of patients with Duchenne muscular dystrophy: effect of age and left ventricular systolic function. *J Cardiovasc Magn Reson.* 2013;15:107.

46. Florian A, Ludwig A, Engelen M, et al. Left ventricular systolic function and the pattern of late-gadolinium-enhancement independently and additively predict adverse cardiac events in muscular dystrophy patients. *J Cardiovasc Magn Reson.* 2014;16:81.

47. Spirito P, Autore C, Formisano F, et al. Risk of sudden death and outcome in patients with hypertrophic cardiomyopathy with benign presentation and without risk factors. *Am J Cardiol.* 2014;113(9):1550-1555.

48. Maron BJ, Spirito P, Shen WK, et al. Implantable cardioverter-defibrillators and prevention of sudden cardiac death in hypertrophic cardiomyopathy. *JAMA.* 2007;298(4):405-412.

49. Green JJ, Berger JS, Kramer CM, Salerno M. Prognostic value of late gadolinium enhancement in clinical outcomes for hypertrophic cardiomyopathy. *JACC Cardiovasc Imaging.* 2012;5(4):370-377.

50. Chan RH, Maron BJ, Olivotto I, et al. Prognostic value of quantitative contrast-enhanced cardiovascular magnetic resonance for the evaluation of sudden death risk in patients with hypertrophic cardiomyopathy. *Circulation.* 2014;130(6):484-495.

51. Kramer CM, Appelbaum E, Desai MY, et al. Hypertrophic cardiomyopathy registry: the rationale and design of an international, observational study of hypertrophic cardiomyopathy. *Am Heart J.* 2015;170(2):223-230.

52. Giri S, Chung YC, Merchant A, et al. T2 quantification for improved detection of myocardial edema. *J Cardiovasc Magn Reson.* 2009;11:56.

53. Thavendiranathan P, Walls M, Giri S, et al. Improved detection of myocardial involvement in acute inflammatory cardiomyopathies using T2 mapping. *Circ Cardiovasc Imaging.* 2012;5(1):102-110.

54. Grun S, Schumm J, Greulich S, et al. Long-term follow-up of biopsy-proven viral myocarditis: predictors of mortality and incomplete recovery. *J Am Coll Cardiol.* 2012;59(18):1604-1615.

55. Eitel I, von Knobelsdorff-Brenkenhoff F, Bernhardt P, et al. Clinical characteristics and cardiovascular magnetic resonance findings in stress (takotsubo) cardiomyopathy. *JAMA.* 2011;306(3):277-286.

56. Hulten E, Aslam S, Osborne M, Abbasi S, Bittencourt MS, Blankstein R. Cardiac sarcoidosis-state of the art review. *Cardiovasc Diagn Ther.* 2016;6(1):50-63.

57. Murtagh G, Laffin LJ, Beshai JF, et al. Prognosis of myocardial damage in sarcoidosis patients with preserved left ventricular ejection fraction: risk stratification using cardiovascular magnetic resonance. *Circ Cardiovasc Imaging.* 2016;9(1):e003738.

58. Patel MR, Cawley PJ, Heitner JF, et al. Detection of myocardial damage in patients with sarcoidosis. *Circulation.* 2009;120(20):1969-1977.

59. Crouser ED, Ono C, Tran T, He X, Raman SV. Improved detection of cardiac sarcoidosis using magnetic resonance with myocardial T2 mapping. *Am J Respir Crit Care Med.* 2014;189(1):109-112.

60. Birnie DH, Sauer WH, Bogun F, et al. HRS expert consensus statement on the diagnosis and management of arrhythmias associated with cardiac sarcoidosis. *Heart Rhythm.* 2014;11(7):1305-1323.

61. Rassi Jr A, Rassi A, Marin-Neto JA. Chagas heart disease: pathophysiologic mechanisms, prognostic factors and risk stratification. *Mem Inst Oswaldo Cruz.* 2009;104 Suppl 1:152-158.

62. Torreao JA, Ianni BM, Mady C, et al. Myocardial tissue characterization in Chagas' heart disease by cardiovascular magnetic resonance. *J Cardiovasc Magn Reson.* 2015;17:97.

63. McLaughlin VV, Shah SJ, Souza R, Humbert M. Management of pulmonary arterial hypertension. *J Am Coll Cardiol.* 2015;65(18):1976-1997.

64. Warnes CA, Williams RG, Bashore TM, et al. ACC/AHA 2008 guidelines for the management of adults with congenital heart disease: a report of the American College of Cardiology/American Heart Association Task Force on Practice Guidelines (Writing Committee to Develop Guidelines on the Management of Adults With Congenital Heart Disease): developed in collaboration with the American Society of Echocardiography, Heart Rhythm Society, International Society for Adult Congenital Heart Disease, Society for Cardiovascular Angiography and Interventions, and Society of Thoracic Surgeons. *Circulation.* 2008;118(23):e714-e833.

65. Baumgartner H, Bonhoeffer P, De Groot NM, et al. ESC guidelines for the management of grown-up congenital heart disease (new version 2010). *Eur Heart J.* 2010;31(23):2915-2957.

66. Baggen VJ, Leiner T, Post MC, et al. Cardiac magnetic resonance findings predicting mortality in patients with pulmonary arterial hypertension: a systematic review and meta-analysis. *Eur Radiol.* 2016 Nov;26(11):3771-3780.

67. Freed BH, Gomberg-Maitland M, Chandra S, et al. Late gadolinium enhancement cardiovascular magnetic resonance predicts clinical worsening in patients with pulmonary hypertension. *J Cardiovasc Magn Reson.* 2012;14:11.

68. Benza RL, Miller DP, Gomberg-Maitland M, et al. Predicting survival in pulmonary arterial hypertension: insights from the Registry to Evaluate Early and Long-Term Pulmonary Arterial Hypertension Disease Management (REVEAL). *Circulation.* 2010;122(2):164-172.

69. Miller CA, Fildes JE, Ray SG, et al. Non-invasive approaches for the diagnosis of acute cardiac allograft rejection. *Heart.* 2013;99(7):445-453.

70. Bonnemains L, Villemin T, Escanye JM, et al. Diagnostic and prognostic value of MRI T2 quantification in heart transplant patients. *Transpl Int.* 2014;27(1):69-76.

71. Butler CR, Savu A, Bakal JA, et al. Correlation of cardiovascular magnetic resonance imaging findings and endomyocardial biopsy results in patients undergoing screening for heart transplant rejection. *J Heart Lung Transplant.* 2015;34(5):643-650.

72. Bonnemains L, Cherifi A, Girerd N, Odille F, Felblinger J. Design of the DRAGET Study: a multicentre controlled diagnostic study to assess the detection of acute rejection in patients with heart transplant by means of T2 quantification with MRI in comparison to myocardial biopsies. *BMJ Open.* 2015;5(10):e008963.

73. Butler CR, Kim DH, Chow K, et al. Cardiovascular MRI predicts 5-year adverse clinical outcome in heart transplant recipients. *Am J Transplant.* 2014;14(9):2055-2061.

74. Chowdhary VB, Spencer B, Gao Y, et al. Prognostic value of cardiac magnetic resonance T2 quantification in heart transplant patients: a 5-year outcome study. *Circulation.* 2015;132:A16194.

24 RIGHT HEART CATHETERIZATION IN HEART FAILURE

Brent C. Lampert, DO

PATIENT CASE

A 62-year-old man with a history of nonischemic cardiomyopathy presents with worsening shortness of breath, orthopnea, lower extremity edema, and weight gain. He is diagnosed with acute on chronic systolic heart failure. Attempts at diuresis with furosemide 80 mg IV twice daily are unsuccessful and his renal function worsens. Right heart catheterization reveals elevated filling pressures and low cardiac output. He is started on inotropes and continuous furosemide infusion with improvement in his symptoms and renal function.

INTRODUCTION

Right heart catheterization (RHC) can be used for a variety of clinical indications in critically ill patients; use in decompensated heart failure (HF) is among the most common.

- Allows direct measurement of right atrial (RA), right ventricular (RV), and pulmonary artery (PA) pressures.[1]
- Can also estimate left atrial (LA) pressure by measuring the pulmonary capillary wedge pressure (PCWP).
- Cardiac output can be estimated using automated thermodilution techniques or calculated using the Fick method.
- Samples of mixed venous blood can be used to quantify oxygen consumption.
- Value of RHC use in HF remains controversial.[2]
  - Unnecessary in most patients who present with acute decompensated HF, but can provide valuable information in select patients.
  - Randomized ESCAPE trial showed no benefit (or increased risk) of using RHC in mortality or days alive out of the hospital.[3]
  - ESCAPE did not enroll all consecutive patients because many physicians would not enroll and risk a 50% chance of not having pulmonary artery catheter.
- Based on ESCAPE trial, routine RHC in HF is not recommended. However, it can be useful in a subset of advanced HF patients.
- The 2013 ACC/AHA HF guidelines suggest RHC be performed in patients with respiratory distress or impaired systemic perfusion when clinical assessment is inadequate.

PRESSURES

RIGHT ATRIAL PRESSURE

- Filling pressure of the right heart reflecting venous return to the RA during ventricular systole and RV end-diastolic pressure.
- Waveform normally has 3 distinct positive waves and 2 negative descents (Figure 24-1).
  - a wave reflects pressure increase at atrial contraction.
  - x descent reflects fall in pressure during atrial relaxation.
  - c wave (generally small) reflects pressure increase due to bulging of tricuspid valve into the RA during ventricular isovolumetric contraction.
  - v wave is increased atrial pressure from passive blood return to the atria while the tricuspid valve remains closed.
  - y descent reflects fall in atrial pressure as the tricuspid valve opens and blood rushes from the atrium to the ventricle.
  - a wave is usually slightly larger than the v wave.
- Normal RA pressure is 3 to 7 mm Hg (Table 24-1).
- Characteristic RA pressure waveforms:
  - Tricuspid regurgitation can result in tall v waves due to blood regurgitated into the RA during systole (Figure 24-2).
  - Atrial fibrillation results in loss of normal a waves due to lack of organized atrial activity.
  - Atrioventricular (AV) dissociation (seen in complete heart block, ventricular tachycardia, or ventricular pacing) may result in large "cannon" a waves due to contraction of the atrium against a close tricuspid valve.

RIGHT VENTRICULAR PRESSURE

- Usually measured at maximal systolic pressure, minimal early diastolic pressure, and end-diastolic pressure (Figure 24-1).
  - Ventricular systole is characterized by rapid upstroke and downstroke.
  - Ventricular diastole consists of an early rapid filling phase, slow filling phase, and atrial systolic phase.
  - End-diastolic pressure is expressed as the pressure immediately before the onset of ventricular contraction and after atrial contraction.
- Normal systolic RV pressure is 20 to 30 mm Hg and normal diastolic pressure is 3 to 7 mm Hg (Table 24-1).
- Elevated RV pressure is seen in pulmonary hypertension (HTN), pulmonic stenosis, and pulmonary embolism.
- Systolic pressure gradient between the RV and PA is seen in pulmonic stenosis.

PULMONARY ARTERY PRESSURE

- Waveform includes systolic pressure, diastolic pressure, and dicrotic notch, which represents closure of the pulmonic valve (Figure 24-1).

- Normal systolic PA pressure is 20 to 30 mm Hg and normal diastolic pressure is 8 to 12 mm Hg (Table 24-1).

- Elevations of PA pressure are seen with decompensated left HF or a range of conditions in which pulmonary vascular resistance is elevated.

PULMONARY CAPILLARY WEDGE PRESSURE

- Obtained by gently inflating a balloon at the distal end of the catheter obstructing blood flow and creating a static column of blood between the catheter tip and left atrium.

- Assuming no obstruction to flow between the PA and left ventricle, the PCWP estimates the left ventricular end-diastolic pressure (LVEDP) (ie, the left heart "filling pressure").[4,5]

- Normal PCWP is 8 to 12 mm Hg (Table 24-1).

- Waveform is similar to that seen in the RA (Figure 24-1).
  - a wave reflects pressure increase at atrial contraction.
  - x descent reflects fall in pressure during atrial relaxation.
  - c wave (often not seen) reflects pressure increase due to bulging of the mitral valve into the LA during ventricular isovolumetric contraction.
  - v wave is increased atrial pressure from passive blood return to the atria while the mitral valve remains closed.
  - y descent reflects fall in atrial pressure as the mitral valve opens and blood rushes from the atrium to the ventricle.
  - v wave is usually slightly larger than the a wave.

- PCWP may be lower than the LVEDP in conditions with decreased LV compliance (diastolic dysfunction, positive pressure ventilation, myocardial ischemia, or cardiac tamponade)[6] or other situations associated with premature closure of the mitral valve such as aortic stenosis.

- PCWP may be greater than the LVEDP when there is hypoxia or pulmonary disease due to constriction of small pulmonary veins.

- PCWP should be recorded at end expiration (which can differ considerably from mean PCWP).

- PCWP should be measured at the a wave to avoid large v waves confounding the interpretation.

- PCWP position should be confirmed by fluoroscopy, waveform inspection, and confirming that oxygen saturation from blood drawn distal to the balloon is consistent with systemic arterial saturations.

- Characteristic PCWP waveforms:
  - Conditions of increased resistance to LV filling, such as mitral stenosis, left-sided volume overload, or decreased LV compliance, can result in elevations of the a wave.
  - Mitral regurgitation may lead to tall v waves.
  - The height of the v wave does not accurately reflect the degree of mitral regurgitation and elevated v waves are neither sensitive nor specific for the diagnosis of mitral regurgitation.[7-10]

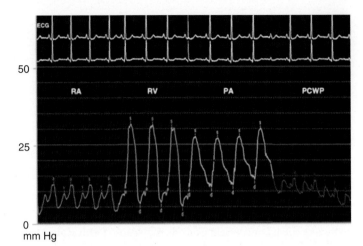

FIGURE 24-1 Normal hemodynamic recordings during RHC. From left to right: right atrium (RA), right ventricle (RV), pulmonary artery (PA), and pulmonary capillary wedge pressures (PCWP) are shown. Note in the arterial tracings, a and v waves can be seen immediately following the P and T waves of the electrocardiogram, respectively. (Reproduced with permission from Kasper DL, Fauci AS, Hauser D, et al. *Harrison's Principles of Internal Medicine*. 19th ed. New York, NY: McGraw-Hill Education; 2015. Figure 272-1.)

Table 24-1 Normal Pressure Measurements

Chamber	Pressure (mm Hg)	
	Average	Range
RA	5	±2
RV	25/5	±5 / ±2
PA	25/10	±5 / ±2
LA (PCWP)	10	±2

Abbreviations: LA, left atrium; PA, pulmonary artery; PCWP, pulmonary capillary wedge pressure; RA, right atrium; RV, right ventricle.

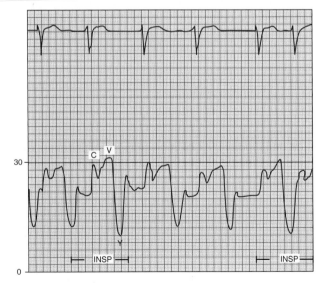

FIGURE 24-2 Right atrial tracing showing broad v (or cv) waves and prominent y descents consistent with tricuspid regurgitation. (Reproduced with permission from Hall JB, Schmidt GA, Wood LDH. *Principles of Critical Care*. 3rd ed. New York, NY: McGraw-Hill Education; 2005:152. Figure 13-21.)

CARDIAC OUTPUT

- Measured by Fick method or indicator dilution method.

FICK METHOD

- Uses amount of oxygen extracted by the body, as measured by the arterial – venous oxygen difference, to estimate cardiac output.
- Fick cardiac output = *Estimated oxygen consumption/10 (ateriovenous oxygen difference)*
  - Oxygen consumption can be directly measured using exhaled breath analysis, but is typically estimated from a nomogram based on age, sex, height, and weight.
  - *Ateriovenous oxygen difference* = $(1.36)(Hgb\ concentration)(SaO_2 - SvO_2)$
  - SaO_2 = arterial oxygen saturation measured from arterial blood
  - SvO_2 = mixed venous oxygen saturation measured from the PA. If there is a left-to-right shunt present, calculated by $MvO_2 = [3*SVC\ saturation + IVC\ saturation] / 4$
- Advantages
  - More accurate if heart rate (HR) or rhythm is irregular (ie, atrial fibrillation).
  - More accurate in low output states (lower cardiac output results in higher A – V O_2 difference).
  - Total error is 10% to 15%.
- Disadvantages
  - Difficult to obtain direct measure of oxygen consumption, so this is typically estimated.
  - Cannot detect rapid changes in cardiac output, so not useful in patients undergoing interventions such as valvuloplasty.

INDICATOR DILUTION METHOD[11]

- Typically consists of injecting a bolus of cold saline in the proximal port of catheter where it mixes with blood.
- Temperature of interventricular blood is lowered.
- Blood flows past the distal thermistor port, which records the temperature change over time and creates a temperature-time curve.
- Area under the temperature-time curve is inversely proportional to cardiac output.
- Continuous thermodilution catheters correlate well with bolus thermodilution methods,[12] but are more expensive and have not been shown to improve outcomes.[13]
- Advantages:
  - More accurate in high output states.
  - Simple to perform.
  - Ability to perform repeated measures to evaluate reproducibility.
- Disadvantages
  - Inaccurate with irregular HRs or rhythms.
  - Falsely low measures when there is tricuspid regurgitation that causes the fluid to be recycled back and forth across the tricuspid valve producing a prolonged, low-amplitude curve.
  - Falsely elevated measures in the setting of right-to-left and left-to-right shunts.
  - Measures can vary by 15% to 20%. Serial measures that differ by >10% should be considered unreliable.

PULMONARY ARTERY SATURATION MIXED VENOUS SATURATION)

- Can be used for an overall estimate of cardiac output in the absence of a shunt, hypoxia, or profound anemia.
- Saturation >80% indicates high output.
- Saturation <65% indicates low output.

OTHER MEASUREMENTS

SYSTEMIC VASCULAR RESISTANCE

- Once cardiac output is determined, systemic vascular resistance (SVR) can be estimated.
- SVR = 80* [*Mean arterial pressure (mm Hg) – right atrial pressure (mm Hg)]/systemic blood flow (cardiac output; L/min)*
- Least accurate of all RHC values—dependent on both direct measures (ie, pressures) and indirect measures (cardiac output), each of which have sources of error.

TRANSPULMONARY GRADIENT

- Transpulmonary gradient (TPG) = mean PA pressure – PCWP
- Normal value ≤12 mm Hg

PULMONARY VASCULAR RESISTANCE

- Pulmonary vascular resistance (PVR) = *TPG/CO*
- Normal value is <3 Wood units (or 240 dynes-sec-cm-5).

INTERPRETING HEMODYNAMICS (TABLE 24-2)

ACUTE HEART FAILURE

- Characterized by elevated PCWP.
- RA pressure normal or elevated.
- Cardiac output may be depressed.

ELEVATED PULMONARY PRESSURE

- Pulmonary arterial hypertension (PAH) is defined as mean PA pressure ≥25 mm Hg and PCWP ≤15 mm Hg.
- Pulmonary HTN associated with HF creates a diagnostic challenge.
  - Pulmonary HTN in proportion to HF occurs when the TPG remains ≤12 mm Hg and PVR is <3 Wood units. Patients should be diuresed to PCWP <15 before considering PAH-specific therapy (ie, pulmonary vasodilators).
  - PH out of proportion to HF occurs when the TPG is >12 mm Hg.

Table 24-2 Interpreting Hemodynamics

	Heart Failure	PAH	PH Associated with HF	
			In Proportion	Out of Proportion
RA (mm Hg)	Normal or ↑	Normal or ↑	Normal or ↑	Normal or ↑
RV (mm Hg)	Normal or ↑	↑	↑	↑
Mean PA (mm Hg)	Normal or ↑	≥25	≥25	≥25
PCWP (mm Hg)	>15	≤15	>15	>15
CO (L/min)	Normal or ↓	Normal or ↓	Normal or ↓	Normal or ↓
TPG (mm Hg)	Normal	>12	≤12	>12
PVR (Wood units)	Normal	>3	<3	>3

Abbreviations: CO, cardiac output; PA, pulmonary artery; PCWP, pulmonary capillary wedge pressure; PVR, pulmonary vascular resistance; RA, right atrium; RV, right ventricle; TPG, transpulmonary gradient.

- ○ Patients may benefit from PAH-specific therapy with guidance from a PAH specialist.
- ○ If the PCWP is >25 mm Hg, PH should be considered "in proportion" to HF regardless of TPG and patient should be completely diuresed before considering PAH-specific therapy.

ACUTE VASODILATOR TESTING

- Useful to determine possible reversibility of elevated PAs.
- Patients with chronic HF often develop "reactive" pulmonary HTN due to chronic elevations of the LVEDP.
- Chronically elevated LVEDP can lead to PA remodeling and irreversible PAH.
- Basis of vasodilator challenges is that the PA pressure will rapidly fall when the left heart is "unloaded."
- Can be performed with a variety of agents, including nitroprusside, nitroglycerin, inhaled nitric oxide, or IV epoprostenol.
- Positive response is considered a PVR reduced to <2.5 with systolic blood pressure remaining >85 mm Hg.
- PAH is considered as a relative contraindication to cardiac transplantation when the PVR is >5 Wood units or the TPG exceeds 16 to 20 mm Hg despite vasodilator challenge.[14]

CARDIAC TAMPONADE

- Diagnosis of tamponade can be confirmed by RHC.
- RA, PA diastolic pressure, and PCWP are all elevated (usually between 10 and 30 mm Hg) and are equal within 4 to 5 mm Hg of each other (Figure 24-3).
- RA and PCWP have attenuated or absent Y descent.
- Cardiac output is reduced and SVR is elevated.
- Definitive treatment involves removal of pericardial fluid.

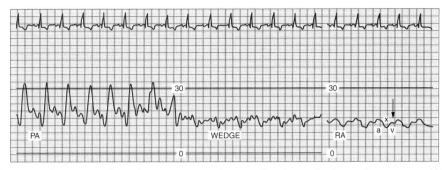

FIGURE 24-3 Pericardial tamponade. Tracings show characteristic equalization of wedge and right atrial pressures and blunting of the y descent (*arrow*). (Reproduced with permission from Sharkey SW. Beyond the wedge: clinical physiology and the Swan-Ganz catheter. *Am J Med.* 1987;83:111.)

ERRORS IN DATA ACQUISITION

- Dampened waveforms appear as rounded contours with delayed upstrokes and downstrokes and are often due to air bubbles within the catheter or tubing.
- Catheter "whip" results in an erratic waveform with highly variable pressures and can be resolved by repositioning the catheter or flushing the system.
- Zero level is set at the midchest with the transducer typically connected by a fluid-filled tube to the zero level fixed at the table or IV pole (Figure 24-4).
  - When transducer is raised above the 0 level, pressure is lower.
  - When transducer is lower than the 0 level, pressure is higher.
- Overwedging results from excessive inflation of the balloon.
  - Produces dampened waveform and leads to inaccurate values.
  - Increases the risk of PA rupture, a potentially fatal complication.
  - Usually corrects with partial deflation of the balloon.
- Underwedging results from incomplete occlusion of the PA.
  - Results in artificial elevation of PCWP.
  - Frequently occurs in patients with high PA pressures, likely due to poor compliance of their pulmonary vasculature.
  - Can deflate balloon and slowly reinflate until catheter wedges more completely or catheter can be withdrawn to the main PA and manipulated into a different PA branch.

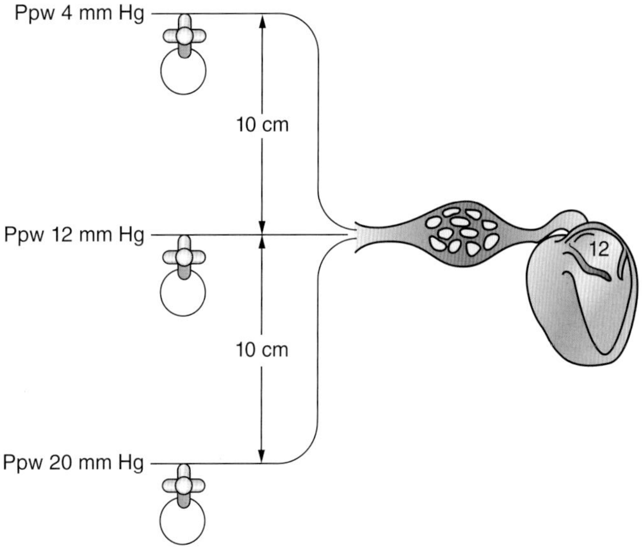

COMPLICATIONS

- Complications related to vascular access can include bleeding, arterial puncture, and pneumothorax.
- Ventricular ectopy is common when passing through the RV, but typically resolves when catheter is advanced into PA.
- Transient right bundle branch block can occur in up to 5% of catheterizations.[15]
- PA rupture can occur as a direct result of catheter-induced vascular injury.
  - Rare complication occurring in 0.06% to 0.2% of catheterizations.[16,17]
  - Patients develop frank onset of hemoptysis.

FIGURE 24-4 Effect of incorrect zero level on pressure measurements. In this example, PCWP is 12 mm Hg. Movement of the transducer above the left atrial plane falsely lowers PCWP reading to 4 mm Hg and movement below the left atrial plane results in falsely elevated reading of 20 mm Hg. (Reproduced with permission from Hall JB, Schmidt GA, Wood LDH. *Principles of Critical Care.* 3rd ed. New York, NY: McGraw-Hill Education; 2005:142. Figure 13-2.)

- Mortality rate exceeds 30% and management often involves emergent thoracotomy.[18]
- Risk factors include pulmonary HTN, advanced age, mitral valve disease, hypothermia, and anticoagulation.[19]
- Avoiding distal catheter placement and overinflation of the balloon decreases the risk.
- Balloon may be reinflated to occlude the bleeding vessel or to temporarily obstruct the feeding artery.

REFERENCES

1. Swan HJ, Ganz W, Forrester J, et al. Catheterization of the heart in man with use of a flow-directed balloon-tipped catheter. *N Engl J Med*. 1970;283:447-451.

2. Stevenson LW. Are hemodynamic goals viable in tailoring heart failure therapy? Hemodynamic goals are relevant. *Circulation*. 2006;113:1020-1033.

3. Binanay C, Califf RM, Hasselblad V, et al. Evaluation study of congestive heart failure and pulmonary artery catheterization effectiveness: the ESCAPE trial. *JAMA*. 2005;294:1625-1633.

4. Walston A, Kendall ME. Comparison of pulmonary wedge and left atrial pressure in man. *Am Heart J*. 1973;86:159-164.

5. Lappas D, Lell WA, Gabel JC, Civetta JM, Lowenstein E. Indirect measurement of left atrial pressure in surgical patient's pulmonary capillary wedge and pulmonary artery diastolic pressures compared with left atrial pressures. *Anesthesiology*. 1973;38:394-397.

6. Raper R, Sibbald WJ. Misled by the wedge? The Swan-Ganz catheter and left ventricular preload. *Chest*. 1986;89:427-434.

7. Pichard AD, Kay R, Smith H, Rentrop P, Holt J, Gorlin R. Large V waves in the pulmonary wedge pressure tracing in the absence of mitral regurgitation. *Am J Cardiol*. 1982;50:1044-1050.

8. Fuchs RM, Henser RR, Yin FCP, Brinker JA. Limitations of pulmonary wedge V waves in diagnosing mitral regurgitation. *Am J Cardiol*. 1982;49:849-854.

9. Schwinger M, Cohen M, Fuster V. Usefulness of onset of the pulmonary wedge V wave in predicting mitral regurgitation. *Am J Cardiol*. 1988;62:646-648.

10. Snyder RW 2nd, Glamann DB, Lange RA, et al. Predictive value of prominent pulmonary arterial wedge V waves in assessing the presence and severity of mitral regurgitation. *Am J Cardiol*. 1994;73:568-570.

11. Ganz W, Donoso R, Marcus HS, Forrester JS, Swan HJ. A new technique for measurement of cardiac output by thermodilution in man. *Am J Cardiol*. 1971;27:392-396.

12. Yelderman ML, Ramsay MA, Quinn MD, et al. Continuous thermodilution cardiac output measurement in intensive care unit patients. *J Cardiothorac Vasc Anesth*. 1992;6:270-274.

13. London MJ, Moritz TE, Henderson WG, et al. Standard versus fiberoptic pulmonary artery catheterization for cardiac surgery in the Department of Veterans Affairs: a prospective, observational, multicenter analysis. *Anesthesiology*. 2002;96:860-870.

14. Mehra MR, Kobashigawa J, Starling R, et al. Listing Criteria for Heart Transplantation: International Society for Heart and Lung Transplantation Guidelines for the Care of Cardiac Transplant Candidates—2006. *J Heart Lung Transplant*. 2006;25:1024-1042.

15. Putterman CE. The Swan-Ganz catheter: a decade of hemodynamic monitoring. *J Crit Care*. 1989;4:127-146.

16. Boyd KD. A prospective study of complication of pulmonary artery catheterizations in 500 consecutive patients. *Chest*. 1983;84:245-249.

17. Shah KB, Rao TLK, Laughlin S, et al. A review of pulmonary artery catheterizations in 6245 patients. *Anesthesiology*. 1984;61:271-275.

18. Kearney TJ, Shabot MM. Pulmonary artery rupture associated with the Swan-Ganz catheter. *Chest*. 1995;108:1349-1352.

19. Voyce SJ, Urbach D, Rippe JM. Pulmonary artery catheters. In: Rippe JM, Irwin RS, Alpert JS, Fink MP, eds. *Intensive Care Medicine*. Boston: Little Brown; 1991:66.

25 DIET IN HEART FAILURE

Eloisa Colin-Ramirez, BSc, MSc, PhD
JoAnne Arcand, PhD, RD
Justin A. Ezekowitz, MBBCh, MSc

PATIENT CASE

A 56-year-old woman was brought to the cardiologist office for routine clinical examination. The patient showed signs of peripheral edema, denied dyspnea, New York Heart Association functional class II, and was on the following cardiac medications: angiotensin-converting enzyme (ACE) inhibitors, beta blockers, statins, mineralocorticoid receptor antagonists, and furosemide. Her focused past cardiac history is that of a prior myocardial infarction, coronary artery bypass surgery, prior heart failure hospitalizations, and a known ejection fraction of 35%. She also notes medical compliance but not dietary compliance and does not feel that her muscle strength is being maintained. Serum electrolytes were: sodium, 140 mmol/L; potassium ranges from 4.9 to 5.8 mmol/L; and creatinine, 62 μmol/L. The woman's weight was 80 kg; height was 169 cm; body mass index (BMI) was 28 kg/m². She and her clinical team wonder if a better focus on diet may play a role.

EPIDEMIOLOGY OF HEART FAILURE

Chronic heart failure (HF) is a major and growing public health problem, with a tremendous impact on patients' quality of life and a broader economic burden. Approximately 5.7 million Americans ≥20 years of age have HF, and prevalence has been projected to increase 46% from 2012 to 2030 as patients survive acute myocardial infarction, live to an older age, and have best medical and nonpharmacologic care available. Survival after HF diagnosis has improved over time; however, HF carries a 5-year mortality rate of ~50% after diagnosis, and total direct medical cost of HF was estimated to be $21 billion in 2012.

ETIOLOGY AND PATHOPHYSIOLOGY

HF is a clinical syndrome that can result from any structural or functional cardiac disorder that impairs the ability of the ventricle to fill with or eject blood.[1] The most common etiologies are ischemic heart disease, hypertension (HTN), and diabetes. Less common causes of HF are cardiomyopathies, infections (eg, viral myocarditis, Chagas disease), toxins (eg, alcohol, cytotoxic drugs), valvular disease, and prolonged arrhythmias.[2]

HOW DOES DIET PLAY A ROLE IN HEART FAILURE?

HF may be associated with reduced cardiac output, which leads to a decrease in mean arterial pressure and diminished renal perfusion and causes to neurohormonal activation characterized by an overexpression of the sympathetic nervous system and the renin angiotensin aldosterone system to maintain optimal tissue perfusion to vital organs. This set of complex compensatory mechanisms causes vasoconstriction and renal sodium and water retention. Chronic neurohormonal activation exacerbates the hemodynamic abnormalities present in HF, producing further remodeling and neurohormone release and progressive cardiac impairment, causing excessive sodium and fluid retention.[2,3] This pathophysiologic process is in part responsible for HF signs and symptoms such as dyspnea and fatigue, which may limit exercise tolerance, and fluid retention, which may lead to pulmonary congestion and peripheral edema, all of which affect functional capacity and quality of life.[1]

DIETARY ASPECTS OF HEART FAILURE

DIETARY SODIUM INTAKE

Patients with chronic HF often have exacerbations requiring an emergency department visit and/or a hospital admission—often precipitated by excess sodium intake.[4] Recognizing the importance of achieving sodium balance in HF, dietary sodium restriction has been suggested as a major component of self-care management in HF. Dietary sodium recommendations for HF management typically call for a reduction in dietary sodium, because most individuals consume excessive amounts of dietary sodium. However, there is a lack of consistency for dietary sodium intake recommendations among the major guidelines for the management of HF.[1,5-10] Recommendations provided by the Canadian Cardiovascular Society (CCS),[5] the Heart Failure Society of America (HFSA),[6] the National Heart Foundation of Australia, and the Cardiac Society of Australia and New Zealand,[8] range from less than 2000 mg to 3000 mg per day, without identifying any safe lower level of consumption; whereas the National Institute for Health and Care Excellence (NICE),[7] the European Society of Cardiology (ESC),[9] and the American College of Cardiology and the American Heart Association (ACC/AHA),[1] on their most recent guidelines for the management of HF, do not provide any precise recommendation for sodium restriction.

Inconsistency in dietary sodium recommendations for HF is due to a lack of conclusive evidence on the impact of decreased dietary sodium on clinical events in the HF population.[3,11] Additionally, it has been suggested that a low-sodium diet may have detrimental effects in patients with HF due to its association with further neurohormonal activation in these patients.[11]

Clinical Studies on Sodium Restriction in Heart Failure

During the last decade, both observational and experimental studies evaluating the effects of sodium restriction in HF population have shown mixed results.[3] A small clinical trial suggested that a sodium intake less than 1500 mg/day may have a beneficial impact on B-type natriuretic peptide (BNP) levels and quality of life in ambulatory patients with chronic HF on optimal medical treatment.[12] However, 3 of the largest randomized controlled trials (RCTs)[13-15] testing the effects of sodium restriction on outcomes in HF showed that among patients with systolic HF, a low-sodium diet (80 mmol [1800 mg] sodium/day) was associated with higher mortality and readmission rates compared with a moderate-sodium diet (120 mmol [2800 mg] sodium/day) in combination with an aggressive diuretic regimen (250-1000 mg/day of furosemide) and fluid restriction (1 L/day). Though these trials tested the effect of dietary sodium restriction, the concomitant treatments administered make it challenging to elucidate the independent effects of dietary sodium on clinical outcomes. The aggressive doses of loop diuretics and fluid restriction likely also resulted in hypovolemia, which explains the adverse outcomes observed.

Overall, there are limitations to the quality of clinical and observational data that limit their use in developing evidence-based clinical practice guidelines. These include clinical studies that have small sample sizes and that administered aggressive cointerventions that prohibit the independent analysis of the effect of sodium restriction on clinical outcomes, making it challenging to compare data and draw definitive conclusions. However, a sodium restriction between 2000 and 3000 mg/day appears to be safe in this patient population, based on expert consensus. Further reduction to less than 1500 needs to be tested in large pragmatic RCTs.[3]

How Do We Assess Sodium Intake in Heart Failure?

Sodium restriction is a recommended dietary strategy for patients with symptomatic HF to reduce congestive symptoms.[1,9] Therefore, estimating dietary sodium intake is a key component of the dietary assessment in the clinical setting of HF to effectively implement appropriate dietary interventions for sodium reduction and monitor adherence to the dietary treatment. Current available sodium intake assessment methods include 24-hour urine collection, spot urine collections, multiple-day food records, food recalls, and food frequency questionnaires. Some of these methods have questionable validity at estimating individual intakes (ie, spot urine collection), require moderate to high participant burden, and do not provide timely feedback to guide dietary counseling in the clinical setting. Importantly, HF-related factors, such as the use of loop diuretics, may impede the utility of 24-hour urinary sodium excretion for estimating sodium intake in this patient population, and its use should be discouraged in the context of patients with HF on diuretics.[16,17] The use of high-quality dietary surveys, such as 3-day food records, might be an alternative to overcome this issue. Future research in this area is needed in order to identify the best method to assess dietary sodium intake in patients with HF.

WHAT ABOUT FLUID INTAKE?

Routine strict fluid restriction in all patients with HF regardless of symptoms or other considerations does not appear to result in significant benefit. Fluid restriction of 1.5 to 2 L/day may be considered in patients with severe HF, especially in those with hyponatremia, to relieve symptoms and congestion.[1,9]

ARE THERE OTHER DIETARY STRATEGIES TO CONSIDER BEYOND SODIUM?

Energy and Protein

Total energy expenditure in healthy subjects is the sum of resting energy expenditure (REE) and energy expenditure induced by physical activity. In patients with chronic HF, compared to healthy subjects, the REE is initially increased about 10% due to hypermetabolism,[18] which should be considered when estimating energy requirements in these patients; however, it is important to consider that physical activity may also be decreased in these same patients.

Negative calorie and nitrogen balances have been reported in patients with chronic HF, despite having similar calorie and nitrogen intakes, as compared to controls, suggesting that HF is a hypercatabolic state requiring increased calorie and protein needs. Therefore, it has been recommended that clinically stable malnourished patients with chronic HF have a daily intake of at least 31.8 kcal/kg + 1.37 grams protein/kg, and normally nourished patients a daily intake of at least 28.1 kcal/kg + 1.12 grams protein/kg in order to preserve their body weight and lean body mass, limiting the effects of hypercatabolism.[19]

Fats

The relationship of dietary fats to clinical outcomes or biochemical measures in patients with HF is scarce. Given that one of the most important risk factors for HF is coronary heart disease (CHD), the general dietary recommendations to reduce saturated fat intake for CHD risk reduction may be extrapolated to the HF population.[20] Current American Heart Association recommendation for saturated fat intake for cardiovascular risk reduction is to aim for a dietary pattern that achieves 5% to 6% of calories from saturated fat.[21] Additionally, there is increasing interest on the effects of omega-3 polyunsaturated fatty acids (n-3 PUFAs) in patients with HF. Results of the GISSI-HF trial, the larger clinical trial assessing the effects of n-3 PUFAs in HF, suggested a modest survival advantage from dietary supplementation with 1 g/day of n-3 PUFAs on mortality and cardiovascular hospital admission in patients with HF.[22,23] However, recent clinical trials and meta-analysis have not shown clear evidence of benefit from the supplementation with n-3 PUFAs on mortality in patients at risk for or with established cardiovascular disease (CVD).[24,25] Therefore, even though its supplementation seems to be reasonable as adjunctive therapy in patients with chronic HF, there is still a need to better define optimal dosing and formulation of omega-3 PUFA supplements.[1]

Micronutrients

There is concern that micronutrient needs may be higher in patients with HF compared to the general population due to oxidative stress.[26] Also, use of prescribed HF medications, such as loop diuretics, may alter the requirements of certain nutrients due to increased urinary excretion of thiamine, potassium, magnesium, and calcium.[27] It is important to consider that if a potassium-losing diuretic is used in combination with an ACE inhibitor and a mineralocorticoid receptor antagonist (MRA) or an angiotensin receptor blocker (ARB), potassium replacement is usually not required. Also, serious hyperkalemia may occur if potassium-sparing diuretics or supplements are taken in addition to the combination of an ACE inhibitor (or ARB) and MRA.[9]

In order to prevent serious micronutrient deficiencies, it is important to ensure that patients meet the Dietary Reference Intake (DRI) for micronutrients,[28,29] especially for those most likely to be deficient in patients with HF, as described below (Table 25-1). Currently, the most recent ACC/AHA guidelines do not recommend nutritional supplements in the treatment of HF.[1]

Table 25-1 Dietary Reference Intake for Adults (≥19 years old) for Relevant Micronutrients in Patients with Heart Failure

	Dietary Reference Intake[28,29,52]		
	Males	Females	Dietary Sources
Calcium (mg/day)	1000 >70 years old: 1200	1000 ≥51 years old: 1200	Milk, cheese, yogurt, kefir, sardines and salmon with bones, Swiss chard, spinach, almonds, beans, calcium-fortified orange juice
Magnesium (mg/day)	19-30 years old: 330 >30 years old: 350	19-30 years old: 255 >30 years old: 265	Spinach, Swiss chard, nuts and seeds, fish (salmon, halibut, mackerel, pollock), bran cereals and wheat germ, soybeans, beans, lentils
*Potassium (mg/day)	4700	4700	Bananas, papaya, potato, dark leafy greens, squash, avocado, tomato juice, oranges, orange juice, milk, yogurt, dried beans, nuts and seeds
Zinc (mg/day)	9.4	6.8	Seafood (oysters), beef, lamb, pork, chicken, wheat germ, pumpkin and squash seeds, nuts, beans, chickpeas, cheese (cheddar, Swiss, gouda, brie, mozzarella)
Thiamin (mg/day)	1	0.9	Fish (trout, salmon, tuna), pork, sunflower seeds, bread (wheat), macadamia, soybean sprouts, edamame, green peas, squash (acorn)
Folate (µg/day)	320	320	Beans, lentils, peas (chickpeas, black-eyed, pigeon), enriched grain products, spinach, asparagus, broccoli, Brussels sprouts, lettuce, avocado, papaya, orange juice
Vitamin E (mg/day)	12	12	Nuts and seeds, dark leafy greens, avocado, wheat germ, egg, oily fish, vegetable oil
Vitamin D (IU/day)	600 >70 years old: 800	600 >70 years old: 800	Cod liver oil, milk, egg yolk, oily fish, pork

*Some patients may also need to reduce potassium intake sometime during the disease course because of the use of potassium-sparing cardiac medications and/or the coexistence of renal disease.

MICRONUTRIENT DEFICIENCY IN HEART FAILURE

Dietary inadequacies (eg, calories, protein, and several vitamins and minerals) are common in patients with HF.[30-36] It has been shown that more than 50% of HF patients have inadequate dietary intakes of several nutrients, including calcium, magnesium, potassium, folate, vitamin E, vitamin D, and zinc.[30,37] Factors associated with deceased food intake in this patient population include decreased hunger sensations, fatigue, shortness of breath, nausea, anxiety, sadness, and medically recommended diet restrictions.[38,39]

A dietary sodium consumption of <2000 mg/day has also been linked to poor overall nutrient intake in these patients.[40,41] A sodium-restricted diet is often described as unpalatable and subsequently related to decreased appetite, leading to higher risk of poor nutritional intake.[38] It was reported that among patients who were prescribed a <2000 mg/day sodium-restricted diet for 1 week, a 49% reduction in dietary sodium (3626-1785 mg/day) was associated with a significant reduction in calorie, carbohydrate, calcium, thiamine, and folate intakes. Also, there was a decrease in saturated fat.[42] However, results of a recent study suggested that dietary sodium reduction in these patients may be achieved without greatly compromising overall dietary intake and nutritional status when an individualized dietary approach, considering the whole diet, is used. Nonetheless, calcium intake was still negatively affected.[43]

Additionally, beyond factors related to a reduced food intake, other aspects need to be taken into consideration when evaluating the risk of nutrient deficiency in HF, such as the possibility of increased nutrient needs due to oxidative stress, hypercatabolic status, and use of loop diuretics, as noted previously, but also an inadequate nutrient absorption. Abdominal and gut edema with dysfunctional intestinal barriers and consequently increased permeability, exposure to endotoxins, and chronic inflammation may impair mucosa function and nutrient uptake, contributing to nutrient deficiency.[44]

Does Replacing Micronutrients Improve Clinical Outcomes in Heart Failure?

It has been proposed that micronutrient deficiency would be associated with adverse health outcomes in patients with HF. However, among 3340 participants in the Women's Health Initiative (WHI) with incident HF hospitalization, intakes of calcium, magnesium, and potassium were not significantly associated with subsequent mortality.[45] Similar results were observed in a study of 116 patients with HF, where an increased consumption of saturated fatty acids was associated with a higher risk of all-cause mortality and dietary polyunsaturated fatty acids consumption was associated with lower all-cause mortality, but no other dietary micronutrient or macronutrient was found to have this association.[20] Conversely, a study involving 113 consecutive outpatients with HF reported that calcium, magnesium, and vitamin D were the most common micronutrient deficiencies, and that micronutrient deficiency was independently associated with worse health-related quality of life, whereas the number of micronutrient deficiencies independently predicted cardiac event-free survival.[37]

Currently, no single clinical trial on single-nutrient or multivitamin supplementation has reported improved outcomes or survival in patients with HF, nor have there been reports of adverse outcomes. Therefore, aside from a pragmatic clinical approach to replenishment of documented deficiencies in the setting of HF, nutritional supplements are not recommended for the treatment of HF.[1,44]

CARDIAC CACHEXIA

EPIDEMIOLOGY AND ETIOLOGY

Malnutrition has been diagnosed in 20% to 70% of patients with HF and is believed to further complicate this clinical syndrome.[44] Cardiac cachexia, one of the most important malnutrition syndromes in HF, is a clinical entity that often occurs at the end-stage of chronic HF.[46] The prevalence of cardiac cachexia is reported to be 5% to 15% and the annual mortality rate of cachexia is 20% to 30%.[18] The pathophysiology of cardiac cachexia is a complex and multifactorial process including catabolic and anabolic imbalance, inadequate protein intake, poor enteral nutrient absorption, immune and neurohormonal disturbance, and physical inactivity.[18,46] Cardiac cachexia is unlikely to develop as a consequence of an inadequate protein or energy intake per se; however, combined micronutrient and macronutrient deficiency may contribute to disease progression. Additionally, even though the REE in patients with HF is initially increased (REE increase about 10%) due to hypermetabolism, which is probably the beginning of the pathway to weight loss, once cachexia has developed, the REE drops below the value of healthy individuals and physical activity is greatly limited; thus the total daily energy expenditure is reduced by 25% compared to healthy subjects and 20% compared to patients with chronic HF without cachexia.[18]

DIAGNOSIS

Malnutrition syndrome is associated with poor prognosis in this patient population, though it tends to be underdiagnosed and often unrecognized until late stages.[18] A consensus panel developed a set of diagnostic criteria to allow clinicians and researchers to make a definitive diagnosis of cachexia. The key component is at least a 5% loss of edema-free body weight during the previous 3 to 12 months or a BMI of <20.0 kg/m^2 in cases where a history of weight loss cannot be documented. In addition to the presence of a weight loss indicator, diagnosis of cachexia requires the presence of at least 3 of the following diagnostic criteria: decreased muscle strength, fatigue, anorexia, low muscle (fat-free) mass, and biochemical abnormalities characteristic of inflammation, anemia, or hypoalbuminemia.[47]

TREATMENT

The treatment of cardiac cachexia remains challenging; because it is a multifactorial disorder, no single agent is fully effective in its treatment.[46] Promising results in the treatment of cachexia have been reported with ghrelin receptor agonists (anamorelin), selective androgen receptor modulators (enobosarm), and some beta blockers (espindolol), while efficacy of myostatin antagonists for treating cardiac cachexia is under investigation.[18] Regarding nutritional therapy, it has been found to have no effect on the underlying catabolic process of cachexia when used alone. However, there is increasing evidence that protein supplementation may improve muscle synthesis with an increased effect when used in conjunction with exercise.[46] It has been suggested that the supplementation with 1 to 1.5 g/kg of high-quality protein may be effective to restore muscle mass in persons with sarcopenia.[48] Additionally, increased calorie intake through nutrient-dense foods or nutritional supplements in cachectic HF patients seems to contribute to enhanced weight and improved quality of life. Likewise, there is some evidence of improved skeletal muscle function and exercise duration with chronic oral carnitine administration, though there is no evidence of improved cardiac function. Other nutritional interventions such as eicosapentaenoic acid, β-hydroxy-β-methylbutyrate, and resveratrol may positively affect body wasting and muscle loss in animal models, without proved effects in humans.[46] Among all investigated therapies, aerobic exercise training is the most proved to have a beneficial effect on skeletal muscle wasting and is recommended by treatment guidelines for HF.[1,9]

OBESITY AND WEIGHT LOSS IN HEART FAILURE

Obesity is an important risk factor for HF. Observational studies have suggested that an obesity paradox may exist in patients with established CVD, where overweight and mildly obese patients with most CVD have a better short- and medium-term prognosis than do leaner patients. This obesity paradox seems most apparent in those patients with low levels of cardiorespiratory fitness, whereas those with preserved cardiorespiratory fitness have a good prognosis, regardless of weight and body composition.[49] To date, there are no large-scale studies of the safety or efficacy of weight loss with diet, exercise, or bariatric surgery in obese patients with HF;[1] however, it is reasonable to manage obesity to keep a healthy weight,[9] avoiding the use of hypocaloric diets because they are associated with increased body protein breakdown.[19] Additionally, because muscular strength is associated with better CVD risk factors and lower mortality, resistance and aerobic exercise training are important during weight loss and maintenance in order to preserve or increase muscle mass and muscular strength.[49]

PATIENT EDUCATION

Most of the sodium in Western diets comes from processed and prepared foods; therefore dietary sodium reduction should focus on reducing frequency of consumption of processed/packaged foods and restaurant meals.[50] Patients should also be counseled to avoid adding salt while cooking or at the table (Figures 25-1 through 25-3).

Prior to providing advice, is important to determine the primary source of sodium in the diet. Importantly, patients frequently misreport the amount of sodium in their diets because they may not be aware of the amount of sodium in certain food. Online tools such as the Sodium Calculator, included in the "Patient and

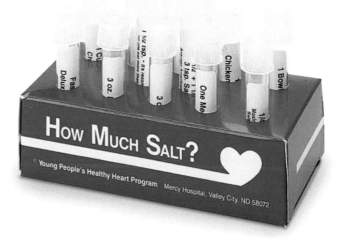

FIGURE 25-1 How Much Salt? This test tube display set by NASCO displays the amount of salt our body needs daily, the average amount Americans eat, the amount listed in the Dietary Goals, as well as the amount of salt (in milligrams) in the following foods: potato, potato chips or tortilla chips, canned chicken noodle soup, homemade soup, pork chop, ham, fast food quarter pound cheeseburger, a typical picnic meal, and ramen noodles. Because patients are familiar with salt, sodium values have been converted to salt for display in the test tubes. (© All rights reserved. *Nutrition Fact Tables.* Health Canada, modified: 2018. Adapted and reproduced with permission from the Minister of Health, 2018.)

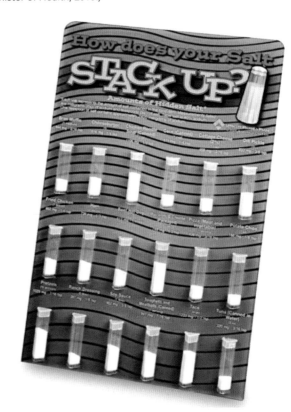

FIGURE 25-2 The Salt Case by NASCO represents the sodium content in 18 popular foods, including cheeseburger, macaroni and cheese, fried chicken, and potato chips. Teaspoons of salt in each item are shown in clear plastic tubes. (© All rights reserved. *Nutrition Fact Tables.* Health Canada, modified: 2018. Adapted and reproduced with permission from the Minister of Health, 2018.)

Provider Resources" section, may be useful to screen for patients' habitual sodium intake. Also, asking patients quick questions about frequency of consumption of main sources of dietary sodium may help clinicians identify patients with a high sodium intake. Some suggested questions are the following:

- How many times per week do you eat bacon or processed/luncheon/deli meat?

- How many times per week do you eat canned or prepackaged soups, chili, or pasta with sauces or fast food?

- How many times per week do you eat frozen food such as frozen pizza or frozen dinners?

- How many times per week do you eat pickles, olives, or sauerkraut?

- How many times per week do you eat a meal in a restaurant?

- Do you regularly use salt in your cooking or salty condiments such as salad dressing, soy sauce, hot sauce, or bouillon cubes?

NUTRITION FACTS LABELS READING

It is important to consider that high amounts of sodium may seem hidden in packaged food, particularly when a food does not taste salty. Reading Nutrition Facts tables on food products is a good strategy to identify how much sodium is in packaged foods and to compare between products, which may help patients to be able to make informed decisions when selecting foods (eg, while grocery shopping) (Figure 25-4). Most packaged foods contain a Nutrition

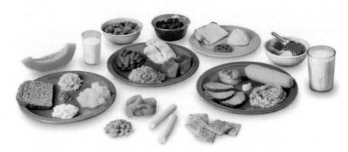

FIGURE 25-3 Food replicas by NASCO bring nutrition education to life, add the sense of touch, and help people retain knowledge. Using food replicas is possible to show how to accomplish appealing, varied, and healthy meals. (© All rights reserved. *Nutrition Fact Tables.* Health Canada, modified: 2018. Adapted and reproduced with permission from the Minister of Health, 2018.)

Cracker A

Nutrition facts	
Per 9 crackers (23 g)	
Amount	**% Daily value**
Calories 90	
Fat 4.5 g	7%
Saturated 2.5 g + Trans 0 g	13%
Cholesterol 0 mg	
Sodium 280 mg	12%
Carbohydrate 12 g	4%
Fiber 1 g	4%
Sugars 0 g	
Protein 3 g	

Vitamin A	0%	Vitamin C	0%
Calcium	2%	Iron	8%

Cracker B

Nutrition facts	
Per 4 crackers (20 g)	
Amount	**% Daily value**
Calories 90	
Fat 2 g	3%
Saturated 0.3 g + Trans 0 g	2%
Cholesterol 0 mg	
Sodium 90 mg	4%
Carbohydrate 15 g	5%
Fiber 3 g	12%
Sugars 1 g	
Protein 2 g	

Vitamin A	0%	Vitamin C	0%
Calcium	2%	Iron	8%

FIGURE 25-4 Comparing labels. Cracker A has 9 crackers per serving and weighs 23 g. Cracker B has 4 crackers per serving and weighs 20 g. Because the weights are similar, you can compare these Nutrition Facts tables. Read the percent daily values (DVs). Because you are comparing crackers, you may want to look at the % DVs for saturated and trans fats, sodium, and fiber. Cracker A has 13% DV for saturated and trans fats, 12% DV for sodium, and 4% DV for fiber. Cracker B has 2% DV for saturated and trans fats, 4% DV for sodium, and 12% DV for fiber. Remember, 5% DV or less is a little and 15% DV or more is a lot. In this case, Cracker B would be a better choice if you are trying to eat less saturated and trans fats, less sodium, and more fiber as part of a healthy lifestyle. (© All rights reserved. *Nutrition Fact Tables.* Health Canada, modified: 2018. Adapted and reproduced with permission from the Minister of Health, 2018.)

Facts table. Table 25-2 provides some relevant considerations that the patient may need to be aware of when reading labels.

TIPS TO REDUCE DIETARY SODIUM INTAKE

- In cooking and at the table, flavor foods with lemon juice, vinegar, herbs, spices, garlic, or onions instead of salt. Switch to seasonings with no added salt.
- Cook foods from fresh, rather than buying prepared, packaged, canned, or frozen foods.
- Rinse canned vegetables and fish.
- Choose low-sodium or no-salt-added breads and cereals (eg, natural oats instead of instant oatmeal).
- Choose unsalted butter and nuts.
- Avoid or limit the use condiments such as mustard, ketchup, salad dressings, soy sauce, and teriyaki sauce. Reduced-sodium versions of soy sauce and teriyaki sauce are also not recommended as these are still high in sodium.
- Avoid cured foods (eg, bacon, ham, sausage, luncheon meats, pickles, olives, and sauerkraut).
- Choose home-prepared foods more often; limit restaurants meals.
- Restaurants may have nutrition information on their menus or online. Take a look at the healthy meals; there may be low-sodium options. Also, most restaurants are willing to accommodate requests.
- Pay attention to potassium-containing salt substitute, especially in patients on potassium-sparing cardiac medications and/or with coexistent renal disease.

Additionally, counseling by a dietitian or nutritionist has shown to further significantly reduce sodium intakes.[51] A dietitian is able to provide nutritional counseling according to patients' individual needs, as well as alternatives to the not recommended foods and examples of healthy foods, which may improve adherence to a low-sodium diet and improve quality of the overall diet.

RESOLUTION TO INTRODUCTORY PATIENT CASE

A review of a 3-day food record completed during the previous week to the clinical appointment identified the following food item as the main sources of sodium in the diet of the patient:

- Cheddar biscuits, 5 pieces 1 of the 3 days recorded
- White bread, 4 slices 1 of the 3 days recorded
- Salted butter, 4 tablespoons/day on average
- Processed cheese, 4 slices/day on average
- Canned beans, one-half can 1 of the 3 days recorded
- Salad dressing, 2 tablespoons/day on average
- Packaged dinner, 1 package 1 of the 3 days recorded
- Restaurant meals, 1 night dined out (bowl of soup, pasta dish, cheesecake)

Patient was advised to reduce her frequency of intake of processed cheeses and opt for those with less sodium content such as Swiss cheese, switch to unsalted butter, and try to prepare dinner at

Table 25-2 Considerations for Reading Food Labels[53,54]

a. The Nutrition Facts table lists the percent daily value (%DV) of sodium in 1 serving of a food.

b. The %DV for sodium listed in the table is based on a 100% of a recommended amount of sodium, which is <2400 mg/d.

c. The %DV listed is for 1 serving, but many packages contain >1 serving. Look at the serving size and how many servings you are actually consuming—if you eat 2 servings you get twice as much sodium (or double the %DV).

d. The %DV tells you whether a food contributes a little or a lot to your total daily diet.

- 5%DV (120 mg) or less of sodium per serving is considered low
- 15%DV (360 mg) or more of sodium per serving is considered high

e. Check the front of the food package to quickly identify foods that may contain less sodium. For example, look for foods with claims such as:

- Free of sodium or salt → <5 mg of sodium per serving
- Low sodium → 140 mg of sodium or less per serving or per 100 g of the food if it is a prepackaged meal
- Reduced sodium → At least 25% less sodium than in the original product
- Lower in sodium → A food contains 25% less sodium compared to a similar food product
- Light in sodium or lightly salted → At least 50% less sodium than the regular product
- No added sodium or salt (or unsalted) → No salt is added during processing, but not necessarily sodium-free. Check the Nutrition Facts table to be sure!

home from fresh, instead of using canned or packaged foods. When eating out, patient was advised to avoid soups, ask for low-sodium preparations, and use olive oil and vinegar on the salad instead of regular dressings. Also, increasing vegetable intake was recommended because it seemed to be low according to the information recorded in the food record.

Importantly, the patient reported to eat 1 banana per day and tomato juice two times a week. Due to her potassium levels (ranges from 4.9 to 5.8 mmol/L), she was advised to reduce intake of those foods. Patient denied used of potassium-containing salt substitutes.

The patient was referred to the dietitian for further nutritional counseling to reduce sodium and potassium intake, and improve quality of the overall diet.

PATIENT AND PROVIDER RESOURCES

Sodium Calculator: https://www.projectbiglife.ca/sodium/

Heart and Stroke Foundation—Healthy Eating: http://www.heartandstroke.ca/get-healthy/healthy-eating

Centers of Disease Control and Prevention—Salt: http://www.cdc.gov/salt/index.htm

Canadian Food Inspection Agency—Food Labeling for Consumers: http://www.inspection.gc.ca/food/labelling/food-labelling-for-consumers/eng/1400426541985/1400455563893

Health Canada—The % of Daily Value: http://www.hc-sc.gc.ca/fn-an/label-etiquet/nutrition/cons/dv-vq/index-eng.php

Canadian Food Inspection Agency—Specific Nutrient Content Claim Requirements, Sodium (Salt) Claims: http://www.inspection.gc.ca/food/labelling/food-labelling-for-industry/nutrient-content/specific-claim-requirements/eng/1389907770176/1389907817577?chap=9#s7c9

KEY POINTS

- Dietary sodium restriction has been suggested as a main component of self-care management in HF.

- A sodium restriction between 2000 and 3000 mg/day appears to be safe in this patient population. The effects of further restriction need to be elucidated.

- Fluid restriction of 1.5 to 2 L/day may be considered in patients with severe HF, especially in those with hyponatremia, to relieve symptoms and congestion.

- It is essential to consider the whole diet when counseling patients with HF in order to ensure appropriate intake of energy, protein, and micronutrients.

- Aside from a pragmatic clinical approach to replenishment of documented deficiencies in the setting of HF, nutritional supplements are not recommended for the treatment of HF.

- Consulting a registered dietitian is especially helpful for patients with recent HF exacerbations or for patients with multiple comorbidities who may need to follow several dietary restrictions.

REFERENCES

1. Yancy CW, Jessup M, Bozkurt B, et al. 2013 ACCF/AHA guideline for the management of heart failure: executive summary: a report of the American College of Cardiology Foundation/American Heart Association Task Force on practice guidelines. *Circulation.* 2013;128(16):1810-1852.

2. Kemp CD, Conte JV. The pathophysiology of heart failure. *Cardiovasc Pathol.* 2012;21(5):365-371.

3. Colin-Ramirez E, Ezekowitz JA. Salt in the diet in patients with heart failure: what to recommend. *Curr Opin Cardiol.* 2016;31(2):196-203.

4. Fonarow GC, Abraham WT, Albert NM, et al. Factors identified as precipitating hospital admissions for heart failure and clinical outcomes: findings from OPTIMIZE-HF. *Arch Intern Med.* 2008;168(8):847-854.

5. Malcom J, Arnold O, Howlett JG, et al. Canadian Cardiovascular Society Consensus conference guidelines on heart failure-2008 update: best practice for the transition of care of heart failure, and the recognition, investigation and treatment of cardiomyopathies. *Can J Cardiol.* 2008;24(1):21-40.

6. Lindenfeld J, Albert NM, Boehmer JP, et al. Executive summary: HFSA 2010 Comprehensive Heart Failure Practice Guideline. *J Card Fail.* 2010;16:475-539.

7. National Institute for Health and Care Excellence. Chronic heart failure: management of chronic heart failure in adults in primary and secondary care. 2010.

8. National Heart Foundation of Australia and the Cardiac Society of Australia and New Zealand (Chronic Heart Failure Guidelines Expert Writing Panel). Guidelines for the prevention, detection and management of chronic heart failure in Australia. Updated October 2011.

9. McMurray J, Adamopoulos S, Anker SD, et al. ESC guidelines for the diagnosis and treatment of acute and chronic heart failure 2012. The Task Force for the Diagnosis and Treatment of Acute and Chronic Heart Failure 2012 of the European Society of Cardiology. Developed in collaboration with the Heart Failure Association (HFA) of the ESC. *Eur J Heart Fail.* 2012;14:803-869.

10. Colin-Ramirez E, Arcand J, Ezekowitz JA. Estimates of dietary sodium consumption in patients with chronic heart failure. *J Card Fail.* 2015;21(12):981-988.

11. Gupta D, Georgiopoulou V, Kalogeropoulos A, et al. Dietary sodium intake in heart failure. *Circulation.* 2012;126:479-485.

12. Colin-Ramirez E, McAlister FA, Zheng Y, Sharma S, Armstrong PW, Ezekowitz JA. The long-term effects of dietary sodium restriction on clinical outcomes in patients with heart failure. The SODIUM-HF (Study of Dietary Intervention Under 100 MMOL in Heart Failure): a pilot study. *Am Heart J.* 2015;169(2):274-281.

13. Parrinello G, Di Pasquale P, Licata G, et al. Long-term effects of dietary sodium intake on cytokines and neurohormonal activation in patients with recently compensated congestive heart failure. *J Card Fail.* 2009;15(10):864-873.

14. Paterna S, Gaspare P, Fasullo S, Sarullo FM, Di Pasquale P. Normal-sodium diet compared with low-sodium diet in compensated congestive heart failure: is sodium an old enemy or a new friend? *Clin Sci.* 2008;114(3):221-230.

15. Paterna S, Parrinello G, Cannizzaro S, et al. Medium term effects of different dosage of diuretic, sodium, and fluid administration on neurohormonal and clinical outcome in patients with recently compensated heart failure. *Am J Cardiol.* 2009;103(1):93-102.

16. Arcand J, Floras JS, Azevedo E, Mak S, Newton GE, Allard JP. Evaluation of 2 methods for sodium intake assessment in cardiac patients with and without heart failure: the confounding effect of loop diuretics. *Am J Clin Nutr.* 2011;93(3):535-541.

17. Colin-Ramirez E, Arcand J, Ezekowitz JA. Estimates of dietary sodium consumption in patients with chronic heart failure. *J Card Fail.* 2015;21(12):981-988.

18. Griva M. Cardiac cachexia – Up-to-date 2015. *Cor et vasa.* 2015.

19. Aquilani R, Opasich C, Verri M, et al. Is nutritional intake adequate in chronic heart failure patients? *J Am Coll Cardiol.* 2003;42(7):1218-1223.

20. Colin-Ramirez E, Castillo-Martinez L, Orea-Tejeda A, Zheng Y, Westerhout CM, Ezekowitz JA. Dietary fatty acids intake and mortality in patients with heart failure. *Nutrition.* 2014;30(11-12):1366-1371.

21. Eckel RH, Jakicic JM, Ard JD, et al. 2013 AHA/ACC guideline on lifestyle management to reduce cardiovascular risk: a report of the American College of Cardiology/American Heart Association Task Force on Practice Guidelines. *Circulation.* 2014;129(25 Suppl 2):S76-S99.

22. Tavazzi L, Maggioni AP, Marchioli R, et al. Effect of n-3 polyunsaturated fatty acids in patients with chronic heart failure (the GISSI-HF trial): a randomised, double-blind, placebo-controlled trial. *Lancet.* 2008;372(9645):1223-1230.

23. Masson S, Marchioli R, Mozaffarian D, et al. Plasma n-3 polyunsaturated fatty acids in chronic heart failure in the GISSI-Heart Failure Trial: relation with fish intake, circulating biomarkers, and mortality. *Am Heart J.* 2013;165(2):208-215.

24. Rauch B, Schiele R, Schneider S, et al. OMEGA, a randomized, placebo-controlled trial to test the effect of highly purified omega-3 fatty acids on top of modern guideline-adjusted therapy after myocardial infarction. *Circulation.* 2010;122(21):2152-2159.

25. Kotwal S, Jun M, Sullivan D, Perkovic V, Neal B. Omega 3 fatty acids and cardiovascular outcomes: systematic review and meta-analysis. *Circ Cardiovasc Qual Outcomes.* 2012;5(6):808-818.

26. Shetty PM, Hauptman PJ, Landfried LK, Patel K, Weiss EP. Micronutrient deficiencies in patients with heart failure: relationships with body mass index and age. *J Card Fail.* 2015;21(12):968-972.

27. Weber KT. Furosemide in the long-term management of heart failure: the good, the bad, and the uncertain. *J Am Coll Cardiol.* 2004;44(6):1308-1310.

28. Institute of Medicine, Food and Nutrition Board. *Dietary Reference Intakes: The Essential Guide to Nutrient Requirements.* Washington, DC: National Academies Press; 2006.

29. Institute of Medicine, Food and Nutrition Board. *Dietary Reference Intakes for Calcium and Vitamin D.* Washington, DC: The National Academies Press; 2011.

30. Arcand J, Floras V, Ahmed M, et al. Nutritional inadequacies in patients with stable heart failure. *J Am Diet Assoc.* 2009;109(11):1909-1913.

31. Price RJ, Witham MD, McMurdo ME. Defining the nutritional status and dietary intake of older heart failure patients. *Eur J Cardiovasc Nurs.* 2007;6(3):178-183.

32. Catapano G, Pedone C, Nunziata E, Zizzo A, Passantino A, Incalzi RA. Nutrient intake and serum cytokine pattern in elderly people with heart failure. *Eur J Heart Fail.* 2008;10(4):428-434.

33. Lourenco BH, Vieira LP, Macedo A, Nakasato M, Marucci Mde F, Bocchi EA. Nutritional status and adequacy of energy and nutrient intakes among heart failure patients. *Arq Bras Cardiol.* 2009;93(5):541-548.

34. Lemon SC, Olendzki B, Magner R, et al. The dietary quality of persons with heart failure in NHANES 1999-2006. *J Gen Intern Med.* 2010;25(2):135-40.

35. Hughes CM, Woodside JV, McGartland C, Roberts MJ, Nicholls DP, McKeown PP. Nutritional intake and oxidative stress in chronic heart failure. *Nutr Metab Cardiovasc Dis.* 2012;22(4):376-382.

36. Son YJ, Song EK. High nutritional risk is associated with worse health-related quality of life in patients with heart failure beyond sodium intake. *Eur J Cardiovasc Nurs.* 2013;12(2):184-192.

37. Song EK, Kang SM. Micronutrient deficiency independently predicts adverse health outcomes in patients with heart failure. *J Cardiovasc Nurs.* 2017;32(1):47-53.

38. Lennie TA, Moser DK, Heo S, Chung ML, Zambroski CH. Factors influencing food intake in patients with heart failure. A comparison with healthy elders. *J Cardiovasc Nurs.* 2006;21(2):123-129.

39. Song EK, Moser DK, Kang SM, Lennie TA. Association of depressive symptoms and micronutrient deficiency with cardiac event-free survival in patients with heart failure. *J Card Fail.* 2015;21(12):945-951.

40. Grossniklaus DA, O'Brien MC, Clark PC, Dunbar SB. Nutrient intake in heart failure patients. *J Cardiovasc Nurs.* 2008;23(4):357-363.

41. Frediani JK, Reilly CM, Higgins M, Clark PC, Gary RA, Dunbar SB. Quality and adequacy of dietary intake in a southern urban heart failure population. *J Cardiovasc Nurs.* 2013;28(2):119-128.

42. Jefferson K, Ahmed M, Choleva M, et al. Effect of a sodium-restricted diet on intake of other nutrients in heart failure: implications for research and clinical practice. *J Card Fail.* 2015;21(12):959-962.

43. Colin-Ramirez E, McAlister FA, Zheng Y, Sharma S, Ezekowitz JA. Changes in dietary intake and nutritional status associated with a significant reduction in sodium intake in patients with heart failure. A sub-analysis of the SODIUM-HF pilot study. *Clin Nutr ESPEN.* 2016;11:e26-e32.

44. Trippel TD, Anker SD, von HS. The role of micronutrients and macronutrients in patients hospitalized for heart failure. *Heart Fail Clin.* 2013;9(3):345-57, vii.

45. Levitan EB, Shikany JM, Ahmed A, et al. Calcium, magnesium and potassium intake and mortality in women with heart failure: the Women's Health Initiative. *Br J Nutr.* 2013;110(1):179-185.

46. Loncar G, Springer J, Anker M, Doehner W, Lainscak M. Cardiac cachexia: hic et nunc: "hic et nunc"—here and now. *Int J Cardiol.* 2015;201:e1-e12.

47. Evans WJ, Morley JE, Argile's J, et al. Cachexia: a new definition. *Clin Nutr.* 2008;27(6):793-799.

48. Bauer J, Biolo G, Cederholm T, et al. Evidence-based recommendations for optimal dietary protein intake in older people: a position paper from the PROT-AGE study group. *J Am Med Dir Assoc.* 2013;14(8):542-559.

49. Lavie CJ, De SA, Parto P, et al. Obesity and prevalence of cardiovascular diseases and prognosis—the obesity paradox updated. *Prog Cardiovasc Dis.* 2016;58(5):537-547.

50. Colin-Ramirez E, McAlister FA, Woo E, Wong N, Ezekowitz JA. Association between self-reported adherence to a low-sodium diet and dietary habits related to sodium intake in heart failure patients. *J Cardiovasc Nurs.* 2015;30(1):58-65.

51. Arcand J, Brazel S, Joliffe C, et al. Education by a dietitian in patients with heart failure results in improved adherence with a sodium-restricted diet: a randomized trial. *Am Heart J.* 2005;150(4):716.

52. Institute of Medicine. *Dietary Reference Intakes for Water, Potassium, Sodium, Chloride, and Sulfate.* Washington, DC: The National Academies Press; 2005.

53. Health Canada. The % of Daily Value. http://www.hc-sc.gc.ca/fn-an/label-etiquet/nutrition/cons/dv-vq/index-eng.php. Accessed March 7, 2016.

54. Canadian Food Inspection Agency. Specific Nutrient Content Claim Requirements. Sodium (Salt) Claims. http://www.inspection.gc.ca/food/labelling/food-labelling-for-industry/nutrient-content/specific-claim-requirements/eng/1389907770176/1389907817577?chap=9#s7c9. Accessed March 7, 2016.

26 DIGOXIN USE IN HEART FAILURE

Mariko W. Harper, MD, MS
Zachary D. Goldberger, MD, FACC, FAHA, FHRS

INTRODUCTION

In 1785, Sir William Withering first described the leaves from the common foxglove plant, *Digitalis purpurea*, as a treatment for heart failure (HF) and arrhythmia in his monograph "An Account of the Foxglove and Some of Its Medicinal Uses."[1] More than 200 years later, digoxin remains in contemporary use for the treatment of HF with reduced systolic function, albeit with increasing scrutiny and controversy. In 1997, the landmark Digitalis Investigation Group (DIG) trial showed that while digoxin did reduce total and HF-related hospitalizations, there was no survival benefit.[2] Over the next decade, a change in practice patterns would lead to a significant reduction in digoxin use, but ultimately no change in the burden of digoxin-related adverse events.[3,4] In patients with persistently symptomatic heart failure with reduced ejection fraction (HFrEF) on guideline-directed medical therapy, the addition of digoxin may help ameliorate signs and symptoms of HF, improve quality of life, and reduce overall and HF-specific hospitalizations. Thus, the 2013 American College of Cardiology/American Heart Association (ACC/AHA) guideline for the management of HF recommends digoxin as an adjuvant agent in select patient populations.[5]

MECHANISM OF ACTION

Digoxin is a purified steroid cardiac glycoside. Cardiac glycosides directly and reversibly inhibit the sodium-potassium-activated adenosine triphosphate transporter (Na^+K^+-ATPase) on the plasma membrane of the cardiac myocyte, preventing the influx of potassium and expulsion of intracellular sodium (Figure 26-1).[6] The net increase in intracellular sodium disrupts the sodium-calcium antiporter (Na^+Ca^{2+} exchange), effectively increasing intracellular calcium concentrations, and as a result, increases cardiac contractility and augments systolic function.[6]

In addition to augmentation of cardiac inotropy, cardiac glycosides also have an important role in neurohormonal regulation, having effects on both vascular smooth muscle tone and the sympathetic nervous system.[6] In patients with advanced systolic HF, digitalis has been shown to reduce plasma renin concentrations and promote peripheral vasodilation, likely due to down-regulation of hypersensitized baroreceptors.[7] By increasing vagal tone and attenuating the sympathetic nervous system, cardiac glycosides also work to slow conduction through the SA and AV nodes.[7] The increased intracellular calcium levels also work to shorten cardiac repolarization time, increasing the propensity for automaticity and arrhythmias.[7] In the setting of cardiac glycoside toxicity, one can

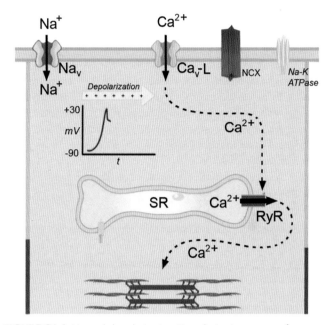

FIGURE 26-1 Normal depolarization. Depolarization occurs after the opening of fast Na+ channels; the increase in intracellular potential opens voltage-dependent Ca^{2+} channels, and the influx of Ca^{2+} induces the massive release of Ca^{2+} from the sarcoplasmic reticulum, producing contraction. (Reproduced with permission from Hoffman RS, Howland MA, Lewin NA, et al. *Goldfrank's Toxicologic Emergencies*. 10th ed. New York, NY: McGraw-Hill Education; 2015. Figure 65-1A.)

see that these dual effects of increased automaticity and nodal block can create dangerous exit blocks and arrhythmias.

KINETICS AND DRUG INTERACTIONS

Digitalis is primarily renally cleared. Due to its large molecular weight and volume distribution, hemodialysis or other methods of extracorporeal elimination are generally ineffective. Digoxin also serves as a substrate for the P-glycoprotein efflux pump, which excretes select drugs into the intestine or proximal renal tubule in exchange for increasing the serum concentration of digoxin.[8] Common classes of drugs that inhibit the P-glycoprotein pump and significantly increase digoxin concentrations include antiarrhythmics such as amiodarone and quinidine (the latter rarely used in contemporary clinical practice), nondihydropyridine calcium channel blockers, as well as certain antibiotics. Care should always be taken to monitor for potential drug interactions when prescribing digoxin. Recommendations are to reduce the dose of digoxin by at least 50% when using these agents.[9]

CLINICAL EVIDENCE FOR DIGOXIN USE IN HEART FAILURE WITH REDUCED SYSTOLIC FUNCTION

Digoxin is the only inotrope that has not been associated with long-term mortality when used in chronic HF.[10,11] While there is a significant risk of adverse events when used at higher doses or in the setting of drug-drug interactions, digoxin can be a safe medication when used within a narrow therapeutic window. While digoxin itself does not cause renal dysfunction or electrolyte abnormalities, the presence of either condition can dangerously potentiate the effects of digoxin.

THE DIGITALIS INVESTIGATION GROUP TRIAL

The Digitalis Investigation Group (DIG) trial was the first randomized controlled trial designed to investigate the impact of digoxin on mortality and morbidity in patients with chronic HF.[2] Published in 1997, this large double-blind randomized controlled trial enrolled almost 6800 ambulatory adult patients with HFrEF (<45% in the trial), and normal sinus rhythm, who were randomized to receive digoxin or placebo.[2] The study failed to reach its primary endpoint, showing no statistically significant effect on all-cause mortality (34.8% in the digoxin arm vs 35.1% in the placebo group; RR 0.99 p = 0.8), although there was a 28% reduction in hospitalizations in the digoxin arm.[2] While this study has had an undeniable impact on contemporary practice patterns in the management of HFrEF, it should be cautioned that this study occurred in an era prior to the use of beta blockers and aldosterone-receptor antagonists for HFrEF, thus impacting its generalizability to current HF management.

There have been multiple post hoc analyses from the DIG trial suggesting that certain subgroups within the digoxin arm may experience a greater benefit from the use of digoxin. For example, patients with more advanced HF, with New York Heart Association (NYHA) class III to IV functional class, left ventricular ejection fraction (LVEF) less than 25%, or cardiomegaly had a modest survival benefit (HR 0.88, P = 0.012) with digoxin use compared to placebo.[12] Similarly, a subgroup analysis of various serum digoxin concentrations (SDCs) in the DIG trial found a 6.8% reduction in mortality among patients with an SDC of 0.5 to 0.9 ng/mL compared to placebo, whereas patients with an SDC of 1.2 to 2 ng/mL had an 11.8% absolute increase in mortality compared to patients receiving placebo.[13] The study authors hypothesized that a lower SDC may predominantly affect neurohormonal modulation, whereas higher plasma concentrations may have more inotropic effects that may lead to increased myocardial oxygen demand and the promotion of arrhythmic complications.[13] Based on these findings, the current AHA/ACC guidelines recommend maintaining SDC between 0.5 and 0.9 ng/mL when using digoxin in the treatment of HFrEF.[5]

DIGOXIN USE IN WOMEN

It should be noted that only 22% of patients enrolled in the DIG trial were women and fewer women had serum digoxin levels drawn during the study.[2,13-14] In a post hoc analysis of sex-based differences in the DIG trial, digoxin was associated with an increased risk of all-cause mortality in women but not in men.[14] A subgroup analysis of SDC among women in the DIG trial was insufficiently powered to determine if there is a safe therapeutic range for digoxin use in women.[13] To date, there is insufficient evidence to support the use of digoxin in women and further studies are needed to evaluate the effect of digitalis on women with chronic HF.

DIGOXIN USE IN HEART FAILURE AND ATRIAL FIBRILLATION

Almost one-third of patients with HF with reduced systolic function have atrial fibrillation (AF).[11,15] Digoxin may help control the rate of ventricular response in AF by increasing vagal tone; however, this effect may be best seen in resting well-compensated HF states with minimal adrenergic stimulation.[16] While the DIG trial excluded patients with AF, subsequent smaller studies have found that the combined use of digoxin and a beta blocker leads to improved rate control, systolic function, and NYHA functional class compared to either agent alone.[17,18] A recent retrospective study of AF in a non-HF population found an increased risk of death among patients taking digoxin, once again raising the controversy of contemporary digoxin use.[19]

DIGOXIN USE IN HEART FAILURE WITH PRESERVED LEFT VENTRICULAR SYSTOLIC FUNCTION

While HFpEF accounts for approximately half of all patients hospitalized in the United States with decompensated HF syndromes,[20-22] there is a paucity of evidence to suggest that these patients demonstrate similar benefits from medical therapy as patients with reduced ejection fraction. All 3 randomized controlled trials with digoxin including patients with HFpEF were considered negative trials for the primary endpoint.[21-23] In the DIG-Ancillary trial, there was no statistically significant difference in survival or hospitalizations in patients with HFpEF who were prescribed digoxin, although there was a modest trend toward reduced HF hospitalizations.[21] In the CHARM-preserved study, evaluating digoxin use combined with candesartan versus candesartan alone in patients with HFpEF, subjects in the digoxin arm had an 11% relative risk reduction in the combined endpoint of cardiovascular death or HF hospitalization, but at the expense of increased hypokalemia, hypotension, and acute kidney injury.[22]

THERAPEUTIC RANGES AND INITIATION OF THERAPY

Current ACC/AHA guidelines suggest a narrow therapeutic SDC between 0.5 and 0.9 ng/mL for subjects being treated for chronic HF.[5] These serum concentrations can typically be achieved with daily doses of 0.125 to 0.25 mg; there is no need for loading doses in the treatment of chronic HF. In the DIG trial, patients prescribed 125 μg of digoxin had mean serum levels of 0.76 ng/mL versus 0.89 ng/mL in patients taking 250 μg.[2,13]

It is suggested that patients at higher risk for developing digoxin toxicity, such as those above the age of 70 years, those with impaired renal function, or those with reduced lean body mass be started at doses of 125 μg daily or every other day.[5] It is also reasonable for such patients to have SDCs obtained at approximately 14 to 21 days after initiation of digoxin therapy, with levels drawn no sooner than 8 hours after the last dose.[11] It is also important to caution that even within these recommended plasma concentrations there is the possibility of digoxin intoxication in certain circumstances, such as with the use of certain concomitant medications or with electrolyte abnormalities.[24]

Current recommendations for SDC are based on several retrospective analyses of digoxin withdrawal, noting that lower plasma concentrations of digoxin were equivalent in preventing HF progression compared to higher digoxin levels.[24,25] In a post hoc analysis of the DIG trial, where the prespecified therapeutic ranges for SDC were 0.5 to 2 ng/dL based on an intention to avoid toxicity, study authors found that subjects in the lowest tertile of digoxin levels (0.5-0.8 ng/mL) had a 6.3% reduction in all-cause mortality versus subjects taking placebo, whereas those with the highest tertile of SDC (1.2-2 ng/mL) had a relative increase in mortality of 11.8%.[13] It is important to note that these findings are all retrospective based on subgroup analysis and that there are no prospective, randomized trials evaluating the relative efficacy or safety of varying SDCs.

Historically, the goal SDC has been between 0.8 and 2.0 ng/mL based on a small study of 39 patients evaluated for toxicity based on electrocardiographic (ECG) abnormalities.[25,26] In this study, significant risk of toxicity increased when SDCs were above 2 ng/mL and almost certainly when concentrations were >4 ng/dL.[26]

TOXICITY

Because of its narrow therapeutic window, digoxin toxicity accounts for one-third of hospital admissions for adverse drug reactions in the elderly.[27] Despite changes in practice patterns and an overall reduction of digoxin use in HF patients in the post DIG trial era, the incidence of digoxin toxicity remains largely unchanged.[4,5] In a recently published study evaluating reported adverse drug events in U.S. emergency departments, digoxin toxicity accounted for more than 3% of emergency department visits and 5.9% of hospitalizations in elderly patients over 85 years in the United States, with relatively constant incidence during the study duration of 2005 to 2010.[4] The annual incidence of digoxin toxicity has been estimated at 4% to 5% with an associated cost of $6500 per event.[28,29]

CLINICAL PRESENTATION

Digoxin toxicity is a clinical diagnosis based on patient history, physical examination, and characteristic ECG findings. Early signs of digoxin toxicity may be nonspecific. Patients frequently describe fatigue and gastrointestinal symptoms including nausea, anorexia, and abdominal pain. With escalating toxicity patients may go on to manifest neurologic or cardiac sequelae. Neurologic manifestations include headache, lightheadedness, and delirium.[25] There is a classic association between digoxin toxicity and xanthopsia, a retrobulbar optic neuritis that causes a yellow halo within the visual field.[30] Xanthopsia is often described as a van Gogh effect referring to Vincent van Gogh's frequent painting of yellow halos within his landscape portrayals during his so-called Yellow Period.[31] (It has been speculated that the famous painter may have suffered from digoxin toxicity during this era.[31])

Digitalis toxicity can cause a variety of cardiac arrhythmias because of its ability to increase both central sympathetic activity as well as peripheral vagal tone. The former promotes myocardial automaticity and increased ventricular and atrial ectopy (Figure 26-2). The latter causes a suppression of normal pacemaker cell function in the sinus and atrioventricular nodes. This collective effect can lead to pathognomonic ECG findings of combined arrhythmia and conduction block, which may manifest in the classic pattern of atrial tachycardia with 2:1 block (enhanced automaticity with vagotonic block) (Figure 26-3).[25,30] Other ECG patterns that should raise suspicion for digoxin toxicity include accelerated junctional rhythm; slow, regularized AF (or AF with complete heart block); and bidirectional ventricular tachycardia (Figure 26-4).

A frequently encountered ECG finding associated with digoxin use is a scooping reverse tick morphology of the ST-T wave segment in the lateral leads—this so-called digitalis effect does not imply toxicity and can be seen in patients taking digoxin at any dose. Digoxin causes PR prolongation due to its vagotonic effects on the AV node as well as QT shortening with secondary repolarization changes reflected in the T wave. It is important to note that this finding is associated with chronic digoxin use but not necessarily with digitalis toxicity.[24,30]

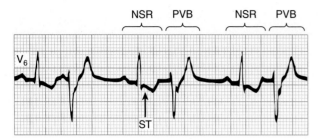

FIGURE 26-2 Electrocardiographic record showing digitalis-induced bigeminy. The complexes marked *NSR* are normal sinus rhythm beats; an inverted T wave and depressed ST segment are present. The complexes marked *PVB* are premature ventricular beats and are the electrocardiographic manifestations of depolarizations evoked by delayed oscillatory afterpotentials.

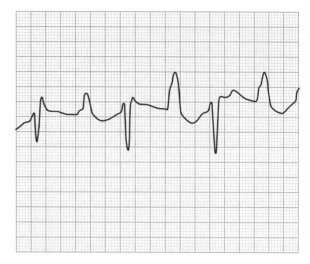

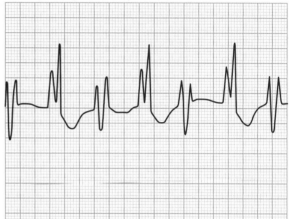

FIGURE 26-4 Digoxin toxic bidirectional fascicular tachycardia. (Reproduced with permission from Longo DL, Fauci AS, Kasper DL, et al. *Harrison's Principles of Internal Medicine.* 18th ed. New York, NY: McGraw-Hill Education; 2012. Figure 233-15.)

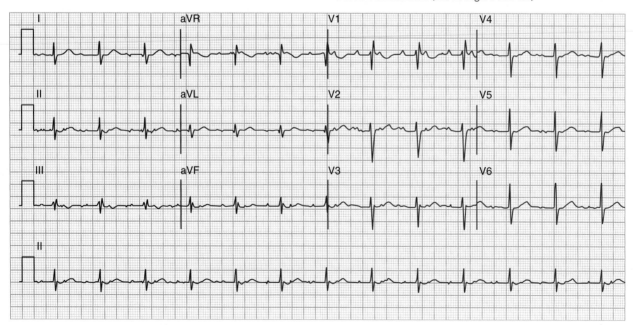

FIGURE 26-3 Atrial tachycardia with 2:1 block. P-wave rate is about 150/min, with ventricular (QRS) rate of about 75/min. The nonconducted ("extra") P waves just after the QRS complex are best seen in lead V₁. Also, note incomplete RBBB and borderline QT prolongation. (Reproduced with permission from Kasper DL, Fauci A, Hauser Stephen, et al. *Harrison's Principles of Internal Medicine.* 19th ed. New York, NY: McGraw-Hill Education; 2015. Figure 278e-11.)

MANAGEMENT

When digoxin toxicity is suspected, it is important to establish intravenous access, obtain a serum chemistry panel and digoxin level, and perform a 12-lead ECG. In acute digoxin toxicity, hyperkalemia can be prevalent because of digoxin's inhibition of the Na-K-ATPase and increase in extracellular potassium. Hyperkalemia has been associated with increased mortality in acute digoxin overdose.[32] With chronic digoxin use, however, hypokalemia, hypomagnesemia, and hypocalcemia are more likely to potentiate toxicity. In patients with chronic HF, concomitant use of loop and thiazide diuretics elevates the risk for these electrolyte derangements.

Mild digoxin poisoning can be treated conservatively with correction of electrolyte abnormalities, stopping digoxin, and avoiding other drugs that may potentiate digoxin's effects. In the presence of life-threatening arrhythmia, multiorgan injury, or hemodynamic instability, digoxin-specific antibodies (Fab fragments) are available and should be administered. For critical bradyarrhythmias, atropine can be administered as a temporizing measure.[24,25]

KEY POINTS

- Digoxin has been used in the treatment of HF for more than 2 centuries.
- Digoxin's narrow therapeutic range and potential for life-threatening toxicity make it a challenging medication to use in patients with chronic HF.
- When used in a carefully selected patient population, it may improve quality of life and reduce total and HF-associated hospitalizations.
- When used, digoxin should be used as an adjuvant to guideline-directed medical therapy for HFrEF, including beta blockers and angiotensin-converting enzyme (ACE) inhibitors.
- The landmark DIG trial showed no survival benefit with digoxin use in patients with chronic HFrEF and normal sinus rhythm, although digoxin use was associated with a modest reduction in hospitalization.
- Current AHA/ACC guidelines recommend SDC between 0.5 and 0.9 ng/mL. Plasma concentrations >1.2 ng/mL have been associated with increased mortality.
- There are a multitude of cardiac, gastrointestinal, and neurologic symptoms associated with digoxin toxicity. Digoxin antibodies (Fab) are available in the case of critical overdoses presenting with life-threatening arrhythmias, hemodynamic instability, or multiorgan failure.

REFERENCES

1. Withering W. An Account of the Foxglove and Some of Its Medicinal Uses: With Practical Remarks on Dropsy, and Other Disease. Birmingham, England: M Swinney; 1785.

2. Digitalis Investigation Group. The effect of digoxin on mortality and morbidity in patients with heart failure: the Digital Investigation Group. *NEJM*. 1997;336:525-533.

3. Hussain Z, Swindle J, Hauptman PJ. Digoxin use and digoxin toxicity in the post-DIG trial era. *J Card Fail*. 2006;12(5):343.

4. See I, Shehab N, Kegler SR, et al. Emergency department visits and hospitalizations for digoxin toxicity: United States, 2005-2010. *Circ Heart Fail*. 2014 Jan;7(1):28-34.

5. Yancy CW, Jessup M, Bozkurt B, et al. 2013 ACCF/AHA guideline for the management of heart failure. *JACC*. 2013;62(16):e147-e239.

6. Rocco TP, Fang JC. Pharmacotherapy of congestive heart failure. In: Brunton LL, Lazo JS, Parker KL, eds. *Goodman & Gilman's The Pharmacological Basis of Therapeutics*. 11th ed. New York, NY: McGraw-Hill: 2006:869.

7. Ribner HS, Plucinski DA, Hsieh AM, et al. Acute effects of digoxin on total systemic vascular resistance in congestive heart failure due to dilated cardiomyopathy: a hemodynamic-hormonal study. *Am J Cardiol*. 1985;56:896.

8. Drescher S, Glaeser H, Murdter T, et al. P-glycoprotein-mediated intestinal and biliary digoxin transport in humans. *Clin Pharmacol Ther*. 2003;73(3):223.

9. Singh BN. Amiodarone: the expanding antiarrhythmic role and how to follow a patient on chronic therapy. *Clin Cardiol*. 1997;20:608-618.

10. Eichhorn EJ, Gheoghiade M. Digoxin. *Prog Cardiovasc Dis*. 2002;44:251-266.

11. Gheorghiade M, Van Veldhuisen DJ, Colucci WS. Contemporary use of digoxin in the management of cardiovascular disorders. *Circulation*. 2006;113:2556-2564.

12. Gheorghiade M, Patel K, Filippatos G, et al. Effect of oral digoxin in high-risk heart failure patients: a pre-specified subgroup analysis of the DIG trial. *Eur J Heart Fail*. 2013;15(5):551-559.

13. Rathore SS, Curtis JP, Wang Y, et al. Association of serum digoxin concentration and outcomes in patients with heart failure. *JAMA*. 2003;289(7):871-878.

14. Rathore SS, Wang Y, Krumholz HM. Sex-based differences in the effect of digoxin for the treatment of heart failure. *N Engl J Med*. 2002;347:1403-1411.

15. Adams KF, Fonarow GC, Emerman CL, et al, for the ADHERE Scientific Advisory Committee and Investigators. Characteristics and outcomes of patients hospitalized for heart failure in the United States: rationale, design, and preliminary observations from the first 100,000 cases in the Acute Decompensated Heart Failure National Registry (ADHERE). *Am Heart J*. 2005;149:209-216.

16. Zarowitz BJ, Gheorghiade M. Optimal heart rate control for patients with chronic atrial fibrillation: are pharmacologic choices truly changing? *Am Heart J*. 1992;123:1401-1403.

17. Khand AU, Rankin AC, Martin W, Taylor J, Gemmell I, Cleland JG. Carvedilol alone or in combination with digoxin for the management of atrial fibrillation in patients with heart failure? *J Am Coll Cardiol.* 2003;42:1944-1951.

18. Veloso HH, de Paola AA. Beta-blockers versus digoxin to control ventricular rate during atrial fibrillation. *J Am Coll Cardiol.* 2005;45:1905-1906.

19. Turakhia MP, Santangeli P, Winkelmayer WC, et al. Increased mortality associated with digoxin in contemporary patients with atrial fibrillations: findings from the TREAT-AF study. *J Am Coll Cardiol.* 2014;64(7)660-668.

20. Fonarow GC, Abraham WT, Albert N, et al. Organized Program to Initiate Lifesaving Treatment in Hospitalized Patients With Heart Failure (OPTIMIZE-HF): rationale and design. *Am Heart J.* 2004;148:43-51.

21. Ahmed A, Rich MW, Fleg JL, et al. Effects of digoxin on morbidity and mortality in diastolic heart failure: the Ancillary Digitalis Investigation Group Trial. *Circulation.* 2006 Aug 1;114(5):397-403.

22. Yusuf S, Pfeffer MA, Swedberg K, et al. for the CHARM Investigators and Committees. Effects of candesartan in patients with chronic heart failure and preserved left-ventricular ejection fraction: the CHARM-Preserved Trial. *Lancet.* 2003;362:777-781.

23. Massie BM, Carson PE, McMurray JJ, et al. for the I-preserve Investigators. *N Engl J Med.* 2008;359:2456-2467.

24. Goldberger ZD, Goldberger AL. Therapeutic ranges of serum digoxin concentrations in patients with heart failure. *Am J Cardiol.* 2012;109(12):1818-1821.

25. Stucky MA, Goldberger ZD. Digoxin: its role in contemporary medicine. *Postgrad Med J.* 2015;91(1079):514-518.

26. Smith TW, Butler VP Jr, Haber E. Determination of therapeutic and toxic serum digoxin concentrations by radioimmunoassay. *N Engl J Med.* 1969;281:1212-1216.

27. Budnitz DS, Lovegrove MC, Shehab N, et al. Emergency hospitalizations for adverse drug events in older Americans. *N Engl J Med.* 2011;365:2002-2012.

28. Haynes K, Heitjan D, Kanetsky P, et al. Declining public health burden of digoxin toxicity from 1991to 2004. *Clin Pharmacol Ther.* 2008;84:90-94.

29. Gandi AJ, Vlasses PH, Morton DJ, et al. Economic impact of digoxin toxicity. *Pharmacoeconomics.* 1997;12:175-181.

30. Goldberger ZD. ECG image of the month. Withering away. *Am J Med.* 2008;121:1052-1054.

31. Lee TC. Van Gogh's vision digitalis intoxication? *JAMA.* 1981;245:728-729.

32. Bismuth C, Gaultier M, Conso F, et al. Hyperkalemia in acute digitalis poisoning: prognostic significance and therapeutic implications. *Clin Toxicol.* 1973;6(2):153-162.

27 DIURETIC THERAPY IN HEART FAILURE

James Monaco, MD
Garric J. Haas, MD

PATIENT CASE: PART 1

A 51-year-old African American man presents to the emergency department (ED) with a chief complaint of dyspnea and swelling. He has a history of hypertension (HTN) and non-insulin-dependent type 2 diabetes. He works as a long-haul truck driver and reports not having seen a physician in over 3 years due to his work schedule and is no longer taking any home medications. He is saturating 93% on room air, has a pulse rate of 80 bpm, a blood pressure of 194/92 mm Hg, and a temperature of 36.5°C. Examination is remarkable for distention of the jugular veins, diffuse rales on inspiration, and 2+ pitting edema to midthigh. Initial electrocardiogram (ECG) shows left ventricular hypertrophy (LVH) by voltage criteria and left-axis deviation. A chest x-ray shows diffuse interstitial edema. Initial bloodwork is notable for a sodium of 135 mEq/L, creatinine of 1.1 mg/dL, albumin of 3.6 g/dL, hemoglobin of 12.9 g/dL, and brain natriuretic peptide (BNP) of 456 pg/mL. The patient receives oral hydralazine and intravenous (IV) nitroglycerin while in the ED with improvement of his blood pressure to 146/85 mm Hg, but he remains dyspneic with minimal exertion. A transthoracic echocardiogram reveals a hypertrophied left ventricle with moderately depressed left ventricular ejection fraction (LVEF) of 35% to 40% and grade II diastolic dysfunction.

OVERVIEW OF INPATIENT DIURETICS IN ACUTE DECOMPENSATED HEART FAILURE

Acute congestion from volume overload is a major driver of hospitalization in heart failure (HF). Loop diuretics remain the cornerstone of decongestive therapy.[1,2]

Figure 27-1 illustrates the principle behind diuretic therapy in acute HF. An initial clinical evaluation of patients with suspected acute decompensated heart failure (ADHF) should focus on determining fluid status and excluding cardiogenic shock.[1]

In general, patients with cardiogenic shock should be adequately stabilized prior to diuretic therapy.[1] Patients with pulmonary edema despite relatively normal volume status have hemodynamic congestion (eg, hypertensive emergency, acute valvular pathology) but may still benefit symptomatically from adjunctive diuretic therapy, which exhibits acute venodilatory effects.[1] Those patients who are clearly volume overloaded should receive loop diuretics to improve symptoms and functional status. Diuretics should be given intravenously for more rapid onset of action and predictable bioavailability.[1]

The diuretic strategies discussed in this chapter apply to both heart failure with reduced ejection fraction (HFrEF) as well as heart failure with preserved ejection fraction (HFpEF).

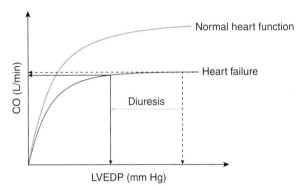

FIGURE 27-1 The principle of diuretic therapy in acute decompensated heart failure (ADHF). The acutely failing heart is functioning in the flat portion of the Frank-Starling curve, where small increases in blood volume result in large increases in left ventricular end-diastolic pressure (LVEDP) without significantly increasing cardiac output (CO). Inversely, decreasing the intravascular volume can significantly decrease the LVEDP and thus relieve congestive symptoms without significantly decreasing CO.

MECHANISMS AND PHARMACOLOGIC PROPERTIES OF LOOP DIURETICS

Commercially available loop diuretics include furosemide, bumetanide, torsemide, and ethacrynic acid. All except ethacrynic acid contain a sulfa moiety. Cross-reaction with allergies to other sulfa drugs is vanishingly rare, however. Ethacrynic acid, which is expensive and has more toxicity, should be used only in patients with documented anaphylaxis to the other loop diuretics.[1,3]

Regarding potency, 40 mg of IV furosemide is equipotent to 20 mg of IV torsemide and 1 mg of IV bumetanide. Further comparisons are shown in Table 27-1.[3,4] The site of action of all loop diuretics is the luminal side of the ascending loop of Henle. Here, the loop diuretics reversibly antagonize the sodium-potassium-2 chloride cotransporter, thus reducing sodium and chloride reabsorption and collapsing the interstitial sodium gradient that allows the kidney to concentrate urine. Because of this, it is the portion of the drug excreted unchanged that produces the desired diuretic effect.[3,5,6]

Figure 27-2 illustrates the sites and actions of several important transporters and receptors within the nephron relevant to diuretic therapy.

The loop diuretics are highly bound to serum proteins. Active secretion of this protein-bound component by proximal tubule cells is the main source of active drug in the urine. Free drug is primarily metabolized to inactive metabolites by glucuronidation and very little enters the urine unchanged.[5,6]

Albumin-bound loop diuretic is unbound and secreted into the proximal tubule by the organic acid transporter, which also mediates renal excretion of urea and uric acid, lactic acid, and many

Table 27.1 Comparison of available loop diuretics

	Furosemide	Bumetanide	Tosemide
Potency relative to furosemide	1:1	1:40	1:2
Bioavailability	20%-70%	80%-100%	80%-100%
Variability of oral absorption	High	Low	Low
Absorption affected by food	Yes	Slight	No
Half-life	2 h	1-1.5 h	3-4 h

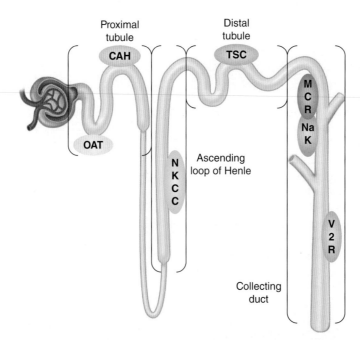

FIGURE 27-2 A diagram of the nephron with locations of relevant transporters. Organic acid transporter (OAT) complexes are found in the proximal tubule and are the main pathway by which diuretics enter the nephron. Carbonic anhydrase (CAH) in the proximal tubule is the target of acetazolamide. NKCCs (Na-K-2Cl cotransporters) in the ascending loop of Henle are the primary target of loop diuretics. Thiazide-sensitive Na-Cl (TSCs) symporters in the distal tubule are the primary target of thiazide diuretics. Mineralocorticoid receptors (MCR)/NaKs respond to aldosterone stimulation by upregulating the presence and activity of sodium-potassium ATPase in the collecting duct. Aldosterone antagonists and potassium-sparing diuretics such as amiloride target this system. V2R (vasopressin antagonists) target type 2 vasopressin receptors, which increase free water absorption through upregulating aquaporins in the collecting duct when stimulated.

other drugs (notably including nonsteroidal anti-inflammatory drugs [NSAIDs]) and endogenous compounds. High doses of loop diuretic may reduce the urinary excretion of these other compounds, and vice versa.[5,6]

The dose-response relationship for the loop diuretics is notable for the presence of an effective threshold dose to achieve diuresis. Doses below the threshold will produce essentially no diuresis, while those above the threshold will quickly hit an effective ceiling response, with further dose increases carrying no additional response.[7]

For a diuretic-naïve patient with normal renal function, a dose of 10 to 20 mg of IV furosemide is generally the threshold dose, and a maximum response is seen with 40 mg. As illustrated in Figure 27-3, the presence of HF tends to increase the threshold and ceiling doses. The presence of intrinsic renal disease will increase the threshold and ceiling doses, while decreasing the responsiveness to an effective dose.[7,8]

INITIAL DOSING OF INTRAVENOUS LOOP DIURETICS

Relevant clinical differences between loop diuretics are primarily related to bioavailability and will be discussed more in Part 2 of this chapter on outpatient diuretic therapy.

When given intravenously, the bioavailability of all loop diuretics is 100% and no significant therapeutic differences have been noted among them. As such, choice of IV diuretic should be driven primarily by local availability and cost.

For patients who are diuretic-naïve with normal renal function, an initial dose of 20 to 40 mg of IV furosemide or equivalent once to twice per day is generally chosen.

For patients who are on home diuretics, each IV dose should be numerically equal to or greater than their home dose. In a randomized controlled trial, patients receiving initial IV doses equal to 2.5 times their oral home dose showed a trend toward faster improvement compared to those receiving the IV equivalent of their home oral dose. Importantly, the high-dose group did not have a greater frequency of complications.[9]

IV diuretics should be given either as boluses or as a continuous infusion. A number of smaller trials have suggested reduced complications and improved diuresis associated with continuous infusion, but the larger and more rigorous DOSE trial did not show a difference between strategies.[9] Both are considered equally valid approaches in the 2013 AHA/ACC guidelines. From a practical standpoint, doses of less than 200 mg of furosemide equivalent per day are usually more simply delivered as boluses. If individual bolus doses exceed 120 mg furosemide equivalent, or need to be given more often than twice daily, continuous infusion may be reasonably considered.[10]

A classically reported method of dose estimation suggests the use of patient age plus serum blood urea nitrogen (BUN) to calculate furosemide dose. Although this has not been clinically verified, it does underscore the role of glomerular filtration rate (GFR) in determining a patient's sensitivity to diuretics and thus the counterintuitive need to give higher doses to patients whose initial serum creatinine is elevated.[11]

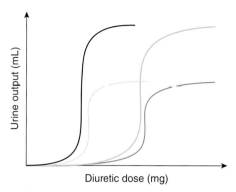

FIGURE 27-3 The S-shaped curve of the response to loop diuretics in different disease states. *Black curve:* A healthy patient. *Yellow curve:* A patient with chronic renal disease has a lower glomerular filtration rate (GFR), and thus has a lower ceiling on his or her response; this patient may also require a higher dose to achieve adequate concentration in the tubule. *Cyan curve:* A patient with chronic heart failure has increased levels of counter-regulatory hormones promoting salt and water retention, and thus requires a higher dose to respond. *Magenta curve:* A patient with cardiorenal syndrome has both a lower ceiling and a higher diuretic requirement to reach it.

The frequency of systemic drug buildup and toxicity is exceedingly rare at the doses of loop diuretics used clinically. In general, bolus doses up to 200 mg and daily doses up to 400 mg will not result in acute or cumulative toxicity.[5,6]

There is no generalized agreement as to the ideal rate of volume removal. Most patients will tolerate 0.5 to 2 L of net volume removal per day. It has been hypothesized that more aggressive volume removal may lead to excessive renin-angiotensin-aldosterone system (RAAS) activation and worse outcomes, but this has not been reliably demonstrated in clinical trials. Diuretic goals should be tailored to the needs of the patient based on symptoms, degree of hypervolemia, and clinical stability.[1,12]

The patient should be closely monitored for response to therapy, with dosing adjustments made frequently if necessary.[1]

It is well documented that measured intake/output and bed weights are fraught with inaccuracies in the hospital environment. Therefore, monitoring of response should be approached holistically, combining intake/output measurements and daily standing weights (preferably on same scales each day) with careful examination and symptom assessment.[13,14]

The majority of the diuresis from an IV bolus of furosemide or bumetanide will occur within the first 2 half-lives of the drug (2-4 hours for furosemide and bumetanide) and will be effectively complete by 6 hours after administration. (Remember, Lasix = LAsts SIX.) Therefore, urine output should be monitored especially closely during this period of time to determine if an effective dose was delivered. An effective dose should produce at least 1 to 2 L of diuresis within this time frame and result in at least 50 mmol of natriuresis. With twice a day dosing, an effective dose will allow a negative fluid and sodium balance if the patient is maintained on a typical inpatient cardiac diet with a 2 L fluid restriction and 2 g (90 mmol) sodium restriction.[15]

Adequate diuretic response can be predicted within the first hour of diuretic administration by a spot test of urine sodium and creatinine, which can be used to predict sodium and volume output for the diuretic bolus according to the validated formulas and examples in Figures 27-4 and 27-5.[15]

If a dose of diuretic fails to achieve a significant response, the subsequent dose should be increased. Remembering the short half-life of the loop diuretics and the need to achieve a threshold concentration in the urine, attempting to stack small doses over the course of several hours is rarely effective. For example, if the patient receives 40 mg of IV Furosemide and has not produced at least 500 mL of urine after 2 hours, the patient should receive 60 or 80 mg for his or her next dose, rather than attempting to add an extra dose of 20 mg right away.

If the patient is achieving adequate response to each dose, but is not achieving net volume loss, then dosing frequency may be increased up to every 6 hours, or changed to continuous infusion at an equivalent rate. Additionally, the patient's sodium and water restrictions should be reviewed to ensure they are adequate.

Be aware of the diuretic braking phenomenon: acutely increased delivery of sodium to the distal tubule of the nephron activates the RAAS causing efferent arteriolar constriction and a decrease in the renal perfusion. This in turn may acutely decrease diuretic sensitivity. An effective diuretic dose on inpatient day 1 may no longer be effective by day 2. Again, careful monitoring and dosing adjustment is required.

$$\text{Sodium output (mmol)} = eGFR \times (BSA/1.73) \times (Cr_{serum}/Cr_{urine}) \times 60 \text{ min/h} \times 3.25 \text{ h} \times (Na_{urine}/1000mL)$$

$$\text{Urine output (mL)} = eGFR \times (BSA/1.73) \times (Cr_{serum}/Cr_{urine}) \times 60 \text{ min/h} \times 3.25 \text{ h}$$

eGFR: GFR by CKD-EPI calculation. BSA: patient's body surface area. Cr: spot creatinine in urine and serum 1 hour after diuretic administration. Na: spot sodium in urine and serum 1 hour after diuretic administration.

These equations take the estimated GFR, then use serum and urine creatinine to determine the re-absorption ratio occurring in the tubules and thus calculate the rate of urine formation. This rate will remain constant for about 2 half lives of the loop diuretic, which for furosemide and bumetanide is about 3.25 hours. The volume of urine can then be multiplied by the concentration of sodium to get a predicted sodium output.

FIGURE 27-4 Equations for predicting diuretic response.

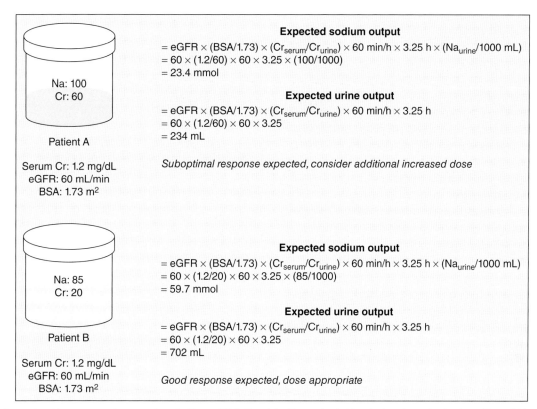

FIGURE 27-5 Example of how to use the equations in Figure 27-4. Consider 2 seemingly identical patients, both given 40 mg IV furosemide. Urine from both patients is sampled 1 hour later, and predicted sodium and urine outputs calculated.

POTENTIAL COMPLICATIONS AND APPROPRIATE MONITORING DURING DIURETIC THERAPY

The potential risks and complications of diuretic therapy have been well documented and include electrolyte imbalance, arrhythmia, alkalosis, renal injury, hemodynamic instability, and gout flare. The majority of these risks can be minimized by careful monitoring.[1]

Patients undergoing IV diuretic therapy should be monitored on telemetry and have serum levels of sodium, potassium, magnesium BUN, and creatinine checked at least once per day. More frequent electrolyte checks may be appropriate if the patient is experiencing very brisk diuresis, has baseline abnormalities in renal function, or consistently shows labile electrolyte levels.[1]

Potassium and magnesium should be supplemented as necessary to maintain a serum potassium between 4.0 and 4.5 mEq/L and a serum magnesium >2 mEq/L.

Numerous influences may cause serum creatinine to rise during diuretic therapy, and not all of them necessitate discontinuation of therapy. Typical activation of the RAAS and competitive antagonism of the organic acid transporter during diuretic therapy can result in increases in serum creatinine and BUN without intrinsic renal injury. Worsening venous congestion may similarly reduce renal perfusion and cause increased creatinine (congestive nephropathy). However, it is only decreased renal perfusion or hypotension related to intravascular volume depletion that results in significant renal injury and that will respond to discontinuation of diuretics. Any change in creatinine must be carefully correlated with clinical findings. A rise in creatinine that occurs in a patient who is clinically volume overloaded and without documented heavy diuretic response within the last 24 hours is unlikely due to overdiuresis.[16]

It is rare for diuresis to cause clinically harmful alkalosis in isolation, and in fact the development of alkalosis may be a marker for effective diuresis. However, it is reasonable to monitor serum bicarbonate and chloride as part of routine labs.[17]

Serum chloride may act as an additional prognostic marker. Low serum chloride in outpatients with HF has been shown to correlate with worse outcomes. However, the exact mechanism of this effect and the utility of trying to maintain a targeted level of serum chloride have not been demonstrated.[18]

Diuretic resistance is suggestive of more severe disease; however, high doses of diuretics are not in and of themselves harmful. Clinicians should not be afraid to increase doses as needed to achieve adequate decongestion.[19]

DETERMINING EUVOLEMIA AND PREPARING FOR DISCHARGE

Failure to fully decongest patients prior to discharge is associated with morbidity and increased re-admission. Therefore, one should strive to achieve optimal volume status prior to discharge.[16,20]

The determination of euvolemia should primarily be made clinically, by observing resolution of the signs and symptoms of acute congestion and hypervolemia.

Clinical findings should be correlated with documented changes in body weight and recorded fluid balance, keeping in mind the limitations of these measurements.

Laboratory evidence of hemoconcentration and volume contraction, specifically mild increase in hemoglobin, bicarbonate, and creatinine has been correlated with more complete diuresis and improved outcomes.[16,17,20-22]

The use of serial natriuretic peptide measurements or invasive pressure monitoring with central or pulmonary artery catheters is not routinely beneficial, and should be reserved for patients in whom symptoms persist and volume status remains uncertain.[1]

The use of a single predischarge natriuretic peptide measurement, however, may help establish postdischarge prognosis and recently received a IIa recommendation by the ACC. Patients whose levels remain high or fail to decrease after diuresis have been shown to have worse outcomes. However, no single diuretic strategy incorporating natriuretic peptide targets has been shown to be beneficial in clinical trials, and thus treatment focus should remain on achieving clinical euvolemia and maximizing tolerated guideline-directed medical therapy (GDMT).[23]

Patients who develop volume overloaded decompensated HF generally require outpatient diuretics in addition to GDMT to remain euvolemic. Although the current body of evidence is not definitive, small trials and retrospective analyses suggest that initiation of oral loop diuretics in patients not previously receiving them is associated with improved outcomes and fewer hospitalizations.[24,25]

In patients who were receiving home diuretics at the time of hospitalization, intensification of the home dosing should be considered if no other correctable cause of their hypervolemia can be identified.

Determining the optimal strategy for transition to oral diuretics depends on local clinical practice, resources, and patient characteristics. In general, monitored inpatient transition to the planned outpatient dose of oral diuretics, followed by rapid outpatient follow-up to reassess volume status should be arranged.

CONCLUSION TO PATIENT CASE: PART 1

The patient received 40 mg of IV furosemide in the ED with appropriate response. Over the next 48 hours he receives IV furosemide 40 mg twice daily and is initiated on GDMT. On day 3 he is felt to be euvolemic and is switched to oral furosemide 40 mg daily. He is extensively counselled on self-care in HF, including adherence to sodium and fluid restrictions and avoidance of harmful drugs such as NSAIDs that promote diuretic resistance. He is scheduled for a visit with the HF transition clinic 7 days after discharge.

PATIENT CASE: PART 2

Six months later, the patient from Patient Case: Part 1 is presenting to the cardiology clinic for general follow-up. At the time of his discharge, the patient was initiated on carvedilol, lisinopril, amlodipine, and 40 mg of Lasix by mouth once daily and appeared to be doing very well at his 1-week follow-up. He has been compliant with therapy but reports that over the last month he is more short of breath with exertion and has developed mild orthopnea. He reports that he does not notice significant increase in urination after taking his furosemide. On examination he has 1+ pitting edema of his shins and jugular venous pressure (JVP) visible 1 cm above the clavicle while upright. His lungs are clear to auscultation, and his vital signs are within normal limits. His lab work is notable for a creatinine of 1.1 mg/dL, sodium of 133 mEq/L, and potassium of 3.8 mg/dL, and a repeat transthoracic echocardiogram (TTE) shows an LVEF of 40% to 45% with grade II diastolic dysfunction.

OUTPATIENT ROLE OF LOOP DIURETICS

The goal of outpatient diuretic therapy is to prevent salt and fluid volume accumulation and the associated morbidity from hypervolemic congestion.

HF patients with evidence of current hypervolemia and those with a history of hospitalization for volume-overloaded decompensation should be maintained on some form of oral diuretic therapy.[1,2]

As with inpatient diuretics, outpatient regimens must be carefully tailored to the patient and monitored and adjusted over time.

SELECTION OF DIURETIC

In contrast to acute IV therapy, the available loop diuretics have clinically relevant differences when delivered orally and chronically. However, all are potentially efficacious and appropriate. Table 27-1 summarizes comparisons between the loop diuretics.

Furosemide is the oldest and most commonly utilized of the loop diuretics. However, it has several well-known limitations compared to the other agents. Its bioavailability is low (50% or less), and highly variable both between patients and within the same patient over time. Bioavailability decreases if taken with a meal. Bioavailability tends to decrease with hypervolemia and with reductions in cardiac output, likely related to gut wall edema, changes in active transport, and reduced splanchnic circulation. The negative feedback loop that can be established by this drop in absorption is frequently cited as a presumed cause of treatment failure.[4,7]

Bumetanide has 80% to 100% oral bioavailability, and more predictable and consistent absorption for patients. Absorption is somewhat reduced when taken with food. However, there is a dearth of clinical evidence to support that these superior pharmacodynamics translate to improved clinical outcomes.[4,7]

Torsemide has 80% to 100% bioavailability and very steady and reproducible absorption. It is not affected by food. Additionally, there is limited evidence suggesting it produces less activation of the RAAS and may in fact act to block uptake of aldosterone by the cardiac myocyte. There is observational evidence and limited clinical trial data to support that clinically meaningful outcomes may be improved with torsemide as compared to furosemide. However, the currently available trials have significant limitations and no professional society has recommended its use over other loop diuretics.[4]

Historically torsemide has been a more expensive option, but currently price differences are small among the 3 drugs. Furosemide is notable for being available on the discount formulary of several national chain pharmacies, which may make it a more attractive option for patients paying out of pocket for their medications. The price difference to the privately insured, Medicare, or Medicaid patient is likely to be negligible or nonexistent.

Ultimately, dosing and monitoring appropriately to confirm efficacy and to avoid complications is more important than choice of diuretic. However, the tendency to default to furosemide as a first agent is based on historical practice patterns and not evidence of clinical superiority. It is not inappropriate to consider bumetanide or torsemide as first-line agents given their potential benefits without significant negatives.

In patients experiencing recurrent treatment failure on furosemide or requiring high doses to respond, a trial of a different loop diuretic is appropriate before trying more intensive interventions.

DOSING, ADJUSTMENT, AND MONITORING OF OUTPATIENT DIURETICS

As with inpatient diuretics, 2 elements are necessary for effective outpatient diuretic therapy: individual doses must produce an effective diuresis, and the total daily natriuresis and diuresis must be equal to the daily salt and fluid intake. During clinic visits, patients should be queried as to whether or not they are obtaining a noticeable diuretic effect, as well as encouraged to avoid excess sodium and fluid consumption.

If patients report responding to their diuretic but remain hypervolemic, frequency of dose should be increased and review of their sodium and fluid intake revisited. If they report no noticeable response, then an increase in the dose is probably necessary.

Because most patients' salt and fluid intake and diuretic responsiveness change significantly over time, required diuretic doses may similarly change.

It is conceptually attractive to involve patients in their own care by providing them with guidelines for adjusting their own diuretic dosing based on home weight measurements and self-assessed signs/symptoms of volume overload (ie, flexible diuretic program). Results of clinical trials on such strategies have been mixed, with meta-analyses suggesting they are potentially beneficial in reducing morbidity if part of a holistic self-care plan. If such a strategy is used, it is important that the patients receive sufficient education as to be confident in their self-care to minimize nonadherence.[26]

Many noninvasive telemonitoring strategies for therapy adjustment have been studied, with mixed results. Reported home weight monitoring and impedance monitoring strategies using commercially available devices have not consistently shown benefit.[27-30]

The use of an implanted pulmonary artery pressure monitor to guide diuretic dosing has proven beneficial, and may be considered in patients with frequent bouts of hypervolemic decompensation that have resulted in hospitalization.[31]

Regardless of strategy chosen, clinical evaluation should be frequent and clinical data should be acted upon.

After any change in diuretic dosing, it is reasonable to obtain follow-up lab work within a short period of time to confirm renal stability and the absence of hypokalemia. Patients with consistent hypokalemia should be supplemented with oral potassium or treated with spironolactone. Aldosterone antagonists (eg, spironolactone, eplerenone) are indicated as part of GDMT in those with HFrEF and symptoms.

CONCLUSION TO PATIENT CASE: PART 2

The patient reported a favorable response to his diuretic; therefore he was increased from once daily to twice a day dosing. He was followed up in 1 week with a brief clinical visit and labs. His signs and symptoms of hypervolemia had resolved, but his potassium had decreased to 3.5. He was therefore initiated on oral potassium supplementation. He received repeat HF self-care education, and began monitoring his weight at home.

PATIENT CASE: PART 3

Ten years later at age 61 years, the same patient is admitted to the hospital directly from the HF clinic for progressive fluid buildup that has been resistant to outpatient interventions. He now has a medical history of chronic kidney disease (CKD) IIIb secondary to diabetic nephropathy with a baseline creatinine of 2.2, and his ejection fraction dropped to 30% after suffering from a STEMI 1 year prior. He has been compliant with GDMT for his HF and usually adheres to a salt-and fluid-restricted diet. His diuretics have been significantly increased over the past year, and he is now taking 50 mg of torsemide twice daily, which had been doubled to 100 mg twice daily for the past 3 days without significant improvement. On admission he is grossly volume overloaded on clinical exam, with 2+ edema to hip height, jugular pulsations at the earlobe while upright, and diffuse rales. His vital signs are notable for a blood pressure of 103/78, a heart rate of 70, and an oxygen saturation of 90% on room air. His admission lab work shows creatinine of 2.9 mg/dL, an albumin of 2.9 g/dL, and a BNP of 1832 pg/mL. He is given an IV bolus of 160 mg of furosemide and initiated on a continuous infusion of furosemide at 10 mg/hour, but after 24 hours has made only 800 mL of urine.

CAUSES OF DIURETIC RESISTANCE

Prior to initiating additional therapies, one should be confident that the patient is in fact volume overloaded. Invasive assessment may be appropriate in diuretic nonresponders with uncertain volume status to confirm that the patient is truly still congested.[1]

A significant portion of patients with decompensated HF will have poor response to loop diuretics and not achieve adequate decongestion despite receiving high doses. This is both a clinical challenge and is prognostically significant, as this subset of patients experiences higher mortality and more frequent hospitalization.[32,33]

There are many causes of diuretic resistance, which are not mutually exclusive. Figures 27-6 and 27-8 summarize the most common causes.

Worsening cardiac function and worsening congestion both lead to decreased perfusion and perfusion pressure at the glomerulus, leading to decreased GFR and decreased delivery of sodium to the loop of Henle. They also result in upregulation of aldosterone and vasopressin, increasing sodium and free water reabsorption.[7]

CKD of any kind decreases the maximum effect of diuretics. Diminished renal perfusion and competitive inhibition of tubular secretion may cause diuretic unresponsiveness. Proteinuria will lead

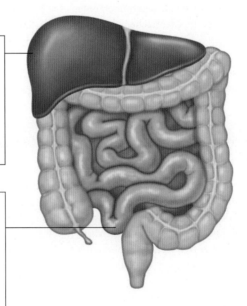

- Decreased albumin synthesis leads to less diuretic secreted into the renal tubules.
- Increased hepatic clearance of diuretic reduces the portion of the dose that reaches the tubules.

- Decreased gut perfusion leads to decreased active uptake of diuretic.
- Congestion and edema lead to decreased passive absorption of diuretic.

FIGURE 27-6 Gastrointestinal mechanisms of diuretic resistance.

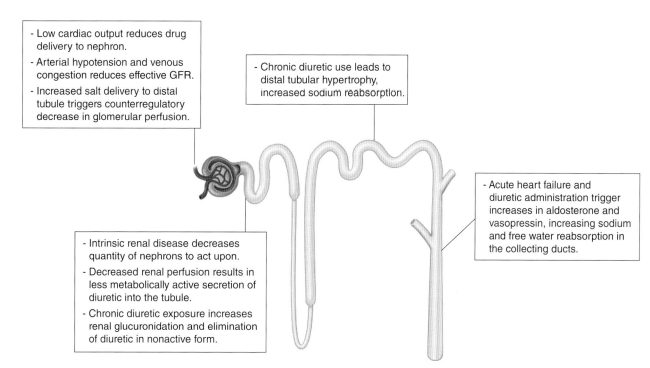

- Low cardiac output reduces drug delivery to nephron.
- Arterial hypotension and venous congestion reduces effective GFR.
- Increased salt delivery to distal tubule triggers counterregulatory decrease in glomerular perfusion.

- Chronic diuretic use leads to distal tubular hypertrophy, increased sodium reabsorption.

- Acute heart failure and diuretic administration trigger increases in aldosterone and vasopressin, increasing sodium and free water reabsorption in the collecting ducts.

- Intrinsic renal disease decreases quantity of nephrons to act upon.
- Decreased renal perfusion results in less metabolically active secretion of diuretic into the tubule.
- Chronic diuretic exposure increases renal glucuronidation and elimination of diuretic in nonactive form.

FIGURE 27-7 Renal mechanisms of diuretic resistance.

to albumin binding of loop diuretic within the tubule, preventing it from binding to its pharmacologic target.[8]

Chronic use of loop diuretics and the resultant increased delivery of sodium to the distal tubule results in hypertrophy of the distal tubule and an increase in the expression of thiazide-sensitive Na-Cl transporters, thus reabsorbing the salt load that was not absorbed in the loop of Henle negating the effect of the loop diuretic.[7]

The hypoalbuminemic state that commonly occurs in advanced HF reduces the amount of albumin-bound loop diuretic in the serum that can be secreted into the proximal tubule, and thus decreases the amount of drug that reaches the active site in the kidney.[5-8]

INPATIENT APPROACHES TO DIURETIC RESISTANCE

If the patient is severely congested or shows evidence of low cardiac output with severely increased systemic resistance, then administration of IV vasodilators such as nitroprusside, nitroglycerin, or nesiritide will acutely improve congestion via improved vascular compliance. These agents have been shown to acutely improve symptoms, and may improve diuretic responsiveness.[1]

If the patient shows evidence of low cardiac output, then inotropic infusions may be necessary to adequately perfuse the kidney and promote a diuretic response. Dopamine in particular receives a IIb recommendation as an adjunct to diuretic therapy in the ACC/AHA guidelines, based on its combined inotropic and renovascular effects.[1]

Combination diuretic therapy is a core approach for the diuretic-resistant patient. The addition of thiazide diuretics will frequently improve response, especially in patients who have been on chronic loop diuretic therapy and thus have distal tubular hypertrophy. This should be a first-line approach to overcoming diuretic resistance, given its low cost and high rate of response.

All thiazides are similarly effective for this purpose. The most commonly used agents are metolazone and chlorothiazide (Diuril). Metolazone has high oral availability and a long half-life, which makes timing of administration less important. Chlorothiazide is available as an IV preparation, although it should be noted that this is rarely necessary—oral chlorothiazide has very high bioavailability, and the IV preparation is extremely expensive.[34,35]

When loop diuretics are combined with thiazides (sequential nephron blockade), the urine produced is more concentrated than when loop diuretics are used alone. Very careful monitoring and replacement of electrolytes is necessary to avoid electrolyte depletion.[34,35]

Acetazolamide is a carbonic anhydrase inhibitor and weak diuretic that decreases sodium and bicarbonate reabsorption in the proximal tubule. There is limited literature suggesting it may have benefit in overcoming diuretic resistance, particularly among patients with alkalosis.[34,36]

Spironolactone reduces reabsorption of sodium in the collecting duct via its antagonism of aldosterone. While many HF patients are on low doses for its cardioprotective effects, natriuretic dosing (50-100 mg twice daily) has been described as an adjunct to overcome resistance to loop diuretics. This is especially effective in patients with concomitant hepatic dysfunction, who have especially elevated aldosterone activity. Careful monitoring is necessary to avoid hyperkalemia.[34,37]

In patients with severe hyponatremia, vasopressin may be markedly upregulated. Such patients can respond well to a vasopressin antagonist (eg, tolvaptan or conivaptan). Randomized studies and clinical experience have demonstrated the short-term safety of these agents in HF as well as their ability to produce acute decongestion in a hyponatremic ADHF population. Their efficacy specifically in the diuretic-resistant population is still under investigation. The recently completed TACTICS trial failed to demonstrate an increased rate of diuretic responsiveness among patients treated with tolvaptan.[34,38,39]

In patients with very low albumin, the combination of concentrated albumin infusion with IV loop diuretics has been shown to increase their delivery to the nephron and increase urine output. However clinically significant benefit has not been demonstrated, and this is generally a minor contributor to diuretic resistance in HF. Combined with the expense of human albumen, this approach is not generally recommended.[5,8,40]

Aquapheresis is a clinically available technology to remove excess fluid volume via ultrafiltration. It has been primarily studied as an alternative to diuretics in the general HF population. In this role, it has not consistently shown superiority to pharmacotherapy and may carry higher risk of renal injury. However, in patients with high-level diuretic resistance, it allows predictable volume and sodium removal regardless of diuretic resistance. As devices and techniques continue to improve, ultrafiltration shows promise as an adjunct or alternative decongestive therapy in carefully selected patients.[34,41-44]

The flowchart in Figure 27-8 outlines a suggested approach to the diuretic-resistant inpatient.

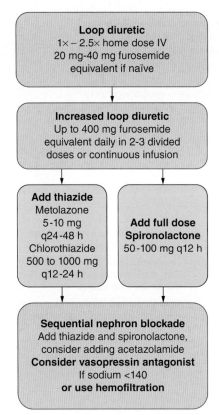

FIGURE 27-8 An example algorithm for stepped intensification of inpatient diuretic therapy. This is based on the author's practice—there is no official guideline-recommended approach to diuretic titration.

OUTPATIENT APPROACHES TO DIURETIC RESISTANCE

Prior to intensifying therapy, patients' medications, diets, and lifestyles should be thoroughly reviewed. If the patient is still on furosemide, he or she should be switched to torsemide or bumetanide to eliminate the possible role of poor gut absorption. All medications, including over-the-counter preparations, should be re-evaluated to ensure that harmful agents, such as NSAIDs, are not being used. A diet inventory should be reviewed to eliminate any possible hidden sources of sodium.

There is evidence that cardiac output and renal perfusion improve in the supine position as compared to the upright position, up to 40%. Having patients remain supine at home for 1 to 2 hours after they take their diuretics may increase diuretic response.[45]

Combination oral diuretics as described in the previous section—especially the use of thiazides—remain a clinically feasible approach as an outpatient. The addition of metolazone is an attractive option as an outpatient, as its long half-life may allow weekly or every-other-day dosing.

Patients on loop diuretics and thiazides should have close monitoring of serum electrolytes and renal function. We would recommend checking a basic metabolic panel no later than 1 week after any intensification of therapy, and at least every 3 months in patients on stable combination diuretic doses.

Patients receiving thiazide-boosted loop diuretics will very likely require scheduled potassium supplementation and/or the further addition of spironolactone.

Some patients will become resistant to oral diuretics due to issues with gut absorption, but have preserved responsiveness to IV loop diuretics. Scheduled or intermittent outpatient administration of IV loop diuretics in the clinic or infusion center has been shown to be safe and may reduce the need for inpatient admissions.[46]

The outpatient use of intermittent ultrafiltration and modified peritoneal dialysis for severely diuretic refractory patients has been evaluated in small feasibility studies. More investigation is required to determine their optimal use, but such techniques might be considered a last resort for patients who cannot be pharmacologically managed but otherwise do not meet criteria for full hemodialysis.[47,48]

CONCLUSION TO PATIENT CASE: PART 3

Returning to this chapter's Patient Case, 10 mg metolazone daily was added to the patient's medical regimen and he was consistently 1 L negative daily over the next 48 hours with improvement in creatinine to 2.2 mg/dL. Due to slow progress, the patient was transitioned to slow continuous ultrafiltration and received 2 L net fluid removal daily for an additional 72 hours. He was then transitioned back to his home oral torsemide with the addition of intermittent metolazone.

REFERENCES

1. Yancy CW, Jessup M, Bozkurt B, et al. 2013 ACCF/AHA guideline for the management of heart failure. *Circulation.* 2013;128:e240-e237.

2. Mentz RJ, Kjeldsen K, Rossi GP, et al. Decongestion in acute heart failure. *Eur J Heart Fail.* 2014;16,471-482.

3. Brunton LL, Lazo JS, Parker KL. *Goodman & Gilman's The Pharmacological Basis of Therapeutics.* New York, NY: McGraw-Hill; 2006.

4. Buggey J, Mentz RJ, Pitt B, et al. A reappraisal of loop diuretic choice in heart failure patients. *Am Heart J.* 2015;169:323-333.

5. Boles Ponto LL, Schoenwald RD. Furosemide (Frusemide) a pharmacokinetic/pharmacodynamic review (part I). *Clin Pharmacokinet.* 1990;18:381-408.

6. Prandota J, Witkowska M. Pharmacokinetics and metabolism of furosemide in man. *Eur J Drug Metab Pharmacokinet.* 1976;4:177-181.

7. Brater DC, Day B, Burdette A, et al. Bumetanide and furosemide in heart failure. *Kidney Int.* 1984;26:183-189.

8. Wilcox CS. New insights into diuretic use in patients with chronic renal disease. *J Am Soc Nephrol.* 2002;13:798-805.

9. Felker GM, Lee KL, Bull DA, Redfield MM, et al. Diuretic strategies in patients with acute decompensated heart failure. *N Engl J Med.* 2011;364(9):797-805.

10. Salvador DRK, Punzalan FE, Ramos GC. Continuous versus bolus injection of loop diuretics in congestive heart failure (review). *Cochrane Database Syst Rev.* 2005;(3):CD003178.

11. Shem S. 7th law of the house of God. In: *The House of God.* Berkley Publishing Group; New York, NY; 1978.

12. Mentz RJ, Stevens SR, DeVore AD, et al. Decongestion strategies and renin-angiotensin-aldosterone system activation in acute heart failure. *JACC Heart Fail.* 2015;3:97-107.

13. Wise LC, Mersch J, Racioppi J, et al. Evaluating the reliability and utility of cumulative intake and output. *J Nurs Care Qual.* 2000;14:37-42.

14. Schneider AG, Baldwin I, Freitag E, et al. Estimation of fluid status changes in critically ill patients: fluid balance chart or electronic bed weight? *J Crit Care.* 2012;27:745.e7-745.e12.

15. Testani JM, Hanberg JS, Cheng S, et al. Rapid and highly accurate prediction of poor loop diuretic natriuretic response in patients with heart failure. *Circ Heart Fail.* 2016;9:e002370.

16. Metra M, Davidson B, Bettari L, et al. Is worsening renal function an ominous prognostic sign in patients with acute heart failure? The role of congestion and its interaction with renal function. *Circ Heart Fail.* 2012;5:54-62.

17. Kahn NNS, Nabeel M, Nan B, et al. Chloride depletion alkalosis as a predictor of inhospital mortality in patients with decompensated heart failure. *Cardiology.* 2015;131:151-159.

18. Grodin JL, Verbrugge FH, Ellis SG, et al. Importance of abnormal chloride homeostasis in stable chronic heart failure. *Circ Heart Fail.* 2016;9:e002453.

19. Mecklai A, Subacius H, Konstam MA, et al. In-hospital diuretic agent use and post-discharge clinical outcomes in patients hospitalized for worsening heart failure. *JACC Heart Fail.* 2016;4(7):580-588.

20. Testani JM, Chen J, McCauley BD, et al. Potential effects of aggressive decongestion during the treatment of decompensated heart failure on renal function and survival. *Circulation.* 2010;122(3):265-272.

21. Vaan der Meer P, Postmus D, Ponikowski P, et al. The predictive value of short term changes in hemoglobin concentration in patients presenting with acute decompensated heart failure. *J Am Coll Cardiol.* 2013;61:1973-1981.

22. Greene SJ, Gheorghiade M, Vaduganathan M, et al. Hemoconcentration, renal function, and post-discharge outcomes among patients hospitalized for heart failure with reduced ejection fraction: insights from the EVEREST trial. *Eur J Heart Fail.* 2013;15:1401-1411.

23. Yancy CW, Jessup M, Bozkurt B, et al. 2017 ACC/AHA/HFSA focused update of the 2013 ACCF/AHA Guideline for the Management of Heart Failure. *J Am Coll Cardiol.* 2017;70:776-803.

24. Faris RF, Flather M, Purcell H, Poole-Wilson PA, et al. Diuretics for heart failure (review). *Cochrane Database of Systematic Reviews.* 2012;2:CD003838.

25. DeVore AD, Hasselblad V, Mentz RJ, et al. Loop diuretic dose adjustments after a hospitalization for heart failure: insights from ASCEND-HF. *Eur J Heart Fail.* 2015;17:340-346.

26. Jonkman NH, Westland H, Groenwold RHH, et al. Do self management interventions work in patients with heart failure? an individual patient data meta-analysis. *Circulation.* 2016;133:1189-1198.

27. Van Veldhuisen DJ, Braunschweig F, Conraads V, et al. Intrathoracic impedance monitoring, audible patient alerts, and outcome in patients with heart failure. *Circulation.* 2011;124:1719-1726.

28. Ong MK, Romano PS, Edgington S, et al. Effectiveness of remote patient monitoring after discharge of hospitalized patients with heart failure: the Better Effectiveness After Transition—Heart Failure (BEAT-HF) Randomized Clinical Trial. *JAMA Intern Med.* 2016;176:310-318.

29. Chaudhry SI, Mattera JA, Curtis JP, et al. Telemonitoring in patients with heart failure. *N Engl J Med.* 363:2301-2309.

30. Pandor A, Gomersall T, Stevens JW, et al. Remote monitoring after recent hospital discharge in patients with heart failure: a systematic review and network meta-analysis. *Heart.* 2013;99:1717-1726.

31. Adamson PB, Abraham WT, Stevenson LW, et al. Pulmonary artery pressure-guided heart failure management reduces 30-day readmissions. *Circ Heart Fail.* 2016;9:e002600.

32. Testani JM, Brisco MA, Turner JM, et al. Loop diuretic efficiency a metric of diuretic responsiveness with prognostic importance in acute decompensated heart failure. *Circ Heart Fail.* 2014;7(2):261-270.

33. Ter Maaten JM, Valente MAE, Damman K, et al. Combining diuretic response and hemoconcentration to predict rehospitalization after admission for acute heart failure. *Circ Heart Fail.* 2016;9(6):e002845.

34. Verbugge FH, Mullens W, Tang WH. Management of cardiorenal syndrome and diuretic resistance. *Curr Treat Options Cardio Med.* 2016;18(2):11.

35. Jentzer JC, DeWald TA, Hernandez AF. Combination of loop diuretics with thiazide-type diuretics in heart failure. *J Am Coll Cardiol.* 2010;56(19):1527-1534.

36. Knauf HH. Sequential nephron blockade breaks resistance to diuretics in edematous states. *J Cardiovasc Pharm.* 1997;29(3):367-372.

37. Eng M, Bansal S. Use of natriuretic-doses of spironolactone for treatment of loop diuretic resistant acute decompensated heart failure. *Int J Cardiol.* 2014;170(3):e68-e69.

38. Konstam MA, Gheorghiade M, Burnett JC Jr, et al. Effects of oral tolvaptan in patients hospitalized for worsening heart failure: the EVEREST outcome trial. *JAMA.* 2007;297(12):1319-1331.

39. Felker GM, Mentz RJ, Cole RT, et al. Efficacy and safety of tolvaptan in patients hospitalized with acute heart failure. *J Am Coll Cardiol.* 2017;69(11):1399-1406.

40. Ter Maaten JM, Rao V, Simon J, et al. Renal tubular resistance, rather than diuretic delivery, is the primary driver for diuretic resistance in acute heart failure patients. *J Am Coll Cardiol.* 2016;67:1544.

41. Costanzo MR, Guglin ME, Saltzberg MT, et al. Ultrafiltration versus intravenous diuretics for patients hospitalized for acute decompensated heart failure. *J Am Coll Cardiol.* 2007;49(6):675-683.

42. Bart BA, Goldsmith SR, Lee KL, et al. Ultrafiltration in decompensated heart failure with cardiorenal syndrome. *N Engl J Med.* 2012;367(24):2296-2304.

43. Costanzo MR, Negoianu D, Jaski BE, et al. Aquapheresis versus intravenous diuretics and hospitalizations for heart failure. *JACC Heart Fail.* 2016;4(2):95-105.

44. Costanzo MR, Ronco C, Abraham WT, et al. Extracorporeal ultrafiltration for fluid overload in heart failure. *J Am Coll Cardiol.* 2017, May 16;69(19):2428-2445.

45. Abildgaard U, Aldershvile J, Ring-Larsen H, et al. Bed rest and increased diuretic treatment in congestive heart failure. *Eur Heart J*. 1985;6(12):1040-1046.

46. Buckley LF, Carter DM, Matta L, et al. Intravenous diuretic therapy for the management of heart failure and volume overload in a multidisciplinary outpatient unit. *JACC Heart Fail*. 2016;4(1):1-8.

47. Sheppard R, Panyon J, Pohwani AL, et al. Intermittent outpatient ultrafiltration for the treatment of severe refractory congestive heart failure. *J Card Fail*. 2004;10(5):380-383.

48. Gotloib L, Fudin R, Yakubovich M, Vienken J. Peritoneal dialysis in refractory end-stage congestive heart failure: a challenge facing a no-win situation. *Nephrol Dial Transplant*. 2005;20 Suppl 7:vii32-36.

28 NEUROHORMONAL BLOCKADE IN HEART FAILURE

Waleed Kayani, MD
Anita Deswal, MD, MPH

■ PATIENT CASE

A 55-year-old man with hypertension, diabetes mellitus and recent drug eluting stent placement to left anterior descending (LAD) artery after suffering a myocardial infarction comes to your clinic after being discharged from the hospital. He is able to carry out daily activities with ease but reports getting short of breath on climbing 2 sets of stairs. An echocardiogram done during the hospitalization revealed an left ventricular ejection fraction (LVEF) of 35%-39% with wall motion abnormalities in LAD territory. He mentions compliance with his regimen of Aspirin 81 mg once daily, Clopidogrel 75 mg once daily, Amlodipine 5 mg, Atorvastatin 80 mg and Furosemide 20 mg once daily. On examination his blood pressure is 147/87 and heart rate 76 beats per minute, he appears in no acute distress, JVP is 7 cm H_2O, lungs are clear, heart sounds are regular with no murmurs and no lower extremity edema is noted. He asks about additional therapies to help recover improve his heart function and quality of life.

NEUROHORMONAL BLOCKADE IN HEART FAILURE

Understanding the pathophysiological role of the neurohormonal axis in heart failure (HF) has been a key driver of the paradigm shift of the management of HF from one of only symptom management to that involving strategies aimed at modulating pathologic left ventricular (LV) remodeling and HF-related mortality.

THE NEUROHORMONAL SYSTEM IN HEART FAILURE

A reduction in myocardial function, stemming from any insult, leads to a decrease in cardiac output and blood pressure and, via activation of baroreceptors, leads to activation of the sympathetic nervous system (SNS) and renal hypoperfusion. The SNS primarily mediates its effects via catecholamines.[1] Via stimulation from the SNS as well as intrinsic renal mechanisms, the renin angiotensin and subsequently aldosterone system are activated, collectively referred to as the renin-angiotensin-aldosterone system (RAAS). The combined effect of the 2 systems leads to increased inotropy, chronotropy, sodium and water retention (leading to an increase in preload), and vasoconstriction (causing an increase in afterload). Over the short term, the above compensation helps maintain cardiac output (CO) and blood pressure (BP); however, chronic activation of the same compensatory mechanisms leads to pathologic remodeling of the ventricular myocardium (Figure 28-1).[2] Although described more extensively in patients with HF with reduced ejection fraction

(HFrEF), regardless of the etiology, similar mechanisms may play a role in HF with preserved ejection fraction (HFpEF).

RENIN-ANGIOTENSIN-ALDOSTERONE RECEPTOR BLOCKADE

Therapies aimed at blocking various steps in the RAAS pathway help to mitigate the effect of the chronically overactivated system, and have demonstrated definitive beneficial effects on morbidity and mortality in HFrEF.

ANGIOTENSIN-CONVERTING ENZYME INHIBITORS

Angiotensin-converting enzyme (ACE) inhibitors exert their effect via inhibition of the ACE. The ACE, in addition to its role in converting angiotensin I to angiotensin II, also facilitates the degradation of bradykinin and substance P, both of which are potent vasodilators (Figure 28-2). ACE inhibitor therapy has short-term benefits including improvement of cardiac output, enhancement of natriuresis, and vasodilation, and long-term effects including prevention or delay of LV remodeling as well as causing favorable LV reverse remodeling.[3]

ANGIOTENSIN-CONVERTING ENZYME INHIBITORS IN HEART FAILURE WITH REDUCED EJECTION FRACTION

ACE inhibitors have been evaluated in multiple clinical trials in patients with symptomatic HF, in patients with asymptomatic LV systolic dysfunction, and in patients with post myocardial infarction (MI) HF, with favorable effects. Enalapril and captopril are the best studied ACE inhibitors; however, similar benefits have been observed with other ACE inhibitors as well. Garg and Yusuf conducted a meta-analysis of 32 trials comparing various ACE inhibitors versus placebo in 7105 symptomatic HFrEF patients of ischemic and nonischemic etiology (Table 28-1). A significant reduction in odds of developing the combined endpoint of death or hospitalization for HF, as well as of death—primarily due to a substantial reduction in deaths attributable to progressive HF—was observed with ACE inhibitor use as compared with placebo.[4] The greatest benefit was seen during the first 3 months, but additional benefit was observed during longer-term treatment. Moreover, the lower the EF, the more the benefit observed. An improvement in exercise capacity in patients with HFrEF was noted by Narang et al in their meta-analysis of 33 studies.[5]

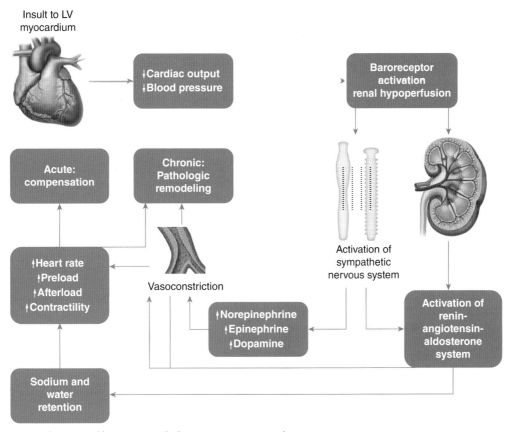

FIGURE 28-1 Short-term adaptive and long-term pathologic responses to cardiac injury.

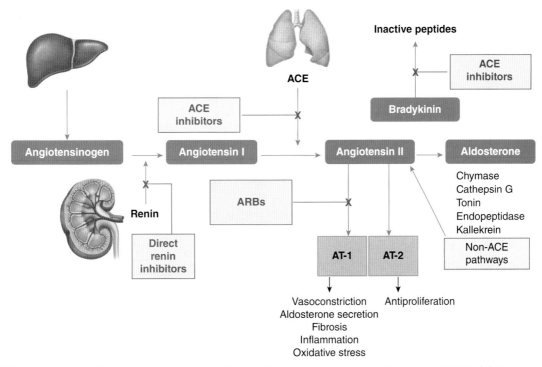

FIGURE 28-2 The renin-angiotensin-aldosterone system and sites of action of angiotensin-converting enzyme (ACE) inhibitors, angiotensin receptor blockers (ARBs), and direct renin inhibitors.

Table 28-1 Beneficial Effects on Outcomes with ACE Inhibitor Therapy vs Placebo in HFrEF[4]

Events	No. of Events/No. of Randomized		OR (95% CI)	P value
	ACE Inhibitor	Controls		
Mortality	611/3870 (15.8)	709/3235 (21.9)	0.77 (0.67-0.88)	<0.001
Mortality or HF hospitalization	854/3810 (22.4)	1036/3178 (32.6)	0.65 (0.57-0.74)	<0.001
Total Mortality or Hospitalization by Different Duration and Subgroups with ACE Inhibitor Therapy				
Subgroup	No. of Events/No. of Randomized		OR (95% CI)	
	ACE Inhibitor	Controls		
90 d or less	239/3810	372/3178	0.53 (0.44-0.63)	
More than 90 d	615/1834	372/3178	0.76 (0.66-0.88)	
Ischemic cardiomyopathy	566/1997 (28.3)	704/1757 (40.1)	0.63 (0.54-0.74)	
Nonischemic cardiomyopathy	263/1132 (23.2)	292/1006 (29.0)	0.72 (0.57-0.91)	

Abbreviations: ACE, angiotensin-converting enzyme; CI, confidence interval; HF, heart failure; HFrEF, heart failure with reduced ejection fraction; OR, odds ratio.

In addition, patients with asymptomatic LV dysfunction comprise a cohort that is at high risk for development of HF and mortality.[6] The Studies of Left Ventricular Dysfunction (SOLVD) prevention trial examined the effect of enalapril on morbidity, mortality, and development of HF in patients with asymptomatic LV systolic dysfunction. Compared with placebo, enalapril significantly reduced the rate of hospitalization for HF and showed a trend toward lower mortality.[7] The salient results from 3 of the landmark clinical trials[7-9] of ACE inhibitors in HFrEF or asymptomatic LV systolic dysfunction are shown in Figure 28-3.

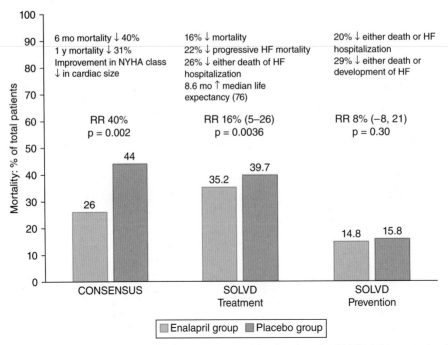

FIGURE 28-3 Benefit of ACE inhibitors on mortality and other key outcomes in 3 landmark trials of ACE inhibitors vs placebo in patients with HFrEF. Abbreviations: CONSENSUS, Cooperative North Scandinavian Enalapril Survival Study[9]; HF, heart failure; RR, % risk reduction; SOLVD, Studies of Left Ventricular Dysfunction.[7,8]

ANGIOTENSIN-CONVERTING ENZYME INHIBITORS IN HEART FAILURE WITH PRESERVED EJECTION FRACTION

There is no convincing evidence to show that ACE inhibitor therapy improves hard endpoints in patients with HFpEF. The Perindopril in Elderly People with Chronic Heart Failure (PEP-CHF) trial studied perindopril in 850 patients with HFpEF and failed to show a significant improvement in the primary outcome (composite of all-cause mortality and unplanned HF-related hospitalization). However, significant improvements were observed favoring ACE inhibitor therapy in some other secondary endpoints, including the proportion of patients in NYHA functional class I and change in 6-minute walk test (6MWT) at 1 year.[10]

OPTIMAL DOSING OF ANGIOTENSIN-CONVERTING ENZYME INHIBITORS

The Assessment of Treatment with Lisinopril and Survival (ATLAS) trial compared the efficacy and safety of low-dose versus high-dose ACE inhibition on mortality and morbidity in chronic symptomatic heart failure with either low-dose (target 2.5-5.0 mg daily) or high-dose (target 32.5-35 mg daily) lisinopril. Compared with the low-dose group, patients in the high-dose group had a nonsignificant 8% lower risk of death ($p = 0.128$) but a significant 12% lower risk of death or hospitalization for any reason ($p = 0.002$) and 24% fewer hospitalizations for HF ($p = 0.002$).[11]

ANGIOTENSIN RECEPTOR BLOCKERS IN HEART FAILURE

Angiotensin II, through its actions on the angiotensin II type I (AT-1) receptor, is a major mediator of vasoconstriction, hemodynamic derangements, adverse remodeling, and symptoms in HF (Figure 28-2).[12] ACE inhibition results in only a partial decrease in the production of angiotensin II, which can also be produced through non-ACE-dependent pathways (Figure 28-2).[13] Angiotensin receptor blockers (ARBs), which block the AT-1 receptor, could theoretically produce more complete blockade of the effects of angiotensin II and could potentially have more favorable effects in HF compared with ACE inhibitors. Moreover, compared to ACE inhibitors, ARBs do not inhibit the breakdown of bradykinin, the substance that causes the adverse effects of cough associated with ACE inhibitor use. ARBs may therefore be better tolerated than ACE inhibitors. Furthermore, it had been hypothesized that concomitant use of ACE inhibitors and ARBs may lead to synergistic effects of RAAS antagonism and could potentially lead to better clinical outcomes. Therefore, several trials evaluated the effects of ARBs compared with ACE inhibitors in HFrEF, as well as the effects of both ACE inhibitors and ARBs used in combination.

ANGIOTENSIN RECEPTOR BLOCKERS IN HEART FAILURE WITH REDUCED EJECTION FRACTION

A head-to-head comparison of ARBs and ACE inhibitors was conducted in New York Heart Association class II to IV HF (LVEF ≤40%) patients in Evaluation of Losartan In The Elderly II (ELITE II) and in high-risk patients after acute MI in the Optimal Trial In Myocardial Infarction with the Angiotensin II Antagonist Losartan (OPTIMAAL) trials, which compared losartan 50 mg daily with captopril 50 mg 3 times daily.[14,15] There was no evidence of superiority of the ARB over the ACE inhibitor. In fact, there was even a trend for better outcomes with the ACE inhibitor in some endpoints. Going 1 step further, the Valsartan in Acute Myocardial Infarction Trial (VALIANT) compared valsartan 160 mg daily, captopril 50 mg 3 times daily, and valsartan 160 mg daily + captopril 50 mg 3 times daily in a 1:1:1 fashion in patients within 10 days post-MI with LV systolic dysfunction and HF.[16] The ACE inhibitor and the ARB were equivalent in terms of the overall mortality as well as fatal and nonfatal cardiovascular (CV) outcomes. Furthermore, VALIANT showed that combined therapy of ACE inhibitor and ARB soon after MI resulted in an increase in adverse events without improving overall survival. Adverse events were less common for monotherapy, with hypotension and renal dysfunction being more common in the ARB group and cough, skin rash, and taste disturbance more common in the ACE inhibitor group.

COMBINED ANGIOTENSIN-CONVERTING ENZYME INHIBITOR AND ANGIOTENSIN RECEPTOR BLOCKER THERAPY IN CHRONIC HEART FAILURE WITH REDUCED EJECTION FRACTION

The Valsartan Heart Failure Trial (Val-HeFT) and the Candesartan in Heart Failure: Assessment of Reduction in Mortality and Morbidity (CHARM)-Added trials evaluated whether the combination of ACE inhibitors and ARBs would be more beneficial than ACE inhibitors alone in symptomatic patients with chronic HFrEF.[17,18] Although a significant decrease in CV mortality and a reduction in HF hospitalization were seen in the CHARM-Added trial with candesartan, Val-HeFT demonstrated only a decrease in HF hospitalizations in the valsartan group. Notably, in Val-HeFT and the CHARM-Added, as well as other studies that have studied concomitant use of ACE inhibitors and ARBs, a higher incidence of hypotension, hyperkalemia, and renal dysfunction has been seen with combination therapy. Therefore, ARBs may be considered in patients who appear to have continuing symptoms of progressive HF and hospitalizations despite therapy with target doses of ACE inhibitors and beta blockers when aldosterone antagonists are not tolerated. However, there is no role for routine combined use of ACE inhibitors, aldosterone antagonists, and ARBs (ACC/AHA Guidelines Class III recommendation).[19]

ANGIOTENSIN RECEPTOR BLOCKERS IN ACE-INTOLERANT PATIENTS

The Candesartan in Heart Failure: Assessment of Reduction in Mortality and Morbidity (CHARM)-Alternative trial addressed the role of ARBs in HF patients intolerant of ACE inhibitors by comparing candesartan with placebo and showing a significant 23% reduction in the composite outcome of CV mortality or HF hospitalizations. Interestingly, the margin of benefit observed with ARBs in the CHARM-Alternative trial was similar to that observed with ACE inhibitors compared to placebo.[20] Therefore, ARBs are now considered to provide equivalent benefit to ACE inhibitors in patients with HFrEF and are often used when patients are unable to tolerate ACE inhibitors due to cough or angioedema.

ANGIOTENSIN RECEPTOR BLOCKERS IN HEART FAILURE WITH PRESERVED EJECTION FRACTION

The effect of ARBs on outcome in HFpEF has been best studied in the Candesartan in Heart Failure: Assessment of Reduction in Mortality and Morbidity (CHARM)-Preserved and the Irbesartan in Heart Failure with Preserved Ejection Fraction (I–PRESERVE) trials.[21,22] A trend toward lower incidence of the primary composite endpoint of CV death or hospital admission for HF was seen in the candesartan arm, driven primarily by a reduction in hospitalizations for HF in CHARM-Preserved. However, the larger I-PRESERVE trial (4128 patients with HFpEF) showed no significant difference in the occurrence of death from any cause or hospitalization for a CV cause (Figure 28-4). Hence, no conclusive data exist to support routine use of ARBs in patients with HFpEF to improve mortality or morbidity outcomes.

ALDOSTERONE ANTAGONISTS

Aldosterone is secreted by the adrenal cortex in response to angiotensin II and other non-RAAS factors, the most potent of which is serum potassium. As the role of ACE inhibitors and ARBs became more prevalent in HF, aldosterone escape, a phenomenon resulting from only partial inhibition of aldosterone by inhibitors of the RAAS and non-RAAS activation of aldosterone, was described.[23] HF is characterized by excess sodium and fluid retention, both of which are enhanced by aldosterone. Moreover, aldosterone increases myocardial and vascular fibrosis and LV hypertrophy (Figure 28-5). As higher levels of circulating aldosterone were found in patients with HF, the role of mineralocorticoid receptor antagonists (MRA) in HF emerged.

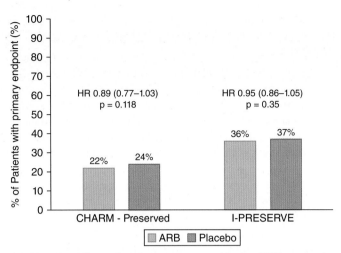

FIGURE 28-4 Effects of angiotensin receptor blocker (ARB) versus placebo on the combined endpoint in HFpEF in 2 clinical trials: CHARM-Preserved = Candesartan in Heart Failure: Assessment of Reduction in Mortality and Morbidity-Preserved trial,[21] and I-PRESERVE = the Irbesartan in Heart Failure with Preserved Ejection Fraction trial.[22] The primary endpoint in CHARM-Preserved was time to cardiovascular (CV) death or HF hospitalization. The primary endpoint for the I-PRESERVE trial was time to death for any cause or CV hospitalization. Abbreviation: HR, hazard ratio.

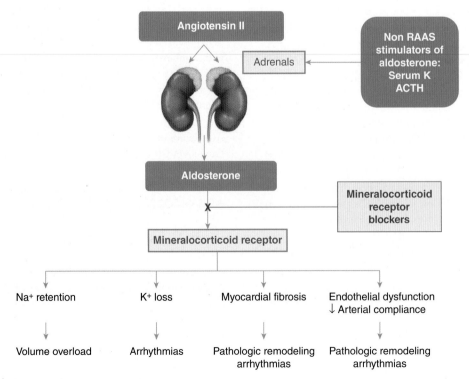

FIGURE 28-5 The aldosterone system.

ALDOSTERONE ANTAGONISTS IN HEART FAILURE WITH REDUCED EJECTION FRACTION

The Randomized Aldactone Evaluation Study (RALES) examined the efficacy of spironolactone 25 mg (titrated to 50 mg daily as tolerated) compared with placebo on a background of standard HF therapy, which at the time of the trial did not routinely use beta blockers in patients with severe HF (NYHA class III-IV).[24] The trial was terminated early when a 30% relative risk reduction in all-cause mortality (95% confidence interval [CI], 0.60-0.82; P <0.001) as well as 29% reduction in sudden death was observed. Incidence of gynecomastia was 10% in the male population and was the major adverse event although leading to discontinuation of the medication in only a very small proportion of patients; but importantly the incidence of serious hyperkalemia (serum potassium ≥6 meq/L) was not significantly higher in the spironolactone group under close potassium-monitoring strategies of the trial. The Eplerenone Post-acute Myocardial Infarction Heart Failure Efficacy and Survival Study (EPHESUS) trial studied eplerenone, a more specific aldosterone antagonist, in patients with LV systolic dysfunction and HF post-MI.[25] Again, a significant reduction in mortality by 15% (P = 0.008) and CV deaths or hospitalizations by 13% (P = 0.002) was observed in the eplerenone group. As expected, incidence of gynecomastia was not higher in the eplerenone group. As aldosterone receptor antagonist use became more prevalent in patients with moderate to severe HF, the Eplerenone in Mild Patients Hospitalization And Survival Study in Heart Failure (EMPHASIS-HF) trial enrolled patients with mild chronic HFrEF on a background of optimal concomitant therapy with nearly 90% of patients being on both beta blockers and ACE inhibitors or ARBs.[26] Once again, results overwhelmingly favored eplerenone. The primary composite outcome of death from CV causes or hospitalization for HF and overall mortality was reduced by 37% (hazard ratio [HR], 0.63; 95% CI, 0.54-0.74; P <0.001) and 24% (HR, 0.76; 95% CI, 0.61-0.94; P = 0.01) in the eplerenone group compared to placebo, respectively. Importantly, incidence of hyperkalemia was not significantly different with eplerenone or placebo (Figures 28-6 and 28-7).

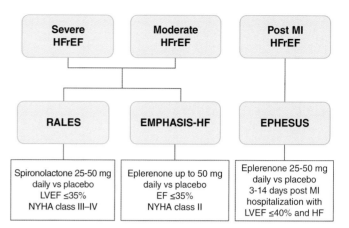

FIGURE 28-6 Trials of aldosterone receptor blockers (eplerenone and spironolactone) in HFrEF with differing severity of HF. AAbbreviations: EF; ejection fraction; EMPHASIS-HF, Eplerenone in Mild Patients Hospitalization And Survival Study in Heart Failure;[26] EPHESUS, Eplerenone Post-Acute Myocardial Infarction Heart Failure Efficacy and Survival Study;[25] HF; heart failure; HFrEF; heart failure with reduced ejection fraction; LVEF; left ventricular ejection fraction; MI; myocardial infarction; RALES, Randomized Aldactone Evaluation Study.[24]

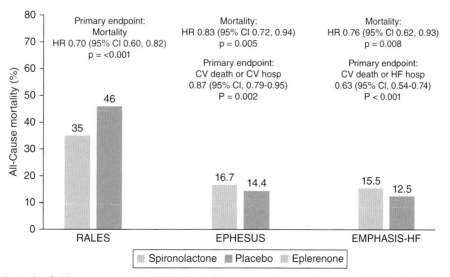

FIGURE 28-7 Results of the trials of aldosterone receptor blockade (eplerenone and spironolactone) in HFrEF with differing severity of HF. Abbreviations: CV, cardiovascular; EMPHASIS-HF, Eplerenone in Mild Patients Hospitalization and Survival Study in Heart Failure;[26] EPHESUS, Eplerenone Post-Acute Myocardial Infarction Heart Failure Efficacy and Survival Study;[25] HF, heart failure; HFrEF, HR, hazard ratio; RALES, Randomized Aldactone Evaluation Study.[24]

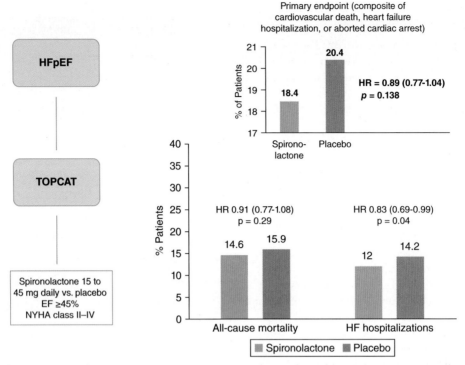

FIGURE 28-8 Results of the Treatment of Preserved Cardiac Function Heart Failure With an Aldosterone Antagonist Trial (TOPCAT) of spironolactone in heart failure with preserved ejection fraction (HFpEF).[27]

ALDOSTERONE ANTAGONISTS IN HFpEF

MRAs have also been studied in HFpEF (Figure 28-8). The Treatment of Preserved Cardiac Function Heart Failure With an Aldosterone Antagonist Trial (TOPCAT) study randomized 3445 patients with symptomatic HF and a left ventricular ejection fraction (LVEF) of 45% or higher to receive either spironolactone (15-45 mg daily) or placebo. Although the study found no difference in the primary endpoint of death from CV causes, aborted cardiac arrest, or hospitalization for HF (HR, 0.89; 95% CI, 0.77-1.04; P = 0.14) for the spironolactone vs placebo group, a reduction in hospitalizations for HF was seen in the spironolactone group (HR, 0.83; 95% CI, 0.69-0.99, P = 0.04) (Figure 28-8).[27] A post hoc analysis of TOPCAT patients enrolled in the Americas versus Russia/Georgia (from where almost 50% of patients were enrolled) demonstrated significant heterogeneity in underlying patient risk and clinical response to spironolactone.[28] In the subgroup enrolled in the Americas, the primary composite endpoint in the placebo arms occurred at ~4 times higher rate in the placebo arm compared with the subgroup enrolled from Russia/Georgia. In the higher-risk subgroup in the Americas, the primary endpoint was reduced by spironolactone compared to placebo (HR, 0.82; 95% CI, 0.69-0.98), but there was no effect in the subgroup enrolled in Russia/Georgia (HR, 1.10; 95% CI, 0.79-1.51). Based on these results, the Canadian Cardiovascular Society updated its HF guidelines to include consideration of spironolactone for HFpEF, with a weak recommendation/low quality of evidence as follows: "In individuals with HFpEF, an elevated natriuretic peptide level, serum potassium <5.0 mmol/L, and an estimated glomerular filtration rate eGFR ≥30 mL/min, an MRA such as spironolactone should be considered with close surveillance of serum potassium and creatinine."[29]

DIRECT RENIN INHIBITORS

The use of ACE inhibitors and ARBs may result in the loss of feedback inhibition and result in higher levels of circulating renin, with subsequent higher levels of angiotensin I. Associated deleterious effects may still occur as follows (Figure 28-9):

1. Angiotensin II production may occur if elevated levels of angiotensin I competitively overcome ACE enzyme inhibition. Angiotensin II production may also occur via ACE-independent escape pathways such as through cathepsin and chymase.[30]

2. The binding of higher levels of renin to the renin receptor may directly result in activation of hypertrophic, apoptotic activity and extracellular matrix remodeling via enhanced mitogen-activated protein kinase 1 and 3 and transforming growth factor-β1 signaling leading to myocardial dysfunction.[31]

Therefore there was interest in the development of direct renin inhibitors, which may alone or in combination with ACE inhibitors or ARBs have greater blockade with resultant benefits in HF compared with use of ACE inhibitors or ARBs themselves.

Aliskiren, a nonpeptide direct renin inhibitor that blocks the active site of both renin and activated prorenin, has been shown to decrease plasma renin activity. The Aliskiren Observation of Heart Failure Treatment (ALOFT) trial compared aliskiren 150 mg daily to placebo in 322 HF patients already on ACE inhibitors and beta blockers.[32] Differences in N-terminal pro-brain natriuretic peptide (NT-proBNP), the primary endpoint, were reduced significantly in the aliskiren group. Moreover, unadjusted results showed an improvement in the echocardiographic measures of LV dysfunction. Subsequently, in the larger Safety and Efficacy of Aliskiren in Post Myocardial Infarction Patients (ASPIRE) trial, which examined aliskiren in comparison to placebo in post-MI patients with LV dysfunction, no differences in the primary endpoint of end-systolic volume change between patients randomized to aliskiren (24.4±16.8 mL) or placebo (23.5±16.3 mL), or in secondary measures of end-diastolic volume, or LVEF were observed. Clinical endpoints were similar between the 2 groups as well.[33] Importantly, in both the ALOFT and ASPIRE trials, a higher incidence of hypotension, renal dysfunction, and hyperkalemia was seen with aliskiren use. Similarly, 2 other trials were halted early given concerns for side effects by their Data Monitoring Safety Boards. Recently, the results of the Aliskiren Trial to Minimize Outcomes in Patients with Heart Failure (ATMOSPHERE) became available. This trial compared the ACE inhibitor enalapril with the renin inhibitor aliskiren (to test superiority or at least noninferiority) and with the combination of the 2 treatments (to test superiority) in patients with HFrEF.[34] However, the addition of aliskiren to enalapril led to more adverse events without an increase in benefit. Noninferiority was also not shown for aliskiren as compared with enalapril (Table 28-2). Therefore, at present there is little role of aliskiren and other direct renin inhibitors over ACE inhibitors or ARBs in patients with HF.

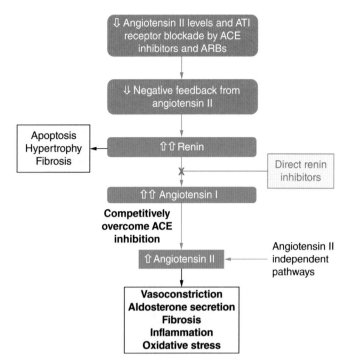

FIGURE 28-9 Suggested mechanisms of benefit with direct renin inhibitors.

Table 28-2 Aliskerin in Heart Failure

Study	Comparison	Population	Key Results
ALOFT[32]	Aliskiren 150 mg daily vs placebo	302 patients NYHA II-IV HF HTN BNP >100 pg/mL Baseline ACE inhibitor/ ARB + beta blockers No LVEF cutoff	25% RRR in primary endpoint of difference in NT-proBNP in favor of aliskiren (95% CI, 0.61-0.94; p = 0.001) ↓ Mitral regurgitation area ↓ Peak early transmitral flow* velocity ↓ E/A ratio ↓ Deceleration time
ASPIRE[33]	Aliskiren up to 300 mg daily vs placebo	820 patients post-AMI LVEF ≤45% Enrolled with 2-8 wk Baseline ACE inhibitor/ ARB + beta blockers	No significant difference in primary endpoint of LV end-systolic volume No significant difference in secondary outcomes of change in LVEF, mortality, or HF hospitalizations
ATMOSPHERE[34]	Aliskiren up to 300 mg daily vs enalapril + aliskiren vs placebo	4676 patients NYHA II-IV HF LVEF ≤35% BNP ≥150 pg/mL or NT-proBNP ≥600 pg/mL or HF hospitalization Baseline ACE inhibitor/ ARB + beta blockers	No significant difference in primary composite endpoint of CV death or HF hospitalization: HR in the combination-therapy vs enalapril group = 0.93 (95% CI, 0.85, 1.03; p = 0.17); aliskiren vs enalapril, HR = 0.99 (95% CI, 0.90, 1.10; p = 0.91 for superiority)

Abbreviations: ACE, angiotensin-converting enzyme; AMI, acute myocardial infarction; ARB, angiotensin receptor blocker; BNP, brain natriuretic peptide; CI, confidence interval; CV, cardiovascular; HF, heart failure; HR, hazard ratio; HTN, hypertension; LVEF, left ventricular ejection fraction; NT-proBNP; N-terminal pro-brain natriuretic peptide.

NEPRILYSIN INHIBITORS

Neural endopeptodase or neprilysin is a metalloproteinase enzyme that is found with the highest concentration in the proximal renal tubule, but is also found in heart and blood vessels. Neprilysin is involved in breakdown of vasoactive peptides such as angiotensin I, bradykinin, and atrial and B-type natriuretic peptides. By augmenting the active natriuretic peptides, neprilysin inhibition increases generation of myocardial cyclic guanosine 3′5 monophosphate, which improves myocardial relaxation and reduces hypertrophy, and stimulates diuresis, natriuresis, and vasodilation (Figure 28-10).[35] These effects may be beneficial in patients with HF. However, with neprilysin inhibition, angiotensin breakdown is decreased too. Indeed, when data from hypertension (HTN) trials involving neprilysin inhibitors emerged, they showed lack of efficacy of this group of agents, suggesting lack of angiotensin II breakdown as the reason.

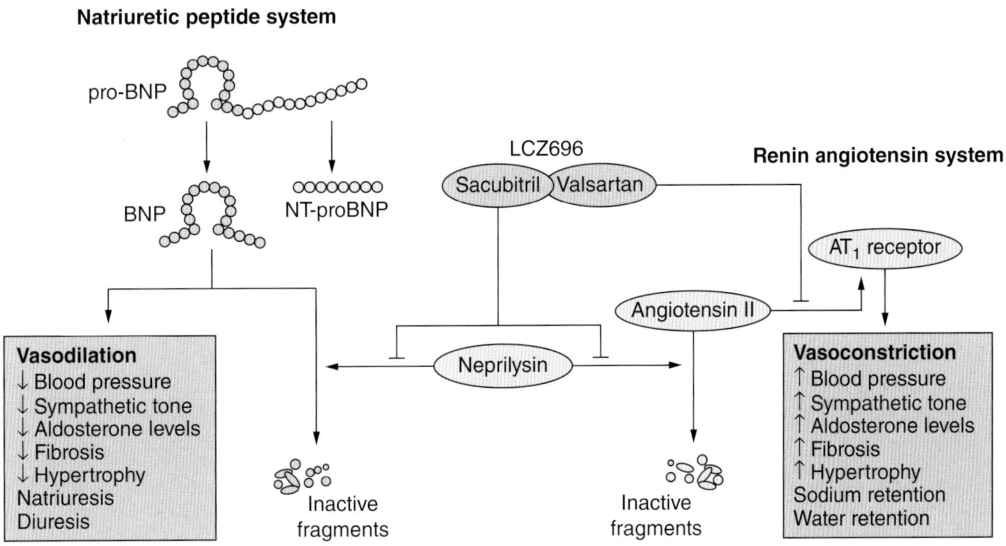

FIGURE 28-10 Mechanisms of action with dual neurohormonal inhibition by LCZ696 (sacubitril/valsartan). (Reproduced with permission from Swedberg K. Heart failure therapies in 2014: mixed results for heart failure therapies. *Nat Rev Cardiology.* 2015;12:73-75).

Emphasis was then toward agents resulting in combined inhibition of neprilysin and ACE, the vasopeptidase inhibitors.

VASOPEPTIDASE INHIBITORS

Omapatrilat was 1 of the vasopeptidase inhibitors that was previously studied in detail in patients with HF. Although it may be effective in patients with HF, the higher incidence of angioedema seen in patients treated with omapatrilat, especially[36-38] in African American patients, led to a halt in further development of vasopeptidase inhibitors for some time. Inhibition of bradykinin, aminopeptidease P, and ACE breakdown by omapatrilat were the proposed mechanisms for the higher incidence of angioedema. Subsequently, combined angiotensin receptor and neprilysin inhibitors have been developed to counteract this adverse effect.

COMBINED ANGIOTENSIN RECEPTOR-NEPRILYSIN INHIBITORS

LCZ696 or valsartan/sacubitril is the first angiotensin receptor-neprilysin inhibitor (ARNI) that comprises the molecular moieties of the neprilysin inhibitor prodrug AHU377 and the ARB, valsartan in 1 compound. Although neprilysin degrades atrial natriuretic peptide (ANP), brain natriuretic peptide (BNP), and C-type natriuretic peptide, NT-proBNP is not cleaved by it (Figure 28-10). In a proof of concept study of 1328 patients for LCZ696 use in treatment of HTN compared with valsartan, Ruilope et al reported no cases of angioedema during the 8 weeks of the study.[39]

The Prospective Comparison of ARNI (Angiotensin Receptor-Neprilysin Inhibitor) with ACE-I to Determine Impact on Global Mortality and Morbidity in Heart Failure (PARADIGM-HF) trial studied the efficacy and safety of LCZ696 200 mg twice daily compared to enalapril 10 mg twice daily in 8458 patients with chronic HF (NYHA class II-IV and EF ≤35%).[40] Based on the recommendations of its Data Monitoring Safety Board, the study

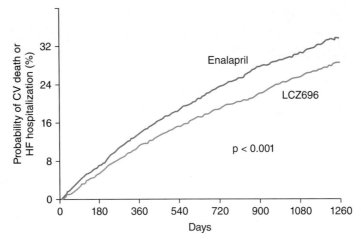

FIGURE 28-11 Benefit of LCZ696 versus enalapril in patients with heart failure with reduced ejection fraction (HFrEF) in the Prospective Comparison of ARNI (Angiotensin Receptor-Neprilysin Inhibitor) with ACE-I to Determine Impact on Global Mortality and Morbidity in Heart Failure (PARADIGM- HF) trial. (Data from McMurray JJ, Packer M, Desai AS, et al. Angiotensin-neprilysin inhibition versus enalapril in heart failure. *N Engl J Med.* 2014;371:993-1004.)

halted recruitment after a median follow-up of 27 months, because of a significant reduction in composite endpoint of CV death or HF hospitalization without a significant increase in adverse events with LCZ696. An absolute risk reduction of 4.8% was seen in the primary endpoint (CV death or hospitalization for HF), (HR, 0.80; 95% CI, 0.73-0.87), p value of <0.001 (Figure 28-11). A similar beneficial effect was seen for CV death (HR, 0.8; 95% CI, 0.71-0.89), hospitalization for HF (HR, 0.79; 95% CI, 0.71-0.89), and death from any cause (HR, 0.84; 95% CI, 0.76-0.93). The number of patients who would need to be treated to prevent 1 primary endpoint is 21, and to prevent 1 CV death is 32. The LCZ696 group had a higher incidence of hypotension and nonserious angioedema but lower incidence of renal impairment, hyperkalemia, and cough than the enalapril group. In a more recent report, the PARADIGM-HF investigators indicated that, in comparison with enalapril, LCZ696 exhibited additional evidence of clinical benefit, including a reduced need for intensification of the treatment for HF, fewer visits to an emergency department for HF, and a lower requirement for intensive care or need for inotropic agents, an HF device, or cardiac transplantation. Progressive symptoms of HF and elevations of NT-proBNP and troponin were also reduced.[41] Overall the results of PARADIGM-HF are robust and promising and may apply to a wide spectrum of patients, even those who are currently receiving the best possible therapy. It must be noted, however, that in the trial patients had an open-label period in which they demonstrated tolerability to enalapril and then to LCZ696 before they were randomized. Therefore, some caution is recommended in determining how patients will tolerate this new medication in clinical practice, especially if it is used as first-line therapy before the patients are stable and tolerating ACE inhibitors or ARBs at moderate doses.

COMBINED ANGIOTENSIN RECEPTOR-NEPRILYSIN INHIBITORS IN HEART FAILURE WITH PRESERVED EJECTION FRACTION

LCZ696 was tested in HFpEF patients in the Prospective Comparison of ARNI with ARB on Management of Heart Failure with Preserved Ejection Fraction (PARAMOUNT) trial, a phase II clinical trial.[42] In this trial, 301 patients with LVEF ≥45%, NYHA class II to III, and NT-proBNP >400 ng/mL were randomized to LCZ696 or valsartan. The primary outcome: NT-proBNP was significantly reduced at 12 weeks in the LCZ696 group compared with the valsartan group. Moreover, a significant improvement was seen in NYHA class and a decrease in echocardiographic parameters such as left atrial width and volume index with LCZ696 at 36 weeks compared with valsartan. However, LVEF, volume, or Doppler parameters of diastolic function did not improve with LCZ696. Given the overall encouraging results, the PARAGON (Prospective Comparison of ARNI with ARB Global Outcomes in HF with Preserved Ejection Fraction) phase III trial has begun. It is intended to enroll 4300 patients with LVEF >45% and will evaluate the effects of LCZ696 on morbidity and mortality endpoints in HFpEF.

BETA BLOCKERS IN HEART FAILURE

As the deleterious effects of chronic overactivation of the SNS in the pathophysiology have been better understood, beta blockers, which were once considered contraindicated in patients with HF, were studied in patients with HF. Activation of the SNS can stimulate renin production and this activation of the RAAS with its associated deleterious effects. Beta blockers act by counteracting the beta-receptor down regulation, altered intracellular coupling of the beta receptors with signaling pathways, as well as downstream inhibition of RAAS and inflammatory cytokines and endothelin (Figure 28-12).[43] Excess catecholamines increase the heart rate and can cause coronary vasoconstriction leading to a reduction in myocardial blood flow; they also lead to a decrease in myocardial contractility at the cellular level, and increase the likelihood of sudden death due to ventricular arrhythmias. Furthermore, catecholamines can also stimulate growth and provoke oxidative stress in cardiac-muscle cells, finally resulting in programmed cell death or apoptosis.

BETA BLOCKERS IN HEART FAILURE WITH REDUCED EJECTION FRACTION

On the basis of several landmark trials, beta blockers now constitute 1 of the most important drug classes of therapy for patients with HFrEF, along with ACE inhibitors, regardless of etiology. Long-term beta-adrenergic blockade halts the progression of cardiac pump dysfunction, improves LV function, and reduces morbidity and mortality rates in patients with HF ranging from asymptomatic LV systolic dysfunction to moderate to severe HF. Unlike ACE inhibitors, which demonstrate a class effect in HF therapy, beta blockers vary in their efficacy in treatment of patients with HF. To date, favorable outcomes in patients with HFrEF have been definitively demonstrated with carvedilol, bisoprolol, and sustained-release metoprolol (succinate).[44-46] Bisoprolol and sustained-release metoprolol (succinate) selectively block beta-1 receptors and carvedilol blocks alpha-1, beta-1, and beta-2 receptors. Overall, beta blocker therapy reduced the rate of hospital admissions and reduced mortality by 34%, when it was added to an ACE inhibitor, diuretic, and digoxin among patients with HFrEF with NYHA class II, III, or IV symptoms.[47] The aforementioned beta blockers have a class I ACC/AHA recommendation in management of patients

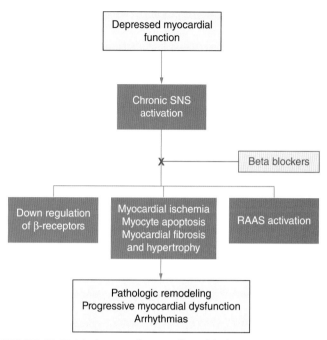

FIGURE 28-12 Mechanism of action of beta blockers in heart failure.

with HFrEF with NYHA class I through IV symptoms.[19] Beta blocker therapy can usually be safely continued in patients with an HF exacerbation; however, cessation of therapy may be necessary in patients with severely decompensated HF that may be resistant to therapy or with evidence of shock or preshock. In patients with HFrEF who are not already on beta blockers, the initiation of beta blockers should be deferred until they are relatively euvolemic.

BETA BLOCKERS IN HEART FAILURE WITH PRESERVED EJECTION FRACTION

Contrary to the established benefit of beta blockers in patients with HFrEF, there is no convincing evidence to support beta blocker use in treatment of patients with HFpEF with a primary goal to reduce mortality and morbidity.[48,49] Beta blockers may be used for the treatment, as indicated, of comorbidities in HFpEF such as atrial fibrillation, angina, post-MI, and HTN.

INCREMENTAL EFFECT OF NEUROHORMONAL THERAPIES IN HEART FAILURE

The proven efficacy and safety of ACE inhibitors, ARBs, beta blockers, and aldosterone antagonists have solidified their role at the forefront of HFrEF therapy. The relative clinical value of each therapy, independent of other therapies, is often questioned. Based on landmark trials, the incremental value of each added guideline-directed therapeutic class of medications on mortality in HFrEF patients can be summarized as shown in Figure 28-13. Although several classes of neurohormonal blockers have demonstrated mortality and morbidity reduction in patients with HFrEF, none of these drug classes has thus far demonstrated definitive benefit on outcomes in patients with HFpEF.

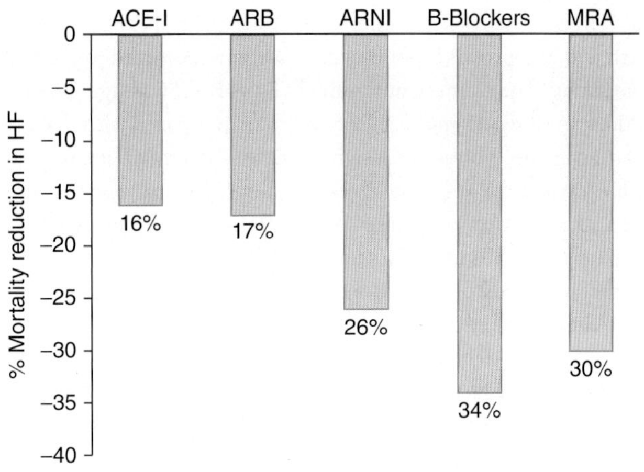

FIGURE 28-13 Summarized mortality reduction with neurohormonal blockers in patients with HFrEF. The mortality reduction is that of the active drug class vs placebo.[8,20,24,26,44-46,50] Abbreviations: ACE-I, angiotensin converting enzyme inhibitor; ARB, angiotensin receptor blocker; ARNI, angiotensin receptor-neprilysin inhibitor; B-Blockers, beta blockers; HF, heart failure; MRA, mineralocorticoid receptor antagonist.

KEY POINTS

ANGIOTENSIN-CONVERTING ENZYME INHIBITORS IN HEART FAILURE

- ACE inhibitors are RAAS blockers that block the conversion of angiotensin I to angiotensin II by inhibition of the ACE.

- ACE inhibitors have shown beneficial effects on mortality and HF hospitalization in patients with symptomatic HFrEF, as well as by reducing the progression to symptomatic HF in patients with asymptomatic LV systolic dysfunction.

- ACE inhibitors are recommended along the entire spectrum of HFrEF from NYHA class I to NYHA class IV.

- The benefit of ACE inhibition is accepted as a class effect across different ACE inhibitors.

- There is no definitive evidence that ACE inhibitor therapy improves clinical outcomes in patients with HFpEF.

ANGIOTENSIN RECEPTOR BLOCKERS IN HEART FAILURE

- ARBs exert their effect through blockade of the angiotensin II type I (AT-1) receptor.
- ARBs are now accepted as having equivalent benefit on mortality and morbidity in HFrEF as compared with ACE inhibitors.
- ARBs are often used in place of ACE inhibitors when patients are intolerant of ACE inhibitors due to cough or angioedema.
- Combined use of ACE inhibitors, aldosterone antagonists, and ARBs is not indicated routinely in patients with HFrEF.
- Data do not support the routine use of ARBs in patients with HFpEF to improve mortality or morbidity.

ALDOSTERONE ANTAGONISTS

- Aldosterone activation in HF promotes sodium and fluid retention, and increases myocardial and vascular fibrosis.
- Aldosterone receptor antagonists are indicated for mortality and morbidity reduction in HFrEF patients with symptomatic HF NYHA class II through IV or in post-MI patients with depressed LVEF and HF, often on a background of ACE inhibitors, beta blockers, and diuretic therapy.
- Because of the risk of hyperkalemia, potassium levels need close monitoring, especially in the initial phase after starting aldosterone antagonists or increasing the dose. Aldosterone antagonists are contraindicated in patients with Cr >2.5 mg/dL (or creatinine clearance <3 mL/min), or serum potassium >5.0 mmol/L.
- ~10% of patients experience gynecomastia with spironolactone use, a side effect not seen with eplerenone.
- Although not definitive, aldosterone inhibitors may provide benefit on reduction of CV events in higher-risk HFpEF patients.

COMBINED ANGIOTENSIN RECEPTOR-NEPRILYSIN INHIBITORS

- ARNIs inhibit angiotensin II type I (AT-1) receptors and augment active natriuretic peptides by inhibiting breakdown of neprilysin.
- ARNIs have recently been proven to have additional morbidity and mortality benefit as compared with ACE inhibitors in symptomatic patients (NYHA class II-IV) with HFrEF who are already on beta blockers and ACE inhibitors/ARBs.
- ARNIs should not be used simultaneously with ACE inhibitors or ARBs. In patients on ACE inhibitors, a minimum washout period of 36 hours from the time of stopping ACE inhibitors to the first dose of ARNI is recommended.
- ARNIs have also shown promising results on biomarkers in patients with HFpEF; larger clinical outcome trials are currently in progress.

BETA BLOCKER THERAPY IN HEART FAILURE

- Beta blockers counteract the beta-receptor down regulation, altered intracellular coupling of the beta receptors with signaling pathways, as well as the downstream activation of the RAAS, and inflammatory cytokines and endothelin that occurs in HF.
- Beta blockers vary in their efficacy in treatment of patients with HF and favorable outcomes in patients with HFrEF have been definitively demonstrated with carvedilol, bisoprolol, and sustained-release metoprolol (succinate).
- Beta blockers reduce morbidity and mortality in HFrEF, and cause an improvement in LVEF, and are recommended for all HFrEF patients with NYHA class I through IV symptoms of nonischemic and ischemic etiology.
- Beta blockers can generally be continued in patients admitted with exacerbation of HFrEF.
- There is no convincing evidence to support beta blocker use to decrease morbidity or mortality in patients with HFpEF.

REFERENCES

1. Triposkiadis F, Karayannis G, Giamouzis G, et al. The sympathetic nervous system in heart failure physiology, pathophysiology, and clinical implications. *J Am Coll Cardiol.* 2009;54:1747-1762.
2. Jessup M, Brozena S. Heart failure. *N Engl J Med.* 2003;348:2007-2018.
3. Brown NJ, Vaughan DE. Angiotensin-converting enzyme inhibitors. *Circulation.* 1998;97:1411-1420.
4. Garg R, Yusuf S. Overview of randomized trials of angiotensin-converting enzyme inhibitors on mortality and morbidity in patients with heart failure. *JAMA.* 1995;273:1450-1456.
5. Narang R, Swedberg K, Cleland JG. What is the ideal study design for evaluation of treatment for heart failure? Insights from trials assessing the effect of ACE inhibitors on exercise capacity. *Eur Heart J.* 1996;17:120-134.
6. Wang TJ, Evans JC, Benjamin EJ, et al. Natural history of asymptomatic left ventricular systolic dysfunction in the community. *Circulation.* 2003;108:977-982.
7. The SOLVD Investigators. Effect of enalapril on mortality and the development of heart failure in asymptomatic patients with reduced left ventricular ejection fractions. *N Engl J Med.* 1992;327:685-691.
8. The SOLVD Investigators. Effect of enalapril on survival in patients with reduced left ventricular ejection fractions and congestive heart failure. *N Engl J Med.* 1991;325:293-302.
9. CONSENSUS Trial Study Group. Effects of enalapril on mortality in severe congestive heart failure: results of the Cooperative North Scandinavian Enalapril Survival Study (CONSENSUS). *N Engl J Med.* 1987;316:1429-1435.
10. Cleland JGF, Tendera M, Adamus J, et al. The perindopril in elderly people with chronic heart failure (PEP-CHF) study. *Eur Heart J.* 2006;27:2338-2345.
11. Packer M, Poole-Wilson PA, Armstrong PW, et al. Comparative effects of low and high doses of the angiotensin-converting

enzyme inhibitor, lisinopril, on morbidity and mortality in chronic heart failure. ATLAS Study Group. *Circulation.* 1999;100:2312-2318.

12. Burnier M, Brunner HR. Angiotensin II receptor antagonists. *Lancet.* 2000;355:637-645.

13. Jorde UP, Ennezat PV, Lisker J, et al. Maximally recommended doses of angiotensin-converting enzyme (ACE) inhibitors do not completely prevent ACE-mediated formation of angiotensin II in chronic heart failure. *Circulation.* 2000;101:844-846.

14. Pitt B, Segal R, Martinez FA, et al. Randomized trial of losartan versus captopril in patients over 65 with heart failure (evaluation of losartan in the elderly study, ELITE). *Lancet.* 1997;349:747-752.

15. Dickstein K, Kjekshus J. Effects of losartan and captopril on mortality and morbidity in high-risk patients after acute myocardial infarction: the OPTIMAAL randomised trial. Optimal Trial in Myocardial Infarction with Angiotensin II Antagonist Losartan. *Lancet.* 2002;360:752-760.

16. Pfeffer MA, McMurray JJ, Velazquez EJ, et al. Valsartan, captopril, or both in myocardial infarction complicated by heart failure, left ventricular dysfunction, or both. *N Engl J Med.* 2003;349:1893-1906.

17. Cohn JN, Tognoni G. A randomized trial of the angiotensin-receptor blocker valsartan in chronic heart failure. *N Engl J Med.* 2001;345:1667-1675.

18. McMurray JJ, Ostergren J, Swedberg K, et al. Effects of candesartan in patients with chronic heart failure and reduced left-ventricular systolic function taking angiotensin-converting-enzyme inhibitors: the CHARM-Added trial. *Lancet.* 2003;362:767-771.

19. Yancy CW, Jessup M, Bozkurt B, et al. 2013 ACCF/AHA guideline for the management of heart failure: a report of the American College of Cardiology Foundation/American Heart Association Task Force on practice guidelines. *Circulation.* 2013;128:e240-e327.

20. Granger CB, McMurray JJ, Yusuf S, et al. Effects of candesartan in patients with chronic heart failure and reduced left-ventricular systolic function intolerant to angiotensin-converting-enzyme inhibitors: the CHARM-Alternative trial. *Lancet.* 2003;362:772-776.

21. Yusuf S, Pfeffer MA, Swedberg K, et al. Effects of candesartan in patients with chronic heart failure and preserved left-ventricular ejection fraction: the CHARM-Preserved Trial. *Lancet.* 2003;362:777-781.

22. Massie BM, Carson PE, McMurray JJ, et al. Irbesartan in patients with heart failure and preserved ejection fraction. *N Engl J Med.* 2008;359:2456-2467.

23. Struthers AD. Aldosterone escape during angiotensin-converting enzyme inhibitor therapy in chronic heart failure. *J Card Fail.* 1996;2:47-54.

24. Pitt B, Zannad F, Remme WJ, et al. The effect of spironolactone on morbidity and mortality in patients with severe heart failure. Randomized Aldactone Evaluation Study Investigators. *N Engl J Med.* 1999;341:709-717.

25. Pitt B, Remme W, Zannad F, et al. Eplerenone, a selective aldosterone blocker, in patients with left ventricular dysfunction after myocardial infarction. *N Engl J Med.* 2003;348:1309-1321.

26. Zannad F, McMurray JJ, Krum H, et al. Eplerenone in patients with systolic heart failure and mild symptoms. *N Engl J Med.* 2011;364:11-21.

27. Pitt B, Pfeffer MA, Assmann SF, et al. Spironolactone for heart failure with preserved ejection fraction. *N Engl J Med.* 2014;370:1383-1392.

28. Pfeffer MA, Claggett B, Assmann SF, et al. Regional variation in patients and outcomes in the Treatment of Preserved Cardiac Function Heart Failure With an Aldosterone Antagonist (TOPCAT) trial. *Circulation.* 2015;131:34-42.

29. Moe GW, Ezekowitz JA, O'Meara E, et al. The 2014 Canadian Cardiovascular Society Heart Failure Management Guidelines Focus Update: anemia, biomarkers, and recent therapeutic trial implications. *Can J Cardiol.* 2015;31:3-16.

30. Schroten NF, Gaillard CA, van Veldhuisen DJ, et al. New roles for renin and prorenin in heart failure and cardiorenal crosstalk. *Heart Fail Rev.* 2012;17:191-201.

31. Nguyen G. Renin and prorenin receptor in hypertension: what's new? *Curr Hypertens Rep.* 2011;13:79-85.

32. McMurray JJ, Pitt B, Latini R, et al. Effects of the oral direct renin inhibitor aliskiren in patients with symptomatic heart failure. *Circ Heart Fail.* 2008;1:17-24.

33. Solomon SD, Shin SH, Shah A, et al. Effect of the direct renin inhibitor aliskiren on left ventricular remodelling following myocardial infarction with systolic dysfunction. *Eur Heart J.* 2011;32:1227-1234.

34. McMurray JJ, Krum H, Abraham WT, et al. Aliskiren, enalapril, or aliskiren and enalapril in heart failure. *N Engl J Med.* 2016;374:1521-1532.

35. Mangiafico S, Costello-Boerrigter LC, Andersen IA, et al. Neutral endopeptidase inhibition and the natriuretic peptide system: an evolving strategy in cardiovascular therapeutics. *Eur Heart J.* 2013;34:886-893c.

36. Packer M, Califf RM, Konstam MA, et al. Comparison of omapatrilat and enalapril in patients with chronic heart failure: the Omapatrilat Versus Enalapril Randomized Trial of Utility in Reducing Events (OVERTURE). *Circulation.* 2002;106:920-926.

37. Kostis JB, Packer M, Black HR, et al. Omapatrilat and enalapril in patients with hypertension: the Omapatrilat Cardiovascular Treatment vs. Enalapril (OCTAVE) trial. *Am J Hypertens.* 2004;17:103-111.

38. Rouleau JL, Pfeffer MA, Stewart DJ, et al. Comparison of vasopeptidase inhibitor, omapatrilat, and lisinopril on exercise tolerance and morbidity in patients with heart failure: IMPRESS randomised trial [see comments]. *Lancet.* 2000;356:615-620.

39. Ruilope LM, Dukat A, Bohm M, et al. Blood-pressure reduction with LCZ696, a novel dual-acting inhibitor of the angiotensin II receptor and neprilysin: a randomised, double-blind, placebo-controlled, active comparator study. *Lancet.* 2010;375:1255-1266.

40. McMurray JJ, Packer M, Desai AS, et al. Angiotensin-neprilysin inhibition versus enalapril in heart failure. *N Engl J Med.* 2014;371:993-1004.

41. Packer M, McMurray JJ, Desai AS, et al. Angiotensin receptor neprilysin inhibition compared with enalapril on the risk of clinical progression in surviving patients with heart failure. *Circulation.* 2015;131:54-61.

42. Solomon SD, Zile M, Pieske B, et al. The angiotensin receptor neprilysin inhibitor LCZ696 in heart failure with preserved ejection fraction: a phase 2 double-blind randomised controlled trial. *Lancet.* 2012;380:1387-1395.

43. Frishman WH. Carvedilol. *N Engl J Med.* 1998;339:1759-1765.

44. CIBIS-II Investigators and Committee. The cardiac insufficiency Bisoprolol Study II (CIBIS-II): a randomised trial. *Lancet.* 1999;353:9-13.

45. Packer M, Coats AJ, Fowler MB, et al. Effect of carvedilol on survival in severe chronic heart failure. *N Engl J Med.* 2001;344:1651-1658.

46. MERIT-HF Study Group. Effect of metoprolol CR/XL in chronic heart failure: Metoprolol CR/XL Randomised Intervention Trial in Congestive Heart Failure (MERIT-HF). *Lancet.* 1999;353:2001-2007.

47. McMurray JJ. Clinical practice. Systolic heart failure. *N Engl J Med.* 2010;362:228-238.

48. Bergstrom A, Andersson B, Edner M, Nylander E, Persson H, Dahlstrom U. Effect of carvedilol on diastolic function in patients with diastolic heart failure and preserved systolic function. Results of the Swedish Doppler-echocardiographic study (SWEDIC). *Eur J Heart Fail.* 2004;6:453-461.

49. Flather MD, Shibata MC, Coats AJ, et al. Randomized trial to determine the effect of nebivolol on mortality and cardiovascular hospital admission in elderly patients with heart failure (SENIORS). *Eur Heart J.* 2005;26:215-225.

50. McMurray J, Packer M, Desai A, et al. A putative placebo analysis of the effects of LCZ696 on clinical outcomes in heart failure. *Eur Heart J.* 2015;36:434-439.

29 AUTONOMIC MODULATION IN HEART FAILURE

Mark J. Shen, MD
Douglas P. Zipes, MD

PATIENT CASE

Mr. K is a 63-year-old Caucasian man with history of coronary artery disease (CAD) with previous coronary interventions of stent implantations in the left anterior descending and circumflex coronary arteries. His most recent left ventricular ejection fraction (LVEF) is 30%. He has an automatic implantable cardioverter defibrillator (AICD) for primary prevention of sudden cardiac death. He has been receiving optimally uptitrated guideline-directed medical therapy (GDMT) for his heart failure (HF) including carvedilol 25 mg twice daily, lisinopril 20 mg daily, and spironolactone 25 mg daily for more than 12 months. His other medications include aspirin 81 mg daily, atorvastatin 40 mg daily, furosemide 40 mg daily, and potassium chloride 40 mEq daily. He denies angina but reports dyspnea while walking less than 2 blocks, which is stable compared to last year. He denies any resting dyspnea or orthopnea. He has had no hospitalizations for HF exacerbation over the past 12 months. He denies any angina. He has been compliant with his medications and adherent to a low-salt diet. On exam, he appears well-nourished and in no acute distress. His heart rate is 65 bpm and regular. Respirations are 16/minute. Blood pressure is 108/65. His cardiac examination reveals a regular rate and rhythm, and a sustained, laterally displaced apical impulse. There were no extra heart sounds or murmurs. His extremities were warm with no edema. His jugular venous pressure appears to be within normal limits and lungs were clear. His electrocardiogram shows sinus rhythm with a narrow QRS complex. Laboratory tests showed both liver and kidney function to be normal. His echocardiography showed LVEF of 30% and LV end-diastolic diameter of 65 mm.

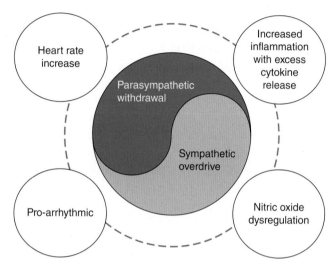

FIGURE 29-1 Autonomic dysfunction in heart failure. An imbalance of a naturally Yin and Yang control of the heart characterized by sympathetic overdrive and parasympathetic withdrawal. The detrimental consequences include, but are not limited to, increase in heart rate, arrhythmogenesis, nitric oxide dysregulation, and proinflammatory state. (From http://www.biocontrol-medical.com.)

MANAGEMENT

PHARMACOLOGICAL

HF, a disease with high mortality and increasing prevalence,[1] is characterized by autonomic imbalance, including decreased parasympathetic tone,[2,3] hyperactive sympathetic tone,[4,5] and impaired baroreflex control of sympathetic activity (Figure 29-1).[6,7] Thus far, the drugs shown to improve survival in systolic HF—beta blockers, angiotensin-converting enzyme (ACE) inhibitors, angiotensin II receptor blockers (ARBs), aldosterone receptor antagonists, and the newest class approved angiotensin receptor-neprilysin inhibitors (ARNIs)—all possess sympatholytic effects and thus help restore autonomic imbalance in patients with systolic HF. For Mr. K, he has already been receiving GDMT and the dosages of his medications are optimally titrated. He is euvolemic on exam ination but still has baseline New York Heart Association (NYHA) class III symptoms.

NONPHARMACOLOGICAL

Although not FDA-approved, several approaches of autonomic modulation at trial level either by implanted devices or interventions have sought to restore the autonomic balance in HF and improve outcomes.[8,9] These measures include spinal cord stimulation, vagus nerve stimulation, baroreceptor activation therapy, and renal sympathetic nerve denervation (Figure 29-2).

Spinal Cord Stimulation

Spinal cord stimulation (SCS) involves the subcutaneous placement of an epidural stimulation lead with distal poles at the level of T_2 to

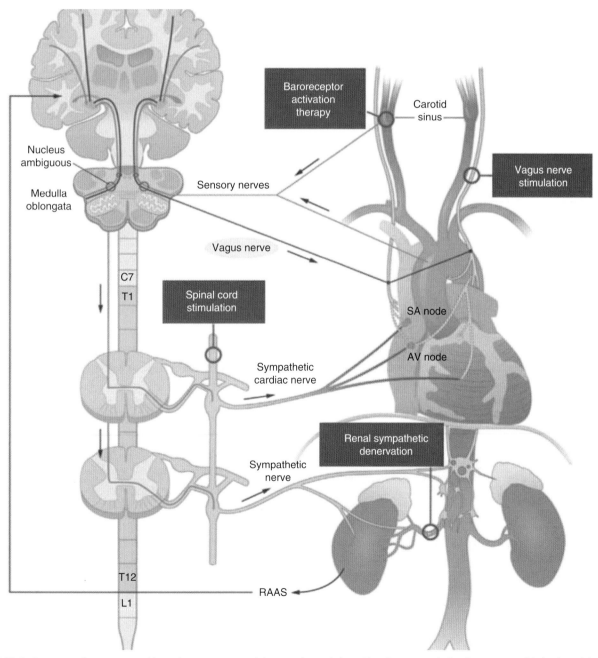

FIGURE 29-2 Overview of interventional-based autonomic modulation in heart failure. This diagram includes the more established modalities of autonomic modulation for heart failure—spinal cord stimulation, vagus nerve stimulation, baroreceptor activation therapy, and renal sympathetic denervation. Abbreviations: AV, atrioventricular; RAAS, renin-angiotensin-aldosterone system; SA, sinoatrial. (Reproduced with permission from Chatterjee NA, Singh JP. Novel interventional therapies to modulate the autonomic tone in heart failure. *JACC Heart Fail.* 2015 Oct;3(10):786-802.)

T$_4$, which is connected to an implanted pulse generator in the paraspinal lumbar region (Figure 29-3). Different stimulation parameters have been used in different trials but it is generally applied at 90% of the motor threshold at a frequency of 50 Hz and a pulse width of 200 ms. SCS is typically applied intermittently with a few hours on and the rest being turned off. Animal studies have demonstrated that SCS works primarily via augmenting vagally mediated effects.[10] SCS was also shown to counteract the heightened sympathetic response during ischemia.[11] An elegant canine study[12] by Lopshire et al showed that SCS was significantly better than optimal medical therapy (carvedilol + ramipril) in improvement of LVEF, reduction of ventricular tachyarrhythmias, and decline in serum norepinephrine and brain natriuretic peptide levels in dogs with rapid pacing-induced HF. A number of clinical trials have taken place to assess the efficacy and safety of SCS in systolic HF patients and report conflicting results. Smaller prospective trials[13,14] have yielded relatively positive results—SCS is safe, feasible, and potentially can improve symptoms, functional status, and LV function in patients with severe, symptomatic systolic HF. However, the largest DEFEAT-HF trial[15]—a multicenter, prospective, randomized (3:2 fashion) control trial enrolling 66 patients with LVEF ≤35%, NYHA class III HF symptoms while on optimal medical therapy, narrow QRS duration and a dilated LV failed to meet the primary endpoint. SCS did not significantly reduce the LV end-systolic volume index. Therefore, DEFEAT-HF does not provide evidence to support a meaningful change in clinical outcomes for HF patients receiving SCS.[16]

Vagus Nerve Stimulation

Vagus nerve stimulation (VNS) utilizes a cuff electrode that is secured around the vagus about 3 cm below the carotid artery bifurcation. A brief stimulation that reduces heart rate by 10% is performed to ensure the correct positioning. The stimulation lead is then tunneled under the skin and over the clavicle to join the intracardiac sensing electrode (placed in the right ventricle, to prevent excessive bradycardia) and the pulse generator in the subcutaneous pocket in the right subclavicular region (Figure 29-4). The stimulation parameter then follows an up-titration protocol to achieve heart rate reduction of 5 to 10 bpm without eliciting adverse reactions.[17,18] Preclinical animal studies have shown that chronic VNS improved LV hemodynamics[19,20] and, more importantly, improved survival in HF.[21] A myriad of mechanisms have been postulated to explain the beneficial effects of VNS—direct inhibition of cardiac sympathetic activities,[22] reduction of the slope of action potential duration restitution curve (and thereby increasing the threshold of ventricular fibrillation),[24] increase in the expression of connexin-43,[19] prevention of mitochondrial dysfunction during ischemia-reperfusion,[25] and also attenuation of systemic inflammation,[20,23] which, theoretically, may be beneficial in preventing coronary artery disease, the leading cause of HF.[26] Two recently published clinical trials have conflicting results. NECTAR-HF failed to demonstrate an improvement in LV end-systolic diameter, the primary endpoint, in 6 months' time.[27] In contrast, Anthem-HF showed that VNS was able to significantly improve LVEF and reduce LV end-systolic diameter in 6 months' time.[28] The same beneficial effects held true in 12 months' extended follow-up.[29] Another much larger trial, INOVATE-HF, with enrollment of 707 patients with similar

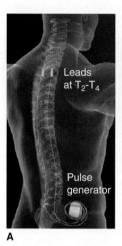
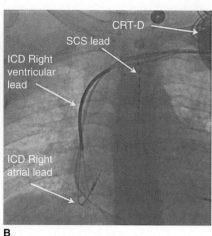

FIGURE 29-3 Spinal cord stimulation (SCS). A. Schematic representation of SCS system. B. X-ray image showing the placement of the SCS lead with concurrent cardiac resynchronization therapy-defibrillator (CRT-D) device and leads. (Reproduced with permission from Torre-Amione G, Alo K, Estep JD, et al. Spinal cord stimulation is safe and feasible in patients with advanced heart failure: early clinical experience. Eur J Heart Fail. 2014;16(7):788-795.)

baseline parameters (LVEF ≤40%, NYHA class III symptoms, and a dilated LV) showed somewhat disappointing results: VNS did not reduce death and HF events. However, the same study did demonstrate a favorable result in terms of quality of life, improvement in NYHA class and exercise capacity associated with VNS treatment.[30,31] The results of this trial will be revealed soon (in 2016 according to its website) and may determine whether VNS is really beneficial in HF.

Baroreceptor Activation Therapy

The implantation of a baroreceptor stimulator entails surgically exposing both carotid sinuses and placing electrodes around the carotid adventitial surface bilaterally. The leads are subcutaneously tunneled and connected to an implantable stimulation device placed in the subclavian subcutaneous position on the anterior chest wall. The newer generation baroreceptor stimulator (Barostim neo, CVRx Inc, Minneapolis, MN, United States) has 1 carotid sinus electrode with smaller size (Figure 29-5). Compared to the previous system, it delivers less power and thus allows easier implant and fewer adverse effects. Its efficacy has been tested in animal models. Chronic baroreceptor activation therapy (BAT) significantly increased LV systolic function and reduced plasma norepinephrine in dogs with ischemic HF.[32] In another study using the canine model of pacing-induced HF, chronic BAT reduced LV filling pressure, decreased plasma norepinephrine, and doubled survival duration.[33] In human patients with LVEF ≤40% and NYHA class III HF symptoms while on optimal medical therapy, BAT was associated with significant improvement in baroreflex sensitivity, LVEF, NYHA class, quality of life, and 6-minute walk test (6MWT), along with significant decrease in muscle sympathetic activity.[34] Barostim HOPE4HF, a recently published, multicenter, randomized control trial that enrolled 146 patients with LVEF ≤40% and NYHA class III HF symptoms while on optimal medical therapy, showed chronic BAT was safe and improved functional status, quality of life, exercise capacity, and N-terminal pro-brain natriuretic peptide (NT-proBNP).[35] BAT was

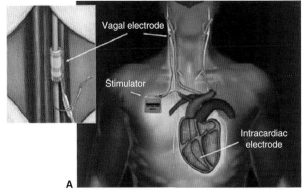

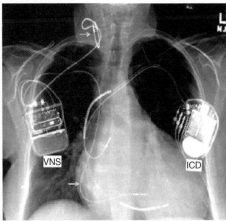

FIGURE 29-4 Vagus nerve stimulation (VNS). A. Schematic representation of VNS system. (From Schwartz PJ, De Ferrari GM, Sanzo A, et al. Long term vagal stimulation in patients with advanced heart failure: first experience in man. *Eur J Heart Fail.* 2008;10(9):884-891; with permission.) B. X-ray image showing the placement of the VNS stimulator with a previously implanted automatic implantable cardioverter defibrillator (AICD). (Reproduced with permission from Singh JP, Kandala J, Camm AJ. Non-pharmacological modulation of the autonomic tone to treat heart failure. *Eur Heart J.* 2014;35(2):77-85.)

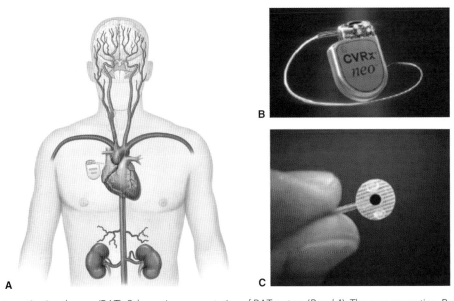

FIGURE 29-5 Baroreceptor activation therapy (BAT). Schematic representation of BAT system (*Panel A*). The new generation, Barostim neo, is shown here with 1 carotid sinus nerve stimulator (*Panel B*) that carries 1 electrode connected to the patch electrode (*Panel C*) that will be fixed to the carotid sinus nerve. (Reproduced with permission from Kuck KH, Bordachar P, Borggrefe M, et al. New devices in heart failure: an European Heart Rhythm Association report: developed by the European Heart Rhythm Association; endorsed by the Heart Failure Association. *Europace.* 2014;16(1):109-128.)

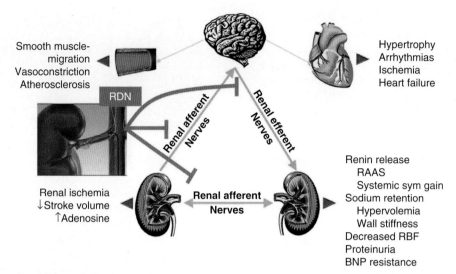

Smooth muscle-
migration
Vasoconstriction
Atherosclerosis

RDN

Renal afferent Nerves

Renal efferent Nerves

Hypertrophy
Arrhythmias
Ischemia
Heart failure

Renal ischemia
↓Stroke volume
↑Adenosine

Renal afferent
Nerves

Renin release
RAAS
Systemic sym gain
Sodium retention
Hypervolemia
Wall stiffness
Decreased RBF
Proteinuria
BNP resistance

FIGURE 29-6 Renal sympathetic nerve denervation (RSDN). Physiological and pathophysiological actions of renal sympathetic afferent and efferent nerves can be blocked by RSDN. Abbreviations: BNP, brain natriuretic peptide; RAAS, renin-angiotensin-aldosterone system; RBF, renal blood flow; RDN, renal denervation. (Reproduced with permission from Krum H, Sobotka P, Mahfoud F, et al. Device-based antihypertensive therapy: therapeutic modulation of the autonomic nervous system. *Circulation.* 2011;123(2):209-215.)

associated with a trend toward reduced HF hospitalization, although it did not meet statistical significance (P = 0.08). A large ongoing randomized trial (BeAT-HF) plans to recruit 800 patients with LVEF ≤35%, NYHA class III HF symptoms and assesses the efficacy of BAT. The study is estimated to complete in 2021 and likely will determine whether BAT is truly beneficial in this group of patients.[36]

Renal Sympathetic Denervation

With a standard femoral artery access, a flexible endovascular electrode catheter connected to a generator is placed within the renal arteries to allow delivery of radiofrequency energy. A series of lesions along each renal artery then are delivered to disrupt the renal nerves located in the adventitia of the renal arteries. For safety reasons, each lesion should be at least 5 mm apart. By ablating the efferent nerves, renal sympathetic denervation (RSDN) decreases the renal norepinephrine spillover by 47%[37] and attenuates the activity of the renin-angiotensin-aldosterone system (RAAS),[38] both important in the pathogenesis of LV remodeling in HF. Afferent RSDN decreases feedback activation to the central nervous system and thereby decreases sympathetic input to the heart (Figure 29-6). In a murine model of ischemic HF, RSDN is associated with reduced LV filling pressure and improved LVEF after 4 weeks of follow-up.[39] In patients with resistant hypertension (HTN), RSDN reduced LV mass and LV filling pressure, shortened isovolumic relaxation time, and increased LVEF.[40] The REACH-Pilot trial enrolled 7 patients with chronic systolic HF and normal blood pressure.[41] Although limited in size, the pilot study showed that there was a trend toward an improvement in symptoms and exercise capacity. Several larger trials[42-46] are ongoing to test whether RSDN is beneficial in patients with HF.

FOLLOW-UP TO INTRODUCTORY PATIENT CASE

Mr. K has systolic HF with LVEF of 30%, and NYHA class III symptoms while on optimal medical therapy. Since FDA approved sacubitril/valsartan (Entresto) in July 2015, his lisinopril was replaced by

Entresto, which compared to ACE inhibitors, reduces risks of death, HF hospitalization, and functional status assessed by Kansas City Cardiomyopathy Questionnaire.[47,48] The dosage of Entresto has been gradually uptitrated to current dose of 97 mg/103 mg twice daily. He felt somewhat improved but still has class III symptoms. It was decided for him to be enrolled in the BeAT-HF trial as he had met all the inclusion criteria of the trial. He is to be followed in our cardiology clinic for re-evaluation of his symptoms and LV function.

REFERENCES

1. Yancy CW, Jessup M, Bozkurt B, et al. 2013 ACCF/AHA guideline for the management of heart failure: executive summary: a report of the American College of Cardiology Foundation/American Heart Association Task Force on practice guidelines. *Circulation.* 2013;128:1810-1852.

2. Newton GE, Parker AB, Landzberg JS, Colucci WS, Parker JD. Muscarinic receptor modulation of basal and beta-adrenergic stimulated function of the failing human left ventricle. *J Clin Invest.* 1996;98:2756-2763.

3. Porter TR, Eckberg DL, Fritsch JM, et al. Autonomic pathophysiology in heart failure patients. Sympathetic-cholinergic interrelations. *J Clin Invest.* 1990;85:1362-1371.

4. Cohn JN, Levine TB, Olivari MT, et al. Plasma norepinephrine as a guide to prognosis in patients with chronic congestive heart failure. *N Engl J Med.* 1984;311:819-823.

5. Hasking GJ, Esler MD, Jennings GL, Burton D, Johns JA, Korner PI. Norepinephrine spillover to plasma in patients with congestive heart failure: evidence of increased overall and cardiorenal sympathetic nervous activity. *Circulation.* 1986;73:615-621.

6. Grassi G, Seravalle G, Cattaneo BM, et al. Sympathetic activation and loss of reflex sympathetic control in mild congestive heart failure. *Circulation.* 1995;92:3206-3211.

7. Ferguson DW, Abboud FM, Mark AL. Selective impairment of baroreflex-mediated vasoconstrictor responses in patients with ventricular dysfunction. *Circulation.* 1984;69:451-460.

8. Shen MJ, Zipes DP. Interventional and device-based autonomic modulation in heart failure. *Heart Fail Clin.* 2015;11:337-348.

9. Chatterjee NA, Singh JP. Novel interventional therapies to modulate the autonomic tone in heart failure. *JACC Heart Fail.* 2015;3:786-802.

10. Olgin JE, Takahashi T, Wilson E, Vereckei A, Steinberg H, Zipes DP. Effects of thoracic spinal cord stimulation on cardiac autonomic regulation of the sinus and atrioventricular nodes. *J Cardiovasc Electrophysiol.* 2002;13:475-481.

11. Garlie JB, Zhou X, Shen MJ, et al. The increased ambulatory nerve activity and ventricular tachycardia in canine post-infarction heart failure is attenuated by spinal cord stimulation (abstract). *Heart Rhythm.* 2012:PO3-P112.

12. Lopshire JC, Zhou X, Dusa C, et al. Spinal cord stimulation improves ventricular function and reduces ventricular

13. Torre-Amione G, Alo K, Estep JD, et al. Spinal cord stimulation is safe and feasible in patients with advanced heart failure: early clinical experience. *Eur J Heart Fail.* 2014;16:788-795.

14. Tse HF, Turner S, Sanders P, et al. Thoracic Spinal Cord Stimulation for Heart Failure as a Restorative Treatment (SCS HEART study): first-in-man experience. *Heart Rhythm.* 2015;12:588-595.

15. Determining the Feasibility of Spinal Cord Neuromodulation for the Treatment of Chronic Heart Failure (DEFEAT-HF) website. http://clinicaltrials.gov/ct2/show/NCT01112579? term=NCT01112579&rank=1. Accessed August 31, 2014.

16. Zipes DP, Neuzil P, Theres H, et al. Determining the Feasibility of Spinal Cord Neuromodulation for the Treatment of Chronic Systolic Heart Failure: the DEFEAT-HF study. *JACC Heart Fail.* 2016;4:129-136.

17. Schwartz PJ, De Ferrari GM, Sanzo A, et al. Long term vagal stimulation in patients with advanced heart failure: first experience in man. *Eur J Heart Fail.* 2008;10:884-891.

18. De Ferrari GM, Crijns HJ, Borggrefe M, et al. Chronic vagus nerve stimulation: a new and promising therapeutic approach for chronic heart failure. *Eur Heart J.* 2010;32:847-855.

19. Sabbah HN, Ilsar I, Zaretsky A, Rastogi S, Wang M, Gupta RC. Vagus nerve stimulation in experimental heart failure. *Heart Fail Rev.* 2011;16:171-178.

20. Zhang Y, Popovic ZB, Bibevski S, et al. Chronic vagus nerve stimulation improves autonomic control and attenuates systemic inflammation and heart failure progression in a canine high-rate pacing model. *Circ Heart Fail.* 2009;2:692-699.

21. Li M, Zheng C, Sato T, Kawada T, Sugimachi M, Sunagawa K. Vagal nerve stimulation markedly improves long-term survival after chronic heart failure in rats. *Circulation.* 2004;109:120-124.

22. Shen MJ, Shinohara T, Park HW, et al. Continuous low-level vagus nerve stimulation reduces stellate ganglion nerve activity and paroxysmal atrial tachyarrhythmias in ambulatory canines. *Circulation.* 2011;123:2204-2212.

23. Calvillo L, Vanoli E, Andreoli E, et al. Vagal stimulation, through its nicotinic action, limits infarct size and the inflammatory response to myocardial ischemia and reperfusion. *J Cardiovasc Pharmacol.* 2011;58:500-507.

24. Ng GA, Brack KE, Patel VH, Coote JH. Autonomic modulation of electrical restitution, alternans and ventricular fibrillation initiation in the isolated heart. *Cardiovasc Res.* 2007;73:750-760.

25. Shinlapawittayatorn K, Chinda K, Palee S, et al. Low-amplitude, left vagus nerve stimulation significantly attenuates ventricular dysfunction and infarct size through prevention of mitochondrial dysfunction during acute ischemia-reperfusion injury. *Heart Rhythm.* 2013;10(11):1700-1707.

arrhythmias in a canine postinfarction heart failure model. *Circulation.* 2009;120:286-294.

26. Ridker PM, Everett BM, Thuren T, MacFadyen JG, Chang WH, Ballantyne C, Fonseca F, Nicolau J, Koenig W, Anker SD, Kastelein JJP, Cornel JH, Pais P, Pella D, Genest J, Cifkova R, Lorenzatti A, Forster T, Kobalava Z, Vida-Simiti L, Flather M, Shimokawa H, Ogawa H, Dellborg M, Rossi PRF, Troquay RPT, Libby P, Glynn RJ. Antiinflammatory Therapy with Canakinumab for Atherosclerotic Disease. *N Engl J Med*. 2017 Sep 21;377(12):1119-1131.

27. Zannad F, De Ferrari GM, Tuinenburg AE, et al. Chronic vagal stimulation for the treatment of low ejection fraction heart failure: results of the neural cardiac therapy for heart failure (NECTAR-HF) randomized controlled trial. *Eur Heart J*. 2015;36(7):425-433.

28. Premchand RK, Sharma K, Mittal S, et al. Autonomic regulation therapy via left or right cervical vagus nerve stimulation in patients with chronic heart failure: results of the ANTHEM-HF Trial. *J Card Fail*. 2014;20(11):808-816.

29. Premchand RK, Sharma K, Mittal S, et al. Extended follow-up of patients with heart failure receiving autonomic regulation therapy in the ANTHEM-HF study. *J Card Fail*. 2016;22(8):639-642.

30. Hauptman PJ, Schwartz PJ, Gold MR, et al. Rationale and study design of the increase of vagal tone in heart failure study: INOVATE-HF. *Am Heart J*. 2012;163:954-962 e1.

31. Gold MR, Van Veldhuisen DJ, Hauptman PJ, Borggrefe M, Kubo SH, Lieberman RA, Milasinovic G, Berman BJ, Djordjevic S, Neelagaru S, Schwartz PJ, Starling RC, Mann DL. Vagus Nerve Stimulation for the Treatment of Heart Failure: The INOVATE-HF Trial. *J Am Coll Cardiol*. 2016 Jul 12;68(2):149-58.

32. Sabbah HN, Gupta RC, Imai M, et al. Chronic electrical stimulation of the carotid sinus baroreflex improves left ventricular function and promotes reversal of ventricular remodeling in dogs with advanced heart failure. *Circ Heart Fail*. 2011;4:65-70.

33. Zucker IH, Hackley JF, Cornish KG, et al. Chronic baroreceptor activation enhances survival in dogs with pacing-induced heart failure. *Hypertension*. 2007;50:904-910.

34. Gronda E, Seravalle G, Brambilla G, et al. Chronic baroreflex activation effects on sympathetic nerve traffic, baroreflex function, and cardiac haemodynamics in heart failure: a proof-of-concept study. *Eur J Heart Fail*. 2014;16(9):977-983.

35. Abraham WT, Zile MR, Weaver FA, et al. Baroreflex activation therapy for the treatment of heart failure with a reduced ejection fraction. *JACC Heart Fail*. 2015;3:487-496.

36. Barostim Therapy for Heart Failure (BeAT-HF) website. https://clinicaltrials.gov/ct2/show/NCT01392196?term=NCT01392196&rank=1. Accessed May 16, 2018.

37. Esler MD, Krum H, Sobotka PA, Schlaich MP, Schmieder RE, Bohm M. Renal sympathetic denervation in patients with treatment-resistant hypertension (The Symplicity HTN-2 Trial): a randomised controlled trial. *Lancet*. 2010;376:1903-1909.

38. Zhao Q, Yu S, Zou M, et al. Effect of renal sympathetic denervation on the inducibility of atrial fibrillation during rapid atrial pacing. *J Interv Card Electrophysiol*. 2012;35:119-125.

39. Nozawa T, Igawa A, Fujii N, et al. Effects of long-term renal sympathetic denervation on heart failure after myocardial infarction in rats. *Heart Vessels*. 2002;16:51-56.

40. Brandt MC, Mahfoud F, Reda S, et al. Renal sympathetic denervation reduces left ventricular hypertrophy and improves cardiac function in patients with resistant hypertension. *J Am Coll Cardiol*. 2012;59:901-909.

41. Davies JE, Manisty CH, Petraco R, et al. First-in-man safety evaluation of renal denervation for chronic systolic heart failure: primary outcome from REACH-Pilot study. *Int J Cardiol*. 2013;162:189-192.

42. Renal Denervation in Patients With Chronic Heart Failure & Renal Impairment Clinical Trial (SymplicityHF) website. https://clinicaltrials.gov/ct2/show/NCT01392196?term=NCT01392196&rank=1. Accessed August 31, 2014.

43. Renal Denervation in Patients With Chronic Heart Failure website. https://clinicaltrials.gov/ct2/show/NCT02085668? term=NCT02085668&rank=1. Accessed August 31, 2014.

44. Denervation of the renAl sympathetIc nerveS in hearT Failure With nOrmal Lv Ejection Fraction (DIASTOLE) website. https://clinicaltrials.gov/ct2/show/NCT01583881?term=NCT01583881&rank=1. Accessed August 31, 2014.

45. Renal Denervation in Heart Failure With Preserved Ejection Fraction (RDT-PEF) website. https://clinicaltrials.gov/ct2/show/NCT01840059?term=NCT01840059&rank=1. Accessed August 31, 2014.

46. Renal Denervation in Heart Failure Patients With Preserved Ejection Fraction (RESPECT-HF) website. https://clinicaltrials.gov/ct2/show/NCT02041130?term=NCT02041130&rank=1. Accessed August 31, 2014.

47. McMurray JJ, Packer M, Desai AS, et al. Angiotensin-neprilysin inhibition versus enalapril in heart failure. *N Engl J Med*. 2014;371:993-1004.

48. Packer M, McMurray JJ, Desai AS, et al. Angiotensin receptor neprilysin inhibition compared with enalapril on the risk of clinical progression in surviving patients with heart failure. *Circulation*. 2015;131:54-61.

30 CARDIAC CARDIOVERTER DEFIBRILLATORS (ICDs) IN HEART FAILURE

Rami Kahwash, MD

PATIENT CASE

A 55-year-old man with past medical history significant for hypertension (HTN), hyperlipidemia, and type 2 diabetes mellitus, was admitted to the coronary care unit 3 months ago with non-ST-elevation myocardial infarction (NSTEMI). Coronary angiography then revealed 95% narrowing in the proximal left anterior descending coronary artery. He underwent successful percutaneous coronary intervention and stent placement with excellent angiographic results and resolution of his symptoms. His left ventricular ejection fraction (LVEF) was 25% by left ventriculography performed at the time of the intervention. He was established on dual antiplatelet therapy, statin, and guideline-directed medical therapy for heart failure (HF). Beta blocker and angiotensin-converting enzyme (ACE) inhibitor were gradually titrated to the maximally tolerated doses during the next few months after discharge. He returned for his 3-month post discharge visit reporting no angina. An echocardiogram in the office revealed an LVEF of 30%. His 12-lead electrocardiogram (ECG) showed normal sinus rhythm (NSR), normal intervals, old septal infarct, and QRS of 110 ms. His medications include carvedilol 25 mg by mouth twice daily, lisinopril 10 mg by mouth twice daily, spironolactone 25 mg by mouth once a day, aspirin 81 mg by mouth once a day, clopidogril 75 mg by mouth once a day, and atorvastatin 80 mg by mouth before bed. He resides in NYHA functional class II. What is the single most important therapy you recommend to improve his survival?

INTRODUCTION

Sudden cardiac death (SCD) is a major public health problem and the cause of death in approximately 500,000 patients every year in the United States. An implantable cardioverter defibrillator (ICD) is a device-based therapy designed to detect and treat lethal ventricular arrhythmias and has shown to decrease mortality in high-risk populations, including those who survived prior cardiac arrests. Among patients without prior history of cardiac arrest or sustained ventricular arrhythmias, the LVEF of 35% or less has been identified as the single best predictor of SCD risks. Several randomized clinical trials have enrolled patients with low ejection fraction, various clinical HF profiles without history of cardiac arrest or sustained ventricular arrhythmias, and shown survival benefits from prophylactic ICD implantation when compared to conventional therapy alone. In this chapter we will discuss the risks of SCD among HF patients, major components and basic functions of the intravenous ICD system, the ICD implant procedure, and possible complications. We will also discuss the clinical trials that led to the introduction of ICD as a lifesaving therapy in certain patient populations and highlight recent indications and contraindications of ICD therapy according to the most recent guidelines.

IMPLANTABLE CARDIOVERTER DEFIBRILLATORS

ICDs are surgically implanted devices with the ability to continuously monitor cardiac rhythm, as well as detect and terminate life-threatening arrhythmias. The ICD system consists of a pulse generator that is implanted subcutaneously in the subpectoral fascia medial to the deltopectoral groove and connected to a single ventricular lead (single-chamber ICD) or dual atrial and ventricular leads (dual-chamber ICD). Leads are introduced to the central venous system through semirigid vascular catheters inserted in the subclavian or axillary veins over a guidewire. In single-chamber ICDs, the lead is advanced to the right ventricular apex and secured into the endocardium. In dual-chamber ICDs, an additional pacing lead can be secured in the right atrium if sequential A-V pacing is desired (Figure 30-1).

When compared to standard pacing devices, the ICD pulse generator is bigger in size, which allows enough space to host a large battery capable of generating high-voltage current during shock delivery. In addition to all pacing microcomponents and software programs included in the standard pacemaker pulse generator, the ICD pulse generator encloses high-voltage capacitors and a very complex system of microprocessors.

The ICD lead distal terminal is equipped with a pacing tip electrode for sensing and pacing purposes, similar to the standard pacing leads. In contrast to pacing leads, the ICD ventricular lead is surrounded by 1 or 2 shock coils that correspond to locations in the right ventricle and superior vena cava when the lead is fully deployed (Figure 30-2). Some leads are designed to be equipped with a single coil only in the right ventricle (single-coil leads).

All ICD devices have pacing capability with features that are comparable to those of traditional pacemakers. Because excessive pacing from the right ventricular apex is proven to be deleterious to the cardiac function, most primary prevention ICDs are generally programmed to minimize ventricular pacing when patients have no pacing indication. Application of a magnet over the ICD pulse generator will disable the ICD detection tachy therapy and leave the pacing capability intact. This is used during urgent surgical procedures to prevent unnecessary shocks from electromagnetic interference.

The ICD's main role is to directly treat cardiac tachydysrhythmia. When the device senses a ventricular rate that is above the programmed threshold, the ICD will attempt to terminate it either by performing antitachycardia pacing (ATP) or defibrillation. With

ATP, the ICD fires a programmed sequential number of rapid pacing impulses (in ramp or burst fashion) in an attempt to terminate the ventricular tachycardia. If ATP was unsuccessful, or if the tachycardia rate fell in the preprogrammed cut-off for ventricular fibrillation (VF), the device will immediately perform a cardioversion/defibrillation. Some device models are capable of performing ATP while charging for defibrillation out of VF (Figure 30-3).

Cardiac resynchronization therapy (CRT) is another device-based therapy that is beginning to occupy a central part in HF management through its proven effects on reducing morbidity and mortality among patients with symptomatic HF with evidence of electrical dyssynchrony, defined as wide QRS > 120 ms with left bundle branch morphology. CRT is delivered by simultaneous pacing of the right and left ventricles (LVs) through an additional lead that is advanced through the coronary sinus (CS) to a posterolateral location of the LV wall. When equipped with CRT functions, a pacemaker device is called a CRT-P and an ICD device is called a CRT-D (Figure 30-4).

At the time of the implant procedure, evaluation of adequate sensing of cardiac intrinsic activities and assessment of the pacing and defibrillation thresholds are usually performed once the system is assembled and the pulse generator is connected to the lead. This is done to confirm device integrity and ensure successful detection and termination of induced VF. Ensuring that the ICD device is sensing adequate R waves is essential to increase device sensitivity to discriminate between intrinsic ventricular activities and other signals (ie, T waves or myopotentials) (Figure 30-5).

The ICD implant procedure is mostly done under moderate sedation with the exception of checking the defibrillation threshold, at which time deep sedation is required. On average, the implant procedure takes 1 to 2 hours and requires an overnight stay for observation. However, there is an increasing trend among operators to discharge patients the same day, especially in low-risk patients who underwent uncomplicated procedures.

The most common complications are hematoma (1.1% of implantations), lead dislodgement (1.0%), and pneumothorax (0.5%); the cumulative major complication rate is 1.5%.[1] The procedure is routinely performed by cardiac electrophysiologists; however, it can also be performed by general cardiologists

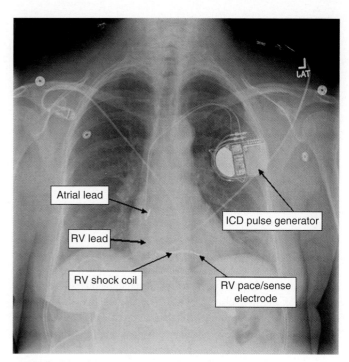

FIGURE 30-1 Major components of the ICD system. Abbreviations: ICD, implantable cardioverter defibrillator; RV, right ventricle; SCV, superior vena cava.

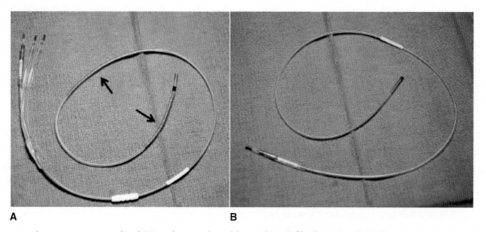

FIGURE 30-2 Compression between a pacing lead (A) and an implantable cardiac defibrillator lead (B). The ICD lead is equipped with high-voltage defibrillation coils (*black arrows*). (Reproduced with permission from McKean SC, Ross JJ, Dressler DD, Scheurer DB. *Principles and Practice of Hospital Medicine.* 2nd ed. New York, NY: McGraw-Hill Education; 2017. Figure 136-2.)

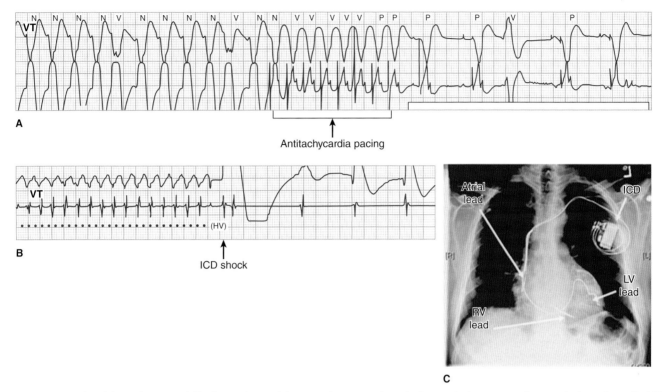

FIGURE 30-3 Implantable cardioverter defibrillator (ICD) and therapies for ventricular arrhythmias. **A.** A monomorphic ventricular tachycardia (VT) is terminated by a burst of pacing impulses at a rate faster than VT (antitachycardia pacing). **B.** A very fast VT is terminated with a high-voltage shock (*arrow*). **C.** The chest x-ray shows the major components of an ICD capable of biventricular pacing (CRT-D). The ICD generator is implanted in the subcutaneous tissue of the left upper chest. Pacing leads terminate in the right atrium and the left ventricular (LV) branch of the coronary sinus (LV lead). A pacing/defibrillating lead terminates in the right ventricle (RV lead). (Reproduced with permission from Kasper D, Fauci A, Hauser S, Longo D, Jameson JL, Loscalzo J. *Harrison's Principles of Internal Medicine.* 19th ed. New York, NY: McGraw-Hill Education; 2015. Figure 277-9.)

and cardiac surgeons who received sufficient training in device implantation and programming.

IMPLANTABLE CARDIOVERTER DEFIBRILLATORS AND SUDDEN CARDIAC DEATH

Secondary prevention is a term commonly used when the indication of ICD is to prevent SCD in patients who already have survived a prior cardiac arrest or in patients with documented long episodes of sustained and hemodynamically unstable ventricular tachycardia (VT). The term primary prevention of SCD, however, is usually used when ICD therapy is used prophylactically against SCD in populations at higher risk for having cardiac arrest because of cardiac disease but who have not yet experienced sustained VT or VF.

Early ICD trials tested the efficacy of device therapy versus antiarrhythmic medications, mostly amiodarone or sotalol, in improving survival among very high-risk populations. These trials evaluated the role of ICDs as secondary preventive measures in patients who either had documented ventricular arrhythmias or cardiac arrest or were post-myocardial infarction (MI) without advanced HF. ICD therapy was proven to be superior to antiarrhythmic medications in this secondary prevention population.

The secondary prevention strategy was founded on the observation of high incidences of VT or VF in patients who survived cardiac arrest. To test the benefits of ICD therapy in this group,

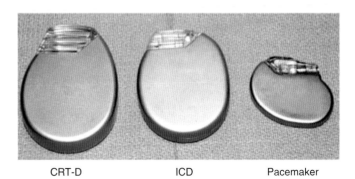

FIGURE 30-4 Images of standard pacemaker devices, implantable cardiac defibrillator (ICD), and cardiac resynchronization therapy with defibrillator (CRT-D). CRT-D and ICD pulse generators are larger than pacemakers. This size difference allows ICD and CRT-D devices to host a high-voltage battery. (Reproduced with permission from McKean SC, Ross JJ, Dressler DD, Scheurer DB. *Principles and Practice of Hospital Medicine.* 2nd ed. New York, NY: McGraw-Hill Education; 2017. Figure 136-1.)

3 secondary-prevention ICD trials were conducted in the late 1980s and early 1990s, including the Antiarrhythmics Versus Implantable Defibrillator (AVID) trial,[2] the Canadian Implantable Defibrillator (CIDS) trial,[3] and the Cardiac Arrest Study Hamburg (CASH) trial.[4] The AVID trial was the first among those 3 trials to show a statistically significant survival benefit for ICD over antiarrhythmic drugs (mostly amiodarone), with an absolute risk reduction of 7% over a follow-up of 2 years.

Following the result of AVID, the CIDS trial was stopped early due to its similar design to AVID. The CASH study was much smaller, and terminated prematurely due to adverse outcomes in 1 of its arms. A meta-analysis of the pooled data from all 3 trials showed a significant survival improvement with the ICD over antiarrhythmic medications (Table 30-1).[5]

Later trials focused on primary prevention in the HF population. Several clinical trials to date have established the efficacy of ICD therapy as primary prevention in HF patients with or without documented ventricular arrhythmias (Table 30-2).[6-9]

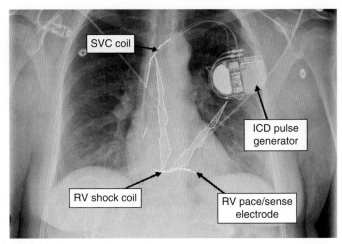

FIGURE 30-5 Schematic view of the defibrillation shock generated by the ICD (*yellow waves*). Each 1 of the device pulse generators cans, SVC high-voltage coil, and RV high-voltage coil can serve as a negative or positive victor for the high-energy current. Some manufacturers will allow a cold can (not active victor), with the high-voltage current generated between SVC and RV coils only. Polarity of those victors can be programmed and reversed to ensure the best defibrillation threshold. Abbreviations: ICD, implantable cardioverter defibrillator; RV, right ventricle; SVC, superior vena cava.

PRIMARY PREVENTION OF SUDDEN CARDIAC DEATH

One of the major challenges in cardiology is attempting to identify high-risk patients for whom treatment with ICD may prevent SCD. In the past few decades, several electrophysiology tests, ECG repolarization parameters, and clinical profiles were developed and tested as possible predictors of SCD. They all lacked adequate sensitivity and specificity and failed to consistently identify patients who are at increased risk. In contrast, low LVEF was found to be a strong predictor of SCD in ischemic and nonischemic dilated cardiomyopathy patients.[10] Based on these concepts, several randomized clinical trials[6-9] have subsequently evaluated ICDs for primary prevention in patients with reduced ejection fraction (< 30%-35%), with some additional risk factors, including nonsustained VT, prior MI, symptomatic HF, and inducible VT by programed stimulation.

Table 30-1   Secondary Prevention Trials of ICD Therapy

Trial	Inclusion	2-Y Total Mortality			
		Control	ICDs	Relative risk reduction	Absolute risk reduction
AVID	VF, VT syncope, VT—EF ≤40%	25%	18%	−27%	−7%
CIDS	Cardiac arrest survivors (VF, VT)	21%	15%	−30%	−6%
CASH	Cardiac arrest survivors (VF, VT)	20%	12%	−37%	−8%

Abbreviations: ICDs, ICD, implantable cardioverter defibrillators; EF, ejection fraction; VF, ventricular fibrillation; VT, ventricular tachycardia.

Table 30-2 Major Primary Prevention ICD Trials

Study	Inclusion	n	Mean EF	Treatment	Mean f/u	Result
MADIT	Post-AMI, NSVT, EF <35%, NYHA class II-III, TV inducible resist, procainamide	196	27%	ICD vs antiarrhythmic agents (80% amiodarone)	27 mo	Reduction in risk of death (54%) with ICD
MADIT II	Post-AMI EF < 30%, >10% ESV/h or paired	1232	23%	ICD vs clinical treatment	20 mo	Reduction in risk of death (31%) with ICD
SCD-HeFT	NYHA class II-III, EF <35%	2521	25%	ICD vs amiodarone vs placebo	45 mo	Reduction in risk of death (23%) with ICD

Abbreviations: AMI, acute myocardial infarction; f/u, follow-up; ICD, implantable cardioverter defibrillator; EF, ejection fraction; ESV, end systolic volume; NSVT, non-sustained ventricular tachycardia.

The Multicenter Automatic Defibrillator Implantation Trials (MADIT)[6,7] evaluated the use of ICDs as primary prevention in high-risk patients with reduced ejection fraction and history of MI. The MADIT-I[6] enrolled 196 patients who were more than 3 weeks post-MI, with ejection fractions ≤35%, documented asymptomatic nonsustained VT, and inducible nonsuppressible sustained VT on electrophysiology (EP) study. Patients were randomized to conventional medical therapy or to an ICD in addition to conventional medical therapy. After a follow-up for 27 months, there was significant survival benefit noted in the ICD group (HR 0.46; 95% CI, 0.26-0.82; P = 0.009). This trial was the first to show mortality benefit with ICD when compared to medical therapy; however, it was criticized for its unbalanced distribution of medical therapy (beta blockers, sotalol, and amiodarone) between the 2 groups, which made the interpretation of the result very challenging. Another concern was raised in regard to the inclusion criteria of requiring sustained VT during EP study that was not suppressible by procainamide. This raised concerns about whether patients in the drug-therapy arm were less responsive to pharmacologic therapy.

The second landmark MADIT (MADIT-II)[7] was a larger trial; it did not require the presence of ventricular arrhythmias in its inclusion criteria. No EP testing was required and the risk of SCD was based on the presence of LV dysfunction and history of MI. In MADIT-II, a total of 1232 patients with reduced LVEF ≤30% and prior MI were randomized to conventional drug therapy or ICD in addition to conventional drug therapy. Patients were required to be at least 40 days post-MI. The 2 groups were well-balanced in regard to their baseline standard medications. The trial was stopped early at 20-month follow up due to a very significant 31% relative reduction in mortality seen in the ICD arm compared to control (P = 0.016), which was wholly related to reduction in SCD. SCD occurred in 10% of the medical-therapy arm compared to 3.8% of the ICD arm (P < 0.01). The rate of nonsudden death was similar in both groups. There was a slight trend toward increased HF hospitalization in the ICD group, which could be related to the deleterious effects of ICD shocks, unnecessary right ventricular apical pacing, or natural progression of pump failure as a result of prolonged survival.

In contrast to the MADIT trials that included post-MI patients and ischemia etiology to their cardiomyopathy, the DEFINITE trial[8] was designed to evaluate the role of ICDs in preventing SCD among patients with a nonischemic cardiomyopathy and moderate to severe LV dysfunction. A total of 484 patients with ejection fraction ≤ 35% were randomized to conventional therapy or ICD. After mean follow-up of 29 months, the ICD arm was associated with significant reduction in arrhythmic death and trend toward reduction in all-cause mortality. ICD prophylaxis resulted in significantly reduced arrhythmic death and a trend toward reduction in the primary endpoint of all-cause mortality. The inclusion of asymptomatic patients could have contributed to the lower mortality rate and underworking of the study as 22% of patients were NYHA class I.

In the Sudden Cardiac Death in Heart Failure Trial (SCD-HeFT),[9] a total of 2520 patients with symptomatic HF in stable NYHA class II or III and an ejection fraction ≤35% were randomized to receiving an ICD, amiodarone therapy, or placebo. At 4-year follow-up, the ICD arm had a 23% reduction in relative mortality compared to placebo. The primary endpoint of all-cause mortality was not improved by amiodarone therapy; furthermore, amiodarone was associated with potential harm in patients with NHYA class III (Figure 30-6). An important aspect of SCD-HeFT was its inclusion of both ischemic and nonischemic etiologies of HFe, with 52% of the study population demonstrating ischemic etiology and 48% demonstrating a nonischemic etiology. The study demonstrated that ICD was an effective therapy in the primary prevention of SCD, regardless of HF etiology. Based on these and other data, the American College of Cardiology, American Heart Association, and Heart Rhythm Society published joint guidelines recommending ICDs for primary prevention in patients with an ejection fraction of less than 30% or 35%, depending on HF etiology and severity.[11,12]

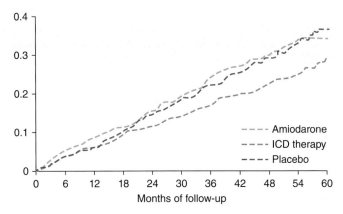

	HR	97.5% CI	P Value
Amiodarone vs placebo	1.06	0.86-1.30	0.53
ICD vs placebo	0.77	0.62-0.96	0.007

FIGURE 30-6 Kaplan-Meier estimates of all-cause mortality in the SCD-HeFT trial. While the empirical use of amiodarone had no effect on outcome, the primary prevention ICD reduced the risk of the primary endpoint by approximately 23%. Abbreviations: CI, confidence interval; HR, heart rate; ICD, implantable cardioverter defibrillator. (Reproduced with permission from Bardy GH, Lee KL, Mark DB, et al. Amiodarone or an implantable cardioverter-defibrillator for congestive heart failure [SCD-HeFT]. *New Engl J Med*. 2005;352:225-237.)

INDICATIONS AND CONTRAINDICATIONS FOR PRIMARY PREVENTION IMPLANTABLE CARDIOVERTER DEFIBRILLATOR

Current HF guidelines recommend[11,12] the use of an ICD as primary prevention of all-cause mortality in well-treated NYHA class II and class III patients with LVEF of ≤30% and either ischemic or nonischemic cardiomyopathy. ICD implantation is also indicated in patients with ischemic cardiomyopathy who are at least 40 days post-MI who have either LVEF ≤30% and are NYHA functional class I, or LVEF ≤35% and are NYHA functional class II. In general, patients with moderate to severe left ventricular systolic dysfunction and symptomatic HF should receive an ICD for prevention of SCD, unless they have a poor chance of survival related to comorbidity such as systemic malignancy or severe renal dysfunction or have a contraindication to the implantation or use of this device, including those with advanced frailty and high risk of nonsudden death.

ICDs are also strongly recommended in patients with a history of sustained VT, VF, and resuscitated cardiac arrest, for the secondary prevention of mortality. ICD implantation is not recommended when certain forms of VT and VF are amenable to catheter ablation in the absence of structural heart disease (ie, atrial arrhythmias with Wolff-Parkinson-White syndrome, idiopathic VT, outflow tract VT, or fascicular VT) (Table 30-3).

KEY POINTS: PRIMARY PREVENTION OF SUDDEN CARDIAC DEATH

- In patients with HF, assessment of LVEF is the most important step in identifying those who are at increased risks of SCD and will benefit from ICD implantation.
- Antiarrhythmic medications have not shown survival benefits in prevention of SCD.

GENERAL APPROACH TO PATIENTS IMPLANTED WITH IMPLANTABLE CARDIOVERTER DEFIBRILLATOR

The indication of ICD has rapidly expanded over the past few decades to include millions of HF patients who became eligible for this device-based therapy for the prevention of SCD. As a result of the surge in ICD prevalence, primary care physicians have become increasingly exposed to patients implanted with these devices. It is very important to establish a systematic way of approaching such patients when taking the medical history.

Knowing the indication of the ICD is perhaps the most important element in the history. Patients with primary prevention devices should be further stratified based on the etiology of their cardiomyopathy and whether it is ischemic or nonischemic, the degree of their LV dysfunction, and their NYHA functional class. Patients with secondary prevention indications should be evaluated thoroughly until a specific etiology is determined, as it is important to know whether their arrhythmia was primary or secondary to structural heart disease or inherited conditions.

It is very important to know the manufacturer of the pulse generator, which can be very helpful in seeking immediate consultation shall any emergency arise. Ensuring the patient is followed by a cardiologist or in a designated device clinic is crucial for frequent surveillance of electrical stability and assessing lead integrity and battery life.

Asking patients about any device-related complaint and examining the surgical site periodically are essential. Thinning of the skin covering the pulse generator or protrusion of wires or hardware through the skin requires immediate attention by a cardiologist to prevent serious complications from impending erosion. Patients who are dependent on the ICD for pacing support should have their device checked every 3 to 6 months or more frequently based on the remaining battery life.

Patients should be asked about any history of ICD shocks and whether they received full device interrogation and clinical evaluation by a specialist following their last reported shock. ICD discharges could be signs of worsening HF, ischemia, or electrolyte disturbances. It is recommended that patients keep a copy of their

Table 30-3 Indications for ICD Therapy

Primary prevention of sudden cardiac arrest

- Ischemic cardiomyopathy, EF <35%, NYHA class II-III, at least 40 d after myocardial infarction
- Ischemic cardiomyopathy, EF <30%, NYHA class I
- Nonischemic cardiomyopathy, EF <35%, NYHA class II-III

Secondary prevention of sudden cardiac arrest

- Survivors of sudden cardiac arrest from VF or sustained VT without reversible causes
- Structural heart disease and sustained VT
- Syncope with inducible hemodynamically significant VT or VF during EP study

Abbreviations: EF, ejection fraction; EP, electrophysiology; ICD, implantable cardioverter defibrillator; VF, ventricular fibrillation; VT, ventricular tachycardia.

last device interrogation with them for future reference. Battery life in most ICDs is between 5 and 7 years. However, this can vary dramatically depending on pacing requirements, capture threshold, and frequency of ICD discharge.

EVALUATION OF AN IMPLANTABLE CARDIOVERTER DEFIBRILLATOR SHOCK

Experiencing an ICD shock is a very traumatic experience especially for patients who remain conscious at the time of shock delivery. The intense level of anxiety surrounding the event and chest soreness trigged by ICD discharge usually prompt most patients to seek immediate medical attention at their primary care physician offices or at emergency departments. The first step in evaluating patients who received ICD shock should be focusing on their clinical status and exploring whether they have been experiencing any recent progression in HF state, development of ischemic symptoms, medication changes, or recent illnesses. Device interrogation by an expert should be performed to examine the stored ECG and evaluate electrical sequences that led to shock delivery (Figure 30-7).

One fundamental step in device evaluation is to determine whether or not the shock was appropriately delivered. A shock is considered appropriate if the device correctly detected a tachyarrhythmia, classified it as VT or VF, and treated it according to a preset tachy therapy algorithm. A shock is considered inappropriate if it was delivered after sensing electrical signals in the detection zone that are not VT or VF. The most common cause of inappropriate

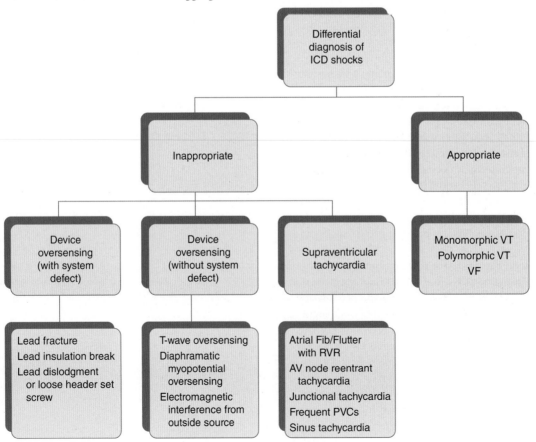

FIGURE 30-7 Differential diagnosis of ICD shock. Abbreviations: AV, atrioventricular; ICD, implantable cardioverter defibrillator; PVC, premature ventricular contraction; RVR, rapid ventricular response; VF, ventricular fibrillation; VT, ventricular tachycardia.

shock is atrial fibrillation or supraventricular tachycardia with rapid ventricular response. If atrial tachycardia is conducted rapidly to the ventricle, the device could interpret the rhythm as VT or VF thus triggering therapies. Historically, tachy therapy algorithms primarily used the ventricular rate to activate shock therapies, which resulted in increased potentials of unnecessary shock when the rapidly conducted ventricular response fell higher than the VT or VF cutoffs. As devices are becoming more sophisticated, programming to distinguish supraventricular tachycardias from VT or VF is becoming more accurate, thus decreasing inappropriate shocks.

When a patient receives multiple shocks, immediate evaluation of both the patient and the device is necessary. Device interrogation can rule out any device integrity and programming issues. As leads age, there is an increased risk of fracture. When a lead fractures, electrical noise can be misinterpreted as VT or VF, initiating therapies. ECG monitoring obtained during patient assessment of those who received multiple shocks can show sustained rhythms that may not be responding to programmed therapies or reoccurring rhythms (eg, VT storm). If a patient presents with multiple shocks and system integrity is ensured, treatment should address the underlying cause (ie, ischemia, HF, drug toxicity especially antiarrhythmic agents, and electrolyte derangement). Treatment for recurrent primary monomorphic VT includes antiarrhythmic drugs or catheter ablation.

Because ICD shocks could be manifestations of worsening cardiac disease, the focus should always remain on optimizing pharmacologic therapy for HF, restoring coronary flow in patients with active ischemia, and eliminating all risk factors. ICD therapy should be viewed as an effective lifesaving therapy against lethal arrhythmias; however, it should not replace adequate implementation of Guideline-Directed Medical Therapy (GDMT) for HF or coronary artery disease.

PREOPERATIVE MANAGEMENT

The main aims at the time of any invasive procedure or surgical operation for patients with ICDs are to maintain appropriate rhythm, avoid electromagnetic interference, and prevent direct damage to or mechanical dislodgement of the ICD leads. If central venous catheter placement is needed for a patient's care, it is recommended that the internal jugular or subclavian veins be accessed in the contralateral side to the device under fluoroscopic guidance, especially in newly placed leads. When patients undergo thoracic or abdominal surgery adjacent to the device, it is recommended that a postoperative interrogation is performed to ensure there was no disruption in the function of the ICD system.

It is not uncommon in preoperative ICD management to encounter circumstances where there needs to be temporary disabling of the tachycardia response of the device to avoid inappropriate shocks triggered by sensing adjacent electrocautery impulses. This is more common if the surgical field is within 6 inches of the pulse generator, especially when monopolar electrocautery is used. While the ICD is disabled intraoperatively, it is crucial to have other ways of monitoring cardiac rhythm and be able to deliver external defibrillation if needed. External defibrillator pads should be placed preoperatively for continuous monitoring and to provide the ability to defibrillate in case of any unstable rhythm.

Generally, if the location of the surgical procedure is below the umbilicus, no preoperative reprogramming is needed for the ICD. For surgeries above the umbilicus, it is advised to disable ICD tachycardia therapy during the procedure and ensure the ability of delivering external defibrillation. Patients with ICDs who are also pacemaker-dependent and having surgery above the umbilicus, should be reprogrammed to an asynchronous mode either via a device representative or by placement of a magnet over the device. For urgent surgeries when the status of the device indication is unknown, it is always recommended to use short bursts of the electrocautery, as short bursts are less likely to interfere with ICD function.[13]

ELECTROMAGNETIC INTERFERENCE

Magnetic resonance imaging (MRI) is an imaging modality that is increasingly used to diagnose a variety of clinical conditions. In general, MRI is contraindicated in patients with ICD because of the risk of damaging the device microcomponents from the MRI's intense electromagnetic field. In recent years, it is becoming feasible to use MRI with certain ICD and lead models that are MRI-compatible if done according to certain protocols. Consulting with specialists is necessary before ordering MRIs in patients with ICDs.

Digital cellular phones can interfere with ICDs, although this rarely happens. It is recommended that cellular phones should be held adjacent to the ear opposite from the side of the ICD. Patients with ICDs should not carry cellular phones in their shirt pockets near their chests.

ICDs are compatible with most electrical appliances that are used routinely in our daily activities, such as radios, televisions, microwave ovens, computers, and vacuum cleaners. Theft-detector gates in stores or at airports emit electrical signals that can potentially interfere with the ICD function. It is safe for patients with ICDs to walk through these gates at a normal speed. However, it is recommended that they should not walk very slowly or stand at or near the gates for longer periods of time. Heavy-duty electrical-powered equipment, such as arc welders, causes disturbances with the ICD and should be avoided (Table 30-4).

MAGNET INHIBITION

Magnets are usually used to temporarily reprogram the pacemaker function of cardiac devices into asynchronous mode when they are placed over the pulse generator. They are also used to determine the longevity of the battery as each device manufacturer has a distinct asynchronous rate for devices at beginning of life (BOL), elective replacement indicator (ERI), and end of life (EOL).

When a magnet is placed over an ICD, it will temporarily turn off defibrillation therapy without changing its pacing capabilities. It is also worth mentioning that most devices have a magnet response feature turned on; however, some devices can be programmed to not respond to magnet application. In such cases, a certified device programmer is needed to change the parameters (Table 30-5).

IMPLANTABLE CARDIOVERTER DEFIBRILLATOR DEACTIVATION

HF is a progressive disease and despite recent advancements in medical- and device-based therapies, a significant number of patients will progress to the end-stage phase (stage D) when goals of care should be modified to a palliative approach. In these advanced HF patients who are more likely to die from pump failure or other comorbidities, an ICD's ability to terminate VT or VF becomes irrelevant and in fact, it will complicate end-of-life care. Disabling the tachy therapy feature of the ICD should be discussed with every patient with advanced HF in order to avoid painful shocks and unnecessary physical and emotional stressors during end-of-life care. Other conditions in which disabling an ICD is warranted is when patients receive recurrent inappropriate shocks or when there is need for external transcutaneous pacing, as this will interfere with ICD functioning (Table 30-6).

PATIENT CASE CONCLUSION

The patient discussed in the case above meets class I indication for a primary prevention ICD implant as an established therapy for the prevention of sudden cardiac death. He has ischemic cardiomyopathy and LVEF remained depressed <30% despite 3 months of guideline-directed medical therapy. ICD is associated with 31% relative risk reduction in sudden cardiac death according to data from the MADIT II trial.

PATIENT EDUCATION RESOURCES

What Is an Implantable Cardioverter Defibrillator? http://www.nhlbi.nih.gov/health/health-topics/topics/icd

Who Needs an Implantable Cardioverter Defibrillator? http://www.nhlbi.nih.gov/health/health-topics/topics/icd/whoneeds

How Does an Implantable Cardioverter Defibrillator Work? http://www.nhlbi.nih.gov/health/health-topics/topics/icd/howdoes

What To Expect During Implantable Cardioverter Defibrillator Surgery: http://www.nhlbi.nih.gov/health/health-topics/topics/icd/during

What To Expect After Implantable Cardioverter Defibrillator Surgery: http://www.nhlbi.nih.gov/health/health-topics/topics/icd/after

What Are the Risks of Having an Implantable Cardioverter Defibrillator? http://www.nhlbi.nih.gov/health/health-topics/topics/icd/risks

How Will an Implantable Cardioverter Defibrillator Affect My Lifestyle? http://www.nhlbi.nih.gov/health/health-topics/topics/icd/lifestyle

PROVIDER RESOURCES

2012 ACCF/AHA/HRS Focused Update of the 2008 Guidelines for Device-Based Therapy of Cardiac Rhythm Abnormalities. A Report of the American College of Cardiology Foundation/American Heart Association Task Force on Practice Guidelines and the Heart Rhythm Society: http://circ.ahajournals.org/content/126/14/1784.long

Table 30-4 ICD Electromagnetic Interferences

- Most home electrical appliances are compatible with ICDs.
- It is recommended that patients hold their cell phones adjacent to the ear on the opposite side of the ICD pulse generator and avoid placing them in chest pockets.
- Passing theft detector gates in stores and airports should be done at a reasonable speed without delay or stopping near the gates.
- High-voltage machinery (eg, arc welders) should be avoided by patients with implantable ICDs.

Abbreviation: ICDs, implantable cardioverter defibrillators.

Table 30-5 Effects of Magnets on Cardiac Devices

- Application of magnet will reprogram pacemakers to a nonsynchronous mode.
- Application of magnet will temporarily disable ICD tachy therapy (detection and treatment of VT and VF) without altering pacing features.

Abbreviations: ICD, implantable cardioverter defibrillator; VF, ventricular fibrillation; VT, ventricular tachycardia.

Table 30-6 Indications for ICD Deactivation

- End-of-life care
- Recurrent inappropriate shocks because of lead failure or SVT/AF with rapid ventricular response
- During transcutaneous pacing
- During surgical procedures requiring the use of electrocautery in close proximity to the ICD pulse generator

Abbreviations: AF, atrial fibrillation; SVT, supra ventricular tachycardia; ICD, implantable cardioverter defibrillator.

2013 ACCF/AHA Guideline for the Management of Heart Failure: Executive Summary. A Report of the American College of Cardiology Foundation/American Heart Association Task Force on Practice Guidelines: http://circ.ahajournals.org/content/128/16/1810.full

The Heart Rhythm Society (HRS)/American Society of Anesthesiologists (ASA) Expert Consensus Statement on the perioperative management of patients with implantable defibrillators, pacemakers and arrhythmia monitors: facilities and patient management. This document was developed as a joint project with the American Society of Anesthesiologists (ASA), and in collaboration with the American Heart Association (AHA), and the Society of Thoracic Surgeons (STS). *Heart Rhythm.* 2011;8:1114-1154. http://www.heartrhythmjournal.com/article/S1547-5271%2811%2900584-4/abstract

REFERENCES

1. Curtis JP, Luebbert JJ, Wang Y, et al. Association of physician certification and outcomes among patients receiving an implantable cardioverter-defibrillator. *JAMA.* 2009;301(16):1661-1670.

2. Antiarrhythmic Versus Implantable Defibrillators (AVID) Investigators. A comparison of antiarrhythmic drug therapy with implantable defibrillators in patients resuscitated from near-fatal ventricular arrhythmias. *N Engl J Med.* 1997;337:1576-1583.

3. Connolly SJ, Gent M, Roberts RS, et al. Canadian implantable defibrillator study (CIDS): a randomized trial of the implantable cardioverter defibrillator against amiodarone. *Circulation.* 2000;101:1297-1302.

4. Kuck KH, Cappato R, Siebels J, Rüppel R, et al. Randomized comparison of antiarrhythmic drug therapy with implantable defibrillators in patients resuscitated from cardiac arrest: the Cardiac Arrest Study Hamburg (CASH). *Circulation.* 2000;102:748-754.

5. Connolly SJ, Hallstrom AP, Cappato R, et al. Meta-analysis of the implantable cardioverter defibrillator secondary prevention trials. AVID, CASH and CIDS studies. Antiarrhythmics vs Implantable Defibrillator study. Cardiac Arrest Study Hamburg. Canadian Implantable Defibrillator Study. *Eur Heart J.* 2000;21:2071-2078.

6. Moss AJ, Hall WJ, Cannom DS, et al. Improved survival with an implantable defibrillator in patients with coronary disease at high risk for ventricular arrhythmia. Multicenter Automatic Defibrillator Implantation Trial Investigators. *N Engl J Med.* 1996;335:1933-1940.

7. Moss AJ, Zareba W, Hall WJ, et al. Prophylactic implantation of a defibrillator in patients with myocardial infarction and reduced ejection fraction. *N Engl J Med.* 2002;346:877-883.

8. Kadish A, Dyer A, Daubert JP, et al. Defibrillators in Non-Ischemic Cardiomyopathy Treatment Evaluation (DEFINITE) Investigators. Prophylactic defibrillator implantation in patients with nonischemic dilated cardiomyopathy. *N Engl J Med.* 2004;350:2151-2158.

9. Bardy GH, Lee KL, Mark DB, et al. Amiodarone or an Implantable Cardioverter-Defibrillator for Congestive Heart Failure (SCD-HeFT). *New Engl J Med.* 2005;352: 225-237.

10. Myerburg RJ. Implantable cardioverter-defibrillators after myocardial infarction. *N Engl J Med.* 2008;359(21):2245-2253.

11. Yancy CW, Jessup M, Bozkurt B, et al. 2013 ACCF/AHA guideline for the management of heart failure: a report of the American College of Cardiology Foundation/American Heart Association Task Force on Practice Guidelines. *J Am Coll Cardiol.* 2013;62:e147-e239.

12. Tracy CM, Epstein AE, Darbar D, et al. 2012 ACCF/AHA/HRS focused update of the 2008 guidelines for device-based therapy of cardiac rhythm abnormalities: a report of the American College of Cardiology Foundation/American Heart Association Task Force on Practice Guidelines and the Heart Rhythm Society. *Circulation.* 2012;126:1784-1800.

13. Crossley GH, Poole JE, Rozner MA, et al. The Heart Rhythm Society (HRS)/American Society of Anesthesiologists (ASA) Expert Consensus Statement on the perioperative management of patients with implantable defibrillators, pacemakers and arrhythmia monitors: facilities and patient management. This document was developed as a joint project with the American Society of Anesthesiologists (ASA), and in collaboration with the American Heart Association (AHA), and the Society of Thoracic Surgeons (STS). *Heart Rhythm.* 2011;8:1114-1154.

31 CARDIAC RESYNCHRONIZATION THERAPY IN THE TREATMENT OF HEART FAILURE

Rami Kahwash, MD

PATIENT CASE

A 55-year-old woman presented to your clinic for a follow-up. She was diagnosed with nonischemic cardiomyopathy diagnosed 9 months ago after she presented to the emergency department (ED) with New York Heart Association (NYHA) class IV heart failure (HF) symptoms. Coronary angiography then revealed no obstructive coronary artery disease (CAD). Echocardiogram at the time of her initial evaluation revealed moderately dilated left ventricle, and global hypokinesis with an ejection fraction of 20%, with no gross valvular abnormalities. Cardiac magnetic resonance imaging (MRI) showed midwall fibrosis consistent with nonischemic cardiomyopathy. During her clinic visit, she reported symptoms of effort intolerance and exertional dyspnea with mild exertion. She denied resting or exertional chest pain. An echocardiogram at the time of her visit showed left ventricular ejection fraction (LVEF) of 25%. Her current medications include carvedilol 25 mg twice daily, lisinopril 10 mg twice daily, aldactone 25 mg by mouth once a day, Lipitor 80 mg by mouth once daily, Aspirin (ASA) 81 mg by mouth once daily, and Plavix 75 mg by mouth once daily. Electrocardiogram showed normal sinus rhythm, left bundle branch block with QRS duration of 155 ms. Blood Pressure is 90/60 mm Hg and heart rate is 70 beats per minute. Her cardiovascular examination was unremarkable.

INTRODUCTION

Cardiac resynchronization therapy (CRT) is a device-based treatment for HF that emerged over the last few decades to be a major contributor to reducing morbidity and mortality. The concept of this therapy is to restore synchronous activation of both ventricles in select patients who had evidence of prolonged depolarization evident by prolongation of the QRS segment on the surface electrocardiogram (ECG). Stimulation of the right ventricle is achieved with the standard transvenous leads used in traditional pacemakers and implantable cardioverter defibrillators (ICDs). Early CRT systems required thoracotomy and epicardial left ventricular (LV) lead placement by open surgical approach. This practice was replaced by a transvenous approach in which implantation of the LV lead is achieved by cannulation of the coronary sinus and targeting a lateral or posterior branch. Given the recent advancement in lead and delivery system technologies, the transvenous approach

has become the standard technique worldwide. The epicardial technique is still used but reserved for patients with difficult venous anatomy or suboptimal target vessels.

CARDIAC DYSSYNCHRONY

Cardiac dyssynchrony has deleterious effects on the heart's performance as a pump. It can occur between the left and right ventricles and within the left ventricle itself.[1] A left bundle-branch blockade (LBBB) with prolongation of the QRS duration ≥120 ms has been used as a universal measure of electrical dyssynchrony in most clinical trials. LBBB is present in approximately one-third of HF patients in whom the septum is activated earlier than the lateral or posterior walls, resulting in paradoxical septal motion and ineffective contraction (Figure 31-1). Furthermore, dyssynchronous contraction increases LV end-systolic and end-diastolic volumes and reduces diastolic filling. Because the onset of LV contraction is delayed, the LV contraction occurs simultaneously with atrial contraction, which leads to reduction in preload and systolic mitral regurgitation through inadequate leaflet closure.

THERAPEUTIC EFFECTS OF CARDIAC RESYNCHRONIZATION THERAPY

CRT benefits can be divided into acute and chronic changes that account for the improvement in patients' symptoms and reduction in HF mortality. Acute CRT benefits include favorable hemodynamic changes such as improved LV systolic function through increased slope of dP/dt and increased stroke volume.[2]

Chronic CRT benefits include restoring normal cardiac chamber size, and reduction in LV end-systolic and end-diastolic volumes with subsequent improvement in ejection fraction.[3] CRT is also capable of producing biventricular pacing that is well synchronized with the atrial activation, which reinstates earlier activation of the left ventricle, restores diastolic filling time, and increases stroke volume. Restoring atrioventricular (AV) delay will also cause reduction in mitral regurgitation and subsequent improvement in LV systolic function. Restoring delays in electrical consequences contributes to the immediate improvement in mitral regurgitation; however, an intermediate and long-term improvement has been observed and is thought to be related to restoring normal chamber geometry seen with chronic CRT.

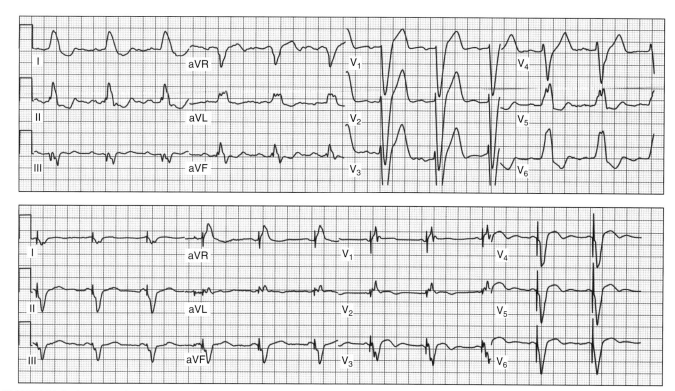

FIGURE 31-1 The top 12-lead electrocardiogram (ECG) illustrates normal sinus rhythm with left bundle-branch block and QRS width of 200 ms. The bottom 12-lead ECG is the same patient after cardiac resynchronization therapy (CRT). It illustrates atrial-sensed biventricular stimulation; note that the paced QRS complex has narrowed significantly from the baseline in response to CRT. (Reproduced with permission from Fuster V, Walsh RA, Harrington RA. *Hurst's The Heart.* 13th ed. New York, NY: McGraw-Hill Education; 2011. Figure 43-19.)

The common long-term benefits seen in responders to CRT is the reverse remodeling of ventricular dilatation, which can be detected within 3 months of CRT[4] and confirmed by several large randomized-controlled trials (Table 31-1).

CLINICAL TRIALS OF CARDIAC RESYNCHRONIZATION THERAPY

The CRT concept was first studied in the early 1990s. Since then, 8 large randomized clinical trials with more than 4000 patients enrolled were completed and established the benefits of CRT in reducing HF's morbidity and mortality with or without an ICD (Table 31-2).

PATH-CHF TRIAL

The Pacing Therapies for Congestive Heart Failure (PATH-CHF) trial[5] was the earliest randomized CRT trial. It studied the acute hemodynamic effects of CRT. PATH-CHF showed that LV and biventricular pacing formed significant acute hemodynamic benefits when compared to right ventricular (RV) pacing alone.

MUSTIC STUDY

The Multisite Stimulation in Cardiomyopathy (MUSTIC) study[6] was a single-blind randomized crossover study that evaluated the safety and efficacy of CRT in moderate HF. The study had a normal sinus rhythm (SR) arm and an atrial fibrillation (AF) arm and enrolled patients with NYHA class III HF and QRS >150 ms. In

Table 31-1 Benefits of Cardiac Resynchronization Therapy

- Improvement in cardiac hemodynamics
- Reverse remodeling of cardiac structures
- Reduction of mitral regurgitation's severity
- Improvement in heart failure symptoms and quality of life
- Prevention of heart failure hospitalizations
- Improvement in survival compared to conventional medical therapy alone in patients with heart failure symptoms and severe left ventricular dysfunction

Table 31-2 Summary of CRT Clinical Trials

Trial	Randomization	Patients	Mean Follow-up	NYHA	LVEF Inclusion Criteria	QRS Inclusion Criteria	Primary Endpoint	Secondary Endpoint	Intervention Group Better?
MUSTIC-SR (2001)	CRT-P/Med crossover	29/29	3	II, III, IV	≤35%	≥150 ms	6 MWT	NYHA, quality of life, peak VO₂, MR, LV improvement, hospitalization, mortality	Yes
PATH-CHF (2002)	RV/LV/CRT-P crossover	41	12	III, IV	NA	≥150 ms	6 MWT, peak VO₂	NYHA, quality of life, hospitalization	Yes
MIRACLE (2002)	CRT-P/Med	228/225	6	III, IV	≤35%	≥130 ms	NYHA, 6 MWT, quality of life	Peak VO₂, LVEDD, MR, LVEF, CCR	Yes
MIRACLE (2003)	CRT-D/ICD	187/182	6	III, IV	≤35%	≥130 ms	NYHA, 6 MWT, quality of life	Peak VO₂, LVV, MR, LVEF, CCR	Yes
CONTAK-CD (2003)	CRT-D/ICD	245/245	6	II, III, IV	≤35%	≥120 ms	NYHA, 6 MWT, quality of life	LVV, LVEF, CCR	Yes
COMPANION (2004)	CRT-D/CRT-P/ICD	617/595/308	15	III, IV	≤35%	≥120 ms	All-cause mortality or hospitalization	Cardiac mortality	Yes/yes
MIRACLE-ICD II (2004)	CRT-D/ICD	85/101	6	II	≤35%	≥130 ms	Peak VO₂	NYHA, quality of life, 6-MWT, LVV, LVEF, CCR	No, but several secondary were met
CARE-HF (2005)	CRT-P/Med	409/404	29	III, IV	≤35%	≥120 ms	All-cause mortality or cardiovascular hospitalization	NYHA, quality of life, LVEF, LVESV, HF hospitalization	Yes
REVERSE (2008)	CRT-P/ICD	419/191	12	I, II	≤40%	≥130 ms	CCR	LVESVi	No, but secondary was met
MADIT-CRT (2009)	CRT-D/ICD	1089, 739	29	I, II	≤30%	≥130 ms	All-cause mortality or HF hospitalization	LVESV, LVEDV, LVEF	Yes
RAFT (2010)	CRT-D/ICD	894/904	40	II, III, IV	≤30%	≥120 ms	All-cause mortality or HF hospitalization	Cardiac death, nonfatal HF hospitalization	Yes

Abbreviations: 6MWT, 6-minute walk test; CCR, clinical composite response; CRT, cardiac resynchronization therapy; HF, heart failure; LV, left ventricular; LVEDD, left ventricular end diastolic dimension; LVEDV, left ventricular end diastolic volume; LVEF, left ventricular ejection fraction; LVESV, left ventricular end systolic volume; LVESVi, left ventricular end systolic volume index; MR, mitral regurgitation; VO₂, oxygen consumption.

each arm, patients were randomized to 3 months of biventricular pacing or the control, followed by a 3-month crossover period, and final programming at 6 months to their preference. The primary endpoint of exercise capacity measured by 6-minute walk test (6MWT) and peak oxygen consumption on metabolic exercise test was significantly improved in both arms who received active CRT. Secondary endpoints of quality of life and NYHA functional class were also significantly improved with active CRT. Fewer hospitalizations were seen with biventricular pacing during a 12-month follow-up period. MUSTIC was the first trial to show clinical benefits with CRT but it was not a mortality trial.

MIRACLE TRIALS

The Multicenter InSync Randomized Clinical Evaluation (MIRACLE)[7,8] was the first prospective double-blind randomized trial that evaluated the benefits of CRT in severe HF patients. It was larger than PATH-CHF and MUSTIC and enrolled patients with NYHA class III and ambulatory class IV HF who were on optimal medical therapy. Patients had to be in normal sinus rhythm (SR) and dyssynchrony was defined as QRS durations ≥130 ms. Patients were assigned to 6 months of biventricular pacing or the control arm of medical therapy alone. Primary endpoints of NYHA class and 6MWT improved significantly with CRT, compared to the control group. There was also statically significant improvement in ejection fraction, oxygen consumption (peak VO_2), and exercise duration in the CRT arm. MIRACLE also demonstrated significant reduction in HF hospitalizations (P = 0.02) among those who received CRT. The study, however, was not powered to assess mortality.

MIRACLE-ICD[9] was a separate trial intended to evaluate the safety and efficacy of devices that combined both CRT and ICD therapies. Patients were randomized to receiving ICD without CRT capacity (n = 182) versus CRT pacing combined with ICD therapies (n = 187). The study demonstrated improvement in quality of life and NYHA functional class at 6 months among patients who received CRT. Mortality at 6 months did not differ between the 2 groups and there was no proarrhythmic effect. The results of MIRACLE-ICD established the safety of combining CRT and ICD therapies.

COMPANION TRIAL

The Comparison of Medical Therapy, Pacing, and Defibrillation in Heart Failure (COMPANION) trial[10] was designed to compare the risks of death and HF hospitalizations in patients who were prospectively randomized to receive medical therapy, resynchronized pacing, and defibrillation. CRT was delivered with and without defibrillator therapy to evaluate whether it had any additive benefits beyond the prevention of sudden cardiac death (SCD) through defibrillation. The trial included patients with NYHA class III and class IV HF on optimal medical therapy, LVEF ≤35%, QRS duration ≥120 ms, and no secondary prevention indication for ICD placement. Patients were randomized in a 1:2:2 ratio into 3 groups. The control group (n = 308) received optimal medical therapy only, group 2 (n = 617) received optimal medical therapy and CRT device without defibrillator capabilities, and group 3 (n = 595) received optimal medical therapy and a CRT device with ICD function.

There was significant (20%) decrease in all-cause mortality and all-cause hospitalizations in both CRT groups compared to the

control group. All-cause mortality alone was significantly reduced by 36% in patients receiving CRT with an ICD (P < 0.003) and trended toward a significant reduction of 24% in patients who received CRT alone (P = 0.06), when compared to the control group.

The COMPANION trial was the first to show survival benefits of combined CRT and defibrillator therapies. It also demonstrated that prophylactic ICD therapy would be beneficial in nonischemic cardiomyopathy before the SCD-HeFT trial, as nearly half of the randomized patients had a nonischemic etiology.

CARE-HF TRIAL

The COMPANION trial showed that CRT alone or in combination with defibrillator therapy would significantly reduce the risks of all-cause mortality and HF hospitalizations in patients with moderate to severe HF, reduced ejection fraction, and prolonged QRS. In order to clear any doubt in regards to the pure effect of CRT alone on the risk of death, the Cardiac Resynchronization Heart Failure (CARE-HF) trial[11,12] was designed. CARE-HF was a multicenter randomized unblended study aimed to evaluate the net effects of CRT without a defibrillator on the risk of death in advanced HF (NYHA class III and class IV). Inclusion criteria included ejection fractions ≤35% if QRS duration was ≥150 ms. If the QRS duration was between 120 and 150 ms, patients had to meet 2 of 3 additional echocardiographic criteria for dyssynchrony: interventricular mechanical delay >40 ms, aortic preejection delay >140 ms, or delayed posterolateral activation. Patients assigned to the control group (n = 404) received optimal medical therapy and those assigned to the treatment arm received CRT devices without defibrillation capabilities (n = 409). One of the unique aspects of CARE-HF is that control patients did not receive a device implant. This helped illustrate the effect of CRT as a whole, incorporating potential risks related to the implant at procedures.

Most enrolled patients were classified as NYHA class III HF (94%) and the majority (63%) of them had nonischemic etiologies of their HF. After an average follow-up of 29.4 months, a significant reduction of 37% (P < 0.001) in the primary endpoint (death from any cause or unplanned hospitalization for a major cardiac event) was found in the CRT group compared to the control group. All-cause mortality was also significantly reduced by 36% in the CRT group (P < 0.002). CARE-HF also showed that CRT significantly reduced all-cause mortality combined with HF hospitalization by 46% and HF hospitalization alone by 52%.

PROSPECT TRIAL

The Predictors of Response to Cardiac Resynchronization Therapy (PROSPECT) trial[13] was designed to address whether a variety of echocardiographic measures of LV mechanical dyssynchrony could predict CRT response. CRT response was defined as either clinical or echocardiographic improvement after 6 months of CRT. Clinical response was founded on a composite score of both subjective and objective measures, including HF hospitalization, HF mortality, improvement in NYHA class, and a patient global assessment score. Echocardiographic response was defined as a reduction in LV end-systolic volume of at least 15%. The study enrolled 426 patients meeting standard CRT indications with QRS ≥130 ms.

Overall, the study demonstrated very low predictive value to the 12 echocardiographic measures evaluated. Those parameters had a low sensitivity and specificity; therefore, the PROSPECT trial did not establish a role for echocardiographic dyssynchrony parameters in CRT patient selection beyond current guidelines.[14]

REVERSE TRIAL

CRT has well-established benefits in reducing HF morbidity and mortality in patients with moderate to severe HF. It was hypothesized that the effects of CRT will benefit milder forms of HF by delaying structural progression through reverse remodeling. The Resynchronization Reverses Remodeling in Systolic Left Ventricular Dysfunction (REVERSE) trial[15] was designed to test this hypothesis and address the benefit of CRT on HF morbidity in mild HF patients when compared to optimal medical therapy alone.

The study enrolled 610 patients with NYHA class I and class II HF, QRS ≥120 ms, LVEF ≤40%, and LVEDD ≥55 mm. All study patients received a CRT device ± ICD. ICD indication was based on class I or class II recommendations according to current guidelines. Among the study population, 191 patients were assigned to standard of care with optimal medical therapy (CRT off) and 419 patients were assigned to the CRT group (CRT on) combined with optimal medical therapy. The primary endpoint was the clinical composite HF score; "unchanged" and "improved" were considered beneficial responses to CRT.

At 12-month follow-up, the percentage with worsened HF scores was not significantly different in the CRT treatment group compared to the control (21% vs 16%, P = 0.10). However, a significant benefit of CRT was seen with improvement in ventricular structural remodeling and function parameters assessed by LV end-systolic volume index, LV end-diastolic volume index, and LV ejection fraction (P < 0.0001). HF morbidity was also significantly improved with a 53% relative risk reduction in the time to first HF hospitalization (HR 0.47, P = 0.03).

The most noticeable finding in the REVERSE trial is the reduction in nonfatal HF events in the prespecified group of patients with QRS ≥150 ms. It was also the first large randomized, multicenter trial to demonstrate a potential CRT effect on slowing the progression of HF through reverse remodeling in mild or asymptomatic HF patients.

MADIT-CRT TRIAL

The Multicenter Automatic Defibrillator Implantation Trial with Cardiac Resynchronization Therapy (MADIT-CRT) trial[16] was a multicenter, randomized clinical trial designed to address the potential effects of CRT in lowering the rate of death and nonfatal HF events in mild HF patients.

The trial randomized 1820 patients to CRT combined with an ICD, or ICD only, in patients with ejection fraction ≤30%, QRS ≥130 ms, and NYHA class I or class II HF (ischemic etiology in functional class I or II, or nonischemic in class II). The average follow-up was 2.4 years.

The rate of death or nonfatal HF events was significantly lowered by 34% (17.2% vs 25.2%, P = 0.001) in the CRT+ICD group compared to the ICD-only group. This was mostly driven by a 41% reduction in HF events. CRT was beneficial in both ischemic and nonischemic etiology; however, women with QRS ≥150 ms showed greater benefits than men.

MADIT-CRT is notable for showing that preventive CRT-ICD therapy can decrease the risk of HF events in both ischemic and nonischemic HF with milder symptoms and a wide QRS duration.

THE RAFT TRIAL

The Resynchronization-Defibrillation for Ambulatory Heart Failure Trial (RAFT)[17] was designed to determine if the addition of CRT to ICD on a background of optimal medical therapy would reduce the mortality and HF hospitalizations in patients with class II and III HF, reduced ejection fraction ≤30%, and wide QRS ≥120 ms. The study demonstrated significant (25%) relative risk reduction in all-cause mortality and hospitalizations for HF among those who received CRT-D compared to ICD alone. Notable for RAFT is that most study patients (80%) were in NYHA class II. The trial has many similarities to MADIT-CRT; however, RAFT enrolled patients with functional class II and III whereas MADIT-CRT enrolled patients in functional class I and II. RAFT had longer follow-up and a more traditional definition of HF and differed from MADIT-CRT in showing significant reduction in all-cause mortality.

RAFT, along with the MADIT-CRT and REVERSE trials, added to our understanding of the benefits of CRT in reducing morbidity and mortality in milder HF classes. These studies also expanded the indication of CRT to include NYHA class II according to the most recent guidelines.[14]

CARDIAC RESYNCHRONIZATION THERAPY DEVICE AND PROCEDURE COMPLICATIONS

The LV lead in the early trials was attached to the epicardium through a limited surgical procedure that required lateral thoracotomy under general anesthesia. This technique was suboptimal because epicardial placement was associated with higher capture thresholds, and because general anesthesia presents risks in this population, which tends to have several comorbidities.

Transvenous placement of the LV lead has replaced the epicardial technique in recent years. However, epicardial placement is still used in technically difficult transvenous cases and in patients with challenging anatomy that will not allow optimal targets. The transvenous technique involves obtaining access to a lateral or posterior branch of the coronary sinus via a technique that is similar to standard pacing or defibrillator lead placement (Figure 31-2).

Success rates for LV lead placement range from 88% to 95% in early clinical trials. As delivery catheter designs and cannulation techniques have evolved to address most technical challenges, most recent trials exhibited a success rate in excess of 95% (Figure 31-3).[12,15,16]

Challenges in cannulating the coronary sinus can be related to tortuosity of the coronary sinus itself or deformation of the ostium as a result of structural changes that take place in severe dilated cardiomyopathy. Deflectable electrophysiology catheters have been used to locate the coronary sinus ostium by voltage mapping. Using the over-the-wire technique has also helped in providing support for the lead to gain access to smaller and tortuous venous branches. There are several lead options that vary in the shape of their tips and sizes of their diameters; those are designed to provide the operator with alternatives to perfectly fit to any anatomical variant (Figure 31-4).

Specific to the CRT procedure, coronary sinus dissection or perforation is one of the most dreaded complications. It occurs in approximately 0.4% to 4% of patients during LV lead placement. It may result in cardiac tamponade and hemodynamic compromise. However, in most cases, it is self-limited and does not require any further intervention as most bleeding will be self-sealed due to the low-pressure system (Figure 31-5).

Other complications during CRT implantation are similar to those seen in standard dual-chamber pacemaker placement, such as bleeding, infection, lead dislodgement, device infection, pneumo-thorax, and pocket erosion.

LV lead dislodgment happens more often in cases where anatom-ical challenges were encountered, such as very tortuous coronary sinus anatomy forcing the operator to pass the lead in sharp angu-lations. Lead dislodgements are classified as macrodislodgement when they can be detected by post procedure chest x-rays, or as microdislodgements when leads appear at a stable location on chest x-rays but changes in capture thresholds are noted (Figure 31-6).

Phrenic nerve stimulation is another problem that is commonly seen during the implant procedure and needs to be addressed as it could be bothersome to patients. The phrenic nerve runs parallel to the lateral LV free wall, which is the same area desired for optimal LV lead placement. In some occasions, phrenic nerve stimulation can be absent during the implant but will later develop due to changes in body position. When facing this problem, several solu-tions can be used. One solution is changing the pacing configura-tion to one that secures adequate capture thresholds with enough safety margin that does not cause diaphragmatic stimulation. This has become much easier with the development of newer leads that are equipped with multiple pacing sites allowing numerous pacing configurations. In rare occasions when the problem persists despite exhausting all pacing configurations, lead repositioning will be the ultimate solution.

NONRESPONDERS TO CARDIAC RESYNCHRONIZATION THERAPY

It is estimated that one-fourth of patients receiving CRT devices do not exhibit any clinical or functional improvement. Those patients are defined as nonresponders.[18] Subgroup analysis of major clini-cal trials showed that female gender, nonischemic etiology of HF, prolonged QRS duration, and LBBB pattern are favored markers of CRT response (Figure 31-7).

Most major CRT trials enrolled patients based on electrical characterization of dyssynchrony defined by conduction delay; however, not all patients with prolonged QRS durations exhibit mechanical dyssynchrony on echocardiography. In one study[19] only 75% of HF patients with QRS >120 ms had tissue Doppler evidence of dyssynchrony. This mismatch between electrical and

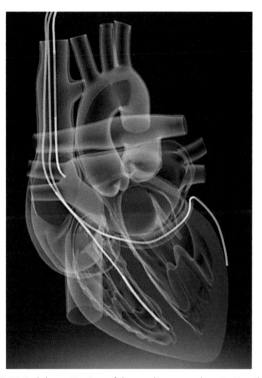

FIGURE 31-2 Schematic view of the cardiac resynchronization therapy (CRT) system in relation to major cardiac vascular structure. The left ventricular (LV) lead is extended through the coronary sinus (CS) to a lateral position. (Quartet, IsoFlex, Optim, ShockGuard, Unify Assura, and St. Jude Medical are trademarks of St. Jude Medical, Inc. or its related companies. Reprinted with permission of St. Jude Medical, © 2018. All rights reserved.)

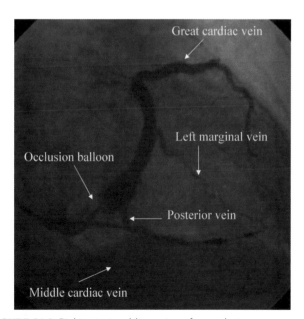

FIGURE 31-3 Right anterior oblique view of an occlusive venogram of the great cardiac vein and the other branches of the coronary sinus (left marginal vein, left posterior vein, and the middle cardiac vein). (Reproduced with permission from Fuster V, Walsh RA, Harrington RA. *Hurst's The Heart.* 13th ed. New York, NY: McGraw-Hill Education; 2011. Figure 43-17.)

mechanical dyssynchrony could explain the absence of response to CRT in nearly one-fourth of patients who meet the electrical criteria but lack associated mechanical dyssynchrony.

One of the main causes of lack of CRT response is suboptimal lead placement either in an area that is not dyssynchronous or placement in a nonlateral position. The anterior wall of the left ventricle is the site of early activation; therefore, placement of the LV lead at the anterior wall leads to further widening intraventricular dyssynchrony with subsequent worsening in hemodynamics.[20]

Maintaining a high percentage of biventricular pacing >95% is the key to ensuring benefit from the therapy. Absence of response or sudden deterioration in patients' symptoms after a period of response should alarm caring physicians to the possibility of significant reduction in biventricular pacing. Possible causes include elevation in ventricular capture thresholds, lead dislodgement, prolonged AV delay, atrial arrhythmias that are conducted rapidly to the ventricles, or frequent premature ventricular contractions.[21]

Other possible causes include LV lead placement at a site of diffuse scarring from prior cardiac injury. This could explain why patients with ischemic etiology of HF tend to be less responsive to CRT. Setting the AV and ventricular-ventricular (VV) timing too short or too long can compromise cardiac performance and could be a modifiable cause of CRT nonresponse. Factory settings of the AV delays are often short, in the 100 to 120 ms range, and this may reduce atrial contribution to LV filling. Most device manufacturers have developed a programmed algorithm installed in the device software, which can be turned on for automatic optimizing of AV and VV delay. Echocardiographic-based optimization is done in a clinic setting and often used in patients who remained nonresponsive to CRT after ruling out all other possibilities. In fact, individual optimization of pacing delays in CRT devices was reserved for nonresponders only, but data support its use in all CRT patients due to proven acute hemodynamic benefits (Figure 31-8).[22]

OPTIMIZATION OF ATRIOVENTRICULAR AND INTERVENTRICULAR DELAYS

The goal of AV and VV optimization is to adjust atrial-to-ventricular pacing and ventricular-to-ventricular pacing delays to optimal settings that ensure adequate cardiac filling and contractile efficacy. The optimal AV interval is decided by prolonging the duration of LV relaxation but yet allowing full atrial contribution. This interval is determined echocardiographically by recording the mitral inflow and assessing the E and A wave morphology. Optimal AV delay is the one that allows separation of these waves with the terminal portion of the A wave falling before the closure of the mitral valve. Adjustment of interventricular or VV delay can be done in the same manner. Optimal sequential ventricular activation can be achieved by changing the activation time of either the right or the left ventricle while measuring the aortic outflow velocity time integral (VTI) as a surrogate of cardiac output. VV delay can be set at the interval that allows the maximal VTI (Figures 31-9 and 31-10).

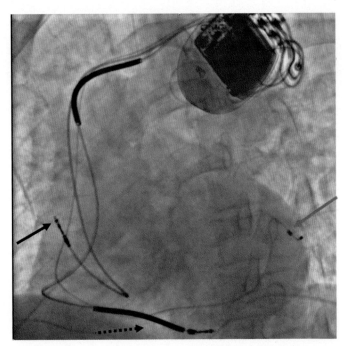

FIGURE 31-4 X-ray view of biventrocilar implantable cardioverter defibrillator (ICD) system and leads. *Red arrow* points to the tip of the left ventricle (LV) lead, *black arrow* points to tip of the atrial lead, *dashed black arrow* points to shocking coil of the right ventricle (RV) lead.

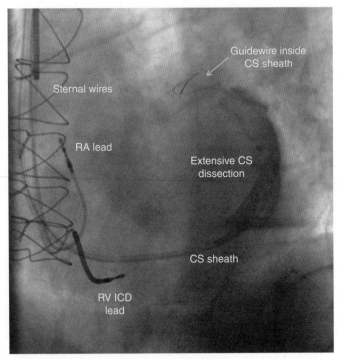

FIGURE 31-5 Coronary sinus lead dissection. Note the extravasation of contrast from the coronary sinus (CS) to the pericardial space.

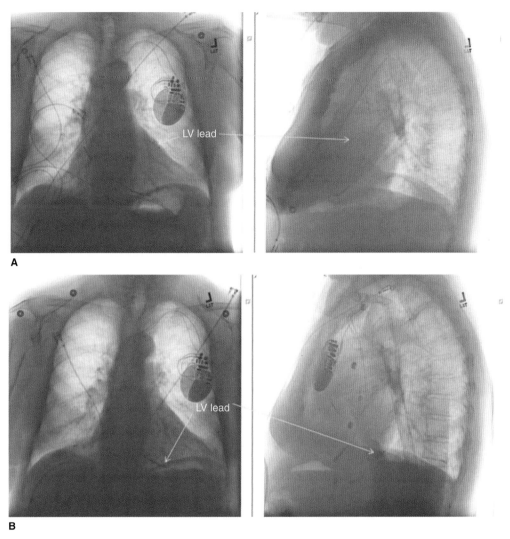

FIGURE 31-6 A. Posteroanterior (PA) and lateral x-rays in the immediate post device implant period. Note that the coronary sinus lead tip is located in an expected posterolateral branch. **B.** PA and lateral x-rays of the same patient 24 hours post device implant. Note coronary sinus lead has retracted proximally due to lead dislodgement.

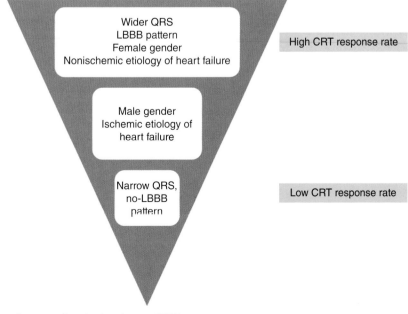

FIGURE 31-7 Predictors of cardiac resynchronization therapy (CRT) response.

RECOMMENDATIONS FOR CARDIAC RESYNCHRONIZATION THERAPY

Prior HF guidelines recommend CRT for patients with LVEF less than or equal to 35%, normal SR, and NYHA functional class III or ambulatory class IV symptoms despite recommended optimal medical therapy, who have ventricular dyssynchrony defined as QRS prolongation of at least 120 ms, unless contraindicated. After the release of the MADIT-CRT, REVERSE, and RAFT trials, which studied the benefit of CRT in milder HF, the ACCF/AHA guidelines[14] were updated to include patients with mild HF (class II) and QRS ≥150 ms (Figure 31-11).

CONTRAINDICATIONS TO CARDIAC RESYNCHRONIZATION THERAPY

CRT is not indicated in HF patients with NYHA functional class I and II with non-LBBB pattern and QRS duration less than 150 ms. It is also not recommended for patients with significant comorbidities and expected survival less than 1 year.

CARDIAC RESYNCHRONIZATION THERAPY IN SPECIFIC POPULATIONS

CARDIAC RESYNCHRONIZATION THERAPY WITH IMPLANTABLE CARDIOVERTER DEFIBRILLATOR

The combined use of CRT and ICD devices has been studied in several clinical trials (MIRACLE ICD, CONTAK-CD, and COMPANION). The current guidelines[14] recommend the use of combined devices in patients who meet the indications for both an ICD and a CRT device. The COMPANION trial results support the use of CRT-ICD device in ambulatory NYHA class IV patients.

CARDIAC RESYNCHRONIZATION THERAPY IN CHRONIC RIGHT VENTRICULAR PACING

Chronic RV pacing is known to negatively affect cardiac function and clinical outcomes in HF; furthermore, it can also provoke trial arrhythmias, which can further worsen cardiac hemodynamics.[23] Those deleterious effects are believed to be mediated by electrical and mechanical dyssynchrony. Over the past few decades, efforts have been made to maintain intrinsic conduction as much as possible in the treatment of bradyarrhythmias, and all device manufacturers have developed programmable features designed to minimize RV pacing. However, circumstances still exist when patients are dependent on RV pacing for the maintenance of adequate heart rate. Because CRT is capable of providing more physiological conduction to both ventricles than RV pacing alone, CRT was hypothesized to be a superior pacing modality in patients with reduced ejection fraction who are expected to be pacer-dependent, and do not, otherwise, have conventional indications for CRT. The Block-HF trial[24] was designed to test this hypothesis and included 691 patients with class I or IIa indications for pacemaker placement including high-grade AV block, permanent arrhythmias, and intrinsic AV block, or those undergoing AV nodal ablation. Patients received biventricular pacers and were randomized to either CRT

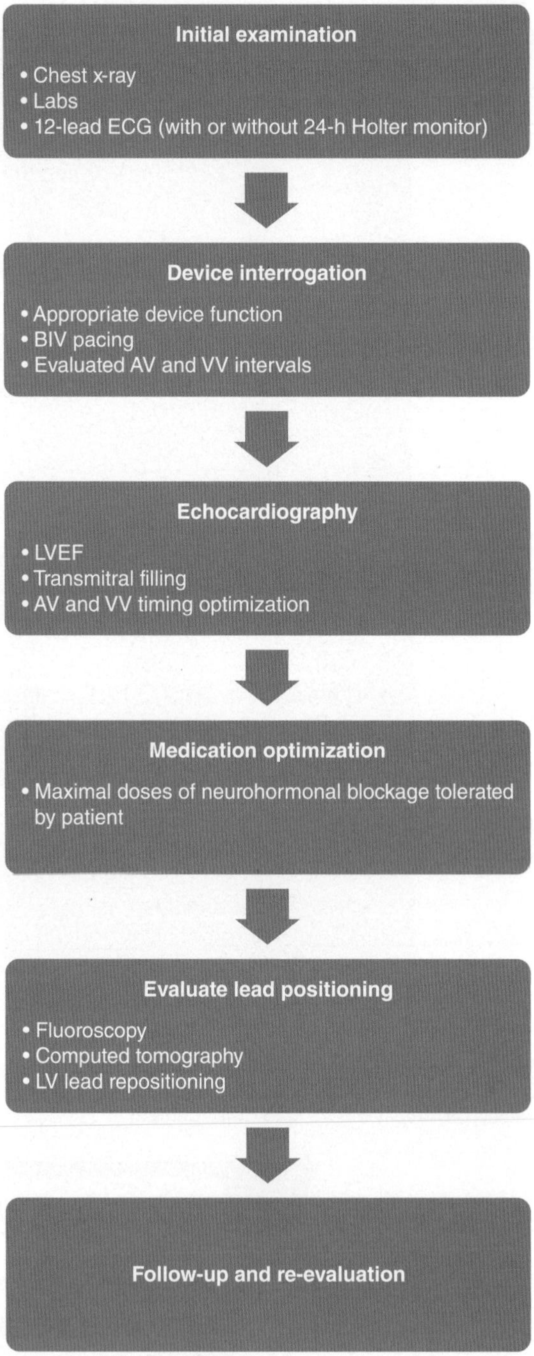

Initial examination
- Chest x-ray
- Labs
- 12-lead ECG (with or without 24-h Holter monitor)

↓

Device interrogation
- Appropriate device function
- BIV pacing
- Evaluated AV and VV intervals

↓

Echocardiography
- LVEF
- Transmitral filling
- AV and VV timing optimization

↓

Medication optimization
- Maximal doses of neurohormonal blockage tolerated by patient

↓

Evaluate lead positioning
- Fluoroscopy
- Computed tomography
- LV lead repositioning

↓

Follow-up and re-evaluation

FIGURE 31-8 Stepwise approach to CRT nonresponse. Abbreviations: AV, atrioventricular; BIV, biventricular; CRT, cardiac resynchronization therapy; ECG, electrocardiogram; LV, left ventricle; LVEF, left ventricular ejection fraction; VV, ventricular-ventricular.

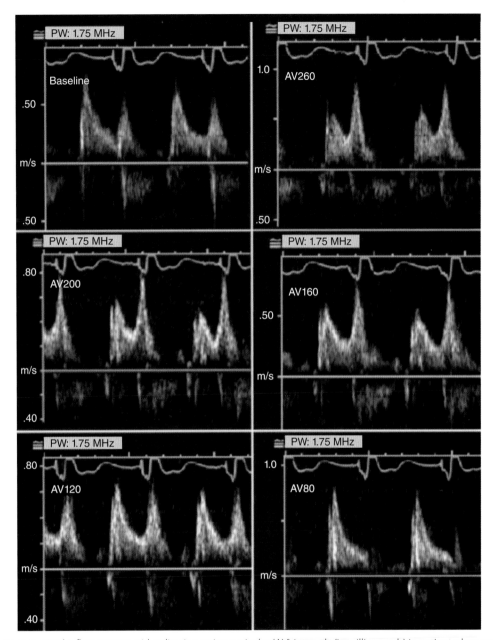

FIGURE 31-9 Variations in mitral inflow pattern with adjusting atrioventricular (AV) intervals (in milliseconds) in patient who received cardiac resynchronization therapy (CRT) device. (Reproduced with permission from Kumbala D, Jacob S, Kamalesh M, et al. *Indian Pacing Electrophysiol J.* 2008 Jul-Sep;8(3):218-221.)

or RV pacing. The study showed significant reduction in time to first death from any cause, decreased urgent care visits for HF, and less worsening in LV dimension defined by increase in LV end-systolic volume by 15%. The study was published after the most recent update to the ACCF/AHA guidelines.[14] However, the guidelines did indicate that CRT may be useful in patients who have LVEF of 35% or less and are undergoing placement of a new device or replacement device with anticipated >40% ventricular pacing.

CARDIAC RESYNCHRONIZATION THERAPY AND NON-LEFT BUNDLE-BRANCH BLOCKADE

In patients with non-LBBB pattern, CRT can be useful for those in NSR, those with LVEF of 35% or less, those with QRS duration of

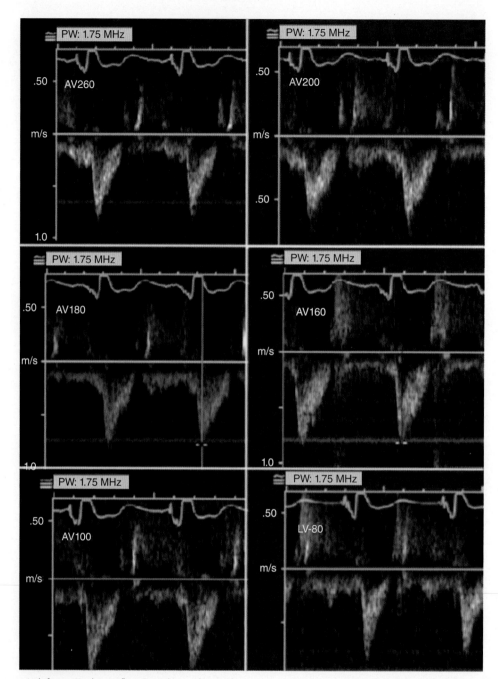

FIGURE 31-10 Change in left ventricular outflow Doppler profiles with changing atrioventricular (AV) intervals (in milliseconds) in patient who received cardiac resynchronization therapy (CRT) device. (Reproduced with permission from Kumbala D, Jacob S, Kamalesh M, et al. *Indian Pacing Electrophysiol J.* 2008 Jul-Sep;8(3):218-221.)

150 ms or greater, and those with NYHA class III and IV symptoms. CRT may be considered if QRS duration is between 120 and 149 ms.

CARDIAC RESYNCHRONIZATION THERAPY AND ATRIAL FIBRILLATION

CRT can be useful in patients with atrial fibrillation, and LVEF ≤35% if (1) they require ventricular pacing or otherwise meet CRT criteria, and (2) AV nodal ablation or pharmacological rate control will permit 100% vernacular pacing with CRT.

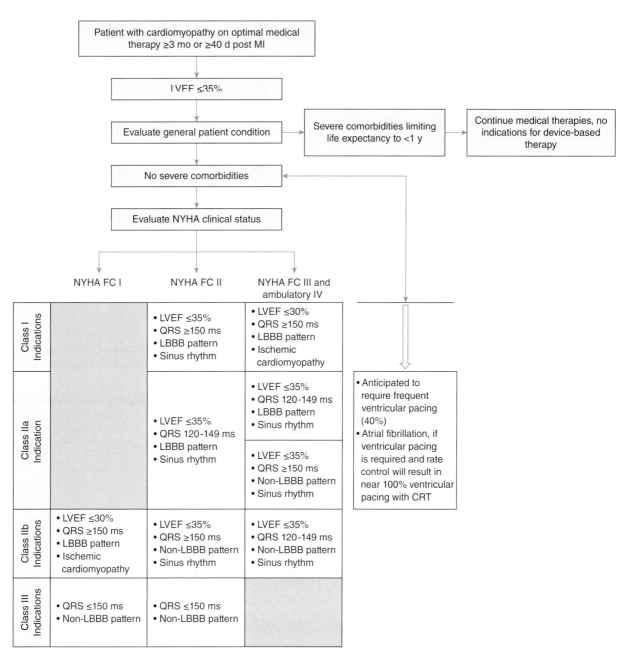

FIGURE 31-11 Indications of cardiac resynchronization therapy. Abbreviations: CRT, cardiac resynchronization therapy; LBBB, left bundle-branch blockade; LVEF, left ventricular ejection fraction; MI, myocardial infarction.

PROVIDER RESOURCES

2012 ACCF/AHA/HRS Focused Update of the 2008 Guidelines for Device-Based Therapy of Cardiac Rhythm Abnormalities. A Report of the American College of Cardiology Foundation/American Heart Association Task Force on Practice Guidelines and the Heart Rhythm Society: http://circ.ahajournals.org/content/126/14/1784.long

2013 ACCF/AHA Guideline for the Management of Heart Failure: Executive Summary. A Report of the American College of Cardiology Foundation/American Heart Association Task Force on Practice Guidelines: http://circ.ahajournals.org/content/128/16/1810.full

The Heart Rhythm Society (HRS)/American Society of Anesthesiologists (ASA) Expert Consensus Statement on the perioperative management of patients with implantable defibrillators, pacemakers and arrhythmia monitors: facilities and patient management. This document was developed as a joint project with the American Society of Anesthesiologists (ASA), and in collaboration with the American Heart Association (AHA), and the Society of Thoracic Surgeons (STS). *Heart Rhythm*. 2011;8:1114-1154. http://www.heartrhythmjournal.com/article/S1547-5271%2811%2900584-4/abstract

REFERENCES

1. Auricchio A, Abraham WT. Cardiac resynchronization therapy: current state of the art: cost versus benefit. *Circulation*. 2004;109:300-307.

2. Auricchio A, Stellbrink C, Block M, et al. Effect of pacing chamber and atrioventricular delay on acute systolic function of paced patients with congestive heart failure. The Pacing Therapies for Congestive Heart Failure Study Group. The Guidant Congestive Heart Failure Research Group. *Circulation*. 1999;99:2993-3001.

3. St John Sutton MG, Plappert T, Abraham WT, et al. Effect of cardiac resynchronization therapy on left ventricular size and function in chronic heart failure. *Circulation*. 2003;107:1985-1990.

4. Yu CM, Chau E, Sanderson JE, et al. Tissue Doppler echocardiographic evidence of reverse remodeling and improved synchronicity by simultaneously delaying regional contraction after biventricular pacing therapy in heart failure. *Circulation*. 2002;105:438-445.

5. Auricchio A, Stellbrink C, Sack S, et al. The Pacing Therapies for Congestive Heart Failure (PATH-CHF) study: rationale, design, and endpoints of a prospective randomized multicenter study. *Am J Cardiol*. 1999;83:130D-135D.

6. Cazeau S, Leclercq C, Lavergne T, et al. Effects of multisite biventricular pacing in patients with heart failure and intraventricular conduction delay. *N Engl J Med*. 2001;344:873-880.

7. Abraham WT. Rationale and design of a randomized clinical trial to assess the safety and efficacy of cardiac resynchronization therapy in patients with advanced heart failure: the Multicenter InSync Randomized Clinical Evaluation (MIRACLE). *J Card Fail*. 2000;6:369-380.

8. Abraham WT, Fisher WG, Smith AL, et al. Cardiac resynchronization in chronic heart failure. *New Engl J Med*. 2002;346:1845-1853.

9. Young JB, Abraham WT, Smith AL, et al. Combined cardiac resynchronization and implantable cardioversion defibrillation in advanced chronic heart failure: the MIRACLE ICD Trial. *JAMA*. 2003;289:2685-2694.

10. Bristow MR, Feldman AM, Saxon LA. Heart failure management using implantable devices for ventricular resynchronization: Comparison of Medical Therapy, Pacing, and Defibrillation in Chronic Heart Failure (COMPANION) trial. COMPANION Steering Committee and COMPANION Clinical Investigators. *J Card Fail*. 2000;6:276-285.

11. Cleland JG, Daubert JC, Erdmann E, et al. The CARE-HF study (CArdiac REsynchronisation in Heart Failure study): rationale, design and end-points. *Eur J Heart Fail*. 2001;3:481-489.

12. Cleland JG, Daubert JC, Erdmann E, et al. The effect of cardiac resynchronization on morbidity and mortality in heart failure. *N Engl J Med*. 2005;352:1539-1549.

13. Chung ES, Leon AR, Tavazzi L, et al. Results of the Predictors of Response to CRT (PROSPECT) trial. *Circulation*. 2008;117:2608-2616.

14. Yancy CW, Jessup M, Bozkurt B, et al. 2013 ACCF/AHA guideline for the management of heart failure: executive summary: a report of the American College of Cardiology Foundation/American Heart Association Task Force on practice guidelines. *Circulation*. 2013;128:1810-1852.

15. Linde C, Abraham WT, Gold MR, et al. Randomized trial of cardiac resynchronization in mildly symptomatic heart failure patients and in asymptomatic patients with left ventricular dysfunction and previous heart failure symptoms. *J Am Coll Cardiol*. 2008;52:1834-1843.

16. Moss AJ, Hall WJ, Cannom DS, et al. Cardiac-resynchronization therapy for the prevention of heart-failure events. *N Engl J Med*. 2009;361:1329-1338.

17. Tang AS, Wells GA, Talajic M, et al. Cardiac-resynchronization therapy for mild-to-moderate heart failure. *N Engl J Med*. 2010;363:2385-2395.

18. Fox DJ, Fitzpatrick AP, Davidson NC. Optimisation of cardiac resynchronisation therapy: addressing the problem of "non-responders." *Heart*. 2005;91:1000-1002.

19. Yu CM, Lin H, Zhang Q, Sanderson JE. High prevalence of left ventricular systolic and diastolic asynchrony in patients with congestive heart failure and normal QRS duration. *Heart*. 2003;89:54-60.

20. Butter C, Auricchio A, Stellbrink C, et al. Effect of resynchronization therapy stimulation site on the systolic function of heart failure patients. *Circulation*. 2001;104:3026-3029.

21. Wang P, Kramer A, Estes NA 3rd, Hayes DL. Timing cycles for biventricular pacing. *Pacing Clin Electrophysiol*. 2002;25:62-75.

22. Porciani MC, Dondina C, Macioce R, et al. Echocardiographic examination of atrioventricular and interventricular delay optimization in cardiac resynchronization therapy. *Am J Cardiol*. 2005;95:1108-1110.

23. Sweeney MO, Hellkamp AS, Ellenbogen KA, et al. Adverse effect of ventricular pacing on heart failure and atrial fibrillation among patients with normal baseline QRS duration in a clinical trial of pacemaker therapy for sinus node dysfunction. *Circulation*. 2003;107:2932-2937.

24. Curtis AB, Worley SJ, Adamson PB, et al. Biventricular pacing for atrioventricular block and systolic dysfunction. *N Engl J Med*. 2013;368:1585-1593.

32 PERCUTANEOUS VENTRICULAR SUPPORT FOR ACUTE HEART FAILURE

Akira Wada, MD
Scott M. Lilly, MD, PhD

INTRODUCTION

The use of mechanical support in acute left ventricular failure can provide temporary circulatory support and is most commonly utilized in the setting of acute myocardial infarction (MI) complicated by cardiogenic shock. The main purpose of a ventricular assist device (VAD) is to unload the failing heart and maintain circulation to vital organs. These devices were initially developed to serve as temporary support to allow the heart to recover or as a bridge to transplant. Currently there are 3 types of FDA-approved percutaneous VADs that can be categorized as follows:

- Counterpulsation devices (intra-aortic balloon pump)
- Left ventricular assist devices (Impella and TandemHeart)

INTRA-AORTIC BALLOON PUMP

The intra-aortic balloon pump (IABP) was developed in the 1960s as a relatively simple and quick system to provide left ventricular assistance (Figure 32-1). The IABP is a catheter-based system that can be placed at the bedside or in the catheterization laboratory. It consists of a polyethylene balloon mounted on a catheter that is placed in the descending aorta. It is typically inserted percutaneously from the femoral artery with the distal tip positioned 2 to 3 cm from the left subclavian artery. The balloon is inflated with helium and deflated in a 1:1 ratio with the cardiac cycle, though lower ratios (1:2, 1:3, 1:4) are frequently employed during weaning and prior to IABP removal. Inflation of the balloon can be triggered by the electrocardiogram (ECG), systolic upstroke, or a pacemaker spike. Because the timing of balloon inflation and deflation is dependent on the cardiac cycle, tachycardia and irregular rhythms such as atrial fibrillation can cause less than ideal augmentation.

The balloon is inflated at the start of diastole, which augments diastolic pressure and improves coronary blood flow. The balloon deflates just prior to the onset of systole, reducing central aortic pressure and consequently early afterload on the left ventricle (Figure 32-2). The 4 main effects of the IABP are:

1. increase in aortic flow,
2. reduction of systolic left ventricular pressure due to phasic deflation of the balloon,

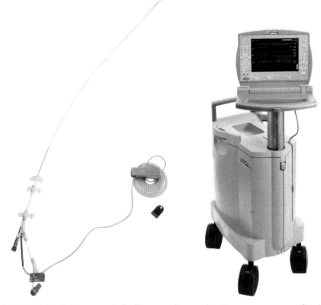

FIGURE 32-1 Intra-aortic balloon and console. (Image courtesy of Teleflex Incorporated. © 2018 Teleflex Incorporated. All rights reserved.)

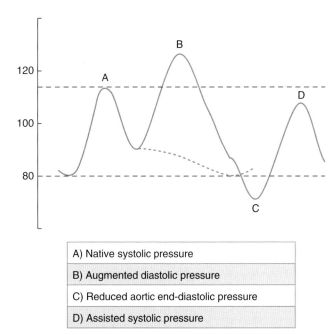

| A) Native systolic pressure |
| B) Augmented diastolic pressure |
| C) Reduced aortic end-diastolic pressure |
| D) Assisted systolic pressure |

FIGURE 32-2 IABP waveform demonstrating both native (unassisted) and assisted systolic pressures. Note the augmentation in diastolic pressure corresponding to balloon inflation as well as the decrease in the end-diastolic pressure.

Table 32-1 Contraindications and Potential Complications Associated with Percutaneous Ventricular Assist Devices

	Contraindications	Potential Complications
Intra-aortic balloon pump	• Severe aortic valve insufficiency • Abdominal/aortic aneurysm • Aortic dissection • Severe calcific aortoiliac disease	• Injury to an atherosclerotic aortoiliac arterial segment • Arterial dissection • Limb ischemia • Anemia and thrombocytopenia
Impella	• Mechanical aortic valve • Aortic valve stenosis/calcification (aortic valves are of 1.5 cm^2 or less) • Severe calcific aortoiliac disease	• Aortic insufficiency • Aortic valve injury • Arrhythmia • Bleeding • Hemolysis and thrombocytopenia • Perforation • Vascular injury • Thrombotic vascular complication
TandemHeart	• Severe aortic valve insufficiency • Aortic dissection • Severe calcific aortoiliac disease • Bleeding diathesis	• Bleeding • Dislodgement of the cannula • Femoral arteriovenous fistula • Thromboembolism • Atrial-septal defect (ASD) • Limb ischemia

3. diastolic aortic pressure augmentation, and

4. increase in coronary flow due to inflation of the balloon.

The combined augmentation of diastolic coronary filling and reduction in ventricular afterload with IABP results in decreased ventricular end diastolic pressure, reduced systemic vascular resistance, and increased cardiac output in both ischemic and nonischemic heart failure (HF).[1]

Current indications for IABP placement include cardiogenic shock due to acute MI, intractable angina, acute mitral regurgitation, and adjunctive therapy in high-risk percutaneous coronary angioplasty (Table 32-1). It also has favorable hemodynamic effects among those with decompensated HF from a nonischemic etiology, also has favorable hemodynamic effects among those with decompensated HF from a nonischemic etiology.

There have been several randomized trials that address the efficacy of IABP support. The largest of these is IABP-SHOCK II. In this trial, patients with acute MI complicated by cardiogenic shock were randomized to IABP support or standard care. At 30 days, there was no difference in the rate of all-cause mortality, although

IABP use was not associated with increased bleeding or vascular complications.[2]

After placement of an IABP, anemia is common and thrombocytopenia is nearly universal due to the mechanical hemolysis. Due to the thrombogenic nature of the catheter system, patients are frequently anticoagulated with heparin, particularly when the augmentation ratio is less than 1:1. In a small randomized trial comparing the use of heparin and no heparin in patients requiring IABP, there was no significant difference in the incidence of limb ischemia; however, the incidence of bleeding was significantly increased (14.1% vs 2.4%) in the heparinized group.[3]

IMPELLA AND TANDEM HEART

Percutaneous continuous-flow VADs have been developed for use in patients who require acute circulatory support. These continuous-flow left ventricular assist devices can support either the right ventricle (RVAD), left ventricle (LVAD), or both (BiVAD). The initial pumps were pulsatile and used positive displacement to provide circulation, similar to the action of the heart. Currently, continuous-flow VADs are more widely utilized due to their small size and proven durability. The principle behind these devices is based on centrifugal or axial flow. Electromagnets are used to provide propulsion to a central rotor that in turn accelerates blood through a cylindrical outflow cannula.

Paracorporeal VADs, such as the Impella 2.5 or Impella CP from Abiomed, function as an axial flow pump. The Impella is typically inserted percutaneously via the femoral artery into the ascending aorta. The distal end of the device is passed through the aortic valve and positioned into the left ventricle. The spiral-shaped cannula is 12F with a 45° angle to contour the left ventricular outflow tract and ascending aorta. The cannula is attached to an encapsulated motor. The Impella motor draws blood out of the ventricle and passes it into the proximal port, which resides in the ascending aorta. The Impella 2.5 can provide up to 4 L/min of flow at peak output (Figure 32-3).

Currently the Impella 2.5 is indicated for partial circulatory support for periods up to 6 hours (Figure 32-3). It can also be used as hemodynamic support during procedures such as high-risk percutaneous coronary angioplasty or complex ablation of ventricular tachyarrhythmias. O'Neill et al (2013) showed that in patients with cardiogenic shock complicating acute MI, initiation of mechanical circulatory support with an Impella 2.5 prior to percutaneous coronary intervention (pre-PCI) compared to post-PCI was associated with a better survival to discharge compared to patients in the post-PCI group (65.1% vs 40.7%, P = 0.003).[4]

The TandemHeart is a percutaneous ventricular assist device (pVAD) developed by CardiacAssist (Figure 32-4). This extracorporeal device is generally inserted in the catheterization laboratory under fluoroscopic and/or ECG guidance. Access is obtained via

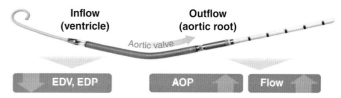

FIGURE 32-3 Impella percutaneous continuous-flow ventricular assist device. (Used with permission from ABIOMED Inc.; Danvers, MA.)

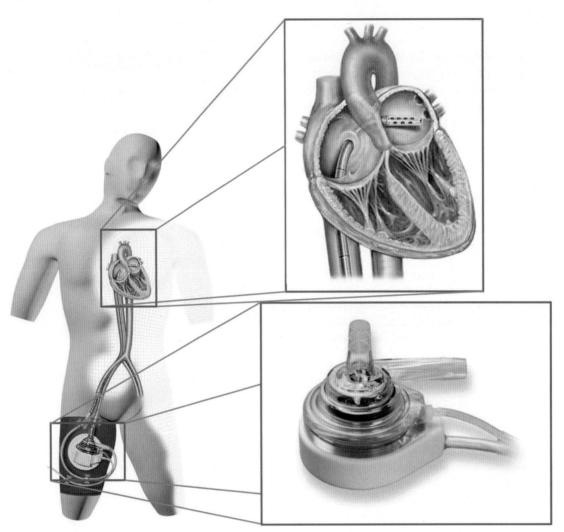

FIGURE 32-4 TandemHeart extracorporeal continuous-flow centrifugal assist device. (Image used with permission from CardiacAssist, Inc. (CAI). © 2018 Tandem Life.)

the femoral vein and a transseptal puncture is performed. The 21F inflow cannula is placed in the left atrium and intravenous heparin is administered. A 15F to 17F outflow cannula is inserted into the femoral artery with the distal tip at the level of the aortic bifurcation. Both cannulas are joined at the pump, and the TandemHeart can provide flows between 4 and 5 L/min.

The TandemHeart can be used in several clinical indications, such as acute HFe and complex percutaneous coronary intervention, and has been employed in emergent and in post-arrest settings. The device is designed to both augment the flow of oxygenated blood as well as to decompress the left ventricle, therefore reducing the workload of the heart. Kar et al (2010) evaluated the use of the TandemHeart in 117 patients in cases of severe refractory cardiogenic shock.[5] These patients, with both ischemic and nonischemic cardiomyopathy, remained in refractory shock despite the use of IABP counterpulsation as well as pharmacological hemodynamic support. After implantation, the cardiac index increased from 0.52 L/min·m^2 to 3.0 L/min·m^2 (p < 0.001).

REFERENCES

1. Feola M, Adachi M, Akers WW, Ross JN Jr, Wieting DW, Kennedy JH. Intraaortic balloon pumping in the experimental animal. Effects and problems. *Am J Cardiol.* 1971;27(2):129-36.

2. Thiele H, Schuler G, Neumann FJ, Hausleiter J, Olbrich HG, Schwarz B, et al. Intraaortic balloon counterpulsation in acute myocardial infarction complicated by cardiogenic shock: design and rationale of the Intraaortic Balloon Pump in Cardiogenic Shock II (IABP-SHOCK II) trial. *Am Heart J.* 2012;163(6):938-45. doi: 10.1016/j.ahj.2012.03.012. Erratum in: *Am Heart J.* 2015;169(1):185.

3. Jiang CY, Zhao LL, Wang JA, Mohammod B. Anticoagulation therapy in intra-aortic balloon counterpulsation: does IABP really need anti-coagulation? *J Zhejiang Univ Sci.* 2003;4(5):607-11.

4. O'Neill WW, Schreiber T, Wohns DH, Rihal C, Naidu SS, Civitello AB, et al. The current use of Impella 2.5 in acute myocardial infarction complicated by cardiogenic shock: results from the USpella Registry. *J Interv Cardiol.* 2014;27(1):1-11. doi: 10.1111/joic.12080. Epub 2013 Dec 13.

5. Kar B, Gregoric ID, Basra SS, Idelchik GM, Loyalka P. The percutaneous ventricular assist device in severe refractory cardiogenic shock. *J Am Coll Cardiol.* 2011;57(6):688-96. doi: 10.1016/j.jacc.2010.08.613. Epub 2010 Oct 14.

33 ULTRAFILTRATION IN HEART FAILURE

Sitaramesh Emani, MD
Maria Rosa Costanzo, MD, FAHA, FACC, FESC

PATIENT CASE

A 61-year-old man with a history of heart failure with reduced ejection fraction (HFrEF) from underlying coronary artery disease (CAD) presents with increasing symptoms of congestion and volume overload. He has a history of difficult-to-maintain volume status requiring high doses of diuretics as an outpatient. Despite increasing his baseline diuretic dosing at home, his symptoms progress and he is admitted for additional therapy. In the setting of high diuretic requirements, he is felt to have diuretic resistance. Instead of initiating therapy with extremely high doses of intravenous loop diuretics, ultrafiltration is initiated for volume management. The patient undergoes successful ultrafiltration over the next few days with return to his baseline volume status. He is subsequently discharged on a standard diuretic regimen with resolution of his symptoms.

EPIDEMIOLOGY

Despite many advances in the therapy of heart failure (HF), hospitalization for worsening HF still accounts for a significant portion of total hospital admissions in the United States. Additionally, rehospitalization after an index HF hospitalization remains a significant challenge in the treatment of HF.[1,2] The risk of rehospitalization is significantly higher when inadequate volume removal occurs during a hospital stay, with up to 50% of patients having little or no weight loss during inpatient treatment.[3,4] Therefore, effective strategies to completely decongest patients are crucial to appropriate HF management.

DIURETIC RESISTANCE

Diuretic resistance occurs when a decrease in diuresis and natriuresis to medical therapy is observed, and is estimated to occur in 25% to 30% of patients with HF.[5] Although variable definitions of diuretic resistance have been proposed, the common themes among criteria are inadequate augmentation of total urine output, urine sodium excretion, weight loss, or symptom relief to large doses of loop diuretics.[6] Although incompletely understood, diuretic resistance may occur either from renal tubular hypertrophy following long-term exposure to loop diuretics or a decreased response to diuretics after the administration of an initial dose (Figure 33-1).[7] The latter phenomenon is likely driven by neurohormonal activation (Figure 33-2), which can lead to a worsening feedback loop in the treatment of HF (Figure 33-3).[8] The use of ultrafiltration allows volume removal without the use of diuretics, and therefore can bypass diuretic resistance and the feedback loop.

ULTRAFILTRATION[9,10]

An ultrafiltration circuit passes blood through an extracorporeal semipermeable membrane that allows passage of plasma water from whole blood in response to transmembrane pressure gradient. The setup of the semipermeable membrane allows for the following features:

- The ultrafiltrate fluid produced is isotonic plasma (in comparison, diuresis from loop diuretics is hypotonic to plasma).
- Ultrafiltration removes more sodium than diuretic therapy.
- Ultrafiltration does not induce electrolyte disturbances (such as hypokalemia seen with diuresis).
- Ultrafiltration has no direct neurohormonal activation.

Two contemporary ultrafiltration circuits are available, and are schematically shown in Figure 33-4.[11]

EFFICACY

Several trials have demonstrated the utility and benefits of ultrafiltration in the treatment of HF. Selected trial results are as follows:

- The EUPHORIA trial showed the use of ultrafiltration prior to IV diuretic use decreased length of stay and readmission for HF for a small group of patients.[12]
- The larger UNLOAD trial showed early ultrafiltration produced greater weight and fluid loss compared to IV diuretics. Additionally, improvements were noted in early rehospitalization rates in patients treated with ultrafiltration. A decreased need for maintenance diuretic dosing was also suggested in patients who received a "diuretic holiday" by undergoing ultrafiltration.[13]
- The CUORE study showed sustained benefits of adjustable rate ultrafiltration through 1 year when used in conjunction with loop diuretics.[14]
- The AVOID-HF trial suggested a greater freedom from a recurrent HF event through 90-days post ultrafiltration, but with an additional risk for ultrafiltration-related adverse events.[15]

Some studies, however, have suggested safety concerns with the use of ultrafiltration. The CARRESS-HF trial results suggested the potential for worsening renal function with ultrafiltration compared to IV diuretic use.[16] In this particular trial, ultrafiltration was conducted at a fixed rate of volume removal, in comparison to medical therapy that was adjusted based on clinical response. In trials that

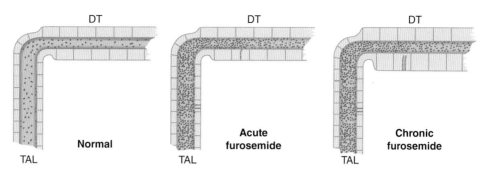

FIGURE 33-1 Mechanisms of diuretic resistance: acute furosemide exposure may cause a diminished response to subsequent doses without changes within the tubule, whereas chronic furosemide exposure leads to distal tubule hypertrophy. Abbreviations: TAL, thick ascending limb; DT, distal tubule.

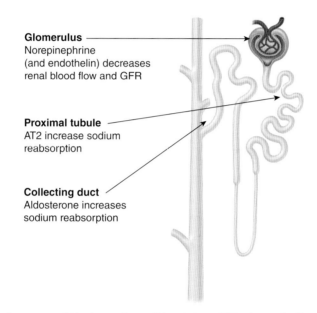

FIGURE 33-2 Effects of elevated neurohormones within the nephron. Abbreviations: GFR, glomerular filtration rate; AT2, angiotensin II.

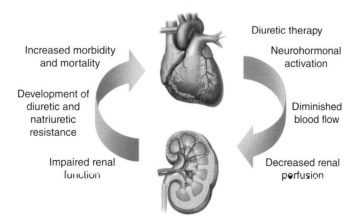

FIGURE 33-3 Negative feedback due to diuretic resistance.

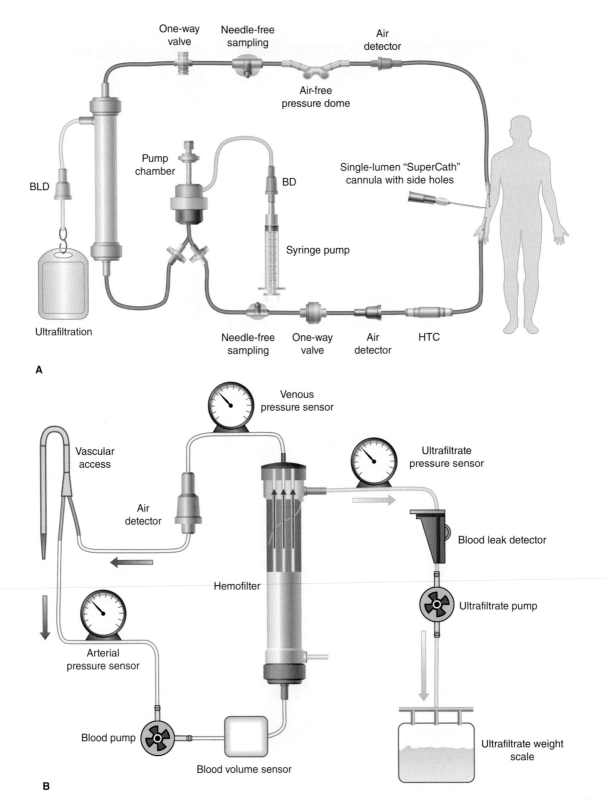

FIGURE 33-4 Contemporary ultrafiltration devices. **A.** The CHIARA device. **B.** The Aquadex System 100. Abbreviations: BLD, Blood Leak Detector; BD, Blood Detector; HTC, hematocrit sensor. (Reproduced with permission from Costanzo MR, Ronco C, Abraham WT, et al. Extracorporeal ultrafiltration for fluid overload in heart failure: current status and prospects for further research. *J Am Coll Cardiol.* 2017;69:2428-2445.)

have shown efficacy, such as CUORE and AVOID-HF, ultrafiltration rates were adjustable based on clinical parameters.

The difference in ultrafiltration rate selection is one of several current unknowns concerning clinical application of extracorporeal volume removal. Others include patient selection, timing of initiation, duration of therapy, and concurrent use of diuretics with ultrafiltration. At present, guidelines endorse the use of ultrafiltration as a method for decongestion, particularly in patients not responding to medical therapy.[17]

SUMMARY

Ultrafiltration is an option to treat acute HF with volume overload. Physiologic benefits exist with the use of ultrafiltration, including decreased activation of neurohormonal factors and bypassing diuretic resistance. Such factors may account for lasting benefits that occur with use of ultrafiltration. Benefits of ultrafiltration should be balanced against the potential for adverse events, including worsening renal function, particularly without rate adjustments. Careful monitoring of patients and thoughtful consideration to ultrafiltration removal rates can potentially reduce adverse events. Ultrafiltration should be considered an option to treat HF patients, particularly when managed by experienced HF teams.

REFERENCES

1. Mozaffarian D, Benjamin EJ, Go AS, et al. Executive summary: Heart disease and stroke statistics—2016 update: a report from the American Heart Association. *Circulation.* 2016;133:447-454.

2. Jencks SF, Williams MV, Coleman EA. Rehospitalizations among patients in the Medicare fee-for-service program. *N Engl J Med.* 2009;360:1418-1428.

3. Jain P, Massie BM, Gattis WA, Klein L, Gheorghiade M. Current medical treatment for the exacerbation of chronic heart failure resulting in hospitalization. *Am Heart J.* 2003;145:S3-S17.

4. Fonarow GC, Horwich TB. Prevention of heart failure: effective strategies to combat the growing epidemic. *Rev Cardiovasc Med.* 2003;4:8-17.

5. Ellison DH. Diuretic therapy and resistance in congestive heart failure. *Cardiology.* 2001;96:132-143.

6. ter Maaten JM, Valente MA, Damman K, Hillege HL, Navis G, Voors AA. Diuretic response in acute heart failure-pathophysiology, evaluation, and therapy. *Nat Rev Cardiol.* 2015;12:184-192.

7. Brater DC. Diuretic therapy. *N Engl J Med.* 1998;339:387-395.

8. Kramer BK, Schweda F, Riegger GA. Diuretic treatment and diuretic resistance in heart failure. *Am J Med.* 1999;106:90-96.

9. Ronco C, Ricci Z, Bellomo R, et al. A novel approach to the treatment of chronic fluid overload with a new plasma separation device. *Cardiology.* 2001;96:202-208.

10. Schrier RW. Role of diminished renal function in cardiovascular mortality: marker or pathogenetic factor? *J Am Coll Cardiol.* 2006;47:1-8.

11. Costanzo MR, Ronco C, Abraham WT, et al. Extracorporeal ultrafiltration for fluid overload in heart failure: current status and prospects for further research. *J Am Coll Cardiol.* 2017;69:2428-2445.

12. Costanzo MR, Saltzberg M, O'Sullivan J, Sobotka P. Early ultrafiltration in patients with decompensated heart failure and diuretic resistance. *J Am Coll Cardiol.* 2005;46:2047-2051.

13. Costanzo MR, Guglin ME, Saltzberg MT, et al. Ultrafiltration versus intravenous diuretics for patients hospitalized for acute decompensated heart failure. *J Am Coll Cardiol.* 2007;49:675-683.

14. Marenzi G, Muratori M, Cosentino ER, et al. Continuous ultrafiltration for congestive heart failure: the CUORE trial. *J Card Fail.* 2014;20(1):9-17.

15. Costanzo MR, Negoianu D, Jaski BE, et al. Aquapheresis versus intravenous diuretics and hospitalizations for heart failure. *JACC Heart Failure.* 2016;4:95-105.

16. Bart BA, Goldsmith SR, Lee KL, et al. Ultrafiltration in decompensated heart failure with cardiorenal syndrome. *N Engl J Med.* 2012;367:2296-2304.

17. Yancy CW, Jessup M, Bozkurt B, et al. 2013 ACCF/AHA guideline for the management of heart failure: a report of the American College of Cardiology Foundation/American Heart Association Task Force on Practice Guidelines. *J Am Coll Cardiol.* 2013;62:e147-e239.

34 INOTROPIC THERAPY IN HEART FAILURE

Randal Goldberg, MD
Shaline Rao, MD
Alexander Reyentovich, MD

▓ PATIENT CASE

A 63-year-old female with a history of diabetes, prior myocardial infarction, and an ischemic cardiomyopathy with a left ventricular ejection fraction of 35% presents to the emergency department with shortness of breath with minimal exertion, as well as three pillow orthopnea, and paroxysmal nocturnal dyspnea. Six months prior to presentation, she was able to walk 3-blocks which has progressively worsened. One month prior she was started on Digoxin 0.125 mg in addition to her regimen of Metoprolol Succinate 25 mg, Lisinopril 2.5 mg, Spironolactone 25 mg, Aspirin 81 mg, and Plavix 75 mg (all daily), in addition to Metformin 1000 mg twice-a-day. In the emergency department, her initial vital signs show her to be afebrile, with a heart rate of 102 beats-per-minute, and a blood pressure of 90/66 mm Hg. Examination notes an elevated jugular venous pressure with a positive hepatojugular reflex. She has bibasilar crackles, an S3 on cardiac auscultation, and 1+ pitting edema with cool lower extremities. Chest x-ray demonstrates pulmonary edema, and an ECG shows sinus tachycardia with q-waves in leads V1-V3 (known from previous), and unchanged intervals and ST segments. Initial labs are notable for a sodium of 130 mmol/L, a serum creatinine of 1.6 mg/dL, a lactate of 3.1 mmol/L, and a troponin I of 0.93 ng/mL that remains unchanged 4-hours later. The managing team was confronted with a series of questions regarding the differential diagnosis, prognosis, and next management steps.

1940s, isoproterenol came to market via researchers in Germany. Isoproterenol quickly became a staple in treating acute cardiac disease. Isoproterenol functioned primarily through changes in chronotropy rather than inotropy. The hope for modified function of isoproterenol led to Ronald Tuttle and Jack Mills removing a side chain hydroxyl group that resulted in an agent with potent inotropic properties, now known as dobutamine (1975).[3] Dobutamine continues to be a vital tool in the treatment of cardiogenic shock and is 1 of the 2 stable inotropes commonly employed in the critical care setting. The road to discovering therapies for HF and cardiogenic shock started many centuries ago, but it is only in the most recent decades that we have seen the advances that truly have allowed the natural history of decompensated HF and cardiogenic shock to change. The advent of inotropes, starting with dobutamine, and more recently, milrinone, has allowed the natural history of acute decompensated HF and cardiogenic shock to be more malleable, with more patients having the opportunity to survive critical cardiac illness either to recovery or to more advanced cardiac therapeutics.

In the following section, the most common inotropes and adjunct vasopressors will be discussed and subsequently will be applied to their appropriate clinical settings, specifically acute decompensated HF and cardiogenic shock.

INTRODUCTION

Modern-day critical care cardiology is predicated on the ready use of hemodynamically active agents including inotropes and vasopressors. Vasoactive medications are far from advents of the 20th century. Ancient Egyptian texts suggest the use of sea onion as a treatment for edema, which was later noted to be a natural cardiac glycoside. Another cardiac glycoside-containing plant, foxglove, was also commonly used as early as the 1500s. Since then, the active ingredient has been extracted, and in 1785, Sir William Withering published his book on the account of foxglove, extolling its ability to treat edematous states, irregular heartbeats, and heart failure (HF). Its modern form is digitalis.[2] In 1893, Dr George Oliver, a British physician, began testing glandular extracts using his son as a research subject. He discovered adrenal extracts caused vasoconstriction. Later efforts on these same extracts led to the first vasopressor, suprarenin, later renamed as epinephrine. As epinephrine quickly became adopted by leading physicians, chemist Helmut Legerlotz synthetized what is now recognized as modern-day phenylephrine (1920s) and, by the

PHARMACOLOGY

The inotropes used in support of patients with HF or cardiogenic shock have different mechanisms of action as well as pharmacologic properties that make them more, or less, ideal in certain situations (Figure 34-1 and Table 34-1). The breadth of evidence in support of these medications varies greatly between the differing classes. In this section, individual inotropes will be discussed as well as the evidence surrounding them (Table 34-2).

Digoxin

Clinical use of digitalis has existed for more than 200 years. Found in the foxglove plant, its properties have been extracted through teas and other formulations.[4] Today it can be given by oral or parenteral routes, and acts by inhibiting the Na-K-ATPase pump in myocardial cells. This causes increased intracellular sodium, promoting greater sodium-calcium exchange, which then causes an increase in intracellular calcium concentration. This increased availability of calcium causes an improved myocyte contractile performance.[5] Digitalis also acts as a vagotonic, upregulating the parasympathetic system. This is

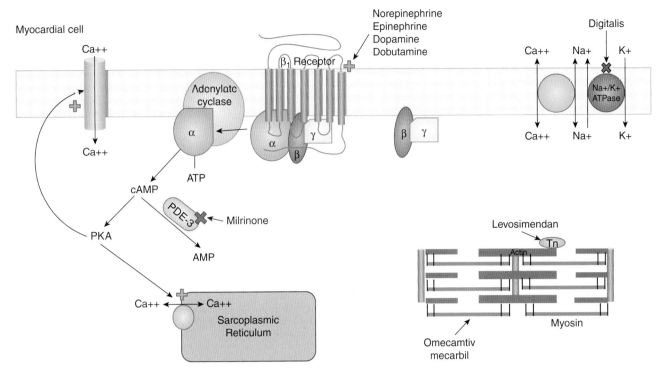

FIGURE 34-1 Diagram of intracellular mechanisms of inotropic agents. Digitalis, the cardiac glycoside in digoxin, acts by blocking sodium/potassium ATPase allowing more calcium to stay intracellularly. Epinephrine, norepinephrine, dopamine, and dobutamine act on the β_1 receptor causing G-protein activation and the adenylate cyclase mediated conversion of ATP to cAMP. cAMP, among other things, activates PKA, which opens the L-type calcium channel via phosphorylation and thus leads to calcium-induced calcium release. cAMP is metabolized by PDE3, which is inhibited by milrinone. Omecamtiv mecarbil is a direct myosin activator. Levosimendan increases the sensitivity of the contractile apparatus to calcium, without increasing calcium influx. Abbreviations: AMP, Adenosine monophosphate; ATP, adenosine triphosphate; Ca++, calcium; cAMP, cyclic adenosine monophosphate; PDE-3, phosphodiesterase 3; PKA, protein kinase A. Adapted from Harrison's and Francis et al.[45,46]

often seen in the reduction of atrioventricular nodal conduction and control of ventricular rates in atrial tachyarrhythmias. Short-term impact of digoxin has been assessed during right heart catheterization of patients in HF. Documented changes include an acute improvement in cardiac output, left ventricular (LV) stroke work index, and a decrease in pulmonary capillary wedge pressure (PCWP) and right atrial pressure both with rest or exercise.[6] Long-term studies show that patients taking digoxin have symptom improvement and improved quality of life, but no meaningful change in mortality.[7] Studies that looked at active removal of digoxin from a medical regimen showed clinical decompensation, suggesting that while survival is not improved, it is reasonable to remain on digoxin for quality of life and symptom control as withdrawal of the medication may result in clinical deterioration.[8] The randomized controlled study (DIG trial) demonstrated no improvement in survival with digoxin though hospitalizations were decreased.[9] In summation, digoxin improves symptoms and quality of life with no improvement in mortality as seen with modern-day neurohormonal blockade.[9] In current practice, it is an adjunct to HF therapy, primarily for patients with systolic dysfunction, persistent symptoms, and atrial arrhythmias.

Dopamine

Dopamine is a vasopressor whose effect varies based upon the dose range administered. While often not a first-line agent, its lower potency allows this agent to be used in transition settings such as step-down units. At doses of 1 to 2 mcg/kg/min, dopamine impacts mostly the dopamine 1 receptors in the renal, mesenteric,

Table 34-1 Pharmacology of Inotropes

Name	Mechanism	Dosing	T ½	Clearance	Comments
Digoxin	Na/K channel blocker	0.125-0.25 mg daily. Lower doses used in certain populations	36-48 h	Renal, requires dose adjustment for renal injury	Weak inotrope compared to other agents, not used for shock states. Can help with atrial tachyarrhythmias as well.
Dopamine	α1, β1, DA1, DA2	2-20 mcg/kg/min	2-20 min	Renal	Different receptor activation at different doses.
Dobutamine	β1, β2, Cardiac α1	2-20 mcg/kg/min	2-3 min	Metabolized by catechol-O-methyl transferase	Increased myocardial oxygen demand, increased risk of arrhythmias. Tachyphylaxis.
Milrinone	PDE inhibitor	0.125-0.75 mcg/kg/min	2.5 h	Renal, requires dose adjustment for renal injury	Effective in presence of beta blockers. Increased risk of hypotension and arrhythmia.
Levosimendan	Ca sensitization	6-24 mcg/kg load and 0.05-0.20 mcg/kg/min	1 h, metabolites 70-80 h	At least partly renal as dialysis prolongs half-life 1.5-fold	Effective in presence of beta blockers.
Omecamtiv mecarbil phase 2 presented at AHA	Cardiac myosin activator	25-50 mg BID	18.5 h	Not published (currently in trials)	Increased contractility without increasing myocardial oxygen demand
Norepinephrine	α1, β1, β2	0.02-2 mcg/kg/min	Duration of action 1-2 min	Metabolized by catechol-O-methyl transferase and monoamine oxidase. Excreted in urine	Inotrope and vasopressor
Epinephrine	α1, β1, β2	0.05-0.5 mcg/kg/min	<5 min	Metabolized by catechol-O-methyl transferase and monoamine oxidase. Excreted in urine	Inotrope and vasopressor

Table 34-2 Review of Trials of Inotropic Agents in Heart Failure[9,14,20,23-25,34-39,41,47,48]

Trial	Population	Study Description	Results
ADHERE (mortality in ADHF on IV vaso-active meds): 2005	Acute decompensated heart failure	Retrospective review of use of nitroglycerin, nesiritide, milrinone, or dobutamine	Nitroglycerin and nesiritide with lower mortality than milrinone/dobutamine
Digitalis Investigation Group: 1997	Chronic HF	RCT: Digitalis vs placebo	No mortality advantage, reduced hospitalizations with digoxin
PROMISE: 1991	Chronic severe HF	Milrinone vs placebo	Milrinone with a 28% increased mortality
VEST 1998	Chronic severe HF	Vesnarinone vs placebo	Dose-related increase in sudden cardiac death
Xamoterol 1990	Chronic severe HF	Xamoterol vs placebo	Increased mortality with xamoterol
PRIME II 1997	Chronic severe HF	Oral ibopramine vs placebo	Increased mortality with ibopramine
PICO II 1996	Chronic HF class II-III	Pimobendan vs placebo	Trend toward increased mortality with pimobendan
RUSSLAN: 2002	AMI with LV failure	Levosimendan vs placebo	Mortality benefit with levosimendan
LIDO: 2002	HF requiring inotropes on admission	Levosimendan vs dobutamine	Levosimendan with improved hemodynamics and lower mortality
PRECEDENT: 2002	Acute decompensated HF (without cardiogenic shock)	Open-label RCT: Nesiritide vs dobutamine	Dobutamine with significantly more ventricular tachycardia compared to nesiritide
REVIVE II: 2013	Acute decompensated HF (SBP >90)	Levosimendan vs placebo	Decreased need for rescue therapy with levosimendan but trend toward increased mortality
SURVIVE 2007	Acute decompensated HF requiring inotropes	Levosimendan vs dobutamine	Similar mortality between groups
ESSENTIALS: 2009	Chronic HF	Enoximone + beta blocker vs placebo	Safe, but no improvement with enoximone
Dobutamine vs milrinone awaiting transplant: 2003	Inotropic dependent HF awaiting cardiac transplant	Dobutamine vs milrinone	Small study, no difference. Milrinone more expensive
DICE: 1999	Severe HF, cardiac index 1.9	Intermit dobutamine vs standard of care	No 6-mo changes, only 38 people
ROSE: 2013	Acute decompensated HF with renal dysfunction	Low-dose nesiritide vs low-dose dopamine vs placebo	Neither more effective than placebo
OPTIME-CHF: 2002	Acute on chronic HF (mostly class III and IV), not requiring inotropes	RCT: Milrinone vs placebo	Similar 60-d hospitalization rate. More hypotension and arrhythmia with milrinone

Abbreviations: AMI, acute myocardial infarction; HF, heart failure; LV, left ventricular; RCT, randomized controlled trial; SBP, systolic blood pressure.

cerebral, and coronary beds. This results in selective vasodilation and urine output may increase via augmentation of renal blood flow, which is greater than the increase in cardiac output achieved from this small dose. Natriuresis is also increased by inhibiting aldosterone and renal tubular sodium transport.[10-12] Despite the promising physiologic studies of dopamine mentioned above, the ROSE HF study showed no additional clinical benefit of adding dopamine to background of diuretics.[13]

As dopamine is further increased, to 5 to 10 mcg/kg/min, dopamine stimulates beta-1 adrenergic receptors and increases cardiac output, primarily by increasing stroke volume. At doses > 10 mcg/kg/min, dopamine stimulates mostly alpha adrenergic receptors resulting in vasoconstriction and increased systemic vascular resistance. As the dose increases, tachyarrhythmias increase as well. In cases of severe HF with evidence of clinical hypoperfusion and hypotension, doses are often started low to take advantage of the increase in inotropy while avoiding the deleterious effects of increased afterload and arrhythmic burden observed at higher doses.

Dopamine was compared with norepinephrine by the SOAP II investigators to help determine the appropriate vasopressor for the initial treatment of shock. In this randomized double-blind study, 1600 patients received either dopamine or norepinephrine for fluid refractory shock.[1] Primary outcome was the 28-day mortality with secondary outcomes including the occurrence of adverse events (arrhythmias, myocardial necrosis, limb ischemia, or infections). While the primary outcome showed no significant differences between the 2 groups, there were more arrhythmias in the dopamine group, specifically atrial fibrillation. Also, in the predefined cardiogenic shock subgroup, mortality was increased with dopamine (Figure 34-2).

Dobutamine

Dobutamine was first developed from modifying isoproterenol by Tuttle and Mills in 1975. The goal was to modify isoproterenol to alter the focused effect on positive chronotropy as well as to redirect the increase in cardiac output toward skeletal muscle due to its vigorous stimulation of beta-2 receptors in the periphery.[3] Their result was a synthetic catecholamine that is both a beta-1 and partial beta-2 agonist. These effects work to increase myocardial contractility and thus, cardiac output, while decreasing left ventricular end diastolic pressure. Its effect on beta-2 receptors in peripheral blood vessels can cause vasodilation, which can be a useful secondary effect of decreasing cardiac afterload. As such, dobutamine has multiple mechanisms to increase cardiac output.

Its use is as a continuous infusion in patients with decompensated HF with signs of end-organ hypoperfusion. Using dobutamine in decompensated patients without end-organ dysfunction is contraindicated, as dobutamine has been associated with increased ventricular arrhythmias and mortality.[14,15] Its short half-life (2-3 minutes) is also ideal for an infusion that needs to reach therapeutic doses quickly. Its pharmacokinetics make it more ideal for patients with renal dysfunction as dosing does not have to be changed based on creatinine clearance.

Dobutamine use may have untoward effects. In patients with severe cardiogenic shock with low systemic blood pressure, the

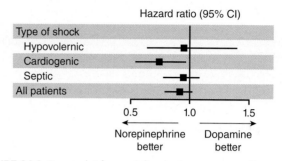

FIGURE 34-2 Forest plot for predefined subgroups according to type of shock (from SOAP II Trial).[1] (Reproduced with permission from De Backer D, Biston P, Devriendt J, et al. Comparison of dopamine and norepinephrine in the treatment of shock. *N Engl J Med.* 2010;362:779-789.)

vasodilatory effects of dobutamine use in isolation of another agent can cause further hypotension and worsened shock. Notably, dobutamine also increases myocardial oxygen demand, which paradoxically may have deleterious consequences in patients with decompensation due to ischemia. Dobutamine is also proarrhythmic, which needs to be considered in a population that already has significant risk factors for atrial and ventricular tachyarrhythmias.[16,17]

Milrinone

Milrinone was derived in the early 1980s as a much more potent inotrope compared to its parent compound, amrinone.[18] It has a unique mechanism of increasing the contractility of the heart more than previously described catecholamines. It is a phosphodiesterase 3 inhibitor, decreasing the degradation of cyclic adenosine monophosphate (cAMP), which in turn increases protein kinase A (PKA) activation, which in turn, causes a downstream increase in the heart's contractility. This allows for cardiac contractile stimulation independent of the beta-1 receptor, on which many other agents rely. Outside of the heart, it is a potent vasodilator and lowers both the pulmonary and systemic vascular resistance.[19]

Milrinone is used for similar purposes to dobutamine, namely in decompensated HF complicated by end-organ hypoperfusion but without systemic hypotension. Its effects on the pulmonary vascular resistance make it possibly more desirable in isolated right HF. It is also used as a continuous infusion, with a markedly longer half-life than dobutamine.

Like dobutamine, milrinone is also proarrhythmic. Its potent vasodilatory effects make it contraindicated in patients with systemic hypotension. Of note, milrinone is renally cleared and thus should be monitored more closely in those with renal failure. It may even have a high risk of toxicity if used in those with marginal renal function.[20]

Levosimendan

Two of the major problems of inotropic agents are their increase in myocardial oxygen demand and their proarrhythmic effects. Some of these effects are thought to be due to the increase in calcium influx in the myocardial cell, which has led to agents, such as levosimendan, that increase the sensitivity of the myocardial contractile system to calcium without increasing the influx.[21] Levosimendan binds to cardiac troponin C to increase calcium sensitization and also opens adenosine triphosphate (ATP)-dependent potassium channels in vascular smooth muscle, inducing vasodilation. It increases contractility and lowers filling pressures while also decreasing vascular resistance.[22] Hypotension is one of the side effects of levosimendan because of its vasodilatory effects.

In 2002, 2 double-blind, randomized control trials were published looking at the effects of levosimendan in different HF populations. The LIDO study assessed hemodynamic improvement in patients with severe HF necessitating inotropic support randomized to a 24-hour infusion of dobutamine or levosimendan. In this study, cardiac output was significantly increased, and PCWP decreased in patients receiving levosimendan. There was also a significant reduction in 30-day and 180-day mortality in the levosimendan group.[23] RUSSLAN compared levosimendan and placebo short-term infusions in patients with left ventricular

failure complicating acute myocardial infarction (MI) who required inotropes for refractory HF symptoms but with systolic blood pressure (SBP) >90 mm Hg. Mortality was significantly reduced with levosimendan as compared with placebo at 14-day and 180-day follow-up. Of note, recruitment was between 1996 and 2000 with only around 15% of patients receiving thrombolytics and no patients receiving revascularization.[24]

The REVIVE I and II trials were randomized, double-blinded trials carried out in 103 centers in the United States, Australia, and Israel with a goal to evaluate the short-term infusion of levosimendan vs placebo in subjective dyspnea and objective signs of deterioration in acute decompensated HF patients with rest dyspnea. While improvement in symptoms and lack of worsening of symptoms both favored levosimendan, the safety profile was not as favorable as with the aforementioned studies. There was significantly increased hypotension, atrial and ventricular arrhythmias, and a trend toward increased mortality.[25] At this time, levosimendan is approved in many countries though not in the United States pending further safety data.

Omecamtiv Mecarbil

Omecamtiv mecarbil acts on the ineffective actin-myosin crossbridge in patients with HF by being a cardiac-specific myosin activator. This increases systolic ejection time and stroke volume without affecting systolic pressure. Due to the increase in systolic ejection time, the heart rate is decreased and there is no change in myocardial oxygen consumption.[26] Omecamtiv mecarbil is currently investigational but does show promise. The COSMIC-HF phase 2 clinical trial presented at AHA Scientific Sessions in 2015 demonstrated increased stroke volume, increased systolic ejection time, and decreased N-terminal pro-BNP at 20 weeks following randomization to omecamtiv mecarbil or placebo.

Istaroxime

Istaroxime is an investigational intravenous agent with both inotropic and lusitropic properties. It works by inhibiting the Na/K ATPase and stimulating sarcoplasmic reticulum calcium ATPase, allowing increased cytosolic calcium during systole and sequestration during diastole.[27] The enhanced intracellular calcium allows for similar effects to digoxin; decreasing heart rate, increasing inotropy, but without proarrhythmic effects while also improving myocardial relaxation.[27,28] The HORIZON-HF study randomized 120 patients admitted with acute systolic HF, with SBP between 90 and 150 mm Hg, HR 60 to 110 bpm, to a 6-hour infusion of differing doses of istaroxime vs placebo with a primary endpoint of a change in PCWP. In this study, PCWP was decreased, whereas SBP was increased.[27] The clinical benefits of this medication need to be further studied.

VASOPRESSORS

Norepinephrine

This vasopressor acts on both alpha-1 and beta-1 adrenergic receptors, resulting in vasoconstriction as well as a mild increase in cardiac output. This agent is preferred in septic shock and can be useful in cases of mixed septic and cardiogenic shock. Systemic vascular resistance is variable in cardiogenic shock[29] and the increase in afterload secondary to alpha-1 stimulation may be deleterious and lead to further decreases in cardiac output. In the SOAP II trial, the subset of patients with a cardiogenic etiology of shock had a mortality benefit with norepinephrine as opposed to dopamine,[1] and it has gained favor as the preferable agent in cardiogenic shock with severe hypotension.[30]

Epinephrine

Related to norepinephrine, this agent is a potent beta-1 adrenergic agonist with moderate beta-2 and alpha-1 adrenergic receptor effects. Low-dose epinephrine can increase cardiac output via beta-1 adrenergic stimulation (increase inotropy and chronotropy). However, as the dose increases, the alpha-1 properties dominate, resulting in a greater increase in systemic vascular resistance. It is used commonly in post cardiotomy patients for hypotension, but typically is not a first-line agent in decompensated HF and cardiogenic shock. Significant splanchnic vasoconstriction and dysrhythmias limit the use of this vasopressor.[31]

Vasopressin

Vasopressin is an antidiuretic hormone, which was originally used in the management of diabetes insipidus and esophageal varices but has been more recently shown to help in the management of vasodilatory shock.[32] In a small retrospective study of cardiogenic shock complicating MI, vasopressin was shown to increase the mean arterial pressure without any negative changes in hemodynamic parameters such as cardiac index and PCWP.[33] It appears to have a role as an adjunct to the treatment of cardiogenic shock with persistently low systemic blood pressures despite inotrope use.[33]

CLINICAL USES OF INOTROPES

CHRONIC HEART FAILURE

Advances in our understanding of adverse remodeling in HF and the role of neurohormonal changes in that process have shepherded highly effective medical therapies in the last 20 years. Beta blockers, angiotensin-converting enzyme (ACE) inhibitors, angiotensin receptor blockers (ARBs), and aldosterone antagonists represent the mainstay of guideline-based therapy and together have a significant mortality and morbidity benefit for patients with systolic HF. In spite of excellent medications for patients with chronic HF, many patients will not improve to NYHA class I or II symptoms. Even with optimized filling pressures documented on right heart catheterization, dyspnea with exertion, poor functional capacity, and difficult-to-control edema all may plague patients despite best efforts to initiate neurohormonal blockade. Decrease in myocardial contractility leads to flattening in the Frank-Starling curve and patients are unable to provide increased cardiac output when they have increased peripheral oxygen consumption. In these patients, it was thought that inotropes could provide a significant improvement in the morbidity of the disease and help improve the hemodynamics closer to baseline.

While pharmacologically appealing, evidence was needed to prove both safety and efficacy of inotropes in chronic HF with

preserved end-organ function (Table 34-2). In 1990, Xamoterol, a partial beta agonist, was compared with placebo and showed a 5.4% increase in absolute risk of mortality in the first 100 days after randomization.[34] After this, the PROMISE trial compared oral milrinone with placebo in 1088 patients with severe HF (NYHA class III or IV) with an ejection fraction (EF) ≤35% for a median follow-up of 6.1 months with a primary endpoint of all-cause mortality. Patients were on standard medical therapy at that time including diuretics, ACE inhibitors, and digoxin. The trial was stopped early due to a relative risk increase of 28% for mortality in the milrinone group (absolute increase of 6%). Milrinone was also worse in all 10 prespecified subgroups.[20] In the PICO trial, 317 patients with stable HF were randomized to pimobendan, a calcium sensitizer and partial phosphodiesterase 3 (PDE3) antagonist, or placebo for at least 24 weeks. There was a significant improvement in exercise tolerance but a nonsignificant trend toward increased mortality with a hazard of death of 1.8 (CI, 0.9-3.5).[35] In the VEST trial in 1998, another PDE3 inhibitor, vesnarinone, was compared with placebo in patients with severe HF and an EF ≤30% and was found to have a dose-responsive increase in mortality, mostly due to sudden cardiac death.[36] Oral ibopramine, a dopamine receptor agonist, was compared to placebo in Prime II. Like PROMISE, this study was also stopped early due to 26% increase in the relative risk of death.[37]

While the above trials demonstrate why inotropes have not gained favor in the treatment of chronic HF, not all agents have demonstrated harmful effects. In 1997, the Digitalis Investigation Group sought to investigate the utility of our oldest inotrope, cardiac glycosides, in the prevention of all-cause mortality as well as cardiac mortality and hospitalization. Approximately 3400 patients were randomized to digoxin or placebo in a population of mostly NYHA class II and III HF with an average EF of 28%. Most patients were on background diuretics and ACE inhibitors, though this was prior to beta blockers being standard of care for heart failure with reduced ejection fraction (HFrEF). There was noted to be no difference in all-cause mortality, with a decrease in the relative risk of hospitalizations of 8%.[9]

At the turn of the 20th century, great advances in the treatment of HF occurred with multiple trials touting the benefits of beta blockers in the treatment of chronic HF. Enoximone, which was already shown to increase mortality in high doses in a 1990 placebo-controlled trial, was to be looked at again in 2009.[38] The ESSENTIAL investigators postulated that the negative outcomes of inotropes may be temporized if patients were on beta blockers during the administration of the inotropes. The ESSENTIAL study randomized patients to enoximone (PDE3 inhibitor) in a double-blind, placebo-controlled trial to patients with NYHA class III or IV symptoms, and an EF ≤30%, who were also on beta blockers. This study had a coprimary endpoint of a composite of mortality and cardiovascular hospitalization, change in 6-minute walk test (6MWT), and the patient global assessment.[39] In a mean follow-up of 16.4 months, enoximone was found to be well tolerated with no increase in mortality. However, it did not provide any benefit in the 3 primary endpoints and caused a rebound effect when the study drug was stopped.

Despite the initial optimism of inotropes, multiple clinical trials have shown the opposite of what was hoped, as increased mortality was replicated with multiple agents. Digoxin is the only inotrope with evidence to suggest it can be beneficial in treatment of chronic HF and has a Class IIa (LOE B) recommendation for the treatment of HFrEF to prevent hospitalizations.[40] Currently, intravenous inotropes are a Class III, LOE B for use in patients with chronic HF if not for palliation or as a bridge to transplant according to ACC/AHA guidelines.[40]

ACUTE DECOMPENSATED HEART FAILURE

HF admissions are an extremely large expenditure for our health care system. The majority of these patients will be admitted with the "warm and wet" profile (Figure 34-3), in which they have signs and symptoms of congestion, without signs of end-organ hypoperfusion. On right heart catheterization, these patients typically will have a preserved cardiac index, with elevated filling pressures. Multiple inotropes have been studied in decompensated systolic HF (Table 34-2).

In 2002, OPTIME-CHF evaluated milrinone for patients with acute decompensated HF in a multicenter, double-blind, placebo-controlled trial of 951 patients. Patients had an EF ≤40%, were admitted within the past 48 hours, and were not felt to require inotropes, have significant arrhythmias, or recent ischemia, or have SBP <80.[41] Treatment was for 48 to 72 hours, and the primary outcome was the total number of days hospitalized within the 60 days after randomization with secondary outcomes looking at worsening HF, all-cause mortality, and hypotension, among others. There was no difference in the primary outcome, but milrinone was associated with significantly increased risk of treatment failure, adverse events, new atrial fibrillation, and sustained hypotension.[41] In 2005, a retrospective analysis of 65,000 patients in the ADHERE registry was published, in which nitroglycerin, nesiritide (balanced arterial and venous dilator), milrinone, or dobutamine were used in acute decompensated HF. With risk factor and propensity score adjustment, in-hospital mortality was similar between nesiritide and nitroglycerin and both were significantly lower than with inotropic agents.[15] In the ROSE trial, 360 patients with acute decompensated HF and renal dysfunction were randomized 1:1:1 to low-dose dopamine, low-dose nesiritide, or placebo to see if there was a benefit in decongestion when added to diuretics over 72 hours. With both dopamine and nesiritide, there was no difference in diuresis when compared to placebo.[13] At this time, it appears there is no role for inotropic therapy in acutely decompensated HF if there are no signs of end-organ hypoperfusion or congestion refractory to diuresis (with an ACC/AHA Heart Failure Guidelines Class III recommendation, LOE B).[40]

CARDIOGENIC SHOCK

Inotropes are the therapeutic backbone in managing cardiogenic shock. Cardiogenic shock is defined as systemic hypoperfusion (and typically hypotension) due to an acute deterioration of cardiac output and/or function. If invasive hemodynamic monitoring is in place, a patient is likely to demonstrate elevated central filling pressures with a diminished cardiac output, and classically are "cold and wet" (Figure 34-3). The landmark SHOCK trial utilized a cardiac index less than 2.2 L per minute per square meter of body-surface area and a PCWP of at least 15 mm Hg in addition to hypotension with end-organ hypoperfusion to define

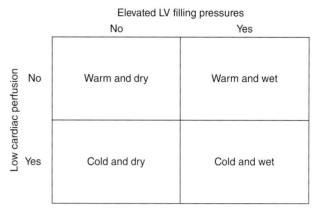

FIGURE 34-3 Four hemodynamic profiles of patients with heart failure.[49] (Data from LW Stevenson. Tailored therapy to hemodynamic goals for advanced heart failure. *Eur J Heart Fail.* 1999;1(3):251-257.)

cardiogenic shock.[42] Echocardiography can confirm biventricular failure or acute valvular disease. MI is the most common precipitant of cardiogenic shock. In the early phases of shock, treatment of the underlying condition may be all that is needed. When stabilization is required before definitive therapy can be undertaken, inotropes are critical for preventing irreversible end-organ dysfunction. Digoxin, though useful for HF in the outpatient setting or for atrial arrhythmias, is not a useful therapeutic in this setting as its effects are not potent enough.

In the 2013 ACC/AHA guideline update on HF, temporary inotropic support was recommended to improve systemic perfusion and preserve end-organ perfusion. As discussed earlier, in cardiogenic shock patients with severe hypotension (defined as SBP <80 mm Hg), norepinephrine should be the first choice for pharmacologic support.[1,30] In patients with a preserved mean arterial pressure who require inotropic support without concomitant vasoconstriction, the 2 primary inotropes used in the United States are dobutamine and milrinone. Dobutamine is often the first-line agent as it has a quicker onset of action. Milrinone, however, is the more stable long-term choice and is reasonable as a first choice in those who have preserved renal function and relatively preserved blood pressure. The 2013 ACC/AHA guidelines endorse the use of pulmonary artery catheter for patients in cardiogenic shock to ensure inotrope dosing is titrated to the level of adequate end-organ perfusion (Class IIA, LOE: C).[40]

ALTERNATE USES OF INOTROPES

While cardiogenic shock remains the best guideline-indicated reason for inotrope use, other situations do lend themselves to requiring inotropic support. For the NYHA class IV, stage D patient, a home inotrope infusion may be necessary as a bridge to transplant or mechanical support. This allows patients to spend more time at home while they await the next definitive step in their advanced HF management. As we see more patients with advanced HF, we will also see more patients having to navigate the transition to end of life. For patients with advanced systolic HF who are not eligible for transplant or left ventricular assist device placement, palliative inotropes should be considered.[43] Palliative inotropes remain a Class IIb LOE B recommendation in the 2013 ACC/AHA guidelines for stage D patients without a pathway to advanced therapies.[40]

CONCLUSION

The utility of inotropes in decompensated HF has been suggested since primitive cardiac glycosides were used to treat "dropsy" centuries ago. In contemporary practice, the short- and long-term use of these agents has not shown clinical benefit and in several studies has demonstrated harm.[14,15,20,25,34,36-38,41] For those patients who do have acute end-organ dysfunction and imminent demise due to insufficient cardiac output (cardiogenic shock), inotropes represent an appropriate first step in management. With the advent of additional support devices, both temporary and durable mechanical support, inotropes are growing in their use as a bridge therapy, expanding beyond their traditional role as a bridge for survival to cardiac transplant. As more of this population ages or nears the advanced stages of their disease, inotropes are providing a supplement to traditional palliative and hospice care to allow greater quality of life from home. Appropriate use of these agents is predicated on an understanding of each agent's unique pharmacology and its window of therapeutic efficacy and harm. In the future, the development of further inotropic support in HF will not only rely on medications with limited side effect profiles, but on utilizing known mechanisms of action to create directed gene therapy that eliminates side effects altogether.[44]

REFERENCES

1. De Backer D, Biston P, Devriendt J, et al. Comparison of dopamine and norepinephrine in the treatment of shock. *N Engl J Med.* 2010;362:779-789.

2. Fisch C. William Withering: an account of the foxglove and some of its medical uses 1785-1985. *J Am Coll Cardiol.* 1985;5:1A-2A.

3. Tuttle RR, Mills J. Dobutamine: development of a new catecholamine to selectively increase cardiac contractility. *Circ Res.* 1975;36:185-196.

4. Gheorghiade M, van Veldhuisen DJ, Colucci WS. Contemporary use of digoxin in the management of cardiovascular disorders. *Circulation.* 2006;113:2556-2564.

5. Smith TW. Digitalis. Mechanisms of action and clinical use. *N Engl J Med.* 1988;318:358-365.

6. Gheorghiade M, St Clair J, St Clair C, Beller GA. Hemodynamic effects of intravenous digoxin in patients with severe heart failure initially treated with diuretics and vasodilators. *J Am Coll Cardiol.* 1987;9:849-857.

7. Arnold SB, Byrd RC, Meister W, et al. Long-term digitalis therapy improves left ventricular function in heart failure. *N Engl J Med.* 1980;303:1443-1448.

8. Packer M, Gheorghiade M, Young JB, et al. Withdrawal of digoxin from patients with chronic heart failure treated with angiotensin-converting-enzyme inhibitors. RADIANCE Study. *N Engl J Med.* 1993;329:1-7.

9. Digitalis Investigation Group. The effect of digoxin on mortality and morbidity in patients with heart failure. *N Engl J Med.* 1997;336:525-533.

10. Bellomo R, Chapman M, Finfer S, Hickling K, Myburgh J. Low-dose dopamine in patients with early renal dysfunction: a placebo-controlled randomised trial. Australian and New Zealand Intensive Care Society (ANZICS) Clinical Trials Group. *Lancet.* 2000;356:2139-2143.

11. Denton MD, Chertow GM, Brady HR. "Renal-dose" dopamine for the treatment of acute renal failure: scientific rationale, experimental studies and clinical trials. *Kidney Int.* 1996;50:4-14.

12. Elkayam U, Ng TM, Hatamizadeh P, Janmohamed M, Mehra A. Renal vasodilatory action of dopamine in patients with heart failure: magnitude of effect and site of action. *Circulation.* 2008;117:200-205.

13. Chen HH, Anstrom KJ, Givertz MM, et al. Low-dose dopamine or low-dose nesiritide in acute heart failure with renal dysfunction: the ROSE acute heart failure randomized trial. *JAMA*. 2013;310:2533-2543.

14. Burger AJ, Horton DP, LeJemtel T, et al; Prospective Randomized Evaluation of Cardiac Ectopy with Dobutamine or Natrecor Therapy. Effect of nesiritide (B-type natriuretic peptide) and dobutamine on ventricular arrhythmias in the treatment of patients with acutely decompensated congestive heart failure: the PRECEDENT study. *Am Heart J*. 2002;144:1102-1108.

15. Abraham WT, Adams KF, Fonarow GC, et al. In-hospital mortality in patients with acute decompensated heart failure requiring intravenous vasoactive medications: an analysis from the Acute Decompensated Heart Failure National Registry (ADHERE). *J Am Coll Cardiol*. 2005;46:57-64.

16. Ruffolo RR Jr. The pharmacology of dobutamine. *Am J Med Sci*. 1987;294:244-248.

17. Vallet B, Dupuis B, Chopin C. [Dobutamine: mechanisms of action and use in acute cardiovascular pathology]. *Annales de cardiologie et d'angeiologie*. 1991;40:397-402.

18. Baim DS, McDowell AV, Cherniles J, et al. Evaluation of a new bipyridine inotropic agent—milrinone—in patients with severe congestive heart failure. *N Engl J Med*. 1983;309:748-756.

19. Colucci WS, Wright RF, Jaski BE, Fifer MA, Braunwald E. Milrinone and dobutamine in severe heart failure: differing hemodynamic effects and individual patient responsiveness. *Circulation*. 1986;73(3 Pt 2):III175-183.

20. Packer M, Carver JR, Rodeheffer RJ, et al. Effect of oral milrinone on mortality in severe chronic heart failure. The PROMISE Study Research Group. *N Engl J Med*. 1991;325:1468-1475.

21. Toller WG, Stranz C. Levosimendan, a new inotropic and vasodilator agent. *Anesthesiology*. 2006;104:556-569.

22. Kivikko M, Lehtonen L. Levosimendan: a new inodilatory drug for the treatment of decompensated heart failure. *Curr Pharm Des*. 2005;11:435-455.

23. Follath F, Cleland JG, Just H, et al; Steering Committee and Investigators of the Levosimendan Infusion versus Dobutamine Study. Efficacy and safety of intravenous levosimendan compared with dobutamine in severe low-output heart failure (the LIDO study): a randomised double-blind trial. *Lancet*. 2002;360:196-202.

24. Moiseyev VS, Poder P, Andrejevs N, et al; RUSSLAN Study Investigators. Safety and efficacy of a novel calcium sensitizer, levosimendan, in patients with left ventricular failure due to an acute myocardial infarction. A randomized, placebo-controlled, double-blind study (RUSSLAN). *Eur Heart J*. 2002;23:1422-1432.

25. Packer M, Colucci W, Fisher L, et al; REVIVE Heart Failure Study Group. Effect of levosimendan on the short-term clinical course of patients with acutely decompensated heart failure. *JACC Heart Fail*. 2013;1:103-111.

26. Greenberg BH, Chou W, Saikali KG, et al. Safety and tolerability of omecamtiv mecarbil during exercise in patients with ischemic cardiomyopathy and angina. *JACC Heart Fail*. 2015;3:22-29.

27. Gheorghiade M, Blair JE, Filippatos GS, et al; HORIZON-HF Investigators. Hemodynamic, echocardiographic, and neurohormonal effects of istaroxime, a novel intravenous inotropic and lusitropic agent: a randomized controlled trial in patients hospitalized with heart failure. *J Am Coll Cardiol*. 2008;51:2276-2285.

28. Micheletti R, Mattera GG, Rocchetti M, et al. Pharmacological profile of the novel inotropic agent (E,Z)-3-((2-aminoethoxy)imino)androstane-6,17-dione hydrochloride (PST2744). *J Pharmacol Exp Ther*. 2002;303:592-600.

29. Hochman JS. Cardiogenic shock complicating acute myocardial infarction: expanding the paradigm. *Circulation*. 2003;107:2998-3002.

30. Reyentovich A, Barghash MH, Hochman JS. Management of refractory cardiogenic shock. *Nat Rev Cardiol*. 2016;13:481-492.

31. Allwood MJ, Cobbold AF, Ginsburg J. Peripheral vascular effects of noradrenaline, isopropylnoradrenaline and dopamine. *Br Med Bull*. 1963;19:132-136.

32. Mutlu GM, Factor P. Role of vasopressin in the management of septic shock. *Intensive Care Med*. 2004;30:1276-1291.

33. Jolly S, Newton G, Horlick E, et al. Effect of vasopressin on hemodynamics in patients with refractory cardiogenic shock complicating acute myocardial infarction. *Am J Cardiol*. 2005;96:1617-1620.

34. Xamoterol in severe heart failure. The Xamoterol in Severe Heart Failure Study Group. *Lancet*. 1990;336:1-6.

35. Lubsen J, Just H, Hjalmarsson AC, et al. Effect of pimobendan on exercise capacity in patients with heart failure: main results from the Pimobendan in Congestive Heart Failure (PICO) trial. *Heart*. 1996;76:223-231.

36. Cohn JN, Goldstein SO, Greenberg BH, et al. A dose-dependent increase in mortality with vesnarinone among patients with severe heart failure. Vesnarinone Trial Investigators. *N Engl J Med*. 1998;339:1810-1816.

37. Hampton JR, van Veldhuisen DJ, Kleber FX, et al. Randomised study of effect of ibopamine on survival in patients with advanced severe heart failure. Second Prospective Randomised Study of Ibopamine on Mortality and Efficacy (PRIME II) Investigators. *Lancet*. 1997;349:971-977.

38. Uretsky BF, Jessup M, Konstam MA, et al. Multicenter trial of oral enoximone in patients with moderate to moderately severe congestive heart failure. Lack of benefit compared with placebo. Enoximone Multicenter Trial Group. *Circulation*. 1990;82:774-780.

39. Metra M, Eichhorn E, Abraham WT, et al; ESSENTIAL Investigators. Effects of low-dose oral enoximone administration on mortality, morbidity, and exercise capacity in patients with advanced heart failure: the randomized, double-blind, placebo-controlled, parallel group ESSENTIAL trials. *Eur Heart J*. 2009;30:3015-3026.

40. Yancy CW, Jessup M, Bozkurt B, et al; American Heart Association Task Force on Practice Guidelines. 2013 ACCF/AHA guideline for the management of heart failure: a report of the American College of Cardiology Foundation/American Heart Association Task Force on Practice Guidelines. *J Am Coll Cardiol.* 2013;62:e147-e239.

41. Cuffe MS, Califf RM, Adams KF Jr, et al; Outcomes of a Prospective Trial of Intravenous Milrinone for Exacerbations of Chronic Heart Failure Investigators. Short-term intravenous milrinone for acute exacerbation of chronic heart failure: a randomized controlled trial. *JAMA.* 2002;287:1541-1547.

42. Hochman JS, Sleeper LA, Webb JG, et al. Early revascularization in acute myocardial infarction complicated by cardiogenic shock. SHOCK Investigators. Should we emergently revascularize occluded coronaries for cardiogenic shock. *N Engl J Med.* 1999;341:625-634.

43. Hershberger RE, Nauman D, Walker TL, Dutton D, Burgess D. Care processes and clinical outcomes of continuous outpatient support with inotropes (COSI) in patients with refractory end stage heart failure. *J Card Fail.* 2003;9:180-187.

44. Greenberg B, Butler J, Felker GM, et al. Calcium upregulation by percutaneous administration of gene therapy in patients with cardiac disease (CUPID 2): a randomised, multinational, double-blind, placebo-controlled, phase 2b trial. *Lancet.* 2016;387:1178-1186.

45. Kasper DL, ed. *Harrison's Principles of Internal Medicine.* 19th ed. New York, NY: McGraw-Hill Education; 2015.

46. Francis GS, Bartos JA, Adatya S. Inotropes. *J Am Coll Cardiol.* 2014;63:2069-2078.

47. Mebazaa A, Nieminen MS, Packer M, et al; SURVIVE Investigators. Levosimendan vs dobutamine for patients with acute decompensated heart failure: the SURVIVE randomized trial. *JAMA.* 2007;297:1883-1891.

48. Oliva F, Latini R, Politi A, et al. Intermittent 6-month low-dose dobutamine infusion in severe heart failure: DICE multicenter trial. *Am Heart J.* 1999;138:247-253.

49. Stevenson LW. Tailored therapy to hemodynamic goals for advanced heart failure. *Eur J Heart Fail.* 1999;1:251-257.

35 ROLE OF REVASCULARIZATION TO IMPROVE LEFT VENTRICULAR FUNCTION

Peter H. U. Lee, MD, PhD, MPH, FACC, FACS

PATIENT CASE

A 65-year-old man with a past medical history of coronary artery disease (CAD), diabetes mellitus, hypercholesterolemia, and hypertension (HTN) presents with a 1-month history of intermittent chest pain and shortness of breath that was associated with exertion. He underwent an exercise stress test that was positive. This was followed by a coronary angiography that demonstrated significant 3-vessel CAD. A transthoracic echocardiogram demonstrated a left ventricular ejection fraction (LVEF) of 30%.

DIFFERENTIAL DIAGNOSIS

It would be reasonable in a patient with multivessel CAD and a significant reduction in left ventricular (LV) function to presume that his/her cardiac dysfunction is directly related to myocardial ischemia resulting from a decrease in coronary blood flow and coronary flow reserve (CFR). Although all of the following are associated with LV dysfunction, whether the myocardium is stunned, hibernating, or infarcted depends on the duration, chronicity, severity, and repetitiveness of the myocardial ischemia (Figure 35-1). These different states of the myocardium can also coexist in different parts of the heart.

- Stunned myocardium—Acute myocardial ischemia can lead to subsequent contractile dysfunction. However, if the myocardium is just stunned and the ischemia is promptly relieved, the contractile function of the myocardium is eventually restored, usually over a period of hours to days.[1] The aberration in a stunned myocardium appears to be predominantly metabolic in nature, not structural.[2,3]

- Hibernating myocardium—In contradistinction to stunned myocardium, when myocardial ischemia persists and becomes chronic, it can lead to an adaptive response of decreasing basal metabolic demand by reducing contractility and cellular activity. This is associated with changes to both cellular and extracellular structures.[4]

- Myocardial infarction—Acute myocardial ischemia that is significant enough to cause myocyte necrosis can lead to myocardial infarction (MI) and subsequent myocardial dysfunction. This can also be a result of extracellular fibrotic changes due to chronic ischemia or repetitive myocardial stunning. Infarcted myocardial tissue does not regain contractile function with revascularization.

- Nonischemic cardiomyopathy—In the setting of proven severe CAD, absent any other obvious diagnoses, a patient's myocardial

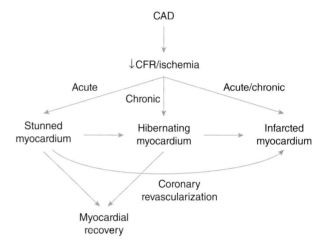

FIGURE 35-1 Ischemia-associated left ventricular dysfunction. Schematic illustration of ischemia-induced myocardial injury. Abbreviations: CAD, coronary artery disease; CFR, coronary flow reserve.

dysfunction is likely due to ischemic cardiomyopathy. However, this does not preclude the possibility that 1 or more of the many nonischemic cardiomyopathy diagnoses is partially or solely responsible for his/her myocardial dysfunction.

MANAGEMENT

In patients with significant CAD and impaired LV function, considerations should be made as to whether they would benefit from coronary revascularization (Figure 35-2). The role of coronary revascularization to improve LV function and ultimately improve mortality has been extensively studied. Although the overall body of evidence appears to support its role and benefits, the topic remains controversial. Three major randomized controlled trials (RCTs) have looked into this and the role of viability testing with mixed results.[5-7] In patients with ischemic cardiomyopathy and significant LV dysfunction, revascularization has been shown to reverse this dysfunction, with patients with the greatest dysfunction and ischemic symptoms benefiting the most.[8,9]

In a 10-year follow-up study of patients with significant ischemic dysfunction (LVEF <35%), the absolute risk reduction in all-cause mortality was 8% in coronary artery bypass grafting (CABG) + optimal medical therapy (OMT) patients compared to patients receiving OMT alone.[10]

- An assessment should be made of the function of the LV. This is most practically done with echocardiography. This will provide not only an assessment of the LVEF, but it can also evaluate the status of all of the valves, any regional wall motion abnormalities, and the size and shape of the heart. In addition to assessing cardiac function, cardiac magnetic resonance (CMR) can also provide a wide range of cardiac information, including cardiac shape, size, wall thickness, volumes, mass, and global and regional wall motion abnormalities. However, CMR is much more costly, is not as readily available, is not well tolerated by patients with claustrophobia, cannot be used in patients with noncompatible implanted hardware, and its use is limited in patients with renal insufficiency because of the use of gadolinium contrast agents.

- Patients require a recent assessment of their coronary anatomy with coronary angiography. This will determine whether they are anatomically candidates for surgical and/or percutaneous coronary interventional (PCI) revascularization.

- Assessment of myocardial viability can be carried out using a variety of means, each having its advantages and disadvantages as determined by its sensitivity and specificity, technical limitations, expense, and availability. These modalities include single-photon emission computed tomography (SPECT), positron emission tomography (PET), late gadolinium enhancement CMR, and dobutamine echocardiography. SPECT, PET, and CMR work by assessing cellular integrity whereas dobutamine echocardiography assesses contractile reserve as a measure of viability by increasing contractility with low-dose dobutamine. Dobutamine can also be used with CMR to assess contractile reserve. Radionuclides used in SPECT imaging include thallium-201 and technetium-99m. See Table 35-1.

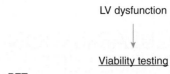

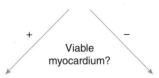

FIGURE 35-2 Management of left ventricular dysfunction and coronary artery disease. Abbreviations: LV, left ventricular; MRI, magnetic resonance imaging; PET, positron emission tomography; SPECT, single-photon emission computed tomography.

Table 35-1 Imaging Modalities to Test Myocardial Viability

	Assessment of Viability	Limitations	Sensitivity (%)	Specificity (%)
^{201}Tl SPECT	Sarcolemmal integrity	Limited spatial resolution. Highest radiation exposure	87	54
^{99m}Tc SPECT	Mitochondrial membrane integrity	Limited spatial resolution	83	65
Cardiac PET	Cellular glucose uptake capacity	Limited spatial resolution. Limited availability	92	63
CMR	Late gadolinium enhancement / Contractile reserve (with dobutamine)	Cannot use in patients with cardiac devices. Limited use with renal insufficiency and claustrophobia. Not widely available.	84	63
Dobutamine echocardiography	Contractile reserve	Limited acoustic windows. Interobserver variability.	80	78

Abbreviations: CMR, cardiac magnetic resonance; PET, positron emission tomography; Tc, technetium; Tl, thallium.

- If a patient with ischemic cardiomyopathy has been determined to have viable myocardium and the coronary anatomy is amenable to surgical revascularization, then a determination should be made regarding the patient's suitability for surgery based on the patient's surgical risk. If the patient is deemed too high-risk, then PCI revascularization should be considered if anatomically favorable. Although controversies still remain, surgical revascularization with CABG appears to be favored over PCI in patients with severe systolic dysfunction.[11-13]

- For patients who are not candidates for coronary revascularization, OMT should be pursued. The mainstay of pharmacological management in these patients includes the use of angiotensin-converting enzyme (ACE) inhibitors, angiotensin receptor blockers (ARBs), beta blockers, aldosterone antagonists, and a combination of hydralazine and isosorbide dinitrate, as these have been shown to reduce mortality in heart failure (HF) patients.[14] The selection of these medications should be individualized based on the patient's cardiac function, clinical symptoms, and other comorbidities.

- Cardiac resynchronization therapy (CRT) should be considered in patients with LVEF less than 35% and QRS greater than 150 ms.[15]

- Those patients who fail OMT and CRT should then be considered for inotropic therapy. End-stage HF patients who have failed all other therapies may be considered for left ventricular assist device (LVAD) implantation or heart transplantation.

PROGNOSIS

The effectiveness of revascularization in ischemic cardiomyopathy has been studied in 3 recent prospective RCTs. Unfortunately, none of these studies provided conclusive evidence of the benefit of coronary revascularization in patients with ischemic

Table 35-2 Randomized Trials of Revascularization in Patients with Severe Ischemic Cardiomyopathy

	PARR-2	HEART	STITCH (Main Trial)	STITCH (Viability Substudy)
Premise	Comparison of FDG-PET-assisted strategy to standard of care for ICM.	Comparison of revascularization to OMT for ICM with viable myocardium.	Comparison of CABG to OMT for ICM with and without viable myocardium.	Comparison of viable to nonviable myocardium in ICM.
Number of patients	430	138	1212	601
Number of centers	9	13	99	99
Viability test	PET	SPECT, PET or dobutamine echo	SPECT, dobutamine echo	SPECT, dobutamine echo
Intervention	CABG or PCI vs OMT	CABG or PCI vs OMT	CABG vs OMT	CABG vs OMT
Endpoints	*Primary*: Composite of cardiac death, MI, or recurrent hospitalization for cardiac cause. *Secondary*: Time to occurrence of primary endpoint and time to cardiac death.	*Primary*: All-cause mortality.	*Primary*: All-cause mortality. *Secondary*: Cardiovascular mortality and composite of all-cause mortality and hospitalization for any cause.	*Primary*: All-cause mortality *Secondary*: Cardiovascular mortality and composite of all-cause mortality and hospitalization for any cause.
Main result	No difference in primary outcome between FDG-PET-assisted strategy and standard of care.	No difference in primary outcome between revascularization and OMT alone.	No difference in primary outcome between CABG and OMT alone in ITT analysis but significant difference in AT analysis. Reduction in cardiovascular mortality and all-cause mortality + cardiac hospitalization with CABG.	Reduced mortality in patients with viable myocardium vs without viable myocardium. But results not significant after adjustment for other baseline variables.
Notable limitations	25% of patients in the FDG-PET group did not undergo recommended revascularization.	The study was underpowered. Only 138 of planned 800 patients enrolled.	Very slow recruitment with concern for selection bias. Significant crossover between groups. Left main patients were excluded.	Viability testing was not randomized so not truly an RCT. Viability testing subject to selection bias. Two different viability tests with variable definitions of viability used.

Abbreviations: AT, as-treated; CABG, coronary artery bypass grafting; ICM, ischemic cardiomyopathy; ITT, intention-to-treat; MI, myocardial infarction; OMT, optimal medical therapy; PCI, percutaneous coronary intervention; PET, positron emission tomography; RCT, randomized control trial.

cardiomyopathy, as these studies did have significant limitations. In many cases, a closer look at the data either showed trends supporting the benefits of revascularization or benefits were seen in subgroup analyses. See Table 35-2.

- The PARR-2 trial randomized 430 patients with an average LVEF of 27% to management based on PET viability testing or standard of care.[6] There was no significant difference in the primary composite endpoint of cardiac death, MI, and 1-year hospitalization. However, 1 of the major limitations of this study is that 25% of the PET group did not undergo the recommended revascularization. But, a subgroup analysis of patients who did undergo revascularization did show a significant decrease in mortality compared to standard of care.[16]
- The HEART trial enrolled patients with an LVEF <35% without angina but viable myocardium. Patients were randomized to CABG or PCI with OMT versus OMT alone.[7] Although no significant difference was seen in the primary endpoint of all-cause mortality, this study was severely underpowered as they recruited only 138 patients of the 800 originally planned.
- The STITCH trial enrolled 121 patients with ischemic cardiomyopathy and LVEF <35%. Patients were randomized to CABG and OMT or OMT alone. After a mean follow-up of 56 months, there was no significant difference in the primary endpoint of all-cause mortality.[5] However, significant limitations included slow recruitment with concerns for selection bias, the exclusion of left main disease patients, and significant crossover in both arms. As-treated analysis did show a significant mortality reduction in CABG patients compared to OMT patients. A subgroup analysis of patients who had undergone viability testing demonstrated no difference in all-cause mortality in those with or without evidence of myocardial viability.[17] However, this was limited by the fact that viability testing was not randomized, leading to selection bias, and that there were inconsistent definitions of viability based on the type of viability study carried out (SPECT vs dobutamine echo).

FOLLOW-UP

Patients with ischemic cardiomyopathy and determined to have hibernating myocardium through viability testing may not see an immediate improvement in contractile function. In fact, hibernating myocardium typically shows delayed recovery after revascularization. Depending on the degree of structural abnormalities, time to functional recovery ranges from as little as 10 days to more than 6 months.[18,19] In 1 study, approximately two-thirds of hibernating segments recovered after 14 months.[20] Therefore, functional assessment of myocardial recovery after revascularization should be made using sound clinical judgment and may not be necessary for several months after the intervention.

PATIENT EDUCATION

Patients should be counseled on the importance of lifestyle modifications and adherence to prescribed medical therapies.

PATIENT RESOURCES

The American Heart Association has patient information on HF. http://www.heart.org/HEARTORG/Conditions/HeartFailure/Heart-Failure_UCM_002019_SubHomePage.jsp

The Heart Failure Society of America has a wide range of patient-oriented resources on its website. www.hfsa.org/patient

PROVIDER RESOURCES

The Heart Failure Society of America has abundant resources for providers, including educational materials and HF guidelines. www.hfsa.org/resources

REFERENCES

1. Chareonthaitawee P, Gersh BJ, Araoz PA, Gibbons RJ. Revascularization in severe left ventricular dysfunction: the role of viability testing. *J Am Coll Cardiol*. 2005;46:567-574.
2. Braunwald E, Kloner RA. The stunned myocardium: prolonged, postischemic ventricular dysfunction. *Circulation*. 1982;66:1146-1149.
3. Lim SP, McArdle BA, Beanlands RS, Hessian RC. Myocardial viability: it is still alive. *Semin Nucl Med*. 2014;44:358-374.
4. Frangogiannis NG. The pathological basis of myocardial hibernation. *Histol Histopathol*. 2003;18:647-655.
5. Velazquez EJ, Lee KL, Deja MA, et al. Coronary-artery bypass surgery in patients with left ventricular dysfunction. *N Engl J Med*. 2011;364:1607-1616.
6. Beanlands RS, Nichol G, Huszti E, et al. F-18-fluorodeoxyglucose positron emission tomography imaging-assisted management of patients with severe left ventricular dysfunction and suspected coronary disease: a randomized, controlled trial (PARR-2). *J Am Coll Cardiol*. 2007;50:2002-2012.
7. Cleland JG, Calvert M, Freemantle N, et al. The Heart Failure Revascularisation Trial (HEART). *Eur J Heart Fail*. 2011;13:227-233.
8. Chatterjee K, Swan HJ, Parmley WW, Sustaita H, Marcus H, Matloff J. Depression of left ventricular function due to acute myocardial ischemia and its reversal after aortocoronary saphenous-vein bypass. *N Engl J Med*. 1972;286:1117-1122.
9. Rahimtoola SH. Coronary bypass surgery for chronic angina—1981. A perspective. *Circulation*. 1982;65:225-241.
10. Velazquez EJ, Lee KL, Jones RH, et al. Coronary-artery bypass surgery in patients with ischemic cardiomyopathy. *N Engl J Med*. 2016;374:1511-1520.
11. Brener SJ, Lytle BW, Casserly IP, Schneider JP, Topol EJ, Lauer MS. Propensity analysis of long-term survival after surgical or percutaneous revascularization in patients with multivessel coronary artery disease and high-risk features. *Circulation*. 2004;109:2290-2295.

12. Hannan EL, Racz MJ, Walford G, et al. Long-term outcomes of coronary-artery bypass grafting versus stent implantation. *N Engl J Med.* 2005;352:2174-2183.

13. Hannan EL, Wu C, Walford G, et al. Drug-eluting stents vs. coronary-artery bypass grafting in multivessel coronary disease. *N Engl J Med.* 2008;358:331-341.

14. Yancy CW, Jessup M, Bozkurt B, et al. 2013 ACCF/AHA guideline for the management of heart failure: a report of the American College of Cardiology Foundation/American Heart Association Task Force on Practice Guidelines. *J Am Coll Cardiol.* 2013;62:e147-e239.

15. Mant J, Al-Mohammad A, Swain S, Laramee P; Guideline Development G. Management of chronic heart failure in adults: synopsis of the National Institute For Health and clinical excellence guideline. *Ann Intern Med.* 2011;155:252-259.

16. Abraham A, Nichol G, Williams KA, et al. 18F-FDG PET imaging of myocardial viability in an experienced center with access to 18F-FDG and integration with clinical management teams: the Ottawa-FIVE substudy of the PARR 2 trial. *J Nucl Med.* 2010;51:567-574.

17. Bonow RO, Maurer G, Lee KL, et al. Myocardial viability and survival in ischemic left ventricular dysfunction. The New England Journal of Medicine 2011;364:1617-1625.

18. Haas F, Jennen L, Heinzmann U, et al. Ischemically compromised myocardium displays different time-courses of functional recovery: correlation with morphological alterations? *Eur J Cardiothorac Surg.* 2001;20:290-298.

19. Vanoverschelde JL, Wijns W, Borgers M, et al. Chronic myocardial hibernation in humans. From bedside to bench. *Circulation.* 1997;95:1961-1971.

20. Bax JJ, Visser FC, Poldermans D, et al. Time course of functional recovery of stunned and hibernating segments after surgical revascularization. *Circulation.* 2001;104:I314-I318.

36 VENOARTERIAL EXTRACORPOREAL MEMBRANE OXYGENATION FOR THE TREATMENT OF ACUTE HEART FAILURE

Arman Kilic, MD
Bryan A. Whitson, MD, PhD, FACS
Ahmet Kilic, MD, FACS

PATIENT CASE

A 55-year-old man with a history of morbid obesity, uncontrolled diabetes mellitus, and smoking presented to the emergency department 48 hours after the onset of chest pain. He was in cardiogenic shock with sinus tachycardia to 120 beats per minute and hypotension with a blood pressure of 87/55 mm Hg. An electrocardiogram (ECG) showed ST elevations and an emergent cardiac catheterization was performed, which demonstrated an occluded left anterior descending artery. The occlusion could not be crossed with a wire and during the procedure the patient went into ventricular fibrillatory arrest. Immediate cardiopulmonary resuscitation was undertaken and despite numerous rounds of pharmacologic therapy and chest compressions, a perfusing rhythm and pressure were not achieved. He was placed on percutaneous venoarterial extracorporeal membrane oxygenation (VA-ECMO) via the femoral vein and femoral artery for acute cardiogenic shock. Over the next 7 days, he was weaned off of VA-ECMO support and was discharged home on optimal medical therapy for his coronary artery disease (CAD).

PATIENT SELECTION

VA-ECMO is typically considered in the setting of continued end-organ hypoperfusion, despite escalating doses of inotropic support with or without the use of an intra-aortic balloon pump for augmentation. In such cases of refractory cardiogenic shock, VA-ECMO is used to bridge patients to recovery, surgical intervention, transplantation, or left ventricular assist device (LVAD). The most common indications for VA-ECMO include fulminant myocarditis, post-cardiotomy support, acute myocardial infarction (MI), and post heart transplant for early graft failure (Table 36-1). Other indications include refractory ventricular tachycardia or ventricular fibrillation unresponsive to conventional therapy, hypothermia, acute anaphylaxis, pulmonary embolism, peripartum cardiomyopathy, sepsis-related cardiac depression, and drug overdose.

There is no standardized and universally accepted list of contraindications to VA-ECMO. Nonetheless, there are several contraindications that we believe many groups would agree upon (Table 36-2). These include advanced age (>75-80 years), active

Table 36-1 Indications for VA-ECMO Support

Indication
Post-cardiotomy support
Acute fulminant myocarditis
Acute myocardial infarction
Post heart transplant for early graft failure
Refractory ventricular tachycardia or ventricular fibrillation unresponsive to conventional therapy
Hypothermia
Acute anaphylaxis
Pulmonary embolism
Peripartum cardiomyopathy
Sepsis-related cardiac depression
Drug overdose

Table 36-2 Contraindications to VA-ECMO Support

Contraindication
Age >75-80 y
Active malignancy with expected survival <1 y
Severe peripheral vascular disease
End-stage renal disease on dialysis
Advanced liver disease
Current intracranial hemorrhage or other contraindication to systemic anticoagulation
Unwitnessed cardiopulmonary arrest with ongoing cardiopulmonary resuscitation
Witnessed cardiopulmonary arrest with cardiopulmonary resuscitation of >30 min without return of spontaneous circulation

malignancy with an expected survival of less than 1 year, severe peripheral vascular disease, end-stage renal disease on dialysis, advanced liver disease, current intracranial hemorrhage or other contraindication to systemic anticoagulation, unwitnessed cardio-pulmonary arrest with ongoing cardiopulmonary resuscitation, and witnessed cardiopulmonary arrest with prolonged cardiopulmo-nary resuscitation (>30 minutes) without return of spontaneous circulation.

VA-ECMO CIRCUIT

The VA-ECMO circuit consists of a pump, a membrane oxygen-ator, a controller, cannulae, and tubing. The pump is usually a centrifugal pump that can generate up to 4000 rotations per minute and flow up to 8 L per minute. The oxygenator functions to elimi-nate carbon dioxide and to oxygenate blood. It is comprised of a polymethylpentene membrane, which is lower in resistance result-ing in less blood consumption, and can be heparin-coated. The con-troller displays and allows for adjustment of rotations per minute and associated flow.

The drainage cannula is inserted into the venous system. It typi-cally has a larger diameter between 21 and 25 French and can be up to 60 cm in length. The venous drainage cannula can be single or multistage drainage. The return cannula is inserted into the arterial system, is typically 15 to 19 French in diameter, and is shorter with lengths of 20 to 25 cm when inserted peripherally.

TECHNIQUE

In establishing access for VA-ECMO, relevant aspects to consider are the indication for which VA-ECMO is being instituted and any anatomic factors that may hinder placement of cannulae in a specific location. In the post-cardiotomy setting of being unable to wean from cardiopulmonary bypass or in the setting of an emergent resternotomy for a post-cardiac surgical patient, patients are typi-cally cannulated centrally, with the arterial cannula placed in the ascending aorta and the venous cannula placed in the right atrium (Figure 36-1). In the latter scenario of emergent resternotomy, some surgeons will immediately proceed to aortotomy and atri-otomy, insert the cannulae with an assistant holding them in place, go on VA-ECMO, and then place purse-string sutures around the cannulae to secure them in place, thereby reducing the amount of time to get the patient on support. If time allows, placing the purse-strings initially with subsequent aortotomy and atriotomy and cannulation in a more controlled sequence minimizes the risk of malpositioning or accidental displacement of the cannulae. With central VA-ECMO, the cannulae are tunneled through the subcuta-neous tissues and away from the midline wound, with the sternum and overlying subcutaneous tissue often left open and an Esmarch dressing sewn in place. A left ventricular vent can also be directly inserted and tunneled away from the midline wound to prevent ventricular distension and Y-ed into the drainage cannulae. After successful weaning from VA-ECMO and decannulation, the purse-strings can be tied and the aortotomy and atriotomy oversewn in usual fashion.

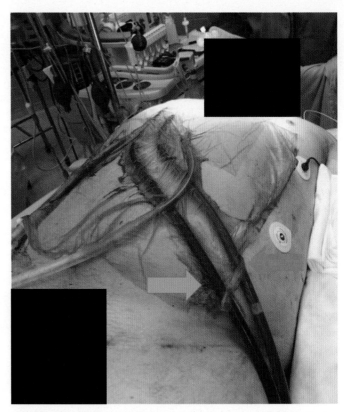

FIGURE 36-1 Central VA-ECMO with the arterial cannula (*red arrow*) inserted in the ascending aorta and the venous cannula (*blue arrow*) inserted in the right atrium.

If a patient is not a post-cardiac surgery patient, peripheral VA-ECMO is typically instituted via the femoral vessels. The initial step should be to evaluate existing access in the patient. If there is an existing femoral venous or femoral arterial line, these can be accessed with a wire, an appropriate sized incision in the skin made, the skin and subcutaneous tissue serially dilated, and the VA-ECMO cannula subsequently inserted. The wire must not be bent, and the cannulae must not be pushed with excessive force. If there is significant resistance, it is often due to inadequate dilatation of the skin or subcutaneous tissue. In addition to utilizing the dilators provided in the cannula kits, some providers have found use in additional, stiffer dilators to allow easier entry of the larger venous cannula as well as stiffer guidewires for placement support. Care should be utilized in the non-image-guided advancement of stiffer guidewires. If an intra-aortic balloon pump is in place, we typically utilize that side for femoral venous access and the contralateral side for femoral arterial access (Figure 36-2).

Multiple configurations can be employed depending on the clinical scenario. One scenario is emergent VA-ECMO in the setting of active cardiopulmonary resuscitation. This scene can often be hectic and the usual helpful measures to gain access and delineate venous versus arterial entry such as palpation of pulses, color of blood return, and pulsatile flow are not reliable. We believe the optimal configuration in this setting is ipsilateral femoral venous and femoral arterial access (Figure 36-3). Although ultrasound-guided cannula placement has been advocated by many as a means to reduce the risk of vascular complications, in the setting of emergent placement during cardiopulmonary resuscitation, retrieving an ultrasound machine may result in a delay of treatment. Therefore, once adequate venous or arterial access is established by the usual anatomic landmarks, then one can use that as a guide on the ipsilateral side to gain access to the other vessel. The patient is commenced on VA-ECMO support after inserting the appropriate cannulae via the Seldinger technique previously described and after administration of systemic anticoagulation. The tip of the venous cannula should be in the distal inferior vena cava by the cavoatrial junction. This position can be confirmed by echocardiography or chest x-ray.

We routinely insert a 7 or 8 French armored (wire wound) catheter in the superficial femoral artery percutaneously by ultrasound guidance in an antegrade manner after the patient has been initiated on VA-ECMO support to reduce lower extremity malperfusion (Figure 36-4). This catheter is then connected to the femoral arterial VA-ECMO cannula to provide antegrade perfusion of the lower extremity. Additionally, the systemic anticoagulation and low-dose nitroglycerin are infused down the distal perfusion cannulae to aid in limb perfusion. Some groups do not routinely place this catheter but rather monitor lower extremity perfusion via oximetry, reserving catheter placement to those patients whose oximetry values decrease in that limb. Fluoroscopy is often helpful in percutaneously cannulating the superficial femoral artery in cases where it cannot be done with ultrasound guidance alone. A surgical incision can be made and the superficial femoral artery dissected out if unable to perform the cannulation percutaneously.

After VA-ECMO support is weaned, decannulation can proceed. If the ipsilateral groin was utilized for both femoral venous and arterial access, a cutdown can be performed, purse-strings placed,

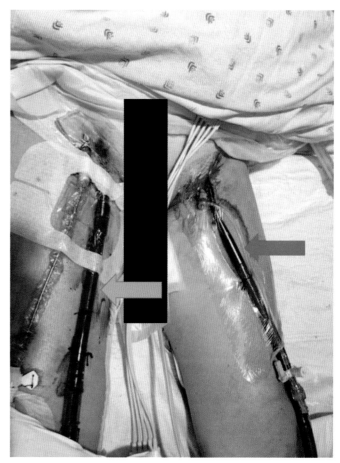

FIGURE 36-2 Peripheral VA-ECMO in a patient with an intra-aortic balloon pump (venous cannula, *blue arrow*; arterial cannula, *red arrow*).

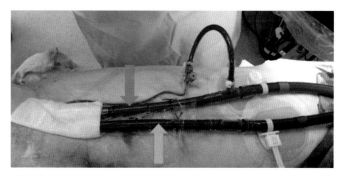

FIGURE 36-3 Peripheral VA-ECMO instituted with venous and arterial cannulae in the ipsilateral femoral vessels (venous cannula, *blue arrow*; arterial cannula, *red arrow*).

and the cannulae removed. It is important to palpate a distal femoral arterial pulse after tying the purse-string to ensure adequate perfusion. If the contralateral groin was utilized, we typically use a cutdown approach for the arterial side but will place a subcutaneous purse-string using a large Vicryl stitch and 2 fragments of red rubber catheters 3 cm in length as bolsters to prevent skin necrosis. This purse-string can then be removed in 1 to 2 days.

OUTCOMES

Several studies have evaluated outcomes of VA-ECMO for refractory cardiogenic shock. According to the Extracorporeal Life Support Organization registry, 56% and 40% of adult patients survived extracorporeal life support for cardiac failure or in the setting of cardiopulmonary resuscitation, respectively.[1] The survival rates to discharge or transfer in these cohorts was 41% and 30%, respectively. A single institution series of 179 patients supported on VA-ECMO demonstrated a 39% survival rate to discharge, with 45% surviving to 30 days.[2] Myocardial recovery was demonstrated in 80% of survivors and 39% were transitioned to a more durable device. Older age and indication for support were predictors of mortality.

In the setting of acute fulminant myocarditis, a multicenter analysis demonstrated cardiac recovery and weaning from VA-ECMO in 76%.[3] Survival to hospital discharge was 72%. A single institution series evaluating outcomes of VA-ECMO in the post-cardiac surgery setting in 233 patients demonstrated a lower survival rate to hospital discharge of 36%.[4] A study comparing outcomes between 321 patients receiving conventional cardiopulmonary resuscitation and 85 patients receiving VA-ECMO in the setting of witnessed cardiac arrest demonstrated significantly improved hospital survival and 6-month survival with none or minimal neurologic impairment in the VA-ECMO group, particularly in cases of cardiac origin.[5] Moreover, survival to discharge was 34% in the VA-ECMO group and 6-month survival with no or minimal neurologic impairment was 28%.

Complications are more common in VA-ECMO than in veno-venous ECMO due to the arterial system being accessed (Table 36-3). Bleeding is a major risk in VA-ECMO and can result from bleeding at the cannulation site, bleeding at a prior operative site, or hemorrhage elsewhere related to anticoagulation. In addition to systemic heparinization, platelet dysfunction and hemodilution of clotting factors contribute to the bleeding risk in patients supported with VA-ECMO. The rate of significant bleeding while supported on VA-ECMO is approximately 40%.[6] Malperfusion can also occur in patients on VA-ECMO. Lower extremity ischemia occurs in 15% to 20% of patients and may be mitigated by the use of superficial femoral artery catheters that provide antegrade perfusion.[6] The need for lower extremity fasciotomy or the development of compartment syndrome occurs in 10%, with a 5% amputation rate.[6] Acute kidney injury occurs in roughly 55% of VA-ECMO patients with 45% requiring renal replacement therapy.[6] Neurologic complications have been reported in 10% to 15% with a stroke rate of 6%.[6] Significant infection complicates 30% of VA-ECMO cases.[6]

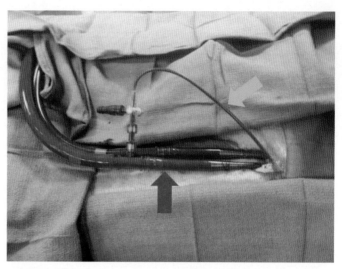

FIGURE 36-4 A superficial femoral artery cannula (*green arrow*) connected to the arterial VA-ECMO cannula (*red arrow*) for antegrade perfusion of the ipsilateral lower extremity.

Table 36-3 Complication Rates of VA-ECMO

Complication	Rate (%)
Major bleeding	40%
Lower extremity ischemia	15%-20%
Lower extremity fasciotomy or compartment syndrome	10%
Lower extremity amputation	5%
Acute kidney injury	55%
Renal replacement therapy	45%
Neurologic complications	10%-15%
Stroke	6%
Major infection	30%

FUTURE DIRECTIONS

VA-ECMO is an important modality in the armamentarium of clinicians who treat patients with acute HF. Despite improvements in technology and patient management, there remains a significant risk of mortality and morbidity in patients supported with VA-ECMO. In coming years, further refinements in treatment algorithms for patients presenting with acute HF will be essential. For example, a disadvantage of VA-ECMO has traditionally been the inability to effectively unload or decompress the left ventricle, which is important in reducing myocardial wall stress and oxygen demand and improving ventricular recovery. Although a left ventricular vent can be directly inserted for this purpose in cases of central VA-ECMO, this presents more of a challenge in cases of peripheral VA-ECMO. More research on outcomes of newer percutaneous ventricular support systems such as the Impella device (Abiomed, Danvers, Massachusetts) in providing ventricular unloading in patients supported on peripheral VA-ECMO is needed.

In addition to clinical advancements, systems-based improvements are needed. A recent study in Germany evaluated the results of a suprainstitutional network for rapid-response mobile VA-ECMO in 115 patients, of which 77% underwent VA-ECMO initiation in the setting of cardiopulmonary resuscitation.[7] The authors demonstrated a 44% survival to hospital discharge and 33% survival at a median follow-up of 1.5 years, suggesting that mobile VA-ECMO may be beneficial to a larger population than expected. Although these results are encouraging, the cost and policy implications of such networks are unknown.[8] Despite the ongoing challenges in improving results of VA-ECMO support, this technology has undoubtedly been responsible for the survival of thousands of critically ill patients who would have likely died otherwise.

REFERENCES

1. Extracorporeal Life Support Organization Registry Report. https://www.elso.org/Registry/Statistics/International Summary.aspx. Accessed March 18, 2016.

2. Truby L, Mundy L, Kalesan B, et al. Contemporary outcomes of venoarterial extracorporeal membrane oxygenation for refractory cardiogenic shock at a large tertiary care center. *ASAIO J.* 2015;61:403-409.

3. Lorusso R, Centofanti P, Gelsomino S, et al. Venoarterial extracorporeal membrane oxygenation for acute fulminant myocarditis in adult patients: a 5-year multi-institutional experience. *Ann Thorac Surg.* 2016;101:919-926.

4. Elsharkawy HA, Li L, Esa WA, Sessler DI, Bashour CA. Outcome in patients who require venoarterial extracorporeal membrane oxygenation support after cardiac surgery. *J Cardiothorac Vasc Anesth.* 2010;24:946-951.

5. Shin TG, Choi JH, Jo IJ, et al. Extracorporeal cardiopulmonary resuscitation in patients with inhospital cardiac arrest: a comparison with conventional cardiopulmonary resuscitation. *Crit Care Med.* 2011;39:1-7.

6. Cheng R, Hachamovitch R, Kittleson M, et al. Complications of extracorporeal membrane oxygenation for treatment of cardiogenic shock and cardiac arrest: a meta-analysis of 1,866 adult patients. *Ann Thorac Surg.* 2014;97:610-616.

7. Aubin H, Petrov G, Dalyanoglu H, et al. A suprainstitutional network for remote extracorporeal life support: a retrospective cohort study. *JACC Heart Fail.* 2016;4:698-708.

8. Shah AS. Cheating death with ECMO: coming soon to a theater near you. *JACC Heart Fail.* 2016;4:709-710.

37 ROLE OF ECHOCARDIOGRAPHY IN SELECTION, IMPLANTATION, AND MANAGEMENT OF PATIENTS REQUIRING LEFT VENTRICULAR ASSIST DEVICE THERAPY

Luca Longobardo, MD
Renuka Jain, MD
Christopher J. Kramer, BA, ACS, RDCS, FASE
Matt Umland, ACS, RDCS, FASE
Concetta Zito, MD, PhD
Scipione Carerj, MD, FESC
Bijoy K. Khandheria, MD, FACP, FESC, FASE, FACC

◼ PATIENT CASE

A 66-year-old man with cardiogenic shock, severe left ventricle (LV) systolic dysfunction, multiorgan failure and rhabdomyolysis caused by influenza B virus infection was admitted to the Intensive Care Unit. He needed circulatory support with veno-arterial extracorporeal life support, intra-aortic balloon pump, inotropes, and vasopressors. In addition, mechanical invasive ventilation and continuous renal replacement therapy were needed to maintain respiratory function, acid-base equilibrium, and fluid electrolyte balance as well as to treat rhabdomyolysis. Antibiotic and antiviral therapies were tailored by culture and serology. However, after seven days, LV systolic function was not improved, the LV was dilating, and filling pressure was increasing. Thus, the patient underwent left ventricular assist device (LVAD) implantation as bridging therapy to recovery or to transplantation. Initially, the LVAD reduced LV filling pressure and volume, and in the following weeks LV systolic function slowly improved. After two months, LV systolic function recovered completely, the LVAD was removed, and the patient was transferred to a peripheral hospital for rehabilitation.

INTRODUCTION

BACKGROUND

Ventricular assist devices (VADs) were introduced in clinical practice in the 1980s as mechanical support for the left ventricle (left ventricular assist device [LVAD]), right ventricle (right ventricular assist devices [RVAD]), or both (biventricular assist device [BiVAD]) in patients with end-stage heart failure (HF) headed to transplant or in patients with temporary cardiac shock who were expected to recover ventricular function. Use of these devices increased in the years that followed, and in 2018, VADs, particularly LVADs, are considered

a pivotal treatment in patients with HF; these devices have several indications, including bridge to transplant, bridge to candidacy, destination therapy, and bridge to recovery. Moreover, LVAD is considered the only valid alternative treatment when there are not enough organs available for transplant to satisfy the growing need. Indeed, the global HF prevalence, currently estimated between 23 and 26 million people, is expected to increase as a result of the population aging and the improved survival rates associated with other forms of heart disease.[1] The huge need for treatment of this population of HF patients easily explains why from 2006 to 2014 more than 15,000 patients in the United States received a VAD implant, with total procedures approaching 2500 per year and with 1- and 2-year survival rates of 80% and 70%, respectively.[2]

LEFT VENTRICULAR ASSIST DEVICE TYPES

LVADs are composed of an inflow cannula, usually placed in the left ventricular (LV) apex; an outflow cannula, usually anastomosed in the ascending aorta; a propulsion pump that moves the blood provided by the inflow cannula to the aorta through the outflow cannula; and an external controller, which receives and processes information from the pump. According to the pumping mechanisms, LVADs can be classified as either pulsatile or continuous flow. Pulsatile LVADs, the first generation of VADs available, were characterized by a pumping mechanism that simulated the pulsatile action of the heart with a rate that could be fixed or self-adjusting according to preload. These VADs, including the Novacor LVAS (Novacor, Salt Lake City, UT), the HeartMate vented electric LVAD (Abbott, Abbott Park, Illinois), and the Abiomed BVS 5000 (Abiomed, Danvers, MA), could be extracorporeal (the pump located outside the body) or intracorporeal (the pump inside the body, usually in the left chest or upper abdomen). All pulsatile LVADs have unidirectional valves in the inflow and outflow cannulae that increase the risk of thrombus formation, are usually large, and are highly dependent on adequate preload. These limitations caused the development of a new generation of LVADs, characterized by pumping mechanisms that guaranteed a continuous flow. These devices are smaller, always intracorporeal, do not require unidirectional valves, and are able to provide higher flows at lower pressures than pulsatile LVADs. Continuous-flow LVADs can be further classified as axial-flow LVADs (MicroMed DeBakey, MicroMed Technology, Houston, TX; HeartMate II, Abbott, Abbott Park, Illinois; Jarvik 2000, Jarvik Heart, New York, NY) and centrifugal-flow LVADs (HeartMate III, Abbott, Abbott Park, Illinois; HeartWare, HeartWare International Inc., Framingham, MA), depending on the mechanical structure of the pump. In both axial- and centrifugal-flow LVADs, preload can be reduced by increasing the speed of the rotor or increased by decreasing the speed of the rotor.

IMPORTANCE OF ECHOCARDIOGRAPHY IN THE MANAGEMENT OF LEFT VENTRICULAR ASSIST DEVICE PATIENTS

Echocardiography commonly is considered the most important diagnostic tool in the selection and management of patients requiring LVAD therapy, as indicated by the International Society for Heart and Lung Transplantation's current guidelines for mechanical circulatory support (2013).[3] Indeed, echocardiography is a commonly available, easy, cheap, and fast diagnostic technique, and it is able to provide all of the information the clinician needs to manage patients with end-stage HF. The fundamental goals of the echocardiographic evaluation of these patients are the identification of eligibility for LVAD implantation, the stratification of the risk profile of the individual patient, the perioperative evaluation of complications that could onset during the implantation, and a serial follow-up to detect eventual device malfunction. Preoperative and follow-up evaluations usually are performed by 2-dimensional (2D) transthoracic echocardiography (TTE), whereas the perioperative assessment is performed by 2D transesophageal echocardiography (TEE). Recently, new technologies, including 3-dimensional (3D) echocardiography and strain measurements, were tested in this setting and shown to provide additional information for the management of these patients.

PREOPERATIVE ECHOCARDIOGRAPHIC ASSESSMENT

PATIENT SELECTION FOR LEFT VENTRICULAR ASSIST DEVICE IMPLANTATION AND RISK STRATIFICATION

Left Ventricle

One of the most important roles of the echocardiographic assessment of patients with end-stage HF is the evaluation of possible eligibility for LVAD treatment. A positive opinion depends on the balance between the advantages conferred by the implant and the risk stratification of the individual patient.

The study of the LV plays a pivotal role in the evaluation of these elements. Several clinical and echocardiographic variables have been tested, and reduced LV ejection fraction (EF), altered LV geometry, and restrictive LV filling pattern, calculated through power Doppler assessment of the mitral inflow pattern, have been shown to have the most powerful ability to identify high-risk patients.[4-6] LV volumes usually are measured using 2D TTE, and EF is calculated by a biplane method of disks summation (modified Simpson's rule), tracing the blood-tissue interface in the apical 4- and 2-chamber views.[7] However, it recently was demonstrated that 3D echocardiography can provide a more accurate estimation of LV volumes and EF because it does not rely on geometric assumptions and is not affected by foreshortening of the LV apex.[8] For this reason, when available, 3D TTE should be considered the technique of choice for the calculation of LV volumes and EF.[7] The use of score systems that combine clinical and echocardiographic variables has been shown to improve risk stratification. A recently proposed score combined 5 TTE variables (end-systolic volume index, left atrial volume index, mitral E-wave deceleration time, tricuspid annular peak systolic excursion, and pulmonary artery systolic pressure) and demonstrated a great ability to predict mortality, the rate of which increased significantly with an increase of the score from 0 to 5, with a 4-fold risk of death in the high-risk subgroup of patients (score 5) compared with the low-risk subgroup.[4]

Recently, new myocardial deformation measurements, such as speckle-tracking echocardiography (STE) strain and strain rate, have provided additional information for further evaluation of this population of patients. STE strain is considered one of the most feasible and sensitive tools in the early diagnosis of cardiac dysfunction; it allows a frame-by-frame tracking of natural acoustic markers within the myocardium, and is angle independent, not influenced by translational movement due to respiration and tethering from adjacent myocardium, and not sensitive to signal noise. Global longitudinal strain (GLS) appeared to be the most sensitive and effective STE parameter for the evaluation of LV function; in patients with end-stage HF, a reduced GLS was more significantly associated with poor outcomes (all-cause mortality, cardiovascular death, heart transplantation, and arrhythmic events)[9] than EF and wall motion score index (WMSI), particularly in patients with a very low EF.[10,11] Moreover, similar results have been obtained using 3D STE. This new technology based on 3D datasets can overcome 2D limitations, such as the significant speckle decorrelation that takes place when out-of-plane motion occurs, and has been shown to be a sensitive and accurate predictor of cardiovascular-related death or hospitalization due to HF.[12,13]

Right Ventricle

The evaluation of right ventricle (RV) function perhaps plays an even more important role than the study of LV function in patients with end-stage HF. Indeed, in this subgroup of subjects, reduced RV function is not only a powerful prognostic tool for the prediction of poor outcomes,[14] it also is a fundamental marker of an increased risk of developing post-LVAD implantation RV failure (RVF),[15-17] one of the most life-threatening post-implant complications.

The echocardiographic assessment of RV size and function is not always easy due to the shape and location of the RV; however, using the apical 4-chamber, parasternal short-axis, and subcostal views, sometimes slightly modifying the angulation or shift of the transducer to better include the entire chamber, it is possible to obtain a fairly detailed evaluation of the RV.[18] Right ventricular ejection fraction (RVEF), when calculated by 2D echocardiography, is not considered a reliable estimation of RV systolic function because the complex RV shape and geometry, with inflow and outflow portions in different planes, make the measurement ineffective. On the other hand, as previously underlined in regard to the LV, 3D echocardiography can overcome these limitations in the quantification of RV volumes and EF, providing a comprehensive, reproducible assessment of the RV chamber that is no longer based on geometric assumptions; thus, it is possible to obtain an accurate and feasible estimation of RV function.[19]

RV systolic function often can be evaluated by 2D echocardiography through several parameters, including tricuspid annular plane systolic excursion (TAPSE), tricuspid annular longitudinal velocity by tissue Doppler imaging (TDI S'), right-sided index of myocardial performance (RIMP), and fractional area change (FAC). Of these measurements, FAC has been shown to be the most reliable for the assessment of RV systolic function, with a good correlation with RVEF estimated by cardiac magnetic resonance.[20] It is calculated in the apical 4-chamber view by obtaining end-diastolic and end-systolic RV areas by planimetry of the endocardial border, and, when reduced, it proved to be an effective predictor of poor outcomes in patients with end-stage HF.[21,22] However, FAC quantification is dependent on image quality, as wrong tracing of the RV area can lead to underestimation or overestimation of RV function. When a reliable estimation of FAC is not possible, TAPSE, a mono-dimensional measure of RV longitudinal function obtained by quantifying the displacement of the lateral portion of the tricuspid annulus in the apical 4-chamber view, has been shown to be a valid alternative to predict outcomes in these patients.[23]

However, the new myocardial deformation measurements, recently tested with great results in the study of RV systolic function, are able to provide additional information about RV systolic function, improving the risk stratification algorithms in use. Two-dimensional STE GLS, the most representative and reproducible strain for the assessment of RV function, recently has emerged as the most accurate and sensitive tool for the evaluation of RV function and as the most powerful independent predictor of severe adverse events in patients with HF.[24,25] RV GLS is obtained only from the apical 4-chamber view, and it could reflect the average value of the RV free wall and septal segments (RV GLS) or of the RV free wall (RV FWLS) alone. In patients with end-stage HF, a more impaired RV strain was associated with increasing New York Heart Association class, greater LV volumes, and worse LV systolic function, and it was able to predict long-term adverse events with an incremental prognostic value to LVEF.[26] These findings reinforce the concept that RV systolic function is a key element in the prediction of poor outcomes in this population.

However, as previously mentioned, RV function also is a fundamental factor in the evaluation of a patient's risk profile for the development of one of the most dangerous post-LVAD implantation complications, RVF. While RVF is more common in patients with pulsatile-flow devices, it still occurs in 13% to 40% of continuous-flow device patients.[27] Several definitions have been provided to indicate RVF; however, the Interagency Registry for Mechanically Assisted Circulatory Support (INTERMACS)[28] defines RVF by the need for an RVAD, inhaled nitric oxide, or inotropic therapy for more than 1 week at any time after LVAD implantation in the presence of symptoms and signs of persistent RV dysfunction, such as central venous pressure >18 mm Hg with a cardiac index <2.3 L/min/m^2 in the absence of elevated left atrial or pulmonary capillary wedge pressure (>18 mm Hg), cardiac tamponade, ventricular arrhythmias, or pneumothorax.

Currently, the pathophysiology of RVF is not completely explained. The main factors include (1) interventricular dependence; (2) the sudden increase of RV preload due to an acute increase in venous return after the restoration of cardiac output, which can determine the dilatation of the RV with an exacerbation of tricuspid regurgitation (TR); and (3) some perioperative events—including suboptimal ventilation, alveolar hypoxia, hyperinflation, acidosis, RV ischemia, bleeding, and transfusions—that could worsen RV function. Evaluation of the patient's risk profile includes assessment of clinical, hemodynamic, and echocardiographic variables. Several different clinical elements have been considered by authors to predict RVF—including laboratory parameters, blood pressure, inotrope dependency, obesity, and so on—and many scores were proposed.[29-33] However, all the schemes perform only modestly when applied to external populations.[34] Therefore, they are not commonly used in clinical practice.

Hemodynamic measurements, including pulmonary vascular resistance (PVR) and pulmonary artery systolic pressure (PASP), can be quantified invasively by catheterization or indirectly by echocardiography. Pulmonary hypertension (HTN) and high PVR seem to be associated with poor outcomes after LVAD implantation,[35] but there is no agreement among authors about the real value of these parameters in the risk stratification for RVF.[31,33]

On the other hand, echocardiography is the most important tool for the evaluation of a patient's risk profile because it is able to provide a large number of measurements noninvasively. Conventional parameters already discussed showed a good ability to predict RVF onset. Dilated RV; reduced systolic function as demonstrated by decreased FAC,[35] TAPSE,[36] and TDI S'; and moderate-to-severe TR[32,37] are the main predictors of RVF and poor outcomes after LVAD implantation. Very interesting results have been obtained using 2D STE parameters. Reduced 2D speckle-tracking strain and strain rate predict a high risk of RVF onset with greater sensitivity compared with conventional parameters,[27,38-41] whereas the improvement of these parameters during follow-up suggests a low-risk profile (Table 37-1).[42,43] These new measurements seem to be the most reliable and accurate elements for the risk stratification of RVF and, unless current data are contradicted by larger future studies, they should be considered essential tools in the echocardiographic preoperative assessment of these patients.

Table 37-1 Role of 2-Dimensional Speckle-Tracking Echocardiography Global Longitudinal Strain in Right Ventricle Failure Risk Stratification

Reference	Number of Patients	Main Findings
Grant AD et al (*JACC* 2012)[27]	117	• Peak strain cutoff of –9.6% predicted RVF with 76% specificity and 68% sensitivity. • RV strain was incremental to the Michigan risk score as a predictor of RVF. • Reduced RV free wall peak longitudinal strain was associated with an increased risk for RVF after LVAD implantation.
Dandel M et al (*Circulation* 2013)[38]	205	• End-diastolic short-/long-axis ratio ≥ 0.6, tricuspid annulus peak systolic velocity < 8 cm/s, and peak systolic longitudinal strain rate < 0.6/s in patients with maximum systolic pressure gradient between RV and right atrium < 35 mm Hg have high predictive values for postoperative RVF. • The same parameters are also predictive for RVF in patients with tricuspid regurgitation grade > 2 and pulmonary arterial pressure < 50 mm Hg.
Kalogeropoulos AP et al (*Eur Heart J Cardiovasc Imaging* 2015)[39]	120	• RV GLS was the most important predictor of RVF among RV function parameters.
Cameli M et al (*J Heart Lung Transplant* 2013)[40]	10	• Patients who presented the lowest free wall RVLS values at baseline showed a progressive decline of RVLS after LVAD implantation, eventually developing RVF.
Kato TS et al (*JACC Heart Fail* 2013)[41]	68	• RV STE longitudinal strain was lower in patients who developed RVF than in patients who did not. • Preoperative TDI S' < 4.4 cm/s, RV-E/E'>10, and RV-strain <−14% discriminated patients who developed RVF at day 14 with a predictive accuracy of 76.5%.
Cameli M et al (*Transplant Proc* 2015)[42]	19	• Patients who presented the lowest RVLS values at baseline presented RVF in the postoperative assessment. • A cutoff value of < 11% was able to identify patients at greater risk of post-implant RVF.
Herod JW et al (*J Card Fail* 2014)[43]	17	• RV systolic strain, systolic strain rate, and RV diastolic strain rate improved after LVAD implantation.

Abbreviations: GLS, global longitudinal strain; LVAD, left ventricular assist device; RV, right ventricle; RVF, right ventricle failure; RVLS, right ventricular longitudinal strain; STE, speckle-tracking echocardiography; TDI S', tricuspid annular longitudinal velocity by tissue Doppler imaging.

GENERAL PREOPERATIVE EVALUATION

Left Ventricle

Patients found to be eligible for LVAD implantation should be evaluated by 2D TTE, with attention focused on the detection of specific elements that can influence the surgical procedure and clinical outcomes. Right-to-left shunting, such as patent foramen ovale and interatrial or interventricular septal defects, should be carefully searched. Indeed, the LV unloading performed by an LVAD causes a drastic reduction in left chamber pressure, whereas right chamber pressure is not significantly modified; this sudden imbalance of pressure can exacerbate a right-to-left shunt or induce reversal of the shunt direction from left to right to right to left, causing hypoxemia and raising the risk of paradoxical embolism.[44] Two-dimensional Doppler TEE should be considered the technique of choice for the detection of intracardiac shunts because it has been shown to be a very accurate and sensitive, although invasive, test. The use of agitated saline contrast agents with the Valsalva maneuver should be avoided in this context because the high LV filling pressure before implantation can make the maneuver useless and result in an underestimated diagnosis.

Another important factor that should be taken into account is the high risk of thrombosis in these patients. Indeed, the very low LVEF that characterizes these subjects is the main risk factor for thrombus formation. The LV, especially the apex, should be carefully examined to find thrombi, which commonly cause inflow cannula obstruction or embolism. Conventional apical views usually allow a good exploration of the left chambers; however, when the image quality is not satisfactory or the presence of clots cannot be excluded safely, the use of intravenous contrast agents or TEE could improve the accuracy of detection.

CARDIAC VALVES AND ASCENDING AORTA

Preoperative evaluation of cardiac valve function plays an important role because the evidence of severe valve dysfunction could modify the surgical procedure. Indeed, some alterations can worsen after LVAD activation or can make the LVAD implant ineffective. The current International Society for Heart and Lung Transplantation guidelines for mechanical circulatory support (2013)[3] recommend surgical repair or valve replacement during device implantation when severe valve dysfunction is detected; however, concurrent valve replacements increase the mortality rate after LVAD implantation[45] and they are an important risk factor for RVF. For these reasons, valve function should be evaluated carefully, using quantitative parameters and, when necessary, improving the accuracy of the measurements using 2D TEE or 3D echocardiography, the gold standard for the evaluation of valve anatomy and function.[46-48]

Aortic stenosis (AS) and mitral regurgitation (MR) usually are not influenced by LVAD activation, nor do they modify outcomes. Indeed, AS is bypassed by the LVAD, which delivers blood from the LV to the ascending aorta, whereas MR, a common finding in patients with a dilated LV, usually improves after LVAD activation because the mechanical unloading of the LV causes a reduction in LV size and filling pressure.

On the other hand, aortic regurgitation (AR), mitral stenosis (MS), and tricuspid regurgitation (TR) can play an important role in hemodynamic equilibrium after LVAD activation and, when severe, can significantly worsen outcomes.

AR might be detected before the surgical procedure, but more often it develops in the medium- to long-term after treatment,[49] especially in patients with pulsatile LVADs, which keep the valve permanently closed. The pathophysiology of de novo AR is not clear, but the main factors considered include pressure overload above the aortic leaflets, aortic root dilatation, and altered leaflet coaptation.[50] When the valve dysfunction is severe, the significant regurgitation volume increases the LVAD preload and decreases the forward flow, creating a closed circle of blood flow that reduces cardiac output despite the high pump flow and the impairment of patient conditions. AR can be quantified by 2D Doppler TTE or

TEE, or 3D TTE, using vena contracta width and, when feasible, the effective regurgitant orifice area (EROA) calculated by the PISA method.[51] AR estimation should be performed, or repeated, during the preoperative assessment, when transvalvular gradients are closer to those to be observed after LVAD insertion; indeed, the high LV filling pressure can partially mask the severity of AR during the preoperative assessment.

MS is a rare finding but, when severe, can obstruct the passage of blood from the left atrium to the LV, reducing LV preload, and increasing pulmonary pressure. MS can be quantified by 2D Doppler TTE or TEE or 3D TTE, using the diastolic pressure gradient derived from the transmitral velocity flow curve and the mitral valve area planimetry obtained by direct tracing of the mitral orifice.[52] Valve replacement with a tissue valve should be considered for more-than-mild mitral valve stenosis.[3]

TR is a common finding in patients eligible for LVAD and, as already discussed, is a risk factor for RVF and poor outcome after implantation. LVAD activation could improve TR because the mechanical LV unloading reduces RV afterload and pulmonary pressures but, at the same time, it can worsen TR because the suddenly increased RV preload can dilate the RV. TR can be evaluated by 2D or 3D Doppler TTE or 2D TEE by using vena contracta width and hepatic vein flow assessment.[51]

The ascending aorta should be evaluated to detect eventual aortic aneurysms or atherosclerotic plaques that could complicate outflow cannula placement. Two-dimensional TTE allows a limited examination of the ascending aorta and aortic arch, but the accuracy of the assessment can be improved by using 2D TEE or, when image quality is not satisfactory or the diagnosis is not clear, computed tomography scan.

All the elements that should be evaluated during the preoperative assessment are listed in Table 37-2.

PERIOPERATIVE ECHOCARDIOGRAPHIC ASSESSMENT

LEFT VENTRICLE

Perioperative echocardiographic assessment, usually performed by 2D TEE, is a fundamental tool for the identification of pathological conditions not detected during the preoperative assessment that could be harmful for the patient. This is necessary to guide the surgical procedure and to prevent complications. The LV, especially the LV apex, where the inflow cannula will be placed, should be carefully evaluated to exclude the presence of clots. The inflow cannula will be oriented within the LV toward the P2 segment of the mitral valve. The echocardiographer will guide the procedure and will test the correct position of the cannula through Doppler measurements: A laminar and unidirectional flow from the ventricle to the device, with a peak velocity of 1 to 2 m/s and a phasic, slightly pulsatile flow pattern, suggests the cannula is well placed, whereas higher velocities and color Doppler aliasing indicate an obstruction that could be due to a thrombus, cannula angulation into the myocardium, or other cannula malposition. The same procedure should be performed for the outflow cannula placement in the ascending aorta. The evidence of laminar flow with low velocities guarantees the good position and function of the cannula.

Table 37-2 Brief Echocardiographic Preoperative Assessment Checklist

LV	RV	Valves and Aorta
➤ LV volumes (2D or 3D TTE)	➤ RV volumes (2D or 3D TTE)	➤ AR
➤ LVEF (2D or 3D TTE)	➤ RVEF (only by 3D TTE)	➤ MS and MR
➤ Left atrial volume	➤ RV function (FAC, TAPSE, RIMP, and TDI S')	➤ TR
➤ Mitral inflow velocities		➤ Ascending aorta aneurysms or atherosclerotic plaques
➤ LV STE global longitudinal strain and strain rate	➤ sPAP, right atrial pressure	
➤ Intraventricular clots	➤ RV STE global longitudinal strain and strain rate	
➤ Intracardiac shunts (2D TEE)		
➤ Pericardial effusion		

Abbreviations: AR, aortic regurgitation; FAC, fractional area change; LV, left ventricle; LVEF, left ventricular ejection fraction; MR, mitral regurgitation; MS, mitral stenosis; RIMP, right-sided index of myocardial performance; RV, right ventricle; RVEF, right ventricular ejection fraction; sPAP, systolic pulmonary artery pressure; STE, speckle-tracking echocardiography; TAPSE, tricuspid annular plane systolic excursion; TDI S', tricuspid annular longitudinal velocity by tissue Doppler imaging; TEE, transesophageal echocardiography; TR, tricuspid regurgitation; TTE, transthoracic echocardiography.

Before LVAD activation, attention should be focused on proper de-airing of the heart chambers and LVAD components. Air bubbles—which could be contained in anastomotic sites, inflow and outflow cannulae, and the anterior interventricular septum—should be carefully detected because they can cause right coronary artery ischemia and the consequent high risk of RVF failure or stroke.[44,53]

After LVAD activation, the main factors that should be considered are (1) the detection of intracardiac shunts and AR, which may previously have been masked by the high filling pressure of the left chambers; (2) evidence of proper LV unloading; and (3) the presence of de novo pericardial effusion.

Right-to-left shunts can sometimes be masked by high filling pressure of the left chambers that obstructs blood passage; when the LVAD is activated, the sudden reduction in left-side pressure can unmask the shunt, which should be closed during the implantation surgical procedure.[3] The same mechanism could provoke the underestimation of AR, which could appear less severe than it is; an accurate staging of AR is fundamental to the ability to compare advantages and risks of a surgical treatment and decide the best option for the patient.

The main goal of LVAD implantation is to obtain an effective mechanical unloading of the LV, which guarantees proper hemodynamic equilibrium. The effectiveness of LVAD therapy is suggested by consistent reduction of left atrial and ventricular filling pressure, size of the left chambers, and pulmonary pressures. Intracardiac and pulmonary pressures should be quantified by cardiac catheterization; however, this is an invasive technique that does not add significant information to what can be found indirectly by echocardiography. The evidence of a mitral ratio of early to late ventricular filling velocities >2, left atrial volume index >33 mL/m^2, systolic pulmonary artery pressure >40 mm Hg, and right atrial pressure >10 mm Hg indicates with high accuracy elevated LV filling pressures.[54] Moreover, a decrease of about 50% in LV volumes and a neutral position or a slight leftward shift of the interventricular septum (IVS) after LVAD activation are suggestive of a proper unloading (Figure 37-1). The IVS position is an important clue in estimating the entity of unloading. A rightward

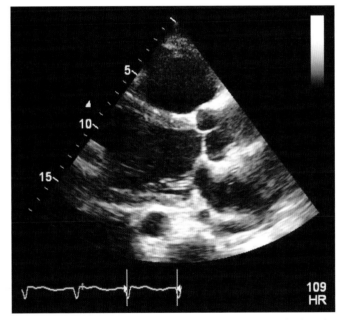

FIGURE 37-1 Normal left ventricular assist device. A properly placed inlet cannula is seen.

Table 37-3 Brief Echocardiographic Perioperative Assessment Checklist

LV	RV	Valves and LVAD Components
➤ De-airing of heart chambers	➤ RV volumes	➤ AR
➤ LV volumes and size	➤ IVS position	➤ MR
➤ IVS position	➤ RV function (FAC, TAPSE, RIMP, and TDI S')	➤ TR
➤ Left atrial volume	➤ sPAP, right atrial pressure	➤ Inflow and outflow cannulae flows (continuous Doppler peak velocities, color Doppler aliasing)
➤ Mitral inflow velocities		
➤ Intraventricular clots		
➤ Intracardiac shunts		
➤ De novo pericardial effusion		

Abbreviations: AR, aortic regurgitation; FAC, fractional area change; IVS, interventricular septum; LV, left ventricle; LVAD, left ventricular assist device; MR, mitral regurgitation; RIMP, right-sided index of myocardial performance; RV, right ventricle; sPAP, systolic pulmonary artery pressure; TAPSE, tricuspid annular plane systolic excursion; TDI S', tricuspid annular longitudinal velocity by tissue Doppler imaging; TR, tricuspid regurgitation.

shift of the IVS with a dilated LV is a common finding before LVAD activation, suggesting high left-side pressures due to an inadequate LV unloading, and requires an increase in rotor speed. A leftward septal shift with a small LV indicates an excessive unloading due to high pump speed that could cause RVF, and therefore should be quickly treated by reducing the rotor speed. A neutral position or a slight leftward shift of the IVS is the goal that should be achieved.

Evaluation for the onset of de novo pericardial effusion is mandatory to early detect one of the most dangerous and challenging-to-diagnose complications after LVAD implantation: cardiac tamponade. It usually occurs with small collections of blood, and it is not easy to find because the assessment of interventricular dependence is no longer possible after LVAD activation. Both 2D TEE and 3D TTE can provide a high level of accuracy in the evaluation of the pericardium using conventional views, provided the physician carefully looks for small effusions (Table 37-3).

RIGHT VENTRICLE

Perioperative assessment of the RV should be focused on RV size and hemodynamic changes caused by LVAD activation. As previously mentioned, LVAD activation can cause 2 opposite responses in the right chambers: the reduced left-side pressure can provoke a decrease in pulmonary pressures and RV afterload, with an improvement of RV systolic function, or, the sudden increase of RV preload, due to the mechanically improved cardiac output, can cause a dilatation of the RV with a worsening of TR and an impairment of RV function, possibly leading to RVF. The positive or negative effect of LVAD is probably determined by the original conditions of the RV before the implant: If the RV has good function with low pulmonary pressures and less-than-moderate TR before the procedure and negative perioperative events do not occur, the risk of RVF onset is very low; on the other hand, when the original RV function is impaired with pulmonary HTN and significant TR, or when RV ischemia or acidosis occurs during the implantation, the risk of severe complications increases.

Another important element that can influence the clinical course is the entity of LV unloading. An excessive rotor speed causes a suction

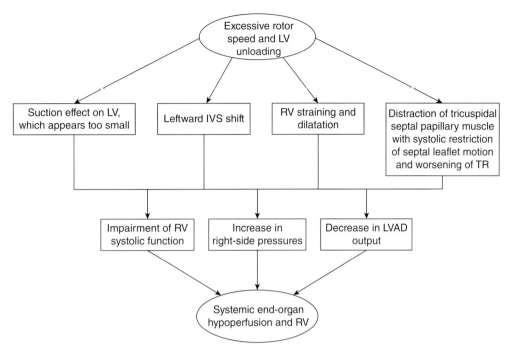

FIGURE 37-2 Effects of excessive mechanical left ventricular unloading. Abbreviations: IVS, intraventricular septum; LV, left ventricle; LVAD, left ventricular assist device; RV, right ventricle; TR, tricuspid regurgitation.

effect on the IVS and the LV, straining and dilating the RV, which can cause the RV to lose part of its contractility. The final effects of this scenario include a decrease of LVAD flow, an increase of right-side pressures, a reduction of RV systolic function, and the development of a systemic end-organ hypoperfusion and RVF (Figure 37-2). Therefore, the RV and IVS should be carefully assessed after LVAD activation to be sure a proper pump speed is set (Table 37-3).

ECHOCARDIOGRAPHIC FOLLOW-UP

A strict echocardiographic follow-up is mandatory after LVAD implantation. Seriate 2D TTEs should be performed to verify the correct functioning of the LVAD and patient hemodynamics, and to eventually improve the device setting. Sonographers and physicians should focus their attention on LV and RV volumes, size, and function; IVS position; hemodynamics; valve diseases; cannula flows; pump speed; and pericardial effusion (Table 37-4).

LVAD implantation improves patient hemodynamics[56,57] and can induce LV reverse remodeling.[58] As previously discussed, a neutral position or a slight leftward shift of the IVS, normal ventricle volumes and size, and low pulmonary pressure suggest a good hemodynamic equilibrium. A very small LV with a marked IVS leftward shift and a dilated RV with worsened TR indicate an excessive pump speed that should be quickly reduced, whereas a dilated LV with a rightward shift of the IVS and high left-side filling pressures require an increase in rotor speed. Measurements should be performed during adjustments of rotor speed to obtain the best performance.

An increased left atrial pressure, a leftward deviation of the IVS, a relatively small LV (<63 mm), an early systolic equalization of RV and right atrial pressure, and RV systolic dysfunction have been shown to be associated with worse midterm outcome.[59,60]

In order to optimize device function and diagnose device malfunctions, several protocols, called ramp tests, were developed by different

Table 37-4 Brief Echocardiographic Follow-up Assessment Checklist

LV	RV	Valves and LVAD Components
➤ LV volumes and size	➤ RV volumes and size	➤ Aortic valve opening
➤ LVEF (after reduction of pump speed)	➤ RVEF (only by 3D TTE)	➤ AR
➤ IVS position	➤ IVS position	➤ MR
➤ Left atrial volume	➤ RV function (FAC, TAPSE, RIMP, and TDI S')	➤ TR
➤ Mitral inflow velocities	➤ sPAP, right atrial pressure	➤ Inflow and outflow cannulae flows (continuous Doppler peak velocities, color Doppler aliasing)
➤ Pericardial effusion	➤ RV STE global longitudinal strain and strain rate	➤ Pump speed

Abbreviations: AR, aortic regurgitation; FAC, fractional area change; IVS, interventricular septum; LV, left ventricle; LVEF, left ventricular ejection fraction; MR, mitral regurgitation; RIMP, right-sided index of myocardial performance; RV, right ventricle; RVEF, right ventricular ejection fraction; sPAP, systolic pulmonary artery pressure; STE, speckle-tracking echocardiography; TAPSE, tricuspid annular plane systolic excursion; TDI S', tricuspid annular longitudinal velocity by tissue Doppler imaging; TEE, transesophageal echocardiography; TTE, transthoracic echocardiography; TR, tricuspid regurgitation.

authors. Currently, recommendations for device speed adjustment include target measures of mean arterial pressure above 65 mm Hg, middle IVS position, and intermittent aortic valve opening while maintaining no more than mild MR to ensure appropriate unloading of the LV.[60] A unique ramp test protocol including the assessment of LV end-diastolic diameter, the frequency of aortic valve opening, valvular insufficiency, blood pressure, and LVAD parameters recorded at increments of 400 rpm from 8000 rpm to 12,000 rpm has been proposed.[61] This protocol showed good effectiveness in pump speed optimization and detection of device malfunction, particularly device thrombosis, and, if the data are confirmed in larger studies, it could be considered a valid tool for the follow-up of these patients.

The evaluation of LV native function is difficult during follow-up, because the LVAD makes LVEF unreliable. Many other measurements have been proposed, eg, the aortic valve opening rate,[62,63] but currently the most-used approach is reducing LVAD pump speed to allow the native LV function to emerge; this procedure, previously considered dangerous and weakly reliable, recently has been revalued and it has been shown to be a safe, accurate, and reproducible method of monitoring myocardial function during LVAD support.[64]

RV volumes, function, and hemodynamics should be carefully evaluated because their alterations are early markers of severe complications. These elements can be assessed by the same parameters already mentioned. The role of 2D STE strain is well established during follow-up,[41] and this measurement should be included in the routine protocol.

The assessment of valve function is an important step in the follow-up echocardiographic assessment. MR and TR should be significantly reduced after LVAD activation, and the evidence of worsened dysfunctions should suggest an inadequate LV unloading. Aortic valve opening should be carefully evaluated. Old pulsatile LVADs caused a permanent aortic valve closure, whereas the continuous-flow devices are associated with intermittent opening of the valve, which could be more or less frequent depending on LVAD pump speed and native LV systolic function. When the valve opening is too frequent, it suggests an inadequate LV unloading or, more rarely, an improvement of LV native function; on the contrary, when the valve is permanently closed, it indicates an excessive LV unloading. According to what is reported, it is mandatory to have certain information about the LVAD type when a patient not known to the clinician has to be evaluated: Evidence of a permanent aortic valve closure is worrisome if the patient has a continuous-flow LVAD, but it is a normal finding if the device is pulsatile.

The aortic valve should be evaluated for regurgitation. As already mentioned, it is not rare to detect the onset of de novo AR or the worsening of dysfunctions already detected before the implantation.

Finally, the inflow and outflow cannula flows should be carefully assessed. Evidence of high peak velocities using Doppler or regurgitation flow suggests the suspicion of cannula obstruction and LVAD pump malfunction, respectively. However, inflow cannula flow is not always detectable because new-generation LVADs can generate a Doppler artifact that confounds the measurements.[65] Sometimes cannula thrombosis can be detected by identifying suspicious masses around the cannulae or in the LV apex. In the assessment of cannula thrombi, 2D TTE and TEE show good accuracy (Figure 37-3), but 3D echocardiography allows a better assessment of all the surrounding structures and can provide additional information when the diagnosis is not clear (Figure 37-4). Evidence of cannula thrombosis is fundamental because the embolic risk is very high and a total occlusion of a cannula can cause acute HF with severe outcomes.

MAIN LEFT VENTRICULAR ASSIST DEVICE DYSFUNCTIONS AND COMPLICATIONS

The most common complications that can occur after LVAD implantation include RVF, pump failure, conditions that cause inadequate LV filling or emptying, and inflow and outflow cannula obstruction.

Pump failure is usually due to pump thrombosis or, rarely, to mechanical malfunction. Pump thrombosis is not an unusual occurrence, particularly in older patients who show a weak compliance with anticoagulation drugs, because LVAD mechanical structure is a good substrate for platelet aggregation and thrombus formation. The diagnosis often is challenging because the LVAD structure reflects ultrasounds. However, a device malfunction could be suggested by evidence of an inadequate LV unloading (dilated LV, rightward deviation of the IVS, MR, permanent opening of the aortic valve) with an increased pump power. Moreover, ramp studies can help to support the diagnosis.[61] This scenario should be distinguished from conditions that cause an inadequate LVAD emptying, which increases afterload, such as outflow cannula obstructions and hypertensive emergencies. These circumstances, reducing the device output despite the high pump power, determine a decrease of LVAD output and an increase of intracardiac pressures, simulating the scenario just described. The evidence of high Doppler velocities at the outflow cannula orifice or the finding of very high blood pressure values without any other echocardiographic pathological finding allows the clinician to obtain the correct diagnosis.

Conditions that reduce the LV preload include RVF, hypovolemia, severe TR, inflow cannula abnormal placement or obstruction (Figure 37-5), and cardiac tamponade.

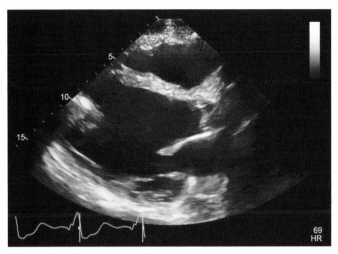

FIGURE 37-3 LVAD thrombus on cannula. The thrombus, identified on the inlet cannula, presents as mobile and with a frondlike appearance on the tip.

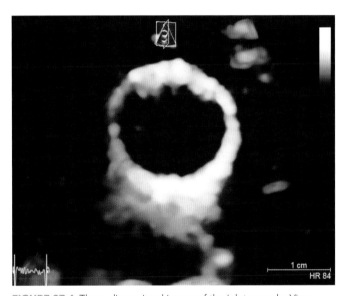

FIGURE 37-4 Three-dimensional image of the inlet cannula. View enface of the inlet cannula looking into the cannula.

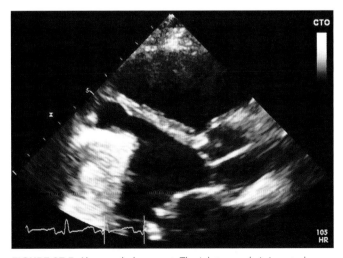

FIGURE 37-5 Abnormal placement. The inlet cannula is inserted deeply into the left ventricle, directed toward the ventricular septum. This causes a "suck down" effect with reduced inflow volume.

RVF pathophysiology, symptoms, and echocardiographic findings were previously discussed; therefore, they will not be repeated here.

These pathological circumstances are all characterized by a reduced LV filling, due to low blood pressure, mechanical obstruction to LV relaxation (cardiac tamponade), or blood passage from the LV to LVAD (inflow cannula obstruction), with a consequent low pump flow despite a normal power. Reduced LV filling causes the decrease in LV size with a leftward deviation of the IVS, whereas the RV is dilated, TR worsens, and right atrial pressure increases. These findings are quite common in RVF or cardiac tamponade, but the scenario is different when an inflow cannula obstruction occurs; in the latter condition, the obstacle to the normal circulation of blood takes place after the LV, which will have increased, and not reduced, volumes and size. Moreover, the evidence of high Doppler velocities at the inflow cannula suggests the correct diagnosis.

A common finding after LVAD implantation is the onset or worsening of AR. When the regurgitation volume is severe, it could reduce the forward pump flow, simultaneously increasing LVAD preload and determining a closed circle that makes the LVAD work ineffectively. Furthermore, increased preload causes an increase of pump speed that, in this case, does not improve cardiac output but causes all those dangerous conditions already mentioned related to a too high pump speed.

REFERENCES

1. Mozaffarian D, Benjamin EJ, Go AS, et al. Heart disease and stroke statistics–2015 update: a report from the American Heart Association. *Circulation.* 2015;131(4):e29-e322. Erratum in: *Circulation.* 2015;131(24):e535.

2. Kirklin JK, Naftel DC, Pagani FD, et al. Seventh INTERMACS annual report: 15,000 patients and counting. *J Heart Lung Transplant.* 2015;34(12):1495-1504.

3. Feldman D, Pamboukian SV, Teuteberg JJ, et al. The 2013 International Society for Heart and Lung Transplantation Guidelines for mechanical circulatory support: executive summary. *J Heart Lung Transplant.* 2013;32(2):157-187.

4. Carluccio E, Dini FL, Biagioli P, et al. The 'Echo Heart Failure Score': an echocardiographic risk prediction score of mortality in systolic heart failure. *Eur J Heart Fail.* 2013;15(8):868-876.

5. Mornoş C, Petrescu L, Ionac A, Cozma D. The prognostic value of a new tissue Doppler parameter in patients with heart failure. *Int J Cardiovasc Imaging.* 2014;30(1):47-55.

6. Ghio S, Temporelli PL, Marsan NA, et al. Prognostic implications of left ventricular dilation in patients with nonischemic heart failure: interactions with restrictive filling pattern and mitral regurgitation. *Congest Heart Fail.* 2012;18(4):198-204.

7. Lang RM, Badano LP, Mor-Avi V, et al. Recommendations for cardiac chamber quantification by echocardiography in adults: an update from the American Society of Echocardiography and the European Association of Cardiovascular Imaging. *J Am Soc Echocardiogr.* 2015;28(1):1-39.e14.

8. Dorosz JL, Lezotte DC, Weitzenkamp DA, Allen LA, Salcedo EE. Performance of 3-dimensional echocardiography in measuring left ventricular volumes and ejection fraction: a systematic review and meta-analysis. *J Am Coll Cardiol.* 2012;59(20):1799-1808.

9. Iacoviello M, Puzzovivo A, Guida P, et al. Independent role of left ventricular global longitudinal strain in predicting prognosis of chronic heart failure patients. *Echocardiography.* 2013;30(7):803-811.

10. Stanton T, Leano R, Marwick TH. Prediction of all-cause mortality from global longitudinal speckle strain: comparison with ejection fraction and wall motion scoring. *Circ Cardiovasc Imaging.* 2009;2(5):356-364.

11. Motoki H, Borowski AG, Shrestha K, et al. Incremental prognostic value of assessing left ventricular myocardial mechanics in patients with chronic systolic heart failure. *J Am Coll Cardiol.* 2012;60(20):2074-2081.

12. Chang SN, Lai YH, Yen CH, et al. Cardiac mechanics and ventricular twist by three-dimensional strain analysis in relation to B-type natriuretic peptide as a clinical prognosticator for heart failure patients. *PLoS One.* 2014;9(12):e115260. Erratum in: *PLoS One.* 2015;10(4):e0123049.

13. Ma C, Chen J, Yang J, et al. Quantitative assessment of left ventricular function by 3-dimensional speckle-tracking echocardiography in patients with chronic heart failure: a meta-analysis. *J Ultrasound Med.* 2014;33(2):287-295.

14. Ghio S, Gavazzi A, Campana C, et al. Independent and additive prognostic value of right ventricular systolic function and pulmonary artery pressure in patients with chronic heart failure. *J Am Coll Cardiol.* 2001;37(1):183-188.

15. Marzec LN, Ambardekar AV. Preoperative evaluation and perioperative management of right ventricular failure after left ventricular assist device implantation. *Semin Cardiothorac Vasc Anesth.* 2013;17(4):249-261.

16. Romano MA, Cowger J, Aaronson KD, Pagani FD. Diagnosis and management of right-sided heart failure in subjects supported with left ventricular assist devices. *Curr Treat Options Cardiovasc Med.* 2010;12(5):420-430.

17. John R, Lee S, Eckman P, Liao K. Right ventricular failure--a continuing problem in patients with left ventricular assist device support. *J Cardiovasc Transl Res.* 2010;3(6):604-611.

18. Rudski LG, Lai WW, Afilalo J, et al. Guidelines for the echocardiographic assessment of the right heart in adults: a report from the American Society of Echocardiography endorsed by the European Association of Echocardiography, a registered branch of the European Society of Cardiology, and the Canadian Society of Echocardiography. *J Am Soc Echocardiogr.* 2010;23(7):685-713; quiz 786-788.

19. Kim J, Cohen SB, Atalay MK, Maslow AD, Poppas A. Quantitative assessment of right ventricular volumes and ejection fraction in patients with left ventricular systolic dysfunction by real time three-dimensional echocardiography versus

cardiac magnetic resonance imaging. *Echocardiography*. 2015;32(5):805-812.

20. Li YD, Wang YD, Zhai ZG, et al. Relationship between echocardiographic and cardiac magnetic resonance imaging-derived measures of right ventricular function in patients with chronic thromboembolic pulmonary hypertension. *Thromb Res*. 2015;135(4):602-606.

21. St John Sutton M, Pfeffer MA, Moye L, et al. Cardiovascular death and left ventricular remodeling two years after myocardial infarction: baseline predictors and impact of long-term use of captopril: information from the Survival and Ventricular Enlargement (SAVE) trial. *Circulation*. 1997;96(10):3294-3299.

22. Zornoff LA, Skali H, Pfeffer MA, et al. Right ventricular dysfunction and risk of heart failure and mortality after myocardial infarction. *J Am Coll Cardiol*. 2002;39(9):1450-1455.

23. Damy T, Kallvikbacka-Bennett A, Goode K, et al. Prevalence of, associations with, and prognostic value of tricuspid annular plane systolic excursion (TAPSE) among out-patients referred for the evaluation of heart failure. *J Card Fail*. 2012;18(3):216-225.

24. Meris A, Faletra F, Conca C, et al. Timing and magnitude of regional right ventricular function: a speckle tracking-derived strain study of normal subjects and patients with right ventricular dysfunction. *J Am Soc Echocardiogr*. 2010;23(8):823-831.

25. Guendouz S, Rappeneau S, Nahum J, et al. Prognostic significance and normal values of 2D strain to assess right ventricular systolic function in chronic heart failure. *Circ J*. 2012;76(1):127-136.

26. Motoki H, Borowski AG, Shrestha K, et al. Right ventricular global longitudinal strain provides prognostic value incremental to left ventricular ejection fraction in patients with heart failure. *J Am Soc Echocardiogr*. 2014;27(7):726-732.

27. Grant AD, Smedira NG, Starling RC, Marwick TH. Independent and incremental role of quantitative right ventricular evaluation for the prediction of right ventricular failure after left ventricular assist device implantation. *J Am Coll Cardiol*. 2012;60(6):521-528.

28. Kirklin JK, Naftel DC, Stevenson LW, et al. INTERMACS database for durable devices for circulatory support: first annual report. *J Heart Lung Transplant*. 2008;27(10):1065-1072.

29. Matthews JC, Koelling TM, Pagani FD, Aaronson KD. The right ventricular failure risk score a pre-operative tool for assessing the risk of right ventricular failure in left ventricular assist device candidates. *J Am Coll Cardiol*. 2008;51(22):2163-2172.

30. Fitzpatrick JR 3rd, Frederick JR, Hsu VM, et al. Risk score derived from pre-operative data analysis predicts the need for biventricular mechanical circulatory support. *J Heart Lung Transplant*. 2008;27(12):1286-1292.

31. Wang Y, Simon MA, Bonde P, et al. Decision tree for adjuvant right ventricular support in patients receiving a left ventricular assist device. *J Heart Lung Transplant*. 2012;31(2):140-149.

32. Atluri P, Goldstone AB, Fairman AS, et al. Predicting right ventricular failure in the modern, continuous flow left ventricular assist device era. *Ann Thorac Surg*. 2013;96(3):857-863; discussion 863-864.

33. Kormos RL, Teuteberg JJ, Pagani FD, et al. Right ventricular failure in patients with the HeartMate II continuous-flow left ventricular assist device: incidence, risk factors, and effect on outcomes. *J Thorac Cardiovasc Surg*. 2010;139(5):1316-1324.

34. Kalogeropoulos AP, Kelkar A, Weinberger JF, et al. Validation of clinical scores for right ventricular failure prediction after implantation of continuous-flow left ventricular assist devices. *J Heart Lung Transplant*. 2015;34(12):1595-1603.

35. Lam KM, Ennis S, O'Driscoll G, Solis JM, Macgillivray T, Picard MH. Observations from non-invasive measures of right heart hemodynamics in left ventricular assist device patients. *J Am Soc Echocardiogr*. 2009;22(9):1055-1062.

36. Puwanant S, Hamilton KK, Klodell CT, et al. Tricuspid annular motion as a predictor of severe right ventricular failure after left ventricular assist device implantation. *J Heart Lung Transplant*. 2008;27(10):1102-1107.

37. Baumwol J, Macdonald PS, Keogh AM, et al. Right heart failure and "failure to thrive" after left ventricular assist device: clinical predictors and outcomes. *J Heart Lung Transplant*. 2011;30(8):888-895.

38. Dandel M, Potapov E, Krabatsch T, et al. Load dependency of right ventricular performance is a major factor to be considered in decision making before ventricular assist device implantation. *Circulation*. 2013;128(11 Suppl 1):S14-S23.

39. Kalogeropoulos AP, Al-Anbari R, Pekarek A, et al. The Right Ventricular Function After Left Ventricular Assist Device (RVF-LVAD) study: rationale and preliminary results. *Eur Heart J Cardiovasc Imaging*. 2015; pii:jev162. [Epub ahead of print]

40. Cameli M, Lisi M, Righini FM, et al. Speckle tracking echocardiography as a new technique to evaluate right ventricular function in patients with left ventricular assist device therapy. *J Heart Lung Transplant*. 2013;32(4):424-430.

41. Kato TS, Jiang J, Schulze PC, et al. Serial echocardiography using tissue Doppler and speckle tracking imaging to monitor right ventricular failure before and after left ventricular assist device surgery. *JACC Heart Fail*. 2013;1(3):216-222.

42. Cameli M, Sparla S, Focardi M, et al. Evaluation of right ventricular function in the management of patients referred for left ventricular assist device therapy. *Transplant Proc*. 2015;47(7):2166-2168.

43. Herod JW, Ambardekar AV. Right ventricular systolic and diastolic function as assessed by speckle-tracking echocardiography improve with prolonged isolated left ventricular assist device support. *J Card Fail*. 2014;20(7):498-505.

44. Patangi SO, George A, Pauli H, et al. Management issues during HeartWare left ventricular assist device implantation and the role of transesophageal echocardiography. *Ann Card Anaesth.* 2013;16(4):259-267.

45. Pal JD, Klodell CT, John R, et al. Low operative mortality with implantation of a continuous-flow left ventricular assist device and impact of concurrent cardiac procedures. *Circulation.* 2009;120(11 Suppl):S215-S219.

46. Vengala S, Nanda NC, Dod HS, et al. Images in geriatric cardiology. Usefulness of live three-dimensional transthoracic echocardiography in aortic valve stenosis evaluation. *Am J Geriatr Cardiol.* 2004;13(5):279-284.

47. Fang L, Hsiung MC, Miller AP, et al. Assessment of aortic regurgitation by live three-dimensional transthoracic echocardiographic measurements of vena contracta area: usefulness and validation. *Echocardiography.* 2005;22(9):775-781. Erratum in: *Echocardiography.* 2006;23(1):table of contents.

48. Agricola E, Oppizzi M, Pisani M, Maisano F, Margonato A. Accuracy of real-time 3D echocardiography in the evaluation of functional anatomy of mitral regurgitation. *Int J Cardiol.* 2008;127(3):342-349.

49. Aggarwal A, Raghuvir R, Eryazici P, et al. The development of aortic insufficiency in continuous-flow left ventricular assist device-supported patients. *Ann Thorac Surg.* 2013;95(2):493-498.

50. Tuzun E, Pennings K, van Tuijl S, et al. Assessment of aortic valve pressure overload and leaflet functions in an ex vivo beating heart loaded with a continuous flow cardiac assist device. *Eur J Cardiothorac Surg.* 2014;45(2):377-383.

51. Lancellotti P, Tribouilloy C, Hagendorff A, et al. Recommendations for the echocardiographic assessment of native valvular regurgitation: an executive summary from the European Association of Cardiovascular Imaging. *Eur Heart J Cardiovasc Imaging.* 2013;14(7):611-644.

52. Baumgartner H, Hung J, Bermejo J, et al. Echocardiographic assessment of valve stenosis: EAE/ASE recommendations for clinical practice. *Eur J Echocardiogr.* 2009;10(1):1-25. Erratum in: *Eur J Echocardiogr.* 2009;10(3):479.

53. Sheinberg R, Brady MB, Mitter N. Intraoperative transesophageal echocardiography and ventricular assist device insertion. *Semin Cardiothorac Vasc Anesth.* 2011;15(1-2):14-24.

54. Estep JD, Vivo RP, Krim SR, et al. Echocardiographic evaluation of hemodynamics in patients with systolic heart failure supported by a continuous-flow LVAD. *J Am Coll Cardiol.* 2014;64(12):1231-1241.

55. Xydas S, Rosen RS, Ng C, et al. Mechanical unloading leads to echocardiographic, electrocardiographic, neurohormonal, and histologic recovery. *J Heart Lung Transplant.* 2006;25(1):7-15.

56. Gupta S, Woldendorp K, Muthiah K, et al. Normalisation of haemodynamics in patients with end-stage heart failure with continuous-flow left ventricular assist device therapy. *Heart Lung Circ.* 2014;23(10):963-969.

57. McDiarmid A, Gordon B, Wrightson N, et al. Hemodynamic, echocardiographic, and exercise-related effects of the HeartWare left ventricular assist device in advanced heart failure. *Congest Heart Fail.* 2013;19(1):11-15.

58. Morgan JA, Brewer RJ, Nemeh HW, et al. Left ventricular reverse remodeling with a continuous flow left ventricular assist device measured by left ventricular end-diastolic dimensions and severity of mitral regurgitation. *ASAIO J.* 2012;58(6):574-577.

59. Topilsky Y, Oh JK, Shah DK, et al. Echocardiographic predictors of adverse outcomes after continuous left ventricular assist device implantation. *JACC Cardiovasc Imaging.* 2011;4(3):211-222.

60. Topilsky Y, Hasin T, Oh JK, et al. Echocardiographic variables after left ventricular assist device implantation associated with adverse outcome. *Circ Cardiovasc Imaging.* 2011;4(6):648-661.

61. Uriel N, Morrison KA, Garan AR, et al. Development of a novel echocardiography ramp test for speed optimization and diagnosis of device thrombosis in continuous-flow left ventricular assist devices: the Columbia ramp study. *J Am Coll Cardiol.* 2012;60(18):1764-1775.

62. Estep JD, Yarrabolu T, Win HK, et al. Median axial flow pump speed associated with cessation of aortic valve opening is an indicator of remission of chronic heart failure in patients supported by a left ventricular assist device (abstract). *J Heart Lung Transplant.* 2008;27:S185.

63. Mancini DM, Beniaminovitz A, Levin H, et al. Low incidence of myocardial recovery after left ventricular assist device implantation in patients with chronic heart failure. *Circulation.* 1998;98(22):2383-2389.

64. George RS, Sabharwal NK, Webb C, et al. Echocardiographic assessment of flow across continuous-flow ventricular assist devices at low speeds. *J Heart Lung Transplant.* 2010;29(11):1245-1252.

65. Lesicka A, Feinman JW, Thiele K, Andrawes MN. Echocardiographic artifact induced by HeartWare left ventricular assist device. *Anesth Analg.* 2015;120(6):1208-1211.

38 EVALUATION OF HEMODYNAMICS IN PATIENTS SUPPORTED BY CONTINUOUS LVADs

Mahwash Kassi, MD
Ashrith Guha, MD, MPH, FACC
Jerry Estep, MD

EVALUATION OF HEMODYNAMICS IN PATIENTS WITH CONTINUOUS FLOW LEFT VENTRICULAR ASSIST DEVICES

INTRODUCTION

End-stage heart failure (HF) is characterized by specific hemodynamic abnormalities. These abnormalities are a result of left ventricular (LV) systolic and diastolic dysfunction. This in turn leads to right ventricular (RV) dysfunction due to secondary pulmonary hypertension (PH). Systolic dysfunction in end-stage HF is manifested by low cardiac output and elevated left ventricular end-diastolic pressure (LVEDP) as measured by pulmonary capillary wedge pressure (PCWP). The elevation of PCWP increases pulmonary arterial pressure and hence increases afterload of the RV. In both ischemic and nonischemic cardiomyopathies, RV often has intrinsic contractile dysfunction and its performance is worsened by increased loading due to secondary PH. Left ventricular assist devices (LVADs) have been shown to decrease left ventricular end-diastolic volume and pressure and, in turn, decrease left atrial pressure (LAP) and pulmonary arterial pressure (PAP), while increasing effective cardiac output (CO).

Currently, the 2 most widely used durable LVADs are HeartMate II (St Jude Medical, Pleasanton, CA) and HeartWare (HVAD, HeartWare Inc., Framingham, MA), both of which are continuous-flow devices (CF-LVAD) (Figure 38-1). Although the 2 devices have a different mechanism of pumping blood—HeartMate II is an axial flow pump and HVAD is an intrapericardial, centrifugal pump—the hemodynamic effects are similar. A newer generation HM III device is currently under investigation.

For simplicity, this chapter will focus on the hemodynamic effects of continuous-flow LVADs. Furthermore, the role of echocardiography in evaluation of device function will be discussed.

HEMODYNAMIC EFFECTS OF VENTRICULAR ASSIST DEVICES

GOALS OF LEFT VENTRICULAR ASSIST DEVICE SUPPORT AND EFFECT ON PRESSURE-VOLUME RELATIONSHIP

Pressure volume loops (PVLs) have played an important role in understanding the hemodynamic effects of LVADs.[1] Figure 38-2A shows the changes in PVL with HF and that of a patient with CF-LVAD. As the name denotes, CF-LVADs continuously unload the heart, irrespective of the cardiac cycle. This results in loss of the isovolumetric phase of the cardiac cycle. The normal PVL is trapezoidal and with loss of the isovolumetric phase, it transforms into a triangular shape. With increasing pump flow rates, the peak LV pressure generation decreases and the LV becomes increasingly unloaded. This causes a shift in the PVL toward the left. This decreases the pressure volume area (PVA) and reflects a decrease in MVO2. As the LV becomes more unloaded, the LAP and the PCWP decrease.

EFFECT OF CONTINUOUS-FLOW LEFT VENTRICULAR ASSIST DEVICE ON BLOOD PRESSURE AND AORTIC VALVE OPENING

With incremental increase in speed of the CF-LVAD, the peak LV pressure decreases and with overall rise in flow rates, the aortic pressure increases. This leads to dissociation between peak LV and aortic pressure (Ao) (Figure 38-2B to E). The aortic valve (AV) opening is dependent on the LV-Ao pressure gradient. As the pump speed increases, the LV-Ao dissociation occurs to a point where the AV no longer opens. This in turn leads to lack of pulsatility. The LV-Ao dissociation is only part of the physiological process that explains opening or closure of the AV. The LV preload and contractility can also play an important role in determining this process.

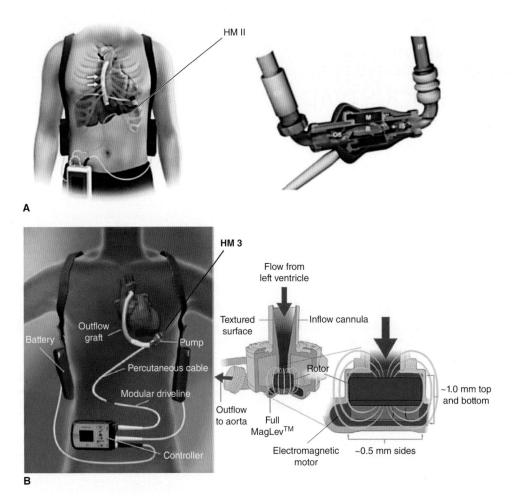

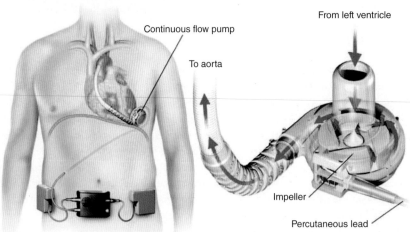

FIGURE 38-1 Drawings and cross-sections of selected continuous-flow left ventricular assist devices (LVADs). **A.** HM II (subdiaphragmatic pump). Arterial blood passes from the left ventricle into the pump through the inflow (IF) conduit; blood flow direction is straightened by the inflow stator (IS); the rotor (R) controlled by the motor (M) spins to generate the needed force for blood to pass through the outflow stator (OS), then through the outflow (OF) conduit. Typical operating speeds are 8800 to 9400 rpm. (Adopted and modified from Stainback et al. *J Am Soc Echocardiogr.* 2015;28:853-909. Heatley et al. *J Heart Lung Transplant.* 2016;35:528-536.) **B.** HM 3 (intrapericardial pump). The rotor is magnetically levitated via electromagnetic coils and rotated via motor drive coils. The levitated rotor produces wide recirculation passages as shown in the magnified schematic on the right side with view of the gaps around the rotor and magnetic fields. (Adopted and modified from Netuka et al. *JACC.* 2015;66(23).) **C.** HVAD (intrapericardial pump). The continuous flow of blood through the centrifugal pump is shown. Blood is conveyed through the pump via an impeller that is suspended by a combination of magnetic and hydrodynamic forces, allowing frictionless rotation at operating speeds of 1800 to 2400 rpm. (Reprinted with permission from Aaronson et al. *Circulation.* 2012;125:3191-3200.)

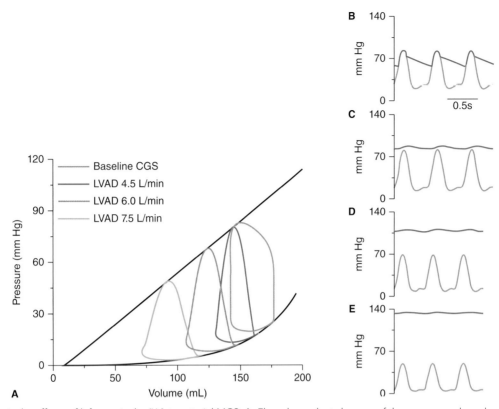

FIGURE 38-2 Ventricular effects of left ventricular (LV)-to-arterial MCS. **A.** Flow-dependent changes of the pressure-volume loop with LV-to-aortic pumping. The loop becomes triangular and shifts progressively leftward (indicating increasing degrees of LV unloading). Corresponding LV and aortic pressure waveforms at baseline **(B)**, 4.5 L/min **(C)**, 6.0 L/min **(D)**, and 7.5 L/min **(E)**. With increased flow, there are greater degrees of LV unloading and uncoupling between aortic and peak LV pressure generation. Abbreviation: LVAD, left ventricular assist device.

As the CF-LVAD speed increases (increased revolutions per minute [RPMs]), the LV preload decreases to a point where there is not enough LV volume to cause ejection. At the bedside, this is evident as the RPMs increase, the pulsatility decreases, to a point where there is no longer a palpable pulse. The speed at which the pulse drop occurs varies from patient to patient. Generally speaking 60% of the patients with CF-LVADs do not have a pulse.

Native contractility of the LV affects AV opening with more pressure generation in the LV cavity. This is particularly true for patients with myocardial recovery, where the AV valve may open at every beat.

BLOOD PRESSURE IN CONTINUOUS-FLOW LEFT VENTRICULAR ASSIST DEVICES

Depending on whether CF-LVAD patients have a pulse, the automatic or manual cuff blood pressure (BP) measurements may be inaccurate. For patients without a palpable pulse, Doppler devices are needed to measure BP accurately. Doppler signals are first heard as the perfusion pressure approaches the mean arterial BP. The mean BP goal in LVAD patients is between 60 and 85 mm Hg. Consistent high BP (defined as mean BP over 90 mm Hg) is associated with higher risks of strokes and bleeding.

EFFECT OF AFTERLOAD ON PUMP FUNCTION

CF-LVADs are sensitive to afterload as pump output depends on the pressure gradient between the pump outflow graft and aorta. Centrifugal flow LVADs are more sensitive to afterload than axial flow pumps. Higher afterload therefore results in decreased flow and in turn decreased LV unloading. Maintaining an effective mean BP is important for appropriate device function of the pump and optimal LV unloading.

EFFECT OF PRELOAD AND PUMP FUNCTION

Optimal preload is important for proper pump function. The preload is determined by 2 factors in patients who are supported by an LVAD: (1) overall volume body status, and (2) native RV function. In conditions where the effective body volume is reduced (such as dehydration and gastrointestinal [GI] bleeding), excess unloading can lead to suction events. The ventricular septum and the lateral free wall can be drawn into the inflow cannula causing both intermittent inflow obstruction and ventricular tachycardia.

EFFECT OF NATIVE VENTRICULAR CONTRACTILITY ON PUMP FUNCTION

Most patients with CF-LVADs do not have much native contractility. Although rare, but with the continuous LV unloading and optimal HF medications, the LV can completely reverse remodel. Increased LV contractility can lead to suction events, which is associated with higher risk of both pump thrombosis and ventricular arrhythmia.

USE OF ECHOCARDIOGRAPHY TO EVALUATE PUMP FUNCTION AND RECOVERY

Echocardiography plays a central role in surveillance of and detection of complications related to LVADs. The recent ASE document provides a comprehensive overview of recommendations regarding acquisition and protocol for surveillance, optimization of device function, troubleshooting complications, and evaluation of myocardial recovery.[2]

SURVEILLANCE ECHOCARDIOGRAPHY

Surveillance echocardiography in patients with CF-LVADs is used to detect the following:

1. Complications related to chronic LVAD support such as thrombosis and right HF, and

2. Pump speed optimization to ensure effective LV unloading.

Particular attention needs to be paid to LV size (and decrement compared to baseline), AV opening, location of the interatrial and interventricular septums, severity of aortic and mitral regurgitation (MR), and RV function. Decreased LV size, impaired AV opening, reduction in MR severity, and reduction of pulmonary

artery systolic pressures (PASPs) are all indices of optimum unloading.

Optimal LVAD hemodynamics, as explained earlier, is a complex interplay of patient characteristics, native heart function, and device settings. Physicians must be cautious when selecting optimum LVAD speed in the perioperative period because preload and afterload conditions are altered by surgery. RV dysfunction often worsens in the postoperative period due to aortopulmonary bypass. However, rare cases may improve postoperatively, which may allow complete LV unloading and an increase in LVAD speed. There is variability among clinicians regarding appropriate speed selection; some physicians advocate partial LV unloading in the immediate postoperative period to avoid acute RV failure due to volume overload, whereas others are more liberal with LVAD speed. A comprehensive table for evaluation of CF-LVAD post implant is shown in Table 38-1.

An LVAD optimization protocol needs to be performed prior to patient discharge to ensure effective unloading. Subsequent surveillance is recommended at 1, 3, 6, and 12 months and every 6 to 12 months thereafter.

Patients with an LVAD may have symptoms of persistent HF. An algorithm delineating optimization of LVAD in patients with persistent HF symptoms is shown in Figure 38-3. Although a right heart catheterization may be useful, echocardiography provides noninvasive means of filling pressure. Figure 38-4 shows tissue Doppler patterns in a clinically stable patient (*panel A*) and 1 with decompensated HF (*panel B*). An algorithm based on right atrial pressure (RAP), pulmonary artery systolic pressure (sPAP), indexed left atrial volume (LAVi), mitral inflow velocities, and tissue Doppler is shown in Figure 38-5. These indices were correlated with invasive hemodynamics and have reasonable sensitivity and specificity to detect high filling pressures.[3]

DETECTION OF COMPLICATIONS

The second major use of echocardiography in patients with LVADs is for detecting complications. In this section we will discuss some of the major complications of LVADs and echocardiographic parameters to assess and predict these complications in light of relevant cases.

PATIENT CASE

A 46-year-old woman with nonischemic cardiomyopathy on home milrinone presented to the hospital for a planned LVAD insertion. The patient was clinically stable postoperatively. Seven days after surgery, the device had low-flow alarms soon after initiation of anticoagulation. Echocardiography was performed to evaluate the

Table 38-1 Continuous-flow LVAD Postimplant Complications and Device Dysfunction Detected by Echocardiography

Pericardial effusion

With or without cardiac tamponade including RV compression. Tamponade: Respirophasic flow changes; poor RVOT SV.

LV failure secondary to partial LV unloading

(by serial examination comparison)

a. 2D/3D: Increasing LV size by linear or volume measurements; increased AV opening duration, increased left atrial volume.

b. Doppler: Increased mitral inflow peak E-wave diastolic velocity, increased E/A and E/e0 ratio, decreased deceleration time of mitral E velocity, worsening functional MR, and elevated pulmonary artery systolic pressure.

RV failure

a. 2D: Increased RV size, decreased RV systolic function, high RAP (dilated IVC/leftward atrial septal shift), leftward deviation of ventricular septum.

b. Doppler: Increased TR severity, reduced RVOT SV, reduced LVAD inflow cannula and/or outflow-graft velocities (ie, <0.5 m/s with severe failure); inflow-cannula high velocities if associated with a suction event. Note: A too-high LVAD pump speed may contribute to RV failure by increasing TR (septal shift) and/or by increasing RV preload.

Inadequate LV filling or excessive LV unloading

Small LV dimensions (typically <3 cm and/or marked deviation of interventricular septum toward LV). Note: May be due to RV failure and/or pump speed too high for loading conditions.

LVAD suction with induced ventricular ectopy

Underfilled LV and mechanical impact of inflow cannula with LV endocardium, typically septum, resolves with speed turndown.

LVAD-related continuous aortic insufficiency

Clinically significant—at least moderate and possibly severe—characterized by an AR proximal jet-to-LVOT height ratio >46%, or AR vena contracta $3 mm; increased LV size and relatively decreased RVOT SV despite normal/increased inflow cannula and/or outflow graft flows.

LVAD-related MR

a. Primary: Inflow cannula interference with mitral apparatus.

b. Secondary: MR-functional, related to partial LV unloading/persistent HF.

Note: Elements of both a and b may be present.

Intracardiac thrombus

Including right and left atrial, LV apical, and aortic root thrombus

Inflow-cannula abnormality

a. 2D/3D: Small or crowded inflow zone with or without evidence of localized obstructive muscle trabeculation, adjacent MV apparatus or thrombus; malpositioned inflow cannula.

b. High-velocity color or spectral Doppler at inflow orifice. Results from malposition, suction event/other inflow obstruction: Aliased color-flow Doppler, CW Doppler velocity >1.5 m/s.

c. Low-velocity inflow (markedly reduced peak systolic and nadir diastolic velocities) may indicate internal inflow-cannula thrombosis or more distal obstruction within the system. Doppler flow velocity profile may appear relatively continuous (decreased phasic/pulsatile pattern).

(Continued)

Table 38-1 Continuous-flow LVAD Postimplant Complications and Device Dysfunction Detected by Echocardiography (Continued)

Outflow-graft abnormality

Typically due to obstruction/pump cessation.

a. 2D/3D imaging: Visible kink or thrombus (infrequently seen).

b. Doppler: Peak outflow-graft velocity $2 m/s* if near obstruction site; however, diminished or absent spectral Doppler signal if sample volume is remote from obstruction location, combined with lack of RVOT SV change and/or expected LV-dimension change with pump-speed changes.

Hypertensive emergency

New reduced/minimal AV opening relative to baseline examination at normal BP, especially if associated with new/worsened LV dilatation and worsening MR. Note: HTN may follow an increase in pump speed.

Pump malfunction/pump arrest

a. Reduced inflow-cannula or outflow-graft flow velocities on color and spectral Doppler or, with pump arrest, shows diastolic flow reversal.

b. Signs of worsening HF including dilated LV, worsening MR, worsened TR, and/or increased TR velocity; attenuated speed-change responses: decrease or absence of expected changes in LV linear dimension, AV opening duration, and RVOT SV with increased or decreased pump speeds; for HVAD, loss of inflow-cannula Doppler artifact.

Adapted from ASE guidelines.

Abbreviations: AR, aortic regurgitation; AV, aortic valve; BP, blood pressure; CW, continuous wave; E/A, early and late diastolic filling; E/e0, tissue Doppler mitral annular velocity; HF, heart failure; HTN, hypertension; IVC, inferior vena cava; LV, left ventricular; LVAD, left ventricular assist device; LVOT, left ventricular outflow tract; MR, mitral regurgitation; MV, mitral valve; RAP, right atrial pressure; RV, right ventricular; RVOT, right ventricular outflow tract; SV, stroke volume; TR, tricuspid regurgitation.

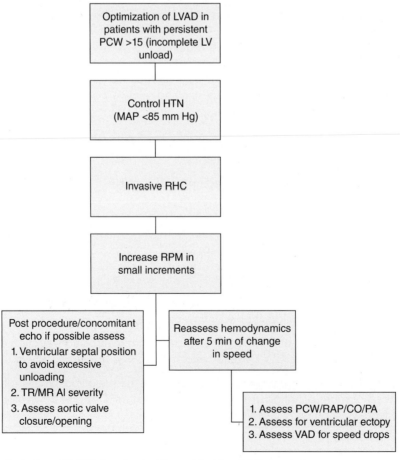

FIGURE 38-3 Algorithm for optimization of LVAD's in patients with persistent heart failure symptoms.

Clinically stable after LVAD   Heart failure during LVAD support

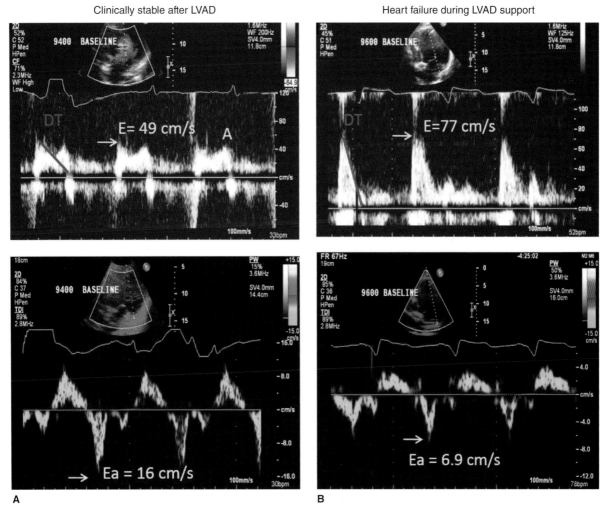

FIGURE 38-4 Echo signs associated with acquired heart failure during long-term continuous-flow LVAD support. **A.** Baseline echo findings in a clinically stable patient on the HeartMate II device (9400 RPM) 1 year after implant. *Upper panel,* peak early diastolic mitral inflow (E)/late (A) velocity (E/A ratio is 1.1), deceleration time (DT) ~154 ms. *Lower panel,* early peak diastolic relaxation velocity (e') measured using tissue Doppler imaging of the lateral mitral valve annulus. **B.** Echo findings 16 months (2.5 years after implant) later in the same patient with acquired clinical left- and right-sided HF in the setting of acquired renal failure with normal device function. *Upper panel,* increased peak E wave velocity, decreased deceleration time (~100 ms) and increased E/A ratio 3.3. *Lower panel,* measured relative decrease in LV relaxation (e') and relative increase in E/e'.

etiology of the low-flow alarms. Anterior echodensity was suggestive of a thrombus compressing the RV (Figure 38-6). A diagnosis of cardiac tamponade was made and the patient's chest was reopened for a washout. After the washout procedure, no further low-flow alarms occurred.

CARDIAC TAMPONADE

Cardiac tamponade is not an uncommon complication after device insertion. It usually occurs in the postoperative period, soon after insertion of the LVAD when anticoagulation is started. Echocardiography may or may not show an obvious effusion. Other hints include LV compression and suction with signs of persistent HF. If no obvious effusion/thrombus is seen, cardiac computed tomography (CT) may be performed to evaluate the etiology of external

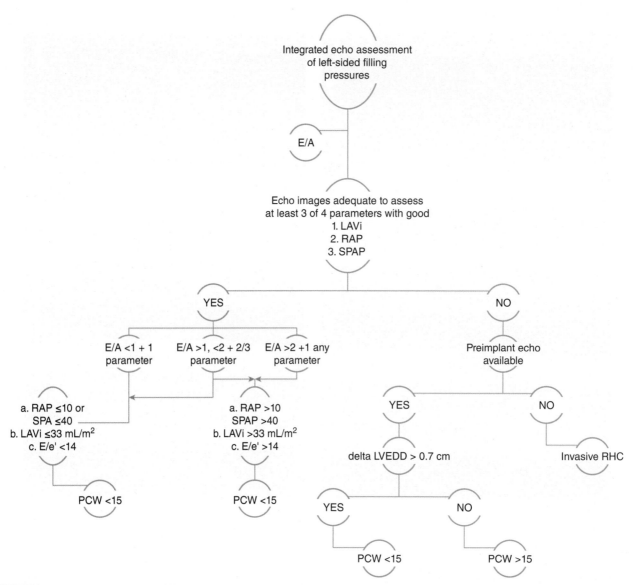

FIGURE 38-5 Non-invasive assessment of filling pressures using echocardiography in patients with left ventricular assist devices. LAVi: Left atrial volume index; RAP: right atrial pressure; SPAP: systolic pulmonary artery pressure; E/A: Mitral inflow E and A velocity ratio; PCW: pulmonary capillary wedge pressure; LVEDD: left ventricular end-diastolic dimension; RHC: right heart catheterization; delta LVEDD = preimplant LVEDD - postimplant LVEDD.

compression. An algorithm for troubleshooting early postoperative LVAD alarms is shown in Figure 38-7.

PATIENT CASE

A 67-year-old man with ischemic cardiomyopathy underwent LVAD placement. An initial echocardiogram showed adequate unloading with a smaller LV size, no AV opening, normal filling pressures, and low tricuspid regurgitation (TR) velocity. However, the patient later presented to the hospital with bilateral edema, abdominal distention, and elevated jugular venous pressure. An echocardiogram showed a large right atrium and ventricle with moderate to severe TR (Figure 38-8). Findings were suspicious for RV failure. A right heart catheterization was performed, which showed high RAP of 20, PA pressures 20/12 mm Hg, and PCWP of 10 mm Hg with a low cardiac index and output. This confirmed the findings of right-sided

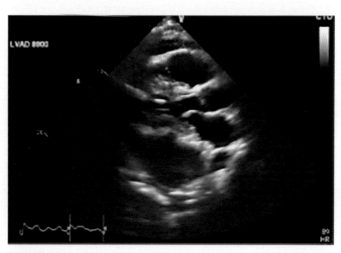

FIGURE 38-6 Echocardiogram parasternal long axis view showing an anterior thrombus compressing the right ventricle.

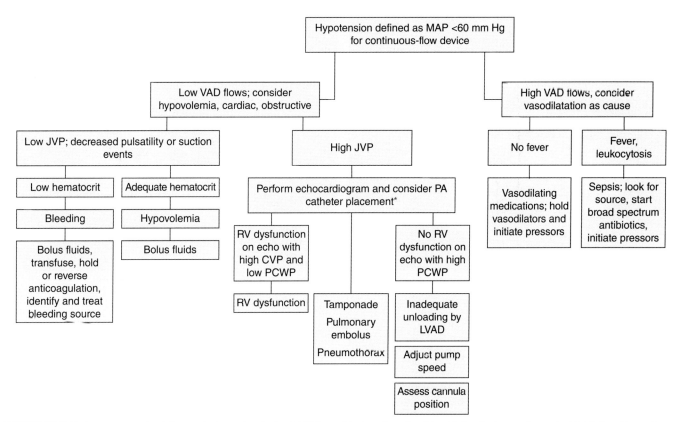

FIGURE 38-7 Early postoperative left ventricular assist device (LVAD) troubleshooting algorithm. Role of echocardiography highlighted by red asterisk to detect (RV) dysfunction, tamponade, inadequate left ventricular (LV) unloading, and inflow cannula position in patients with hypotension on continuous-flow LVAD support. (Reprinted with permission from The 2013 International Society for Heart and Lung Transplantation Guidelines for mechanical circulatory support: Executive summary Feldman, David et al. *The Journal of Heart and Lung Transplantation.* 32(2):157-187.)

HF. Thus, the patient was started on low-dose milrinone and inhaled nitric oxide with rapid transition to heart transplant.

RIGHT VENTRICULAR FAILURE

RV failure is a morbid complication of LVAD implantation. Definitions of early RV failure vary, but the generally accepted definition is CVP greater than 18 mm Hg and cardiac index less than 2 L/min/m² and requiring inotropic or vasodilator therapy or placement of right ventricular assist device (RVAD). Recent studies have emphasized the value of predicting RV failure to evaluate the need for planned biventricular support.

Features that are suggestive of RV failure include high RAP, an enlarged RV resulting in dilated annulus with severe TR, and deviation of the interventricular toward the left side with or without a small LV. When making this diagnosis by echocardiography, clinical correlation is necessary. RV failure occurs in the immediate postoperative period because of deleterious effects of aortopulmonary bypass, volume overload because of the now unloaded LV, blood transfusion, or other metabolic effects. Some of these factors such as acidosis are reversible, and in those situations, reversing the underlying condition may result in recovery. Figure 38-9 shows images of a patient with early postoperative RV failure.

Late RV failure is either a result of ineffective unloading of the LV or persistent and possibly irreversible RV failure. For patients

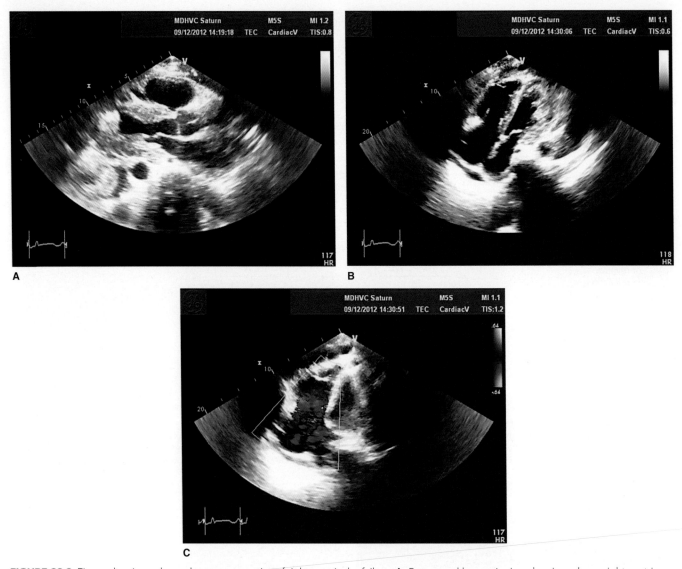

A

B

C

FIGURE 38-8 Figure showing echocardogram suggestive of right ventricular failure. **A:** Parasternal long axis view showing a large right ventricle and small left ventricle. **B:** 4-chamber view showing a large right atrium and right ventricle with septal preference towards the left ventricle. **C:** severe functional tricuspid regurgitation due to dilation of the annulus.

with ineffective unloading, increasing the pump speed will affect RV hemodynamics. Persistent late RV failure in the presence of normal LV filling pressure or PCWP less than 15 mm Hg is usually medically managed with diuretics, inotropes, or even an RVAD, although the patient may eventually need heart transplant.

PATIENT CASE

A 56-year-old woman with nonischemic cardiomyopathy and on HMII LVAD support for 2 years, presented to the hospital with decompensated HF. She was on a stable anticoagulation regimen of aspirin and Coumadin. A few days prior to presentation, she noticed that her urine was darker; in the last day, she had minimal urine output. Her blood work was suggestive of hemolysis with elevated lactate dehydrogenase (LDH) and plasma-free Hb. Urine analysis showed hemoglobinuria. These findings were concerning for pump thrombosis. A speed change echo was performed that

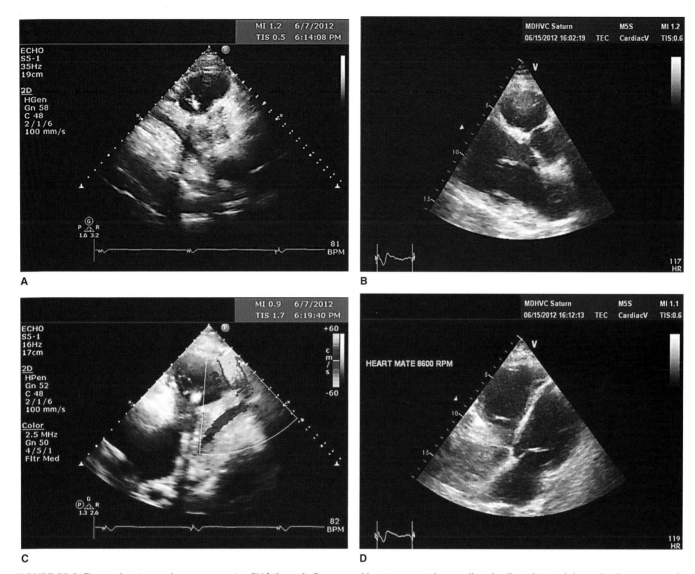

FIGURE 38-9 Figure showing early post-operative RV failure. **A:** Parasternal long image with a small and collpsed LV with large RV, **B:** parasternal long axis view showing a large left and right ventricle. The right ventricle is enlarged and had reduced function with incompletely unloaded left ventricle. **C:** Color flow Doppler showing flow through a small LV **D:** 4 chamber view showing large right atrium and ventricle and septal preference to the left.

showed no change in the left ventricular end-diastolic dimension (LVEDD) with increasing speeds and no AV closure at the highest speed. After LVAD exchange, postoperative findings were consistent with a large thrombus in the device rotor.

PUMP THROMBOSIS

Pump thrombosis is a feared complication of LVADs. A recent study of LVAD patients by Scandroglio et al illustrated 3 types of pump thrombosis, each with different flow patterns and management.[4] The 3 types of pump thrombosis are:

1. Prepump thrombosis: Occurring at the inflow cannula

2. Intrapump thrombosis: Thrombosis within the rotor

3. Postpump thrombosis: Thrombosis or stenosis in the outflow graft.

Studies predicting pump thrombosis in patients with LVADs are rare. The lower LV decrement index (preimplant dimension – optimal set speed dimension ÷ preimplant dimension × 100) <15% was shown to be predictive of pump thrombosis in a recent study (Figure 38-10).[5] A larger angle of the inflow cannula relative to the midline of the mitral valve is also thought to be predictive of pump thrombosis.

Echocardiographic-guided ramp studies are helpful to detect pump thrombosis (Figures 38-11 and 38-12). The protocols include assessment of LVEDD, AV opening, severity of MR and aortic regurgitation (AR), and tricuspid regurgitation velocity and pulmonary artery systolic pressure at each incremental speed. However, there are 2 important caveats when interpreting the results of a ramp study. First, HeartMate II (HM II) and HeartWare (HVAD) do not behave similarly in terms of reduction in LVEDD size. The slope of reduction in HM II is more predictable and linear. However, in HVAD the degree of reduction in LVEDD with incremental pump speed while the AV is open is less than when the AV is closed. With the AV completely closed, a significant reduction in LVEDD is seen with incremental pump speed. This is hypothesized to be a result of the difference in device design. Therefore, a decreased slope of LVEDD in patients with HVADs does not necessarily mean device malfunction. For HVAD patients, we refer readers to the algorithm proposed by Scandogriole, where clinical, echocardiographic, and flow curves from the device were employed to make a diagnosis.[4] Secondly, conditions that cause false-positive ramp studies include elevated mean arterial pressure (MAP) and AR, whereas small thrombus size can cause false-negative tests.

Doppler flow patterns may also help in detecting pump thrombosis. Systolic and diastolic velocities should be measured at the inflow and outflow cannula. A high velocity (2 cm/s) is indicative of obstruction. A high systolic and diastolic (S/D) velocity ratio has

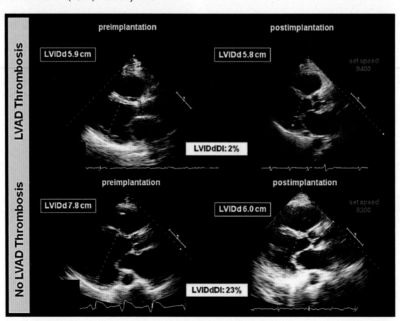

FIGURE 38-10 LV dimension decrement index. LVIDd before and after LVAD implantation at optimal set speed before discharge in a patient who subsequently developed pump thrombosis requiring urgent pump exchange (*top panel*) and a patient without pump thrombosis or other thromboembolic complication after LVAD implantation (*bottom panel*). Derived decrement index (preoperative dimension optimal set speed dimension ÷ preoperative dimension × 100, LVIDdDI) is also shown for each patient. The patient who subsequently developed pump thrombosis is shown to have an LVIDdDI ≤15% at a set speed of 9400 rpm at the end of a routine predischarge speed optimization study. The patient who remained free of this complication at study follow-up time of 26 months is shown with an LVIDdDI >15% at a set speed of 9200 rpm. Adopted with permission.

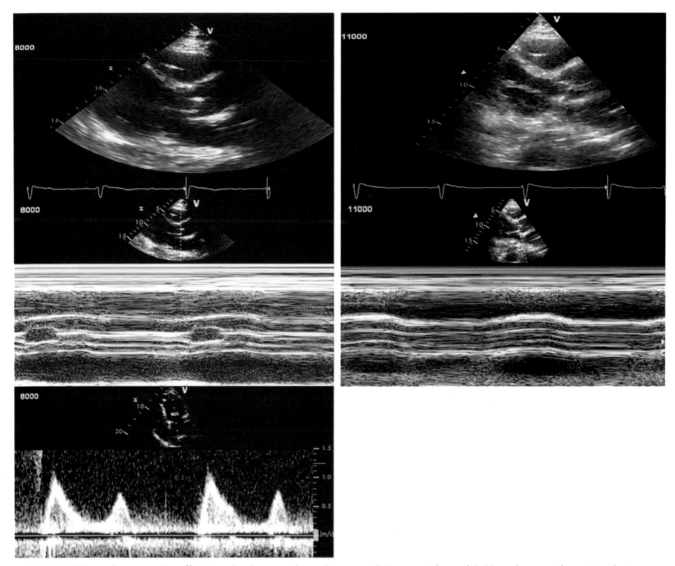

FIGURE 38-11 Figure demonstrating effective unloading on echocardiogram with incremental speed **A:** M-mode across the aortic valve in a parasternal view on echocardiogram showing aortic valve opens every beat at 8000 RPM. **B:** At 11,000 the M-mode does not demonstrate any aortic valve opening. **C:** Mitral inflow pattern suggestive of high filling pressures at 8000 RPM.

shown to be indicative of pump thrombosis. The theory behind a high S/D ratio is as device malfunction ensues the systolic velocity may not be affected as much because of the native heart function but the diastolic velocity drops significantly resulting in high S/D ratio.

As far as post pump thrombosis, echocardiography may not be enough as the true anatomy of the outflow is rarely ever visualized in LVADs. In such situations CT should be performed.

PATIENT CASE

A 36-year-old man with prior history of hemochromatosis was undergoing workup for liver transplant. His pretransplant workup revealed depressed ejection fraction (EF 35%-40%). Cardiac MR was consistent with nonischemic cardiomyopathy secondary to iron overload. A decision to perform LVAD at the time of liver transplant was made. After the transplant, the patient's LV function improved; in 2 years, it returned to normal. At 2-year follow-up an echocardiographic ramp wean protocol was done (Figure 38-13). The patient

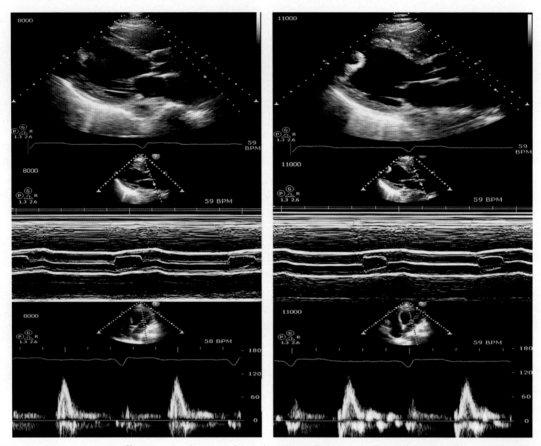

FIGURE 38-12 Figure demonstrating ineffective unloading on echocardiogram with incremental speed **A:** M-mode across the across the aortic valve in a parasternal long axis on echocardiogram at 8000 RPM shows aortic valve opens every beat. **B:** No change is seen at 11,000 RPM and aortic valve continues to open every beat. **C:** Mitral inflow pattern suggestive of elevated filling pressure at 8000 RPM. **D:** The mitral inflow pattern remains unchanged at 11,000 RPM.

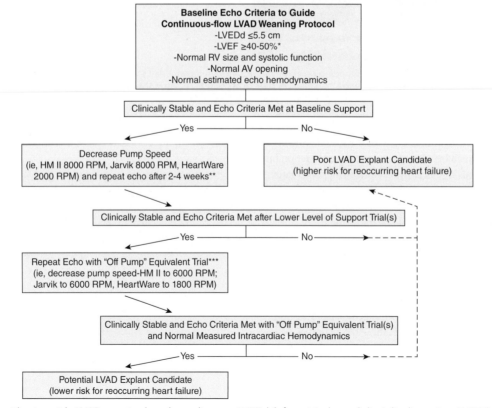

FIGURE 38-13 Algorithm to guide LVAD weaning by echocardiogram. LVEDd (left ventricular end-diastolic dimension, LVEF (left ventricular ejection fraction), RV (right ventricle), AV (aortic valve).

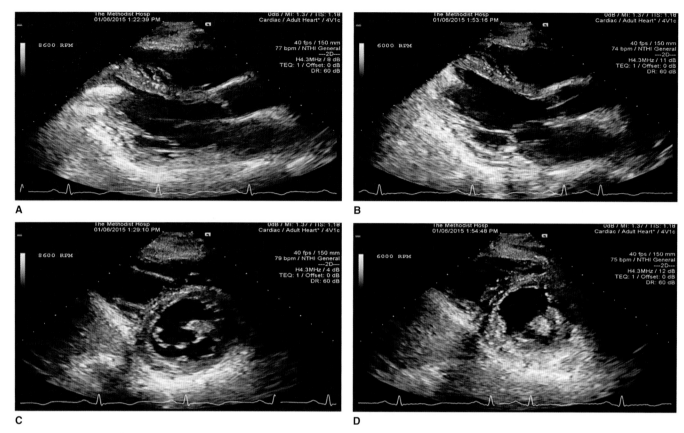

FIGURE 38-14 Figure demonstrating weaning echocardiogram; **A:** At 8000 RPM the left ventricle appears to small and is effectively unloaded. **B:** No change is noted in left ventricular size with decrement in speed to 6000 RPM. **C:** Short axis view again demonstarting a small left ventricular cavity at 8000 RPM. **D:** Short axis view at 6000 RPM demonstarting no change in left ventricular size.

did well with decremental speed and with exercise on minimal speed (6000 rpm). The patient's LVAD subsequently was explanted.

MYOCARDIAL RECOVERY

A small proportion of LVAD patients recover to a point where the LVAD can be explanted. In this situation, echocardiography is used to predict clinical stability after device removal. The parameters that are evaluated for myocardial recovery protocol, as illustrated in Figure 38-14, include LVEDD, LVESD, LVEF, RVEF, and hemodynamic indices. In continuous-flow devices, the major predictors of successful recovery include LVEF of at least 55%, with either LVEDD less than or equal to 55 mm or a history of HF within the last 5 years. Myocardial recovery is more common in younger patients and those with nonischemic cardiomyopathy, shorter duration of HF, and who are on guideline-directed medical therapy. Echocardiography plays an important role in screening for myocardial recovery for LVAD explantation consideration.

CONCLUSION

The hemodynamics of CF-LVADs is a complex interplay of patient characteristics including native heart function and vascular physiology and device parameters. Understanding LVAD hemodynamics is crucial for patient management and for device troubleshooting. This chapter summarizes the various hemodynamic effects in light of invasive and noninvasive hemodynamics with PVLs, right heart catheterization, and echocardiography, respectively.

REFERENCES

1. Burkhoff D, Sayer G, Doshi D, Uriel N. Hemodynamics of mechanical circulatory support. *J Am Coll Cardiol.* 2015;66:2663-2674.

2. Stainback RF, Estep JD, Agler DA, et al. Echocardiography in the management of patients with left ventricular assist devices: recommendations from the American Society of Echocardiography. *J Am Soc Echocardiogr.* 2015;28:853-909.

3. Estep JD, Vivo RP, Krim SR, et al. Echocardiographic evaluation of hemodynamics in patients with systolic heart failure supported by a continuous-flow LVAD. *J Am Coll Cardiol.* 2014;64:1231-1241.

4. Scandroglio AM, Kaufmann F, Pieri M, et al. Diagnosis and treatment algorithm for blood flow obstructions in patients with left ventricular assist device. *J Am Coll Cardiol.* 2016;67:2758-2768.

5. Joyce E, Stewart GC, Hickey M, et al. Left ventricular dimension decrement index early after axial flow assist device implantation: a novel risk marker for late pump thrombosis. *J Heart Lung Transplant.* 2015;34:1561-1569.

39 LEFT VENTRICULAR ASSIST DEVICES

Sitaramesh Emani, MD

PATIENT CASE

A 72-year-old man presents to a heart failure clinic for further evaluation of his progressive fatigue and dyspnea. He has a history of an ischemic cardiomyopathy with a severely reduced ejection fraction (EF <20%), which was originally diagnosed several years ago. He was initially maintained on optimal medical therapy for his cardiomyopathy and resultant heart failure (HF). Despite medical therapy, however, he has noted progressive exertional intolerance as well as several episodes of acutely decompensated HF in the past year requiring admission for intensification of HF medical therapies. After a thorough evaluation, he is felt to be a good candidate for a left ventricular assist device (LVAD). He subsequently undergoes successful implantation of an LVAD as destination therapy.

EPIDEMIOLOGY

It is estimated that more than 5 million Americans have HF with more than 650,000 new patients being diagnosed annually. Of these patients, half are estimated to have heart failure with a reduced ejection fraction (HFrEF).[1] Further estimations suggest 25% to 30% of these patients have either NYHA functional class III or IV HF. Within this subpopulation, approximately 150,000 to 250,000 patients may qualify for advanced HF therapies such as cardiac transplantation or LVAD support.[2] Due to a relative paucity of suitable donor organs, the number of annual transplants performed in the United States has remained stable at around 2000.[3] As such, transplantation does not represent a viable treatment option for the majority of advanced HF patients. This gap has led to the growth of ventricular assist devices (VADs) as standard therapy in the treatment of advanced HF.[1]

ADVANCED HEART FAILURE

Advanced HF can be described qualitatively as persistent significant HF symptoms despite ongoing optimal medical therapy,[1] or more objectively using specific criteria described in detail elsewhere.[4] Additional criteria have been evaluated to identify high-risk HF patients that may benefit from an evaluation for additional therapies.[5-7] Some of these criteria are noted in Table 39-1. Patients categorized with advanced HF are noted by the designation of the ACC stage D heart failure.[1] For patients with an acceptable surgical risk, successful implantation of an LVAD can be expected to improve both survival as well as quality of life.[8-12]

Table 39-1 High-Risk Heart Failure Features

Selected Criteria Used to Identify High-Risk Heart Failure Patients
• HF symptoms that fail to respond to medical therapy (persistent NYHA class III or worse symptoms)
• EF <25%
• Intolerance to HF medications
○ Hypotension
○ Renal dysfunction
○ Bradycardia
• Frequent HF hospitalizations
○ More than 2 in 3 mo
○ More than 3 in 6 mo
• Need for inotropes during hospital stay

Abbreviations: EF, ejection fraction; HF, heart failure.

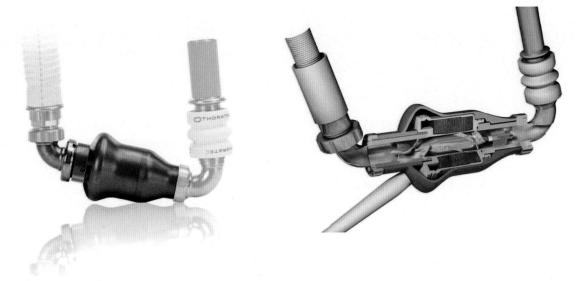

FIGURE 39-1 Two images of the axial-flow HeartMate II VAD. (HeartMate and St. Jude Medical are trademarks of St. Jude Medical, Inc. or its related companies. Reprinted with permission of St. Jude Medical, © 2018. All rights reserved.)

CLINICAL INDICATIONS FOR VENTRICULAR ASSIST DEVICES

Currently, VADs are used for primarily for 1 of 2 indications: bridge to transplant (BTT) or destination therapy (DT).[2] For patients who are eligible for cardiac transplantation but are anticipated to have a long wait for a donor organ, are not immediately eligible for transplant due to relative contraindications, or may not survive the wait for a donor organ, an LVAD can be used until transplantation can occur (BTT indication). Patients for whom cardiac transplant is not an option can receive an LVAD as permanent therapy (DT indication). The majority of LVADs implanted in the United States are done with a DT indication.[13] Rarely, myocardial recovery can occur after LVAD implantation and may lead to explant of the device.[13,14]

TYPES OF VENTRICULAR ASSIST DEVICES

Current-generation LVADs are continuous-flow devices, which can lead to significantly diminished or even absent pulses in supported patients. Two prominent designs currently exist for continuous-flow LVADs: axial-flow pumps and centrifugal pumps. Figures 39-1 and 39-2 show the different styles of pumps; Figure 39-3 shows the pumps and the external equipment as part of the complete system. Although often used relatively interchangeably, the 2 pump designs do have clinically unique flow characteristics due to engineering differences.[15] Figure 39-4 shows chest radiographs with 2 different pump designs.

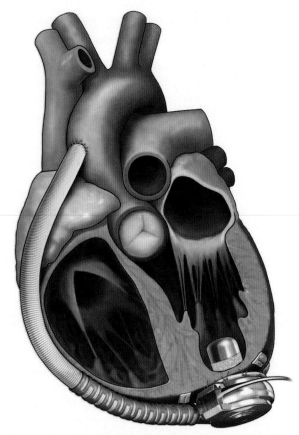

FIGURE 39-2 The centrifugal HVAD system shown, as it would look implanted into the apex of the left ventricle. (Reproduced with permission from Medtronic, Inc.)

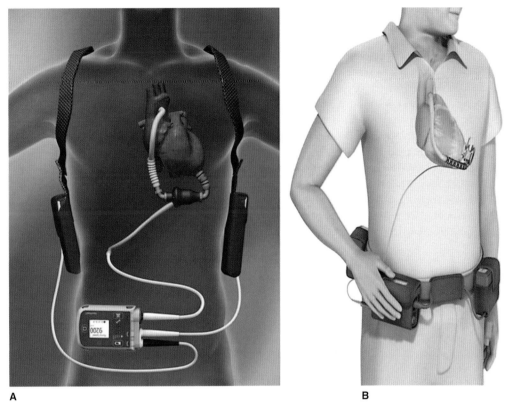

A   **B**

FIGURE 39-3 LVAD systems shown with external equipment. **A.** HeartMate II system (HeartMate and St. Jude Medical are trademarks of St. Jude Medical, Inc. or its related companies. Reprinted with permission of St. Jude Medical, © 2018. All rights reserved.) **B.** HVAD (Reproduced with permission of Medtronic, Inc.). Note both systems have externalized controllers that must be connected at all times to a power source. Here both systems are shown attached to externalized batteries, allowing for patient mobility.

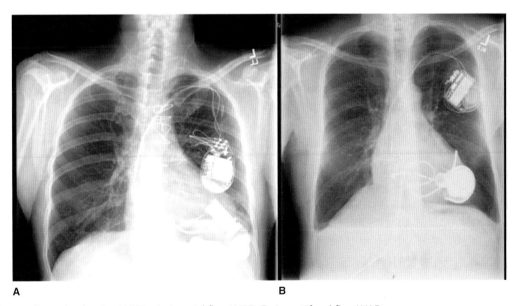

A   **B**

FIGURE 39-4 Chest radiographs showing LVADs. **A.** An axial-flow LVAD. **B.** A centrifugal-flow LVAD.

EVALUATION OF PATIENTS

Specific guidelines have been developed to describe the indications and contraindications to LVAD support.[16] In general, patients with comorbidities likely to limit either survival or quality of life independent of their cardiac disease are not considered candidates for LVAD support. Specific considerations are paramount in the evaluation of a potential LVAD patient. Among these considerations is a thorough evaluation of right ventricular (RV) function; RV dysfunction in the setting of an LVAD is correlated with worse outcomes.[13] Additionally, the ability to tolerate chronic systemic anticoagulation with vitamin K antagonists is crucial. Many of the long-term adverse events associated with LVAD therapy include either significant bleeding or thrombosis formation.[13]

MANAGEMENT

The selection and management of LVAD patients should occur through specialized advanced HF programs that include multidisciplinary experts in LVAD therapy.

REFERENCES

1. Yancy CW, Jessup M, Bozkurt B, et al. 2013 ACCF/AHA guidelines for the management of heart failure: a report of the American College of Cardiology Foundation/American Heart Association Task Force on Practice Guidelines. *J Am Coll Cardiol.* 2013;62:e147-e239.

2. Miller LW, Guglin M. Patient selection for ventricular assist devices: a moving target. *J Am Coll Cardiol.* 2013;61:1209-1221.

3. Lund LH, Edwards LB, Kucheryavaya AY, et al. The Registry of the International Society for Heart and Lung Transplantation: thirtieth official adult heart transplant report—2013; focus theme: age. *J Heart Lung Transplant.* 2013;32:951-964.

4. McMurray JJ, Adamopoulos S, Anker SD, et al. ESC guidelines for the diagnosis and treatment of acute and chronic heart failure 2012: The Task Force for the Diagnosis and Treatment of Acute and Chronic Heart Failure 2012 of the European Society of Cardiology. Developed in collaboration with the Heart Failure Association (HFA) of the ESC. *Eur J Heart Fail.* 2012;14:803-869.

5. Levy WC, Mozaffarian D, Linker DT, et al. The Seattle Heart Failure Model: prediction of survival in heart failure. *Circulation.* 2006;113:1424-1433.

6. Setoguchi S, Stevenson LW, Schneeweiss S. Repeated hospitalizations predict mortality in the community population with heart failure. *Am Heart J.* 2007;154:260-266.

7. Thorvaldsen T, Benson L, Stahlberg M, Dahlstrom U, Edner M, Lund LH. Triage of patients with moderate to severe heart failure: who should be referred to a heart failure center? *J Am Coll Cardiol.* 2014;63(7):661-671.

8. Rose EA, Gelijns AC, Moskowitz AJ, et al. Long-term use of a left ventricular assist device for end-stage heart failure. *N Engl J Med.* 2001;345:1435-1443.

9. Miller LW, Pagani FD, Russell SD, et al. Use of a continuous-flow device in patients awaiting heart transplantation. *N Engl J Med.* 2007;357:885-896.

10. Slaughter MS, Rogers JG, Milano CA, et al. Advanced heart failure treated with continuous-flow left ventricular assist device. *N Engl J Med.* 2009;361:2241-2251.

11. Rogers JG, Aaronson KD, Boyle AJ, et al. Continuous flow left ventricular assist device improves functional capacity and quality of life of advanced heart failure patients. *J Am Coll Cardiol.* 2010;55:1826-1834.

12. Slaughter MS, Pagani FD, McGee EC, et al. HeartWare ventricular assist system for bridge to transplant: combined results of the bridge to transplant and continued access protocol trial. *J Heart Lung Transplant.* 2013;32:675-683.

13. Kirklin JK, Naftel DC, Kormos RL, et al. Fifth INTERMACS annual report: risk factor analysis from more than 6,000 mechanical circulatory support patients. *J Heart Lung Transplant.* 2013;32:141-156.

14. Sun BC, Catanese KA, Spanier TB, et al. 100 long-term implantable left ventricular assist devices: the Columbia Presbyterian interim experience. *Ann Thorac Surg.* 1999;68:688-694.

15. Moazami N, Fukamachi K, Kobayashi M, et al. Axial and centrifugal continuous-flow rotary pumps: a translation from pump mechanics to clinical practice. *J Heart Lung Transplant.* 2013;32:1-11.

16. Feldman D, Pamboukian SV, Teuteberg JJ, et al. The 2013 International Society for Heart and Lung Transplantation Guidelines for mechanical circulatory support: executive summary. *J Heart Lung Transplant.* 2013;32:157-187.

40 CARDIAC TRANSPLANTATION

Ayesha Hasan, MD, FACC

■ PATIENT CASE

A 54-year-old African American woman with nonischemic cardiomyopathy, that is, LMNA-related familial cardiomyopathy, presented for advanced therapy evaluation based on recurrent admissions for volume overload and intravenous diuresis. She was diagnosed over 10 years ago, but ejection fraction declined to 15% on goal-directed medical therapy with carvedilol, valsartan, spironolactone, hydralazine, and nitrates. She was a nonresponder to cardiac resynchronization therapy despite underlying QRS of 140 ms. Hypotension resulted in reducing medication doses during the last few hospitalizations. Primary transplantation was discussed (blood type B), and cardiopulmonary exercise testing revealed a peak VO_2 of 13.1 mL/kg/min, 59% predicted with Ve/VCO_2 30. Right heart catheterization found severe pulmonary hypertension with pulmonary capillary wedge pressure 31 mm Hg, PA 66/44, mean 52 mm Hg, PA sat 38%, and CI 1.5 L/min/m^2 by Fick. She was started on milrinone for inotrope support. However, her pulmonary HTN did not improve significantly despite diuresis, and clinical status was tenuous. Her PVR declined to 4 WU with diuresis despite improvement in cardiac output on milrinone. She was implanted with a Heartmate II left ventricular assist device (LVAD) with the goal of bridging to transplantation until PVR improved. Because of progressive right heart failure and deteriorating renal function after LVAD, percutaneous temporary right heart support helped improve her clinical status and renal function without the need for dialysis. However, she required milrinone as a chronic infusion with her LVAD for RV support. She was listed as a 1A for VAD complication involving right heart failure. Pulmonary hypertension reversed to normal values on LVAD, and PVR was 1.8 WU. She was successfully bridged to heart transplantation approximately 14 months after LVAD with creatinine level of 1.5 mg/dL, and she had an uncomplicated first year post-heart transplantation.

INTRODUCTION

Therapy for refractory heart failure (HF) has advanced both pharmacologically and nonpharmacologically in the past decades. Despite the survival benefit of defibrillators, cardiac resynchronization devices, and medical therapy, morbidity and mortality associated with advanced HF is excessive, up to 50% 5-year mortality and greater than 50% 1-year mortality for those considered end-stage. Such challenges are addressed with cardiac transplantation where the median survival ranges from 10 to 13 years based upon a patient's surviving the first year.[1] Replacement of the heart is standard treatment for select patients with refractory symptoms, whereas mechanical support is the alternative for those who are either not candidates or require more immediate support. The early field of transplantation was plagued by poor survival and refining surgical techniques. Despite the first successful human heart transplant in South Africa in 1967 and the first U.S. case in 1968, survival was limited until the introduction of cyclosporine in the 1980s[2] and continues to improve with refinements in recipient and donor selection, donor management, immunosuppression, and treatment of comorbidities. Estimated annual transplant rates are >4000 cases with the limiting factor being donor availability.

EVALUATING THE TRANSPLANT CANDIDATE

INDICATIONS

Cardiac transplantation is reserved for advanced HF, refractory angina, and intractable ventricular arrhythmias (Table 40-1).[3] Candidates for cardiac transplantation have New York Heart Association (NYHA) class III to IV symptoms despite optimal medical and device therapy, including resynchronization therapy and often surgical treatment of ischemic and/or valvular heart disease. Etiology of HF most commonly involves coronary artery disease (CAD) or nonischemic cardiomyopathy and less often restrictive cardiomyopathy and congenital heart disease (Figure 40-1). Candidates with repeated ventricular arrhythmias despite pharmacologic and ablative treatment are considered for evaluation often on an urgent basis due to the risk of sudden death and hemodynamic intolerance with the arrhythmias. Chronic angina unresponsive to medical therapy and not amenable to further revascularization is also an indication but often in the presence of HF. These indications are the result of end-stage disease failing maximal therapy and reducing quality of life and survival.

CONTRAINDICATIONS

The majority of contraindications to transplant are relative contraindications as opposed to absolute and are weighed according to the patient's comorbidities and clinical status. These contraindications may vary among transplant centers as to absolute or relative in terms of patient candidacy (Table 40-2).

Age

The upper age limit for transplant has increased over the decades with improvement in outcomes in older patients. Previously, patients ≥65 years of age were excluded but current guidelines

Table 40-1 Indications for Heart Transplantation

Advanced systolic heart failure

- NYHA class III-IV symptoms
- Low cardiac output
- CPX testing with peak VO$_2$ max <12 to 14 mL/kg/min or <50% predicted in select patients

Acute heart failure not expected to recover

- Acute myocardial infarction
- Acute myocarditis

Refractory angina in ischemic disease

- Not amenable to percutaneous or surgical revascularization
- Unresponsive to maximal medical therapy

Intractable ventricular arrhythmias

- Maximal anti-arrhythmic therapy and ablative therapy

Advanced diastolic heart failure symptoms in restrictive or hypertrophic cardiomyopathy

Congenital heart disease with refractory symptoms

Abbreviations: CPX, cardiopulmonary exercise test; NYHA, New York Heart Association; Vo$_2$, maximal oxygen uptake.

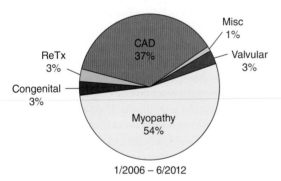

FIGURE 40-1 Etiology of adult heart transplantation indication from January 2006 to June 2012. (Reprinted from Lund LH, Edwards LB, Kucheryavaya AY, et al. The registry of the International Society for Heart and Lung Transplantation: thirtieth official adult heart transplant report—2013. *J Heart Lung Transpl.* 2013;32(10):951-964. Copyright 2013, with permission from Elsevier.)

Table 40-2 Contraindications to Cardiac Transplantation

Fixed pulmonary hypertension

- PVR >5 Woods units
- TPG >15 mm Hg
- PA systolic pressure >50-60 mm Hg or >50% systemic pressure in conjunction with the above parameters
- Inability to reduce PVR <2.5 Woods units with vasodilator or inotrope with systemic BP >85 mm Hg

Advanced age (usually >70 y)

Active infection or malignancy

- Recent malignancy
- Risk of recurrence

Irreversible renal, hepatic, or pulmonary disease unless undergoing dual organ transplantation

Obesity

- BMI >30 kg/m^2 or PIBW >140% (will vary by center)

Diabetes mellitus complications

- Poorly controlled (Hgb A1c>7.5 mg/dL)
- End organ complications (neuropathy, nephropathy, proliferative retinopathy)

Severe peripheral or cerebrovascular disease not amenable to revascularization

Psychosocial factors hindering compliance and/or comprehension of management

- Active or recent substance abuse (alcohol, illicit drugs, tobacco)
- Poor compliance with medical regimen or follow-up
- Poor social support system
- Psychiatric illness that is not well controlled on therapy

Abbreviations: BMI, body mass index; BP, blood pressure; Hgb, hemoglobin; PA, pulmonary artery; PIBW, percent ideal body weight; PVR, pulmonary vascular resistance; TPG, transpulmonary gradient.

survival in older recipients.[6,7] Careful selection of older patients based on comorbidities, especially preoperative renal function, and "physiologic" age is critical. Upper age limit is perhaps one of the more undecided issues in transplantation; centers will determine their comfort zone in terms of age criteria and whether or not an absolute cutoff exists for their individual program based on chronologic age.

Obesity

Obesity in cardiac surgery is associated with adverse outcomes of poor wound healing, infectious risk, and pulmonary and thromboembolic complications with additional studies in transplantation identifying increased risk of rejection, vasculopathy, and mortality.[8] Weight gain is a likelihood posttransplant often related to age and gender,[9] while immunosuppression can also lead to weight gain and worsening blood sugar, which could further impact preexisting comorbidities. Therefore, recipient weight is critical and usually measured as body mass index (BMI, weight in kilograms per height in meters squared) or percent ideal body weight (PIBW) for a given height and gender. Both measurements take into account height as opposed to considering weight only. The International Society for Heart and Lung Transplantation (ISHLT) guidelines recommend a pretransplant BMI <30 kg/m^2 or PIBW <140%, and state it is reasonable to recommend weight loss in candidates who do not meet this criteria due to the association with poor outcomes.[4] Given the prevalence of obesity, many centers accept a higher BMI or PIBW in recipients and an upper limit is usually center-specific.

Active Infection and Malignancy

Both active infection and malignancy (other than nonmelanoma skin cancer) are absolute contraindications to transplantation due to the risk of progression with immunosuppression. Traditionally, 5 years of remission has been utilized as a safety measure, but this is arbitrary and dependent on the type of cancer, response to treatment, and risk of recurrence.[4] Malignancy that is in remission and has a low risk of recurrence will usually be considered after oncology consultation, especially when considering the urgency of the patient clinical presentation. For example, a patient with end-stage HF and prostate cancer within the past few years would be a reasonable candidate based on the "cure" rate and slow-growing nature of this cancer as opposed to a patient who presents with chemotherapy-induced cardiomyopathy a few months after treatment for breast cancer. Pretransplant evaluation includes routine screening for malignancy.

plant infectious disease specialists should be undertaken in these situations.

Irreversible Pulmonary Hypertension

Due to the risk of right HF posttransplant, irreversible pulmonary hypertension (PH) is an absolute contraindication to candidacy.[4] In advanced HF, secondary or venous PH develops as a result of elevated filling pressures, which is usually considered reversible; however, persistent elevation may lead to irreversible or fixed PH as a result of chronic intimal changes and medial hypertrophy in the pulmonary vasculature. A donor heart cannot withstand the high afterload of an elevated pulmonary vascular resistance (PVR), which results in failure of the right ventricle and adverse outcomes including acute cardiogenic shock and mortality.[11] Therefore, routine evaluation of candidates includes invasive assessment of pulmonary pressures, filling pressures, cardiac output, and PVR. When the PVR >5 Woods units, pulmonary artery systolic pressure (PASP) >60 mm Hg, PVR index >6, or a transpulmonary gradient (TPG) >15 mm Hg (difference of the mean PA and wedge pressure), transplant candidacy is usually not considered unless provocative testing with a vasodilator reduces the pressures and PVR to an acceptable level while maintaining a systemic blood pressure >85 mm Hg.[4] Patients with fixed, elevated PVR may also have underlying lung disease, concurrent obstructive sleep apnea, or chronic thromboembolic PH, which should be excluded.

Diabetes Mellitus

Diabetes with end-organ damage (proliferative retinopathy, nephropathy, and neuropathy) or uncontrolled blood sugars is considered a relative contraindication at most institutions; previously, diabetes was considered an absolute contraindication. Single-center data, n = 161, have shown no difference in infection, rejection, and vasculopathy when compared to nondiabetic controls with similar 1-, 5-, and 10-year survival.[12] In contrast, larger reviews by Russo et al[13] and Kilic et al,[14] respectively, found uncomplicated diabetic patients have improved survival when compared to those with complicated diabetes, defined as the collective number of diabetic-related complications, and diabetes was associated with reduced 10-year survival, without mention of severity. Further evidence is lacking to further delineate what degree of end-organ involvement is acceptable, but guidelines recommend considering only those with nonproliferative retinopathy.[4] In select cases of nephropathy, patients might be evaluated for a combined heart and kidney transplant. Consultation

...ly exertion and the anaerobic peak oxygen consumption ...and provides an objective measure in addition to NYHA class) ...jection fraction, blood pressure, heart rate, and other parameters of clinical status. A VO_2 level between 10 and 14 mL/kg/min is associated with a reduced survival; evaluation for transplantation is recommended. Guidelines mention ≤12 mL/kg/min if a patient is on a beta blocker and ≤14 mL/kg/min if not on a beta blocker.[4] It is important that patients have a maximal study and reach anaerobic threshold, where carbon dioxide production exceeds oxygen consumption and is reported as the respiratory exchange ratio (RER) >1.05. Deconditioning often limits reaching the anaerobic threshold and parameters that do not reflect peak exercise should be evaluated, such as the ventilatory response to exercise or the ventilation to carbon dioxide slope (V_E/VCO_2), which can be measured throughout the length of exercise. This slope is higher in patients with low cardiac output, PH, and a higher dead space volume; V_E/VCO_2 >35 is a poor prognostic indicator.

...consider...

...cultural...

...ed is ad...

...or Ca...

...ria es full...

...ent wi...

...ters st...

...includes

...ing and assessment of pro-

...indicate irreversible dysfunction that would

...ria) as th...

not be expected to improve after correcting cardiac function. In a review of 1732 patients, patients with impaired renal function at the time of listing were more likely to develop chronic kidney disease (CKD) with function often deteriorating within the first year after transplantation, progressing from 50% with CKD stage III or higher immediately before transplantation to 77% during the first year.[15] Patients with CKD stage IV and V had a higher mortality rate and progression of renal dysfunction after transplantation. Risk factors for developing CKD included recipient age, female gender, diabetes, and temporary dialysis or hemofiltration perioperatively.[15,16] ISHLT listing criteria state it is reasonable not to consider irreversible renal dysfunction with eGFR <40 mL/min for heart transplantation alone.[4] Dual-organ candidacy should be considered where appropriate.

Peripheral Vascular Disease

Symptomatic cerebral or peripheral vascular disease is considered a contraindication to candidacy if clinically severe or not amenable to revascularization. However, asymptomatic disease will likely be considered, but is specific to individual centers. Retrospective data suggested progression of peripheral vascular disease posttransplant and possible risk factors associated with development include presence of pretransplant ischemic etiology and former smoking.[4] Rehabilitation potential is essential in any candidate with vascular disease.

Psychosocial Factors

A detailed psychosocial assessment of all transplant candidates is a fundamental component in the evaluation process. This includes medication and clinic visit compliance, social support system, psychiatric history, and substance abuse history. Transplant programs have dedicated social workers who perform these assessments and meet with the patient's social network. Often, patients will be referred to psychologists or psychiatrists based on their history and whether any active psychiatric illness is present. Substance abuse of alcohol, illicit drugs, or tobacco is a contraindication to listing and programs require 6 to 12 months of abstinence documented with negative toxicology screens; current alcohol and illicit drug use are absolute contraindications in transplant programs. Based on a patient's history, various rehabilitation or substance abuse programs, counseling, sponsorship, or neurocognitive testing could also be required. Many patients are denied candidacy based on their psychosocial situation, as this has been critical to long-term success.[17] Patients who have demonstrated poor medication compliance are not considered candidates, and dementia is considered a relative contraindication.[4] Comprehensive screening tools are now utilized by many transplant programs in order to standardize this assessment and predict psychosocial outcome.[18]

PRETRANSPLANT WAITLIST MANAGEMENT

LISTING

Patients are waitlisted for heart transplant after decision by a multidisciplinary selection committee consisting of the various team members involved in the evaluation process: cardiac surgeons, HF cardiologists, coordinators, pharmacists, social workers, and subspecialty consultants such as pulmonology, nephrology, and infectious disease. Listing status consists of 3 levels, which from highest to lowest priority are 1A, 1B, and 2. See Table 40-3 for details on listing status.[19] Patients accrue time on the waitlist regardless of status and are matched to available organs based on size, blood type, and medical urgency. The goal of organ allocation is to transplant those who are the most critical and have the shortest survival. Average wait times on the list will vary by region. Patients who are large and blood type O will typically wait longer than those who are smaller and not blood type O. For this reason, ventricular assist devices (VADs) are implanted in those who are less likely to survive the wait for an available organ and are termed bridge to transplantation. Some transplant programs have an alternate list for higher-risk recipients (age >70 years, renal dysfunction, retransplantation) and donors (high-risk behavior, older donors, or presence of CAD).

RIGHT HEART CATHETERIZATION

Routine right heart catheterization (RHC) is performed as part of the transplant evaluation and at 3- to 6-month intervals as part of waitlist management. A vasodilator challenge is indicated when PASP >50 mm Hg and TPG >15 mm Hg or PVR >3 Woods units; commonly utilized agents are nitroprusside or nitroglycerin as an acute vasodilator and milrinone or dobutamine for inotrope support while maintaining systolic blood pressure (SBP) >85 mm Hg. If the patient becomes hypotensive with SBP <85 mm Hg despite an appropriate decline in PVR with a vasodilator challenge, poor outcomes have been associated due to a high risk of right HF and

performed serially on all patients waitlisted for transplant; in our institution, we perform RHC every 3 months if a vasodilator study was required to reverse PH or the patient is on a chronic inotrope infusion and every 6 months for the rest of the patients.

It is critical for transplant success to accurately evaluate hemodynamics and determine reversibility of PH given the risk of right HF and mortality in the setting of PH. Fixed PH and pulmonary arterial hypertension (HTN) are considered contraindications to transplantation due to elevated and nonreversible PVR, but even reversible PH carries a significantly higher risk of mortality post-transplant[11] and a nonsignificant trend to increased mortality in another study[20] emphasizing careful monitoring of these patients pretransplant and posttransplant.

SURGICAL MANAGEMENT OF THE TRANSPLANT PATIENT

DONOR SELECTION AND ORGAN ALLOCATION

Evaluation and management of potential donors is the responsibility of the local organ procurement organization (OPO), and it involves a comprehensive medical and social history; laboratory studies including blood type, infectious serologies (human immunodeficiency virus, hepatitis B and C, and cytomegalovirus); and evaluation of cardiac function with an echocardiogram. Further cardiac studies (ie, coronary catheterization) are recommended based upon donor cause of death or risk factors, especially age. Substantial left ventricular hypertrophy (LVH), obstructive coronary disease, excessive inotrope use, ventricular arrhythmias, or reduced ejection fraction <40% are cardiac abnormalities that in general are not accepted for use in transplantation.[21] Donors with chest trauma should be carefully assessed for any damage to the heart. Donor comorbidities will influence decisions on organ utilization, also. The process of identifying an appropriate donor is not standardized, and data are limited on the impact of concerning donor risk factors on outcomes because these hearts are not usually transplanted.

Donor management optimizes organ function through support of blood pressure, volume resuscitation, oxygenation, and correction of electrolyte and metabolic abnormalities including hormonal imbalances noted in brain death (insulin, corticosteroids, arginine vasopressin, triiodothyronine). The ischemic time, also termed the cold ischemic time, is the total time from organ procurement in the donor to reperfusion in the recipient. Warm ischemic time refers to the duration of implantation or removal of the organ from ice until reperfusion, but the total ischemic time is

to be inpatient)

- LVAD or RVAD with significant device-related complication: Thromboembolism, infection, device failure, ventricular arrhythmias

- IABP, TAH, or ECMO

• Mechanical ventilation

• Inotrope support

- Continuous hemodynamic monitoring plus multiple inotropes or high dose of single inotrope

Status 1AE (by exception): Recertified every 14 d from initial listing as status 1AE

• Urgent clinical status but patient does not meet above criteria (ie, ventricular tachyarrhythmias preventing inotrope use or hemodynamic monitoring)

• Approved by appropriate Regional Review Board

Status 1B

• LVAD, RVAD beyond 30 d without a complication

• Continuous infusion of single inotrope and no hemodynamic monitoring

Status 1B (by exception): Similar criteria as status 1AE

Status 2

• Candidates not meeting status 1A or 1B criteria

Status 7

• Temporarily unsuitable for transplantation

Abbreviations: ECMO, extracorporeal membrane oxygenation; IABP, intra-aortic balloon pump; LVAD, left ventricular assist device; RVAD, right ventricular assist device; TAH, total artificial heart.

utilized when evaluating a potential donor. General recommendations are for an ischemic time between 4 and 6 hours with preference <4 hours for older donor organs.[21] ABO incompatibility is a long-established contraindication in adults due to hyperacute rejection. Size matching is usually within 20% to 30% of recipient body size. An average-size male donor of 70 kg should typically be an appropriate size match for any recipient. Gender mismatching carries increased mortality risk and poor outcomes.[22,23] Size mismatch with a female donor to male recipient is disconcerting in that a female heart tends to be smaller and would be incapable of meeting the demands of a larger male recipient or higher PVR. This was demonstrated in a large UNOS database review of 18,240 transplants between 1999 and 2007 with the lowest 5-year survival in female donors/male recipients and no difference in female recipients of gender-matched or gender-mismatched organs.[23] Male donors/male recipients had the highest 5-year survival at 74.5%. With an endpoint of 10 years rather than 5 years (n = 857 from 1994-2008) in a single-center study, Kittleson et al found a reduced 10-year actuarial survival in both types of gender mismatches suggesting an immunologic effect could also have a role in outcomes (Figure 40-2).[22] There was no difference among the cause of death for gender-matched and gender-mismatched recipients.

Utilization of donor hearts has decreased in the past decade and is around 40% in recent data.[24] Current practice was reviewed by Khush et al within the California Transplant Donor Network from 2001 to 2008 with turndown of 1872 donors. Potential donors who were not accepted were the following: age >50 years, female sex, cerebrovascular accident (CVA) as the cause of death, HTN, diabetes, positive troponin, LV dysfunction with regional wall motion abnormalities, and LVH.[24] Only CVA as the donor cause of death minimally predicted prolonged recipient post-transplant hospitalization (odds ratio, 1.41 [1.00-2.00]), whereas diabetes mellitus was the only donor predictor of reduced recipient survival. Experts have suggested that our current criteria for donor selection are contributing to our shortage of donors due to non-use of potential donors and likely donor characteristics have a small contribution to posttransplant adverse events based on available data.[25] Efforts to expand donor selection and organ perfusion are ongoing, but heart transplantation remains limited by donor availability.

Organs are allocated according to region, status on the waitlist, and matching by size and blood type. The allocation policy changed on June 12, 2006, to concentric 500-mile zones with the goal of prioritizing higher-risk recipients (status 1A and 1B), and increasing the availability of a donor. Prior to this updated policy, organs were offered to all status patients within a UNOS region before they were available to bordering regions (Figure 40-3). Waitlist mortality has decreased significantly from 13.3% to 7.9% up to 180 days (p < 0.001) while waitlist time has increased—maybe partly related to the rise in LVAD bridging, which was found to vary by region.[26] Currently, LVAD patients have 30 days of 1A time regardless of a complication, but discussion is ongoing about the low waitlist mortality of continuous-flow LVAD patients, which is similar to status 2

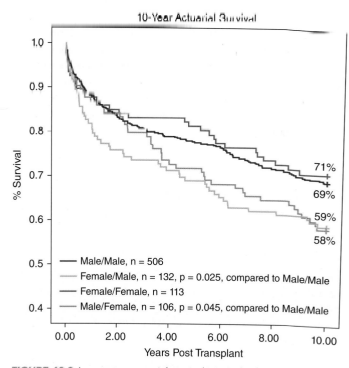

FIGURE 40-2 Long-term actuarial survival in gender-matched and gender-mismatched recipients.[22] There was no difference in survival between male donor/male recipient and female donor/female recipient groups. Significantly reduced survival was noted in both groups with gender mismatching when compared to the male/male group. (Reprinted from Kittleson MM, Shemin R, Patel JK, et al. Donor-recipient sex mismatch portends poor 10-year outcomes in a single-center experience. *J Heart Lung Transpl.* 2011;30(9):1018-1022. Copyright 2011, with permission, from Elsevier.)

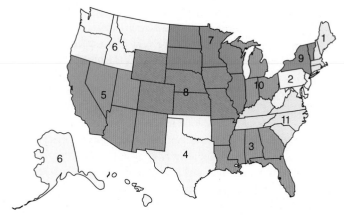

FIGURE 40-3 Organ allocation is regulated by the United Network for Organ Sharing in the United States according to these geographic regions.

SURGERY

Donor procurement is coordinated between the procuring and transplanting teams with the goal of organ preservation and minimizing ischemic time. The organ is placed in a cold cardioplegia solution and transported to the transplanting center (Figure 40-4). Experimental animal models have shown promise in using novel techniques to help reduce ischemia and reperfusion injury: targeted complement inhibition in recipients,[28] cardioplegia solution supplemented with erythropoietin,[29] a hypothermic hydrogen-rich water bath,[30] and ex vivo heart perfusion after cardiocirculatory death.[31] These methods clearly need further investigation before incorporating into standard procedure.

Early transplantation was performed in the orthotopic position by the forefathers of heart transplantation: Norman Shumway, Richard Lower, Adrian Kantrowitz, and Christiaan Barnard. Lower and Shumway described biatrial anastomosis in 1960.[32] Initial anastomosis was biatrial and has progressed to the bicaval technique currently. Biatrial anastomosis involves midatrial transection of both donor and recipient hearts along with transection of the great vessels just above the semilunar valves. This method keeps the pulmonary venous connection to the left atrium intact in the recipient and includes the donor sinoatrial node in the right atrium. Reanastomosis begins with the atrial septum followed by the great vessels. The bicaval technique, first reported in 1991 by Dreyfus et al, differs in that the atria are not resected and anastomosis occurs at the inferior and superior vena cavae and pulmonary veins, which keeps the donor atria intact.[33] An advantage of the biatrial method is fewer connections with only 2 in the atria versus 6 atrial connections in the bicaval method (2 to the vena cavae and 4 to the pulmonary veins), possibly reducing ischemic time.[34] The disadvantages to the biatrial technique are the large geometry of the atria and its possible effect on hemodynamics and arrhythmia risk along with the chance of damaging the sinoatrial node. The purpose of modifying the implantation technique was to reduce atrial size, atrial arrhythmias, tricuspid valve regurgitation, and bradycardia requiring a pacemaker, which were considered to occur with more frequency in the biatrial method. Davies et al reviewed almost 21,000 transplants from 1997 to 2007 with 59.3% biatrial and 38.1% bicaval anastomoses performed; they found bicaval anastomosis less often required postoperative pacemaker implantation and had a significant yet small survival advantage at 30 days and 1, 5, and 10 years.[34] Despite the increasing use of the bicaval anastomosis, tricuspid regurgitation persists after transplantation to a certain extent due to repeated endomyocardial biopsies.

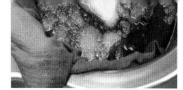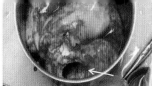

FIGURE 40-4 Donor heart (*left*) compared to excised recipient heart (*right*) with dilated cardiomyopathy and VAD cannula (*arrow*). (Used with permission from the Division of Cardiac Surgery, Ohio State University Wexner Medical Center).

PHYSIOLOGY OF THE TRANSPLANTED HEART

When transplanted, the new heart is surgically denervated without afferent and efferent nerve supply. The afferent supply from the heart to the central nervous system is responsible for angina and is not generally present in transplant patients for this reason. Without angina, patients who are ischemic tend to present with HF symptoms or arrhythmias instead. Loss of the efferent nerve supply from the central nervous system to the heart results in loss of vagal tone leading to a higher resting heart rate often up to 110 beats per minute and lack of response to drugs that rely upon the autonomic nervous system, such as atropine. A blunted response to exercise is a hallmark of transplantation related to efferent denervation because the recipient is now reliant upon circulating catecholamines for chronotropic effect; therefore, a patient's heart rate slowly recovers postexercise as these levels decline. The baroreceptor reflex is not intact in these patients either, due to sympathetic and parasympathetic denervation, which leads to a more sensitive orthostatic response and absent effect of carotid sinus massage. Re-innervation is a phenomenon that tends to transpire with time based on lower resting heart rate and the presence of angina but is not a consistent occurrence as to who, when, or how much.[36]

AFTERCARE OF THE TRANSPLANT PATIENT

IMMUNOSUPPRESSION

Preventing rejection of the graft is the cornerstone of an immunosuppression regimen that consists of multiple drugs with numerous pharmacologic interactions and side effects. The early regimen tends to have the highest intensity because rejection risk is greatest in the early posttransplant period, and maintenance therapy tends to require lower doses as this risk declines with time in the majority of patients. A medical regimen will vary per individual patient based on the patient's crossmatch and sensitization (or pretransplant and posttransplant antibodies), but the overall purpose is to prevent rejection while avoiding chronic over-immunosuppressive complications of infection and malignancy.

INDUCTION

Approximately one-half of transplant centers use induction therapy in the initial postoperative management of a transplant recipient due to the risk of early rejection[1] with the perception that donor antigen expression is spurred immediately by donor brain death, ischemia, and reperfusion, and the trauma of surgery.[37] The resultant immunosuppressive response allows delay of calcineurin antagonists in the setting of acute or worsening CKD during this early postoperative period. Induction therapy includes T cell cytolytic agents such as polyclonal antithymocyte antibodies derived from rabbits (thymoglobulin) or horses (ATGAM) and the monoclonal antibody OKT3 derived from mice. Interleukin-2 (IL-2) antagonists, such as basiliximab and daclizumab, inhibit proliferation of T cells activated through the IL-2 pathway. The decision to induce any patient must weigh infectious and/or malignancy risk of these agents versus rejection risk, leading many centers to treat patients based upon the patients' individual risk profiles rather than inducing all transplant patients. Studies have shown varying results in terms of infectious risk with the choice of induction agent and no major differences in prevention of rejection in small comparison studies.[38-40]

MAINTENANCE THERAPY

Maintenance regimens usually consist of triple therapy in the early transplantation period (calcineurin inhibitor, antimetabolite, and corticosteroids), and usually reduce to 2 drugs if possible as corticosteroids are gradually discontinued. The transplant physician must be familiar with the numerous drug interactions and toxicities of an immunosuppressive regimen. Figure 40-5 demonstrates the multiple targets of the immunologic response when using combination drug therapy.

Corticosteroids

Corticosteroids prevent cytokine production and all types of lymphocyte proliferation (T and B cell, monocytes, granulocytes, and macrophages); given the potency, steroids are used during the first year of transplantation when rejection risk tends to be greatest and for treatment of acute and/or chronic cellular and humoral rejection.[41] Doses are high initially and then tapered during the first year with discontinuation in approximately 50% of patients during this year based on their rejection history. The substantial side effect profile of corticosteroids is the limiting factor in long-term use. These include HTN, poor wound healing, tremors, emotional lability, skin fragility, weight gain, osteoporosis, cataracts, peptic ulcer disease, infectious risk, and myopathy. Adverse metabolic effects include hyperglycemia, fluid retention, salt retention, osteopenia, and hyperlipidemia. Some patients will develop adrenal insufficiency if on chronic steroid doses.

Calcineurin Inhibitors

Calcineurin inhibitors (CNI), cyclosporine and tacrolimus, inhibit transcription of IL-2 and cytokines through binding and prevention of calcineurin activation of this pathway. These drugs represent the foundation of immunosuppressive therapy since the beginning of cyclosporine use in the 1980s due to a significant increase in survival. Tacrolimus utilization has escalated in recent years with some evidence that it is associated with less rejection, although survival is similar.[42-44] Kobashigawa et al found a significantly lower occurrence of grade 3A or higher rejection in both groups treated with tacrolimus and lower median serum triglycerides and creatinine in the tacrolimus/mycophenolate mofetil group (groups were tacrolimus plus mychophenolate or sirolimus and cyclosporine plus

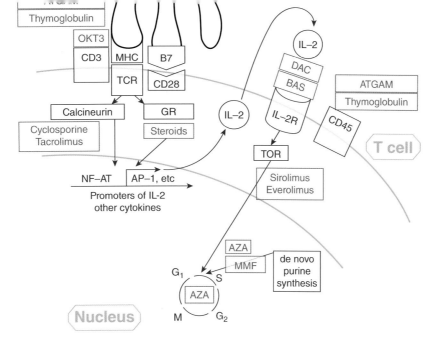

FIGURE 40-5 Immunologic mechanisms leading to graft rejection and sites of action of immunosuppressive drugs. Immunologic mechanisms are shown in *blue*; immunosuppressive drugs and their site of action are shown in *red*. Acute rejection begins with recognition of donor antigens that differ from those of the recipient by recipient APCs (indirect allorecognition). Donor APCs (carried passively in the graft) may also be recognized by recipient T cells (direct allorecognition). Alloantigens carried by APCs are recognized by TCR-CD3 complex on the surface of T cells. When accompanied by costimulatory signals between APC and T cells such as B7-CD28, T cell activation occurs, resulting in activation of calcineurin. Calcineurin dephosphorylates transcription factor NF-AT, allowing it to enter nucleus and bind to promoters of IL-2 and other cytokines. IL-2 activates cell surface receptors (IL-2R), stimulating clonal expansion of T cells (T helper cells). IL-2, along with other cytokines produced by T helper cells, stimulates expansion of other cells of the immune system. Activation of IL-2R stimulates TOR, which regulates translation of mRNAs to proteins that regulate cell cycles. Sites of action of individual drugs (*highlighted in red*) demonstrate multiple sites of action of these drugs, underscoring the rationale for combination therapy. Abbreviations: AZA, azathioprine; BAS, basiliximab; DAC, daclizumab; GR, glucocorticoid receptor; MMF, mycophenolate mofetil. (Reprinted from Lindenfeld J, Miller GG, Shakar SF, et al. Drug therapy in the heart transplant recipient: part II: immunosuppressive drugs. *Circulation.* 2004;110:3858-3865. Copyright 2004, with permission from Wolters Kluwer Health.)

mycophenolate, Figure 40-6).[42] In a meta-analysis of 7 randomized controlled trials (n = 885), similar survival and less rejection for tacrolimus versus cyclosporine microemulsion was confirmed along with the different side effect profile noting a lesser degree of HTN and dyslipidemia and a higher rate of new-onset diabetes for tacrolimus.[44] Nephrotoxicity is associated with both drugs.

Antimetabolite Agents

The most commonly used antimetabolites are azathioprine, use of which has fallen off, and mycophenolate mofetil (MMF). Both inhibit T and B lymphocyte proliferation by inhibiting DNA replication. MMF is more selective in its action on de novo purine synthesis and for this reason, does not have the degree of bone marrow suppression noted with azathioprine, which acts upon both de novo and salvage pathways targeting all cell lines as opposed to lymphocytes only.[41] Comparison of MMF to azathioprine in cardiac transplant patients revealed an improved late survival using an MMF regimen in randomized trials[45] and review of UNOS registry data.[46] Adverse effects of

MMF are primarily gastrointestinal with nausea, vomiting, and diarrhea, and tend to be dose responsive; mycophenolate sodium (MPS) is an enteric-coated, delayed-release formulation with less gastrointestinal upset and therefore fewer dose reductions along with a similar efficacy in maintenance regimens.[47] Fewer dose reductions with MPS were associated with a higher average daily dose of MPS (represented as the % of the recommended dose; 88.4% MPS vs 79.0% MMF, $p = 0.016$) and a significantly lower rate of biopsy proven and treated rejection grade ≥3A (25.4% MPS vs 11.0% MMF, $p = 0.033$).[48]

Proliferation Signal Inhibitors

Also known as mammalian target of rapamycin (mTOR) inhibitors, sirolimus and everolimus prevent T and B lymphocyte proliferation in addition to smooth muscle and endothelial cell proliferation in response to growth factors.[41] The latter explains the beneficial effect of these drugs in preventing transplant coronary allograft vasculopathy (CAV) and possibly tumor regression. Both drugs have been associated with a lower incidence of CAV and rejection when compared to azathioprine.[49,50] Combination therapy with CNI can aggravate CNI-related nephrotoxicity, but evidence suggests that reduced CNI levels plus earlier initiation of mTOR inhibitors preserves renal function without loss of immunosuppressive protection.[51] Major side effects include hypertriglyceridemia, bone marrow suppression, diarrhea, capillary leak, poor wound healing, pneumonitis, and aphthous ulcers; the side effect profile of these agents often limits tolerance and results in withdrawal of treatment.

REJECTION

Acute rejection is more common early after transplant and the risk declines with duration from transplantation. Hyperacute rejection occurs within hours of transplantation and is rare as it is related to ABO incompatibility. Cellular and antibody mediated rejection can be acute or chronic and occur individually or in a mixed scenario. Acute cellular rejection (ACR) is T cell mediated and the most common form of rejection occurring within the first year posttransplant. Diffuse inflammation and myocyte injury, hemorrhage, and necrosis are hallmarks and graded according to the ISHLT grading scale (Table 40-4).[52] Acute antibody mediated rejection (AMR) is B cell related with antibody deposition in the vasculature, complement activation, and endothelial swelling leading to hemodynamic compromise and allograft dysfunction.

Presentation

Symptoms of rejection are nonspecific or even absent in earlier stages and often are not apparent until rejection has progressed to an advanced stage. Patients present with decompensated HF and hypotension, volume overload, or an S_3 gallop. They may have vague symptoms of fatigue, cough, or a low-grade fever. Atrial arrhythmias have also been a presenting sign.

Diagnosis

Surveillance endomyocardial biopsies and RHC are performed in the routine management of heart transplant recipients due to the lack of clear symptoms in early rejection. The purpose is to discover rejection before later stages in order to start appropriate therapy and improve outcomes. Endomyocardial biopsies (EMB) are performed through the right internal jugular vein, preferentially, followed by the

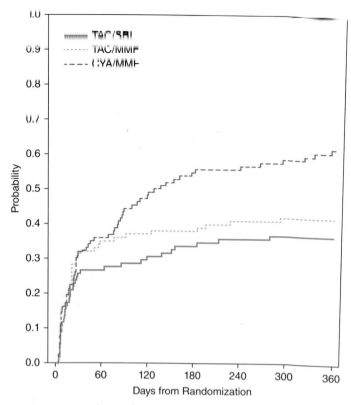

FIGURE 40-6 Incidence of any treated rejection over 1 year was significantly lower in the tacrolimus treated groups ($p < 0.001$). Abbreviations: MMF, mycophenolate mofetil; SRL, sirolimus; TAC, tacrolimus. (Reprinted from Kobashigawa J, Miller LW, Russell SD, et al. Tacrolimus with mycophenolate mofetil (MMF) or sirolimus vs. cyclosporine with MMF in cardiac transplant patients. 1-year report. *Am J Transplant.* 2006;6(6):1377-1386. Copyright 2006, with permission from Wiley and Sons.)

Table 40-4 International Society for Heart and Lung Transplantation Grading System of Cardiac Biopsies for Diagnosis of Rejection

2004		1990	
Grade 0R	No rejection	Grade 0	No rejection
		Grade 1, Mild	
Grade 1R, Mild	Interstitial and/or perivascular infiltrate with up to 1 focus of myocyte damage	A—Focal	Focal perivascular and/or interstitial infiltrate without myocyte damage
		B—Diffuse	Diffuse infiltrate without myocyte damage
Grade 2R, Moderate	2 or more foci of infiltrate with associated myocyte damage	Grade 2, Moderate (Focal)	1 focus of infiltrate with associated myocyte damage
		Grade 3, Moderate	
		A—Focal	Multifocal infiltrate with myocyte damage
Grade 3R, Severe	Diffuse infiltrate with multifocal myocyte damage ± edema, ± hemorrhage ± vasculitis	B--Diffuse	Diffuse infiltrate with myocyte damage
		Grade 4, Severe	Diffuse, polymorphous infiltrate with extensive myocyte damage ± edema, ± hemorrhage ± vasculitis

Adapted from Steward et al.[52] Copyright 2004, with permission from Elsevier.

femoral vein and samples taken from the right ventricular septum using a bioptome. Centers perform EMB with echocardiography or fluoroscopy to identify the appropriate location and avoid sampling the tricuspid valve apparatus and the free wall. Of late, a blood test (AlloMap) that evaluates gene expression in peripheral blood mononuclear cells is available to detect cellular rejection in stable patients at low risk of rejection;[53] such patients underwent significantly fewer biopsies, reducing the risk of biopsy-related complications such as tricuspid regurgitation, arrhythmias, and perforation. Noninvasive testing is an advance in the transplant field as routine use of EMB in stable patients without a clear indication of HF symptoms or allograft dysfunction has been shown to have a low yield beyond 6 months posttransplant; most rejection diagnoses in the stable patient are mild and do not require treatment.[54] Given the risk of rejection in the first year posttransplant, a unique risk score was developed and validated among 14,265 recipients in the UNOS registry with 4 variables demonstrating a strong correlation between observed and predicted rejection rates in the validation cohort ($r^2=0.96$, $p <0.001$); these factors were younger age, female sex, race (Asian < White, Black, Hispanic, and other), and degree of human leukocyte antigen (HLA) matching (4-6 antigen mismatches).[55] Figures 40-7 to 40-9 demonstrate ACR, AMR, and ischemia in early transplant recipients.

Treatment

Therapy is based on clinical presentation, hemodynamic compromise on RHC and/or imaging, and biopsy grade. Low-grade rejection in an asymptomatic patient is typically not treated. In scenarios of graft dysfunction or hemodynamic deterioration, treatment of ACR includes pulse and oral steroids, augmentation of oral

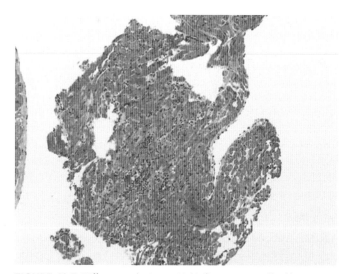

FIGURE 40-7 Diffuse patchy interstitial inflammatory cell infiltrate with associated myocyte injury suggestive of severe acute rejection grade 3R cellular rejection related to noncompliance with immunosuppression regimen. (Used with permission from Ohio State University Wexner Medical Center.)

immunosuppression (CNI, MMF, mTOR inhibitor), changing cyclosporine to tacrolimus, and the addition of antithymocyte antibody or cytolytic antibody. AMR is recognized as a source of allograft dysfunction and is associated with development of cardiac vasculopathy.[56] AMR is particularly challenging in that few randomized studies exist for guidance on therapy; hence, centers have various protocols for treatment rather than a standardized approach. Therapy focuses on the following 4 targets: suppression of T lymphocytes (ATG, CNI, MMF), inhibition of circulating antibodies (intravenous immunoglobulin or IVIG), elimination of circulating antibodies (apheresis), and suppression of B lymphocytes (rituximab).[56] Although more difficult to treat than ACR and escalating immunosuppression does not always result in resolution, a combined approach seems best along with routine follow-up of anti-HLA antibodies. Chronic rejection, both cellular and humoral, can be further treated with total lymphoid radiation, or extracorporeal photopheresis, which requires central access.

Rejection is often precipitated by an infection such as cytomegalovirus (CMV). It is imperative to obtain a detailed history to define the etiology of rejection given that psychosocial factors, noncompliance, and changes in the patient's drug regimen resulting in lower drug levels should be reviewed.

OTHER COMPLICATIONS

Bradycardia

The denervated transplanted heart has a higher heart rate of 110 bpm, and rates under this are considered relative bradycardia, which may be related to sinus node dysfunction, pretransplant negative chronotropic agents such as amiodarone, and possibly the type of anastomosis (Table 40-5).[34,35] These patients are dependent upon chronotropic response to maintain exercise tolerance. In cases of bradycardia with heart rates of 70 bpm or chronotropic incompetence, beta agonists such as terbutaline could increase heart rate or, if persistent, a permanent pacemaker is indicated.

Right Ventricular Dysfunction

Some degree of right ventricular (RV) dysfunction is common after cardiac transplantation, in as much as half of recipients, but acute RV failure is high risk for early mortality.[57] Preoperative PH predisposes to RV dysfunction perioperatively explaining why high or fixed PVR is a contraindication to transplantation. When present, RV dysfunction is treated with inhaled vasodilators such as nitric oxide or epoprostenol and pulmonary afterload reduction and unloading of the RV with milrinone. Inotrope support of the RV with dobutamine or milrinone, volume control (diuretics, dialysis, ultrafiltration), and maintenance of a higher heart rate also support the RV in the setting of failure. If RV dysfunction does not improve, worsening renal failure ensues contributing to a higher volume load on the RV.

Infection

Infection is always a hazard for a chronically immunosuppressed patient and poses the greatest risk during the first year after transplantation due to the higher intensity regimen.[58,59] Early posttransplant infections tend to involve donor- or recipient-derived infection or are associated with surgical complications; nosocomial bacterial infections related to indwelling lines/catheters, pneumonia, and wound

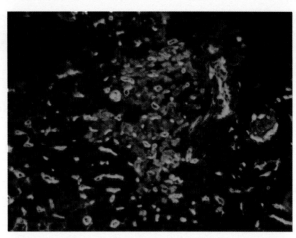

FIGURE 40-8 Antibody-mediated rejection in a heart transplant recipient. Risk factors were younger age and noncompliance with medication regimen. The patient expired 5 years posttransplant due to noncompliance and demonstrated graft dysfunction with chronic AMR despite aggressive therapy on multiple admissions (ATG, apheresis, rituxan, IVIG, photopheresis, and increased immunosuppression maintenance doses). Note the "donut" appearance of the immunofluorescence positivity with C4d in the capillaries. Abbreviations: AMR, antibody mediated rejection; ATG, antithymocyte globulin; IVIG, intravenous immunoglobulin. (Used with permission from Ohio State University Wexner Medical Center.)

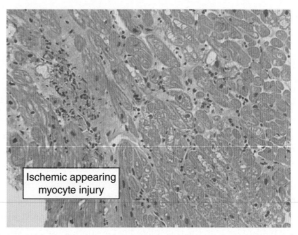

Ischemic appearing myocyte injury

FIGURE 40-9 Ischemia noted in posttransplant patient with vacuolization of myocytes. (Used with permission from Ohio State University Wexner Medical Center.)

Table 40-5 Complications Posttransplant

Bradycardia
Right ventricular dysfunction/failure
Infection
Malignancy
Coronary artery vasculopathy
Hypertension
Hyperlipidemia
Diabetes mellitus
Renal dysfunction
Osteoporosis

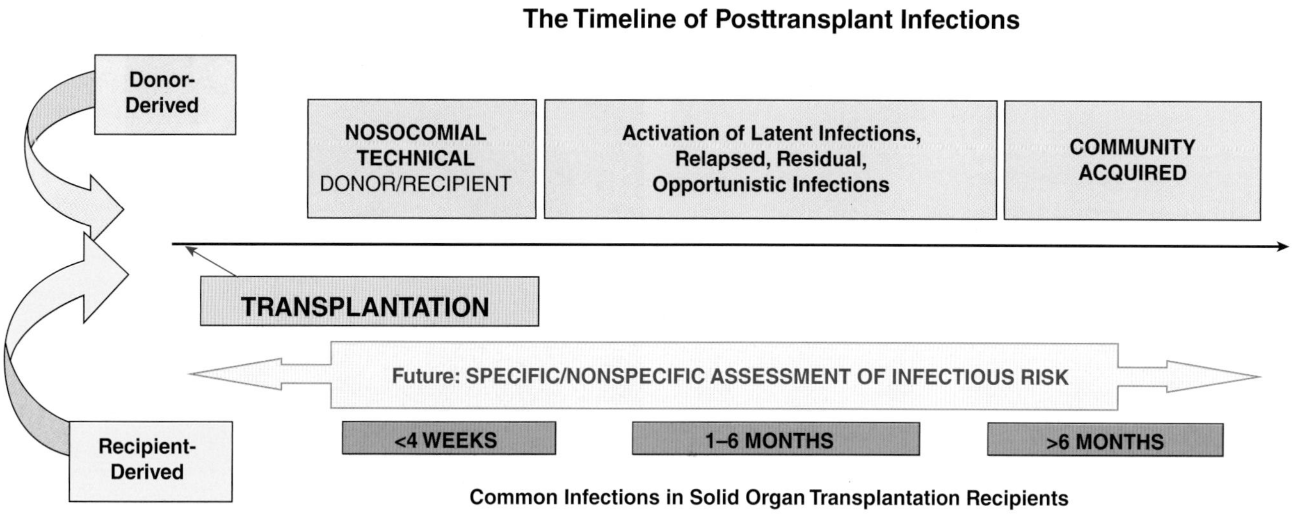

The Timeline of Posttransplant Infections

Donor-Derived

| NOSOCOMIAL TECHNICAL DONOR/RECIPIENT | Activation of Latent Infections, Relapsed, Residual, Opportunistic Infections | COMMUNITY ACQUIRED |

TRANSPLANTATION

Future: SPECIFIC/NONSPECIFIC ASSESSMENT OF INFECTIOUS RISK

Recipient-Derived

| <4 WEEKS | 1–6 MONTHS | >6 MONTHS |

Common Infections in Solid Organ Transplantation Recipients

Antimicrobial-resistant Species:	With PCP and antiviral (CMV, HBV) Prophylaxis:	Community Acquired Pneumonia Urinary Tract Infection
• MRSA • VRE • Candida species (non-albicans) Aspiration Line Infection Wound Infection Anastamotic Leaks/Ischemia *C difficile* colitis **Donor-Derived (Uncommon):** HSV, LCMV, rabies, West Nile **Recipient-Derived (colonization):** Aspergillus, Pseudomonas	• BK Polyomavirus Nephropathy • *C difficile* colitis • Hepatitis C virus • Adenovirus, influenza • *Cryptococcus neoformans* • *M tuberculosis* **Anastamotic complications** **Without Prophylaxis Add:** *Pneumocystis* Herpesviruses (HSV, VZV, CMV, EBV) Hepatitis B virus *Listeria, Nocardia, Toxoplasma* *Strongyloides, Leishmania, T cruzi*	*Aspergillus,* Atypical molds, *Mucor* species *Nocardia, Rhodococcus* species Late Viral: • CMV (Colitis/Retinitis) • Hepatitis (HBV, HCV) • HSV encephalitis • Community acquired (SARS, West Nile) • JC polyomavirus (PML) Skin Cancer, Lymphoma (PTLD)

FIGURE 40-10 Timeline of infection in solid organ transplant recipients. (Reprinted from Fishman JA. From the classic concepts to modern practice. *Clin Microbiol Infect.* 2014;20(S7):4-9. Copyright 2014, with permission from John Wiley and Sons.)

infection are common (Figure 40-10). Such organisms, *Staphylococcus, Pseudomonas, Proteus, Klebsiella, Escherichia coli,* and *Clostridium difficile* colitis commonly occur in the first month. Opportunistic infections usually occur 1 to 6 months after transplant with various sources, viral (CMV), fungal (aspergillus, candida), and parasites (toxoplasmosis, pneumocystis) (Figure 40-11). Beyond 6 months, community-acquired infections are more common given that immunosuppression is tapered. Antiviral (CMV, herpes simplex virus) and pneumocystis carinii prophylaxis are standard protocol in transplant centers; antifungal prophylaxis differs per center.

Malignancy

Malignancy is a common cause of late death ranging from 20% to 24% for patients beyond 3 to 10 years posttransplant.[1] Risk is related to chronic immunosuppression, both intensity and duration, which contributes to decreased immune surveillance for cancer, chronic immune stimulation, and activation of oncogenic viruses such as Epstein-Barr virus (EBV in posttransplant lymphoproliferative disorder, PTLD), human herpes virus 8 (HHV-8 in Kaposi sarcoma), and human papilloma virus (HPV in anogenital cancer). The most common de novo posttransplant malignancy is skin cancer followed by PTLD. Squamous and basal cell cancers

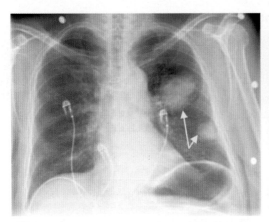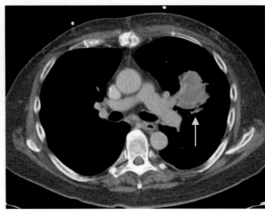

FIGURE 40-11 Cardiac transplant patient diagnosed with pulmonary aspergillus (*arrows*) at 6 months posttransplant. Patient presented with cough, low-grade fever, and night sweats without early rejection and had not been on antifungal prophylaxis. (Used with permission from Ohio State University Wexner Medical Center.)

occur at a much higher rate in the solid organ transplant population and at many sites in a more aggressive manner than in the general population.[60] Although not as excessive, melanoma risk is greater along with Kaposi sarcoma. Breast, lung, prostate, bladder, and colon cancers also occur in transplant recipients although evidence varies in terms of additional incidence in these patients, but may present more aggressively due to immunosuppression. PTLD is the most common noncutaneous malignancy and most cases are related to EBV reactivation or primary infection.

Multiple mechanisms contribute to cancer induction as described above including the different immunosuppressive drugs that can disrupt DNA repair or upregulation of angiogenic growth factors.[61] Treatment first involves prevention and following current recommendations for cancer screening with mammograms, Papanicolaou testing, colonoscopy, and prostate-specific antigen. Careful sun protection and reduced exposure are fundamental precautions in transplant patients, who are also encouraged to seek the care of a dermatologist for regular skin cancer screening. Once diagnosed, immunosuppression is reduced in patients with malignancy, especially in the case of PTLD, and consideration is given to replacing MMF or CNI with sirolimus, which may have antiproliferative properties.[41,61] The pleiotropic benefits of statins could play a role in reducing posttransplant malignancy risk, but need further evaluation.[62] Additionally, future research could focus on malignancy prevention tactics such as biomarkers for tolerance prediction, memory B cell reduction, and naive B cell repopulation.[61]

Renal Failure

Renal dysfunction is a common posttransplant complication and risk factors include older recipient age, female gender, diabetes, temporary dialysis or hemofiltration perioperatively, and impaired renal function pretransplant and early posttransplant.[15] In addition, CNI damages renal function especially in those patients with underlying intrinsic renal disease.[63] Multiple patient-specific factors play a role in the structural development of CKD: acute kidney injury from hypotension, vasoconstrictor use and cardiopulmonary bypass, hypertensive and diabetic nephropathy, ischemic disease, and nephrotoxic medications including CNI with vasoconstrictor effects. In addition to managing comorbidities such as HTN and diabetes, renal sparing immunosuppression regimens are initiated in these patients and include reducing CNI dose/level or converting from CNI to sirolimus maintenance therapy alone or in combination with lower dose CNI.[64-66] The key in converting to proliferation signal inhibitors is earlier utilization because the presence of pro teinuria negates any benefit from these drugs.[66] As previously mentioned, a higher intolerance level has been noted with sirolimus due to the side effect profile and more episodes of acute rejection.[65]

Coronary Vasculopathy

Coronary allograft vasculopathy is present in approximately 50% of recipients at 5 years posttransplant; therefore, it is a major complication limiting posttransplant survival.[1] When it presents early (ie, up to 10% of patients within the first year), CAV is more aggressive and carries a worse prognosis. Clinical presentation is not typical of angina due to denervation although some could experience angina with reinnervation over time; patients present with systolic or diastolic HF, arrhythmias, infarction, or sudden death.[36] Thus, screening angiography is performed routinely with left heart catheterizations.

Detecting CAV with surveillance angiography is challenging due to the unusual features of vasculopathy when compared to nontransplant CAD. Lesions are diffuse rather than focal and have less lipid and calcium deposition in plaque. CAV involves intimal wall thickening of the epicardial vessels resulting in lesions in larger sized vessels and in "distal pruning" preventing intervention on small-caliber vessels (Figure 40-12). Diffuse intimal hyperplasia also affects the microvasculature including intramyocardial arteries (50-20 μm), arterioles (20-10 μm), and capillaries (<10 μm).[67] Diffuse involvement of the vessels is concentric and may extend along the entire length of the vessel, resulting in underestimation of disease by coronary angiography until the use of additional imaging modalities as described in further detail in this section (Figure 40-13). Both immunologic and nonimmunologic mechanisms contribute to endothelial dysfunction and arterial constriction in the development of CAV.[67] HLA compatibility and alloreactive T cells and humoral cells comprise immunologic factors resulting in an inflammatory response stimulating proliferation of smooth muscle cells and mononuclear infiltrate; nonimmunologic factors are older donor age, ischemia-reperfusion time, and traditional risk factors such as hyperlipidemia and diabetes. CMV infection also plays a part in CAV due to a proinflammatory response and adverse effects on the nitric oxide pathway. Intraplaque hemorrhages as a result of endothelial damage may cause rapid increase of stenosis and generate a substrate for plaque destabilization.[68] Histopathology of CAV reveals various phenotypes (inflammatory lesions, lesions rich in smooth muscle cells, and fibrotic lesions) suggesting a relationship to time after transplantation, age at transplantation, occurrence of infection, and amount of atherosclerotic disease.[69]

Detection of CAV is challenging given its characteristic diffuse and concentric nature. Intravascular ultrasound (IVUS) measurements of coronary intimal thickening have significant prognostic endpoints; patients with intimal thickening in the first year posttransplant had a higher incidence of death, graft loss, nonfatal major cardiac events, and angiographic CAV after 5 years.[70] More recently, optical coherence tomography (OCT) is another intravascular imaging modality with a high spatial resolution allowing

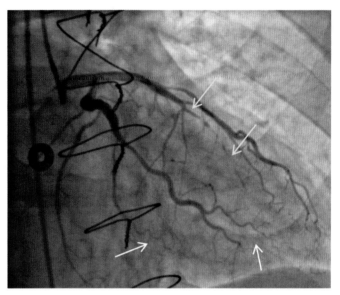

FIGURE 40-12 Extensive coronary allograft vasculopathy in a patient with recurrent cellular rejection and history of CMV viremia approximately 4 years posttransplant. Vasculopathy affected large- and small-caliber vessels in this patient. Arrows (*yellow*): total obliteration of the mid and distal LAD. Arrows (*white*): mild-moderate nonobstructive transplant vasculopathy in the distal portions of the OM₁ and LCX. Abbreviations: CMV, cytomegalovirus; LCX, left circumflex; LAD, left anterior descending artery; OM1, first obtuse marginal. (Used with permission from Ohio State University Wexner Medical Center.)

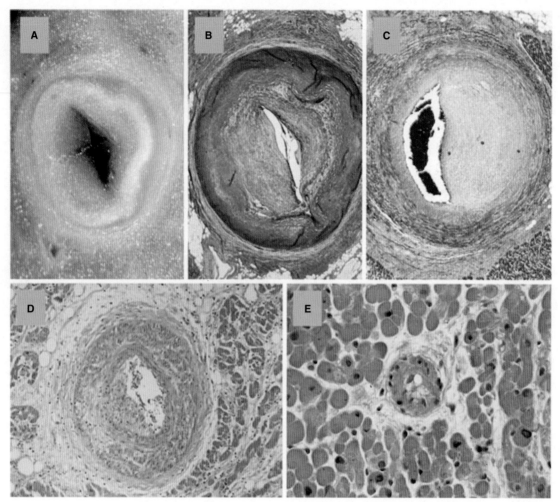

FIGURE 40-13 Pathologic characteristics of transplant coronary allograft vasculopathy. **A.** Gross pathology of concentric diffuse intimal thickening of an epicardial coronary artery. **B.** Concentric lesion, with focal attenuation of tunica media. **C.** Eccentric fibrocellular lesion. **D., E.** Concentric diffuse intimal thickening of the small intramyocardial arteries, with focal attenuation of tunica media in (**D.**). (Reprinted from Angelini A, Castellani C, Fedrigo M, et al. Coronary cardiac allograft vasculopathy versus native atherosclerosis: difficulties in classification. *Virchows Arch.* 2014;464(6):627-635. Copyright 2014, with permission from Springer.)

for detailed evaluation of intimal hyperplasia and possibly early identification of patients with a high intimal-to-media thickness ratio and characterization of atherosclerotic plaque.[71] Given this relatively new imaging method, outcome data on OCT are needed for routine use in CAV screening. Alternative noninvasive imaging includes dobutamine stress echocardiography with a moderate sensitivity and specificity and a more recent promising meta-analysis of coronary computed tomography angiography.[72,73]

As with traditional CAD, treatment of CAV begins with prevention. This includes reducing ischemic times, preventing recurrent rejection and infection, and risk factor modification—HTN, diabetes, smoking, and hyperlipidemia. Pharmacologic management consists of the following: (a) aspirin prophylaxis; (b) statins for lipid lowering and pleiotropic benefits such as anti-inflammatory properties, inhibition of smooth muscle cell proliferation, and improved endothelial function;[74] (c) the antimetabolite agent, MMF;[75] and (d) proliferation signal inhibitors, sirolimus and everolimus, with promising evidence.[49,50,76] Two recent trials suggest that early conversion to a PSI regimen is more effective in preventing CAV progression: a sirolimus-based regimen within the first 2 years and everolimus within the first year posttransplant.[77,78] Although observational, the latter study (n = 143) also found a benefit of statins on early and late progression of CAV while hypertriglyceridemia was a late influence.

The ISHLT has developed standardized definitions of CAV ranging from CAV_0 (no detectable angiographic lesion) to CAV_1 (mild), CAV_2 (moderate), and CAV_3 (severe) based on degree of stenosis, number of vessels affected, and which vessels are involved (left main, primary vessel, or branch vessel).[79] Classification of CAV by this nomenclature at 1 year posttransplant had prognostic significance in predicting major adverse cardiac events (death, acute coronary syndrome, coronary revascularization, HF admission unrelated to an acute rejection episode, and cardiac retransplantation).[80]

Standard revascularization with coronary artery bypass grafting in CAV is limited due to the shortage of proximal and midvessel stenosis with adequate distal anastomotic targets; poor outcomes have been seen in existing evidence.[81] In-stent restenosis with percutaneous coronary intervention is higher when compared to this technique in native coronaries.[82] Database review of drug-eluting stents in CAV found a reduction in in-stent restenosis at 12 months and no significant difference in mortality or major adverse cardiac events when compared to bare-metal stents, but all studies were retrospective in this review.[83] Revascularization in CAV is not straightforward because many patients are asymptomatic and evidence has not clearly defined an association with better outcomes. Retransplantation is the definitive answer for severe CAV, but comorbidities often limit candidacy for a second organ.

Hypertension

HTN is prevalent in transplant patients and for the most part related to CNI therapy, perhaps associated more with cyclosporine than tacrolimus as recognized in a meta-analysis of 7 randomized controlled trials of 885 patients.[44] The majority of patients will be hypertensive, which often requires multiple drug therapy for control, and is a risk factor for development of CAV and renal dysfunction. Patients have a higher ambulatory blood pressure for daytime and nighttime with a diminished nocturnal decrease in BP.[84,85] Beta blockers are traditionally avoided at least in the early posttransplant course due to the recipient's denervation and dependence on circulating catecholamines for chronotropic response and exercise tolerance; for this reason, exercise intolerance and fatigue are often observed when these patients are taking beta blockers.[35] Typical regimens include standard antihypertensive medications: angiotensin-converting enzyme (ACE) inhibitors or angiotensin receptor blockers (ARBs) based on renal dysfunction or hyperkalemia; calcium channel blockers such as amlodipine or diltiazem, which will increase CNI levels; thiazide diuretics; hydralazine; and nitrates.

Diabetes Mellitus

Diabetes is present in up to one-third of heart transplant recipients at 5 years.[86] It is related to the presence of pretransplant diabetes, age, obesity, ethnicity, family history of diabetes, and the immunosuppression regimen—corticosteroids and CNI drugs, tacrolimus more than cyclosporine.[44,84,86] Diabetes has been associated with reduced long-term survival and is associated with comorbidities such as CAV

and renal dysfunction. Complicating effective treatment in this patient population are renal insufficiency that can limit use of metformin and fluid retention as a result of thiazolidinediones. A guideline consensus statement was developed for renal, liver, and heart transplantation to reduce individuals' risk of developing new-onset diabetes and reduce the long-term complications associated with diabetes.[87]

Hyperlipidemia

The immunosuppression regimen is largely responsible for dyslipidemia after heart transplantation due to the use of corticosteroids, CNI, and proliferation signal inhibitors.[84] Development of hyperlipidemia contributes to CAV, peripheral vascular disease, and cerebrovascular disease. Statins, or HMG-CoA reductase inhibitors, are effective in reducing the lipid profile; pravastatin may have a lower incidence of rhabdomyolysis because it is not metabolized by cytochrome enzymes like the other statins. Risk of rhabdomyolysis increases with higher statin doses or the addition of other agents such as fibrates or niacin. When titrating drugs, it is important to recall that statins have a drug interaction with CNI therapy resulting in a greater risk of myalgias and statin-induced rhabdomyolysis. In addition to lipid lowering, the pleiotropic benefits of statins are important in preventing CAV; these include plaque stabilization, reduction in inflammation, inhibition of smooth muscle cell proliferation, and improved endothelial function.[74] Given the association with lower rejection in heart transplant recipients, statins are considered to have an immune-modulating effect and have been associated with a better long-term survival compared to patients who were not on statins (94.6% vs 74.1%; $p < 0.05$). A review of 7 randomized controlled trials of statins in cardiac transplants confirmed a modest survival benefit of statins, low incidence of adverse effects but no difference in rejection episodes.[88]

Osteoporosis

Osteoporosis and fragility fractures are common after solid organ transplantation; corticosteroids exacerbate the risk.[89] Bone metabolism abnormalities leading to bone loss tend to occur within the first year after transplant due to immunosuppression, immobilization, and pretransplant risk factors including chronic disease. Many centers perform bone density studies as part of the pretransplant evaluation. Prevention should include supplementing calcium and vitamin D, bisphosphonates, and weight-bearing exercises.

Psychosocial Factors

Education level and social/economic satisfaction are emerging as critical influences on posttransplant outcomes. Patients who have private insurance/self-pay had a higher 10-year survival when compared to Medicare and Medicaid patients (8.6% and 10% lower survival for Medicare and Medicaid, respectively, in a UNOS database review of >20,000 recipients).[90] College-educated patients had a 7% higher 10-year survival. Multivariable analysis determined that college education decreased mortality risk by 11% while Medicare and Medicaid increased mortality risk by 18% and 33%, respectively ($p \le 0.001$). In a self-reported quality of life assessment, Farmer et al found that a higher level of education and social and economic satisfaction predicted improved survival whereas poor compliance with medical care predicted worse survival.[91] Such psychosocial factors are key in transplant survival due to the necessary frequent follow-up by specialized health care professionals and management of a complicated regimen of immunosuppressive and cardiovascular medications.

RETRANSPLANTATION

The reason for retransplantation plays a role in survival with the worst survival found for acute rejection (32% and 8% at 1 and 5 years, respectively) followed by retransplantation for early graft failure (50% and 39% at 1 and 5 years, respectively).[92] Survival after retransplantation for CAV has reasonable results and is an indication for retransplantation. Nonetheless, retransplantation is limited by patient comorbidities and graft failure.

Risk factors associated with a high risk of graft failure in patients who underwent retransplantation are older recipient age, increasing serum creatinine, and mechanical ventilation. When present alone or in combination, these factors significantly increased 1-year graft failure rates; the effect of multiple risk factors is cumulative as patients with all 3 factors had a 32% higher risk of graft failure within 5 years as compared with patients with no risk factors. Each decade increase in recipient age was associated with a 20% increase in odds of 1-year graft failure and each 1 mg/dL increase in serum creatinine increased odds of graft failure by 58%.[93]

OUTCOMES

In the 30th ISHLT adult heart transplant report, 1- and 5-year survival are 81% and 69%, respectively, with a median survival of 11 years for all and 13 years for those surviving the first year.[1] Survival has improved with successive eras, but the most recent cohort of 2006 to 2011 is similar to 2002 to 2005 (Figure 40-14). Mortality within the first 3 years is predominately related to infection and graft failure, whereas after 3 to 5 years, malignancy, cardiac allograft vasculopathy, and renal failure gradually become more important. Functional status improves to normal activity in almost 90%.[1] The number of older recipients >60 years is increasing, and age is a risk factor for mortality at all follow-up points according to the most recent ISHLT report with a focus theme on age.[1]

Predictors of long-term survival were examined in a multivariate analysis of the UNOS registry in patients surviving a minimum of 10 years from 1987 to 1999 and compared to patients who died within 10 years from the time of transplantation. These factors of survival included recipient age <55 years, shorter ischemic time, younger donor age, white race, and annual center volume >9.[94] Mechanical ventilation and diabetes decreased the probability of long-term survival. The authors noted that each 1-hour reduction in ischemic time improved the odds of long-term survival by 11% (p <0.001) while each decade decrease in donor age had a similar 10% improvement in 10-year survival. Racial differences in several studies have shown a persistently elevated mortality among black recipients and attribute the documented higher rate of graft loss in this patient population to immune-related mechanisms, such as the degree of HLA matching, a need for higher levels of immunosuppression, differential drug absorption, and systemic complications of therapy.[95,96] Along with racial disparities in post-outcome

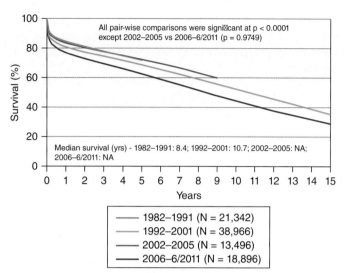

FIGURE 40-14 Kaplan-Meier long-term survival by era for adult heart transplant recipients. Data from the Registry of the International Society for Heart and Lung Transplantation: 30th Official Adult Heart Transplant Report-2013.[1] Survival in the most recent cohort from 2006 to 2011 is similar to those who received transplants in the 2002 to 2005 cohort with an unadjusted 1-year survival of 84%. (Reprinted from Lund LH, Edwards LB, Kucheryavaya AY, et al. The registry of the International Society for Heart and Lung Transplantation: thirtieth official adult heart transplant report—2013. *J Heart Lung Transpl.* 2013;32(10):951-964. Copyright 2013, with permission from Elsevier.)

mortality, evaluation of the waitlist also continues to find divergence with Hispanic and blacks more often listed as an urgent status (1A). Listed Hispanic patients in the United States appear to be at higher risk of dying on the waitlist or becoming too ill for a transplant in comparison with white patients. Black patients had a similar waitlist mortality but had a higher early posttransplant mortality.[97] Further research is necessary to refine and resolve these disparities.

CONCLUSIONS

In summary, cardiac transplantation is the preferred treatment for end-stage HF in select patients. Multiple advances in the recent decades have improved survival and quality of life. Pretransplant bridging with mechanical support continues to increase and has contributed to reduced waitlist mortality if patients remain without a VAD-related complication. Enhancement of immunosuppression regimens has reduced acute allograft rejection episodes, and donor procurement and surgical techniques have contributed to improved donor function. Posttransplant care is complicated involving complex medical regimens, drug interactions, preexisting comorbidities and development of posttransplant comorbidities, all of which affect quality of life and outcomes. Median survival is 10 years and 13 years for those surviving the first posttransplant year; yet, complications of malignancy, infection, rejection, and coronary allograft vasculopathy still limit survival. There remains a shortage of available donors. Clinical and research focus has been in the direction of patient selection, desensitization, expanding the donor pool, and further optimizing immunosuppression to prevent posttransplant complications such as vasculopathy and renal failure. Continued advances in cardiac transplantation will lead to refinement of patient management and long-term outcomes.

REFERENCES

1. Lund LH, Edwards LB, Kucheryavaya AY, et al. The registry of the International Society for Heart and Lung Transplantation: thirtieth official adult heart transplant report—2013. *J Heart Lung Transpl.* 2013;32(10):951-964.

2. Reitz BA, Bieber CP, Raney AA, et al. Orthotopic heart and combined heart and lung transplantation with cyclosporine-A immune suppression. *Transplant Proc.* 1981;13(1):393-396.

3. Macdonald P. Heart transplantation: who should be considered and when? *Int Med J.* 2008;38:911-917.

4. Mehra MR, Kobashigawa J, Starling R, et al. Listing criteria for heart transplantation: International Society for Heart and Lung Transplantation Guidelines for the Care of Cardiac Transplant Candidates—2006. *J Heart Lung Transplant.* 2006;25:1024-1042.

5. Zuckermann A, Dunkler D, Deviatko E, et al. Longterm survival (>10 years) of patients >60 years with induction therapy after cardiac transplantation. *Eur J Cardiothorac Surg.* 2003;24:283-291.

6. Tjang YS, van der Heijden GJ, Tenderich G, Körfer R, Grobbee DE. Impact of recipient's age on heart transplantation outcome. *Ann Thorac Surg.* 2008;85:2051-2055.

7. Marielli D, Kobashigawa J, Hamilton M, et al. Long term outcomes of heart transplantation in older recipients. *J Heart Lung Transplant.* 2008;27:830-834.

8. Lietz K, John R, Burke EA, et al. Pretransplant cachexia and morbid obesity are predictors of increased mortality after heart transplantation. *Transplantation.* 2001;72:277-283.

9. Williams JJ, Lund LH, LaManca J, et al. Excessive weight gain in cardiac transplant recipients. *J Heart Lung Transplant.* 2006;25(1):36-41.

10. Uriel N, Jorde UP, Cotarlan V, et al. Heart transplantation in human immunodeficiency virus-positive patients. *J Heart Lung Transplant.* 2009;28(7):667-669.

11. Butler J, Stankewicz MA, Wu J, et al. Pretransplant reversible pulmonary hypertension predicts higher risk for mortality after cardiac transplantation. *J Heart Lung Transplant.* 2005;24(2):170-177.

12. Morgan JA, John R, Weinberg AD, et al. Heart transplantation in diabetic recipients: a decade review of 161 patients at Columbia Presbyterian. *J Thorac Cardiovasc Surg.* 2004;127(5):1486-1492.

13. Russo MJ, Chen JM, Hong KN, et al. Survival after heart transplantation is not diminished among recipients with uncomplicated diabetes mellitus: an analysis of the United Network of Organ Sharing database. *Circulation.* 2006;114:2280–2287.

14. Kilic A, Weiss ES, George TJ, et al. What predicts long-term survival after heart transplantation? An analysis of 9,400 ten-year survivors. *Ann Thorac Surg.* 2012;93(3):699-704.

15. Thomas HL, Banner NR, Murphy CL, et al. Incidence, determinants, and outcome of chronic kidney disease after adult heart transplantation in the United Kingdom. *Transplantation.* 2012;939(11):1151-1157.

16. Hamour IM, Omar F, Lyster HS, et al. Chronic kidney disease after heart transplantation. *Nephrol Dial Transplant.* 2009;24(5):1655-1662.

17. Rivard AL, Hellmich C, Sampson B, et al. Preoperative predictors for postoperative problems in heart transplantation: psychiatric and psychosocial considerations. *Prog Transpl.* 2005;15(3):276-282.

18. Maldonado JR, Dubois HC, David EE, et al. The Stanford integrated psychosocial assessment for transplantation (SIPAT): a new tool for the psychosocial evaluation of pre-transplant candidates. *Psychosomatics.* 2012;53(2):123-132.

19. United Network for Organ Sharing's Organ Procurement and Transplantation Network Policies: 3.7 Organ Distribution. Allocation of Thoracic Organs. optn.transplant.hrsa.gov/PoliciesandBylaws2/policies/.../policy_9.pdf.

20. Mogollón MV, Gallé EL, Pérez RH, et al. Prognosis after heart transplant in patients with pulmonary hypertension secondary to cardiopathy. *Transpl Proc.* 2008;40(9):3031-3033.

21. Costanzo CR, Dipchand A, Starling R, et al. The International Society of Heart and Lung Transplantation: guidelines for the care of heart transplant recipients. *J Heart Lung Transpl.* 2010:29(8):914-956.

22. Kittleson MM, Shemin R, Patel JK, et al. Donor–recipient sex mismatch portends poor 10-year outcomes in a single-center experience. *J Heart Lung Transpl.* 2011;30(9):1018-1022.

23. Weiss ES, Allen JG, Patel ND, et al. The impact of donor–recipient sex matching on survival after orthotopic heart transplantation: analysis of 18,000 transplants in the modern era. *Circ Heart Fail.* 2009;2(5):401-408.

24. Khush KK, Menza R, Nguyen J, et al. Donor predictors of allograft use and recipient outcomes after heart transplantation. *Circ Heart Fail.* 2013;6(2):300-309.

25. Wittwer T, Wahlers T. Marginal donor grafts in heart transplantation: lessons learned from 25 years of experience. *Transpl Int.* 2008;21(2):113-125.

26. Schulze PC, Kitada S, Clerkin K, et al. Regional differences in recipient waitlist time and pre- and post-transplant mortality after the 2006 United Network for Organ Sharing policy changes in the donor heart allocation algorithm. *JACC Heart Fail.* 2014;2(2):166-177.

27. Wever-Pinzon O, Drakos SG, Kfoury AG, et al. Morbidity and mortality in heart transplant candidates supported with mechanical circulatory support: is reappraisal of the current United Network for Organ Sharing thoracic organ allocation policy justified? *Circulation.* 2013;127(4):452-462.

28. Atkinson C, Floerchinger B, Qiao F, et al. Donor brain death exacerbates complement-dependent ischemia/reperfusion injury in transplanted hearts. *Circulation.* 2013;127:1290-1299.

29. Watson AJ, Gao L, Sun L, et al. Enhanced preservation of the rat heart after prolonged hypothermic ischemia with erythropoietin-supplemented Celsior solution. *J Heart Lung Transplant.* 2013;32:633-640.

30. Noda K, Shigemura N, Tanaka Y, et al. A novel method of preserving cardiac grafts using a hydrogen-rich water bath. *J Heart Lung Transplant.* 2013;32:241-250.

31. White CW, Ali A, Hasanally D, et al. A cardioprotective preservation strategy employing ex vivo heart perfusion facilitates successful transplant of donor hearts after cardiocirculatory death. *J Heart Lung Transplant.* 2013;32:734-743.

32. Lower RR, Shumway NE. Studies on orthotopic homotransplantation of the canine heart. *Surg Forum.* 1960;11:18-19.

33. Dreyfus G, Jebara V, Mihaileanue S, et al. Total orthotopic heart transplantation: an alternative to the standard technique. *Ann Thorac Surg.* 1991;52:1181-1184.

34. Davies RR, Russo MJ, Morgan JA, et al. Standard versus bicaval techniques for orthotopic heart transplantation: an analysis of the United Network for Organ Sharing database. *J Thorac Cardiovasc Surg.* 2010;140(3):700-708.

35. Kittleson MM, Kobashigawa JA. Heart transplantation. In: Baliga RR, ed. *Specialty Board Review: Cardiology.* New York, NY: McGraw-Hill; 2012:743-755.

36. Pham MX, Berry GJ, Hunt SA. Cardiac transplantation. In: Fuster V, Walsh RA, Harrington RA, eds. *Hurst's: The Heart.* 13th ed. New York, NY: McGraw-Hill; 2011:781-797.

37. Lindenfeld J, Miller GG, Shakar SF, et al. Drug therapy in the heart transplant recipient: part I: cardiac rejection and immunosuppressive drugs. *Circulation.* 2004;110:3734-3740.

38. Hershberger RE, Starling RC, Eisen HJ, et al. Daclizumab to prevent rejection after cardiac transplantation. *N Eng J Med.* 2005;3:2705-2713.

39. Carlsen J, Johansen M, Boesgaard S, et al. Induction therapy after cardiac transplantation: a comparison of anti-thymocyte globulin and daclizumab in the prevention of acute rejection. *J Heart Lung Transplant.* 2005;3:296-302.

40. Mullen JC, Kuurstra EJ, Oreopoulos A, et al. A randomized controlled trial of daclizumab versus anti-thymocyte globulin induction for heart transplantation. *Transplant Res.* 2014;3:14. doi: 10.1186/2047-1440-3-14.

41. Lindenfeld J, Miller GG, Shakar SF, et al. Drug therapy in the heart transplant recipient: part II: immunosuppressive drugs. *Circulation.* 2004;110:3858-3865.

42. Kobashigawa Ja, Miller LW, Russell SD, et al. Tacrolimus with mycophenolate mofetil (MMF) or sirolimus vs. cyclosporine with MMF in cardiac transplant patients. 1-year report. *Am J Transplant.* 2006;6(6):1377-1386.

43. Grimm M, Rinaldi M, Yonan NA, et al. Superior prevention of acute rejection by tacrolimus vs. cyclosporine in heart transplant recipients–a large European trial. *Am J Transplant.* 2006;6(6):1387-1397.

44. Ye F, Ying-Bin X, Yu-Guo W, et al. Tacrolimus versus cyclosporine microemulsion for heart transplant recipients: a meta-analysis. *J Heart Lung Transpl.* 2009;28(1):58-66.

45. Eisen HJ, Kobashigawa J, Keogh A, et al; Mycophenolate Mofetil Cardiac Study Investigators. Three-year results of a randomized, double-blind, controlled trial of mycophenolate mofetil versus azathioprine in cardiac transplant recipients. *J Heart Lung Transpl.* 2005;24(5):517-525.

46. Hosenpud JD, Bennett LE. Mycophenolate mofetil versus azathioprine in patients surviving the initial cardiac transplant hospitalization: an analysis of the Joint UNOS/ISHLT Thoracic Registry. *Transplantation.* 2001;72(10):1662-1665.

47. Lehmkuhl H, Hummel M, Kobashigawa J, et al. Enteric-coated mycophenolate-sodium in heart transplantation: efficacy, safety, and pharmacokinetic compared with mycophenolate mofetil. *Transpl Proc.* 2008;40(4):953-955.

48. Segovia J, Gerosa G, Almenar L, et al. Impact of dose reductions on efficacy outcome in heart transplant patients receiving enteric-coated mycophenolate sodium or mycophenolate mofetil at 12 months post-transplantation. *Clin Transplant.* 2008;22(6):809-814.

49. Keogh A, Richardson M, Ruygrok P, et al. Sirolimus in de novo heart transplant recipients reduces acute rejection and prevents coronary artery disease at 2 years. A randomized clinical trial. *Circulation.* 2004;110(17):2694-2700.

50. Eisen HJ, Tuzcu EM, Dorent R, et al. Everolimus for the prevention of allograft rejection and vasculopathy in cardiac transplant patients. *N Engl J Med.* 2003;349(9):847-858.

51. Gonzalez-Vilchez F, Vazquez de Prada JA, Paniagua MJ. Use of mTOR inhibitors in chronic heart transplant recipients with renal failure: calcineurin-inhibitors conversion or minimization? *Int J Cardiol.* 2014;171(1):15-23.

52. Stewart S, Winters GL, Fishbein MC, et al. Revision of the 1990 working formulation for the standardization of nomenclature in the diagnosis of heart rejection. *J Heart Lung Transpl.* 2005;24(11):1710-1720.

53. Pham MX, Teuteberg JJ, Kfoury AG, et al. Gene-expression profiling for rejection surveillance after cardiac transplantation. *New Engl J Med.* 2010;362(20):1890-1900.

54. Orrego CM, Cordero-Reyes AM, Estep JD, et al. Usefulness of routine surveillance endomyocardial biopsy 6 months after heart transplantation. *J Heart Lung Transpl.* 2012;31(8):845-849.

55. Kilic A, Weiss ES, Allen JG, et al. Simple score to assess the risk of rejection after orthotopic heart transplantation. *Circulation.* 2012;125(24):3013-3021.

56. Nair N, Ball T, Uber PA, et al. Current and future challenges in therapy for antibody-mediated rejection. *J Heart Lung Transpl.* 2011;30:612-617.

57. Bozbas H, Karacağlar E, Ozkan M, et al. The prevalence and course of pulmonary hypertension and right ventricular dysfunction in patients undergoing orthotopic heart transplantation. *Transpl Proc.* 2013;45(10):3538-3541.

58. Fishman JA. Introduction: infection in solid organ transplant recipients. *Am J Transpl.* 2009;9(S4):S3-S6.

59. Fishman JA. From the classic concepts to modern practice. *Clin Microbiol Infect.* 2014;20 (S7):4-9.

60. Ajithkumar TA, Parkinson CA, Butler A, et al. Management of solid tumours in organ-transplant recipients. *Lancet Oncol.* 2007;8:921-932.

61. Nair N, Gongora E, Mehra MR. Long-term immunosuppression and malignancy in thoracic transplantation: where is the balance? *J Heart Lung Transplant.* 2014;33:461-467.

62. Frohlich GM, Rufibach K, Enseleit F, et al. Statins and the risk of cancer after heart transplantation. *Circulation.* 2012;126:440-447.

63. Pinney SP, Balakrishnan R, Dikman S, et al. Histopathology of renal failure after hearttransplantation: a diverse spectrum. *J Heart Lung Transplant.* 2012;31:233-237.

64. Arora S, Gude E, Sigurdardottir V, et al. Improvement in renal function after everolimus introduction and calcineurin inhibitor reduction in maintenance thoracic transplant recipients: the significance of baseline glomerular filtration rate. *J Heart Lung Transplant.* 2012;31(3):259-265.

65. Zuckerman A, Keogh A, Crespo-Leiro MG, et al. Randomized controlled trial of sirolimus conversion in cardiac transplant recipients with renal insufficiency. *Am J Transplant.* 2012;12(9):2487-2497.

66. Potena L, Prestinenzi P, Bianchi IG, et al. Cyclosporine lowering with everolimus versus mycophenolate mofetil in heart transplant recipients: long-term follow-up of the SHIRAKISS randomized, prospective study. *J Heart Lung Transplant.* 2012;31(6):565-570.

67. Vecchiati A, Tellatin S, Angelini A, et al. Coronary microvasculopathy in heart transplantation: consequences and therapeutic implications. *World J Transplant.* 2014;4(2):93-101.

68. Angelini A, Castellani C, Fedrigo M, et al. Coronary cardiac allograft vasculopathy versus native atherosclerosis: difficulties in classification. *Virchows Arch.* 2014;464(6):627-635.

69. Hulbers MM, Vink A, Kaldeway J, et al. Distinct phenotypes of cardiac allograft vasculopathy after heart transplantation: a histopathological study. *Atherosclerosis.* 2014;236(2):353-359.

70. Kobashigawa JA, Tobis JM, Starling RC, et al. Multicenter intravascular ultrasound validation study among heart transplant recipients: outcomes after five years. *J Am Coll Cardiol.* 2005;45(9):1532-1537.

71. Khandar SJ, Yamamoto H, Teuteberg JJ, et al. Optical coherence tomography for characterization of cardiac allograft vasculopathy after heart transplantation (OCTCAV study). *J Heart Lung Transplant.* 2013;32:596-602.

72. Sade LE, Sezgin A, Eroglu S, et al. Dobutamine stress echocardiography in the assessment of cardiac allograft vasculopathy in the asymptomatic patient. *Transplant Proc.* 2008;40(1):267-270.

73. Wever-Pinzon O, Romero J, Kelesidis I, et al. Coronary computed tomography angiography for the detection of cardiac allograft vasculopathy: a meta-analysis of prospective trials. *J Am Coll Cardiol.* 2014;63(19):1992-2004.

74. Luo CM, Chou NK, Chi NH, et al. The effect of statins on cardiac allograft survival. *Transplant Proc.* 2014;46(3):920-924.

75. Dandel M, Hetzer R. Impact of immunosuppressive drugs on the development of cardiac allograft vasculopathy. *Curr Vasc Pharmacol.* 2010;8(5):706-719.

76. Kobashigawa JA, Pauly DF, Starling RC, et al. Cardiac allograft vasculopathy by intravascular ultrasound in heart transplant patients: substudy from the Everolimus versus mycophenolate mofetil randomized, multicenter trial. *J Am Coll Cardiol.* 2013;1(5):389-399.

77. Matsuo Y, Cassar A, Yoshino S, et al. Attenuation of cardiac allograft vasculopathy by sirolimus: Relationship to time interval after heart transplantation. *J Heart Lung Transplant.* 2013;32:784-791.

78. Masetti M, Potena L, Nardozza M, et al. Differential effect of everolimus on progression of early and late cardiac allograft vasculopathy in current clinical practice. *Am J Transplant.* 2013;13(5):1217-1226.

79. Mehra MR, Crespo-Leiro MG, Dipchand A, et al. International Society for Heart and Lung Transplantation working formulation of a standardized nomenclature for cardiac allograft vasculopathy—2010. *J Heart Lung Transplant.* 2010;29:717-727.

80. Prada-Delgado O, Estévez-Loureiro R, Paniagua-Martín MJ, et al. Prevalence and prognostic value of cardiac allograft vasculopathy 1 year after heart transplantation according to the ISHLT recommended nomenclature. *J Heart Lung Transplant.* 2012;31(3):332-333.

81. Halle AA, DiSciascio G, Massin EK, et al. Coronary angioplasty, atherectomy and bypass surgery in cardiac transplant recipients. *J Am Coll Cardiol.* 1995;26(1):120-128.

82. Bader FM, Kfoury AG, Gilbert EM, et al. Percutaneous coronary interventions with stents in cardiac transplant recipients. *J Heart Lung Transplant.* 2006;25(3):298-301.

83. Dasari, TW, Hennebry TA, Hanna EB, et al. Drug eluting versus bare metal stents in cardiac allograft vasculopathy: a systematic review of literature. *Catheter Cardiovasc Interv.* 2011;77(7):962-969

84. Lindenfeld J, Page RL, Zolty R, et al. Drug therapy in the heart transplant recipient part III: common medical problems. *Circulation.* 2005;111:113-117.

85. Kotsis VT, Stabouli SV, Pitiriga Vch, et al. Impact of cardiac transplantation in 24 hours circadian blood pressure and heart rate profile. *Transplant Proc.* 2005;37(5):2244-2246.

86. Marchetti P. New-onset diabetes after transplantation. *J Heart Lung Transplant.* 2004;23(5S):S194-S201.

87. Wilkinson A, Davidson J, Dotta F, et al. Guidelines for the treatment and management of new-onset diabetes after transplantation. *Clin Transplant.* 2005;19(3):291-298.

88. Som R, Morris PJ, Knight SR. Graft vessel disease following heart transplantation: a systematic review of the role of statin therapy. *World J Surg.* 2014;38(9):2324-2334.

89. Kulak CAM, Borba VZC, Júnior JK, et al. Bone disease after transplantation: osteoporosis and fractures risk. *Arquivos Brasileiros de Endocrinologia and Metabologia.* 2014;58(5):484-492.

90. Allen JG, Weiss ES, Arnaoutakis GJ, et al. Insurance and education predict long-term survival after orthotopic heart transplantation in the United States. *J Heart Lung Transplant.* 2012;31:52-60.

91. Farmer SA, Grady KL, Wang E, et al. Demographic, psychosocial, and behavioral factors associated with survival after heart transplantation. *Ann Thorac Surg.* 2013;95:876-883.

92. Radovancevic B, McGiffin DC, Kobashigawa JA, et al. Retransplantation in 7,290 primary transplant patients: a 10-year multi-institutional study. *J Heart Lung Transplant.* 2003;22:862-868.

93. Kilic A, Weiss ES, Arnaoutakis GJ, et al. Identifying recipients at high risk for graft failure after heart retransplantation. *Ann Thorac Surg.* 2012;93(3):712-716.

94. Kilic A, Weiss ES, George TJ, et al. What predicts long-term survival after heart transplantation? an analysis of 9,400 ten-year survivors. *Ann Thorac Surg.* 2012;93:699-704.

95. Liu V, Bhattacharya J, Weill D, et al. Persistent racial disparities in survival after heart transplantation. *Circulation.* 2011;123(15):1642-1649.

96. Singh TP, Almond C, Givertz MM, et al. Improved survival in heart transplant recipients in the United States: racial differences in era effect. *Circ Heart Fail.* 2011;4:153-160.

97. Singh TP, Almond CS, Taylor DO, et al. Racial and ethnic differences in wait-list outcomes in patients listed for heart transplantation in the United States. *Circulation.* 2012;125(24):3022-3030.

41 TOTAL ARTIFICIAL HEART

Yazhini Ravi, MD
Emmanuel A. Amulraj, MD
Srihari K. Lella, MD
Mohammed Quader, MD
Chittoor B. Sai-Sudhakar, MD

■ PATIENT CASE

A 55-year-old male with a history of dilated ischemic cardiomyopathy, presented with NYHA Class IV CHF, with worsening SOB. Echo demonstrated biventricular failure. Invasive hemodynamic monitoring suggested low cardiac output with elevated filling pressures including a high CVP and laboratory values were indicative of renal and hepatic dysfunction. Initial trial of therapy with dual inotropes did not lead to an improvement in his clinical status. His ABO blood group was O+. He was considered a candidate for advanced therapies and a TAH was inserted. Following adequate clinical recovery and improvement in his functional and nutritional status, he had a heart transplantation and was discharged in a stable condition.

INTRODUCTION

Heart transplantation is considered the gold standard for the treatment of end-stage heart failure (HF). However, the total number of patients receiving heart transplantation worldwide in the last few decades has remained around 4000 due to the limitations posed by the supply of donor hearts. The rising worldwide epidemic of HF coupled with increasing waitlist times for heart transplantation has made the concept of developing heart assist or heart replacement devices a reality. Total artificial heart (TAH), ventricular assist device (VAD), and cardiopulmonary bypass technologies all share the same lineage, originating in 1934 when Michael Ellis DeBakey described a dual roller pump for blood transfusions. This brought about a new era in cardiac surgery and the dawn of mechanical circulatory support. The critical difference between a VAD and TAH is that the native heart is left in situ during a VAD implantation, whereas implantation of the TAH requires excision of the left and right ventricles of the heart and replacing them with the TAH in the orthotropic position. The majority of patients in New York Heart Association (NYHA) class IV HF can be supported with isolated left VAD (LVAD) only—evidenced by the fact that more than 20,000 LVADs have been implanted worldwide. However, a minority of patients present with biventricular failure or other structural abnormalities of the heart precluding the placement of an isolated LVAD only. The TAH is an excellent therapeutic option under those circumstances. The TAH has been implanted in more than 1400 patients in North America, Europe, Russia, Turkey, Israel, and Australia with nearly all the implants being the SynCardia temporary Total Artificial Heart (SynCardia Systems, Inc.; Tucson, AZ, US).

The objective of this chapter is to give a brief review on the evolution and development of the TAH, its indications, clinical management, outcomes, and the current advances.

A BRIEF HISTORY

A clear start in the history of the TAH can be attributed to some of the scientific incentives advocated by the Kennedy administration in the 1960s. The National Institutes of Health initiated an artificial heart program for the development of partial and complete cardiac replacement devices. Parallel efforts progressed in Baylor College of Medicine in Texas, Cleveland Clinic, Pennsylvania State University, and University of Utah, creating a global race with research programs in the United States, Japan, West Germany, East Germany, Czechoslovakia, and the Soviet Union.

Willem Kolff and his trainees pioneered and laid the foundation for the development of TAH in its current form. The first reported TAH implantation was in a dog in 1957 by Dr Kolff and Tetsuzo Akutsu and circulation was supported for 90 minutes.[1] In 1969, Denton Cooley and Domingo Liotta performed the first human TAH implantation using the Liotta heart designed by Dr Liotta in a 47-year-old patient with ischemic cardiomyopathy, following a ventriculoplasty and an inability to separate from cardiopulmonary bypass. This device provided hemodynamic support for 64 hours. However, the early development of hemolysis and renal failure necessitated heart transplantation and the patient succumbed to sepsis 32 hours following the transplantation.[2] The media attention and controversy generated from this first human TAH implantation hampered its progress. After a long hiatus, a second TAH device (the Akutsu III developed by Dr Akutsu) was implanted in 1981 by Dr Cooley in a 36-year-old male patient in postcardiotomy shock following coronary artery bypass grafting. This procedure was complicated by renal failure and hypoxia and necessitated heart transplantation after 55 hours of TAH support. The patient expired 1 week later from sepsis.[3] In 1962, William DeVries implanted the Jarvik 7 TAH (designed by Robert Jarvik) into Dr Clark, a 61-year-old retired dentist with nonischemic cardiomyopathy.[4] While Dr Clark was supported for 112 days on this device, enthusiasm for further implantations of TAH was dampened because of the complex postoperative course, the adverse publicity generated by significant complications suffered by Dr Clark, and the advances in immunosuppression in the field of heart transplantation that resulted in superior results. After spluttering starts, and a few successes with the Jarvik 7 TAH,[5] a trial of the CardioWest TAH (developed from Jarvik 7) was initiated in 1993 and concluded in 2002. Eighty-one patients were implanted with the device with 79% survival to transplantation and 70% 1-year survival. Based on the encouraging results of the Cardio-West TAH (currently marketed as SynCardia TAH) as a bridge to transplantation, the device was approved by the United States Food and Drug Administration in 2004 and Centers for Medicare and Medicaid Services in 2008.

TECHNOLOGY

A VAD is a pump primarily designed to augment the function of the ventricle. However, with continued clinical use and more familiarity with these devices, its uses have also extended to serve as biventricular support devices, where both ventricles are supported with the devices or the ventricles are excised and completely replaced with 2 of these pumps as first described by O.H. Frazier in 2011.[6]

With advancements in the fields of technology, aerospace, and bioengineering, multiple research teams continued to work on the TAH. Fundamental engineering designs that have evolved are the pneumatic diaphragm pumps as in SynCardia and the centrifugal pump as in AbioCor. In the mid-1980s, the major issues related to the TAH were that artificial hearts were powered by washing-machine-sized pneumatic power sources derived from Alfa Laval milking machines and that 2 sizable catheters had to cross the body wall to carry the pneumatic pulses to the implanted heart, greatly increasing the risk of infection. These limitations were overcome by SynCardia, which designed a more compact compressor and power supply known as the Freedom portable driver. The AbioCor TAH does not require percutaneous cable for power supply; it has both internal and external components. The internal thoracic unit is powered via the transcutaneous energy transfer (TET) coil.

SYNCARDIA TOTAL ARTIFICIAL HEART

SynCardia TAH is an upgraded version of the TAH formerly known as Jarvik 7 (Symbion, Inc.; Salt Lake City), designed by Robert Jarvik. Collectively, research and implantation techniques were pioneered by Denton Cooley, Wihelm Kolff, Robert Jarvik, Clifford Kwan-Gett, William DeVries, Lyle Joyce, Jack Copeland, and Don Olsen. The device consists of 2 polyurethane ventricles each with a stroke volume of 70 mL and a total displacement volume of 400 cc in the chest cavity. It delivers a cardiac output of more than 7 to 9 L /min. The current version in clinical trial is smaller with a stroke volume of 50 mL.[7] Traditionally, an anterior-posterior chest diameter (from the anterior border of T10 vertebra to the posterior table of the sternum) of at least 10 cm by computed tomography and a minimum body surface area of 1.7 m^2 were considered as absolute contraindication for the 70 mL device. Each chamber contains 2 mechanical single leaflet tilting disc valves (Medtronic Hall valves), a 27-mm inflow valve, and a 25-mm outflow valve to regulate direction of blood flow (a total of 4 mechanical valves). The 2 ventricles are pneumatically actuated by drivelines attached percutaneously to an external pump.

IMPLICATIONS

1. Candidates for heart transplantation
   a. Severe biventricular failure
   b. Failing right ventricle while on a LVAD
   c. Infiltrative diseases such as amyloidosis
   d. End-stage hypertrophic cardiomyopathy
   e. Anatomic reasons such as congenital heart disease with single ventricles or a corrected transposition with failing ventricles
   f. Ventricular septal defects
   g. Ventricular rupture
   h. Cardiac tumors (rare)
2. Severe clot burden in the left ventricle
3. Malignant arrhythmias uncontrolled with surgical or medical options
4. Failed allograft posttransplant
5. Complex reoperative surgery
6. Humanitarian reasons for patient as bridge to recovery from an acute cardiac failure and multiorgan failure, who would otherwise be a transplant candidate.

SURGICAL TECHNIQUE

A standard median sternotomy is performed. Two small incisions are made in the left upper abdomen and intramuscular tunnels are created through the left rectus muscle for the TAH drivelines. Mediastinal dissection and mobilization of the great vessels are minimized to maintain dissection planes for subsequent transplantation. The arterial cannulation is done via the aorta and venous cannulation via the superior and inferior vena cava; the aorta is then cross-clamped. The pulmonary artery and aorta are divided and separated at the level of the valve commissures. The left and right ventricles are excised, leaving a 1-cm rim of ventricular muscle around the mitral and tricuspid annulus, but the mitral and tricuspid valve leaflets are excised (Figure 41-1A-C). The coronary sinus is oversewn and the atrial septum is inspected for patent foramen ovale, which is repaired if present. The TAH atrial quick connectors are sutured to the respective valve annuli with 2-0 Prolene sutures over Teflon strips (Figure 41-1D). The aortic and pulmonary artery graft quick connectors are trimmed and sutured to the respective vessels with running 3-0 Prolene sutures. It is important that these are carefully cut to size to avoid both stretching and kinking. The pulmonary artery graft is longer than the aortic graft in order to reach over the aortic graft and connect to the artificial right ventricle.[8] At time of implantation, extra efforts are made to maintain the avascular tissue planes; this dramatically simplifies re-entry for transplantation. The drivelines are passed through the intramuscular tunnels in the left rectus sheet with the Penrose drains. The TAH ventricles are attached to their respective atrial and arterial graft quick connects (Figure 41-2). Routine de-airing maneuvers are done and the left ventricle is started and the aortic cross clamp

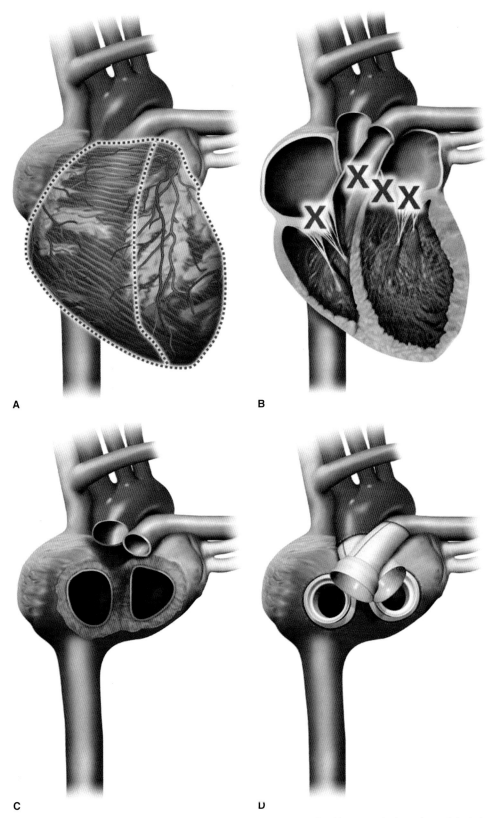

FIGURE 41-1 A. The portions of the heart resected for the implantation of the total artificial heart. Both the right and the left ventricles are replaced. **B.** The portions of the heart resected internal view. **C.** View of native myocardial tissue after the left and right ventricles are excised leaving a 1 cm rim of ventricular muscle around the mitral and tricuspid annulus. **D.** The atrial quick connectors in place with the outflow pulmonary and aortic grafts in place. (Images A through D courtesy of www.syncardia.com.)

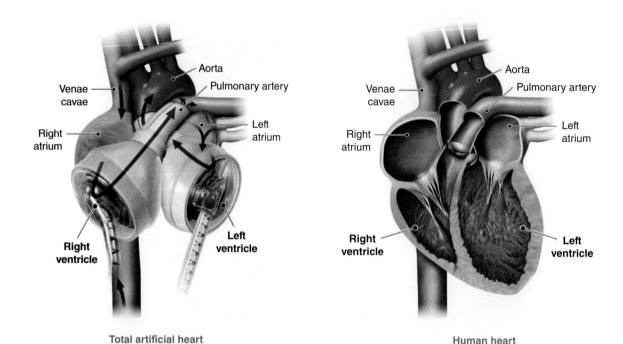

Total artificial heart · Human heart

FIGURE 41-2 A functional and anatomic orientation of the TAH. (Image courtesy of www.syncardia.com.)

is removed. De-airing is confirmed by transesophageal echocardiography. The patient is often readily weaned off cardiopulmonary bypass as TAH support is increased. Usual post bypass TAH parameters are left drive pressure 180 to 200 mm Hg, right drive pressure 30 to 60 mm Hg, HR 100 to 120 bpm, and 50% systole. Vacuum is usually not initiated until the chest is closed.[9] At re-entry for transplantation, during the initial implants, intense inflammatory reaction was observed in the pericardium and the surrounding structures and added to the complexity of the dissection process. To minimize this difficulty, the pericardium is reconstructed at the end of the procedure utilizing Gore-Tex surgical membrane (W.L. Gore & Associates; Flagstaff, AZ). In addition it was also noted that the mediastinum had collapsed around the TAH without leaving enough mediastinal space for the transplanted heart. To overcome this difficulty, a saline implant (Mentor smooth round, Mentor Worldwide LLC; Santa Barbara, CA) is placed at the former cardiac apex and inflated to 150 to 250 mL to maintain the space. This is removed at the time of heart transplantation along with the device and this extra space allows adequate room for the transplanted heart to function effectively.

POSTOPERATIVE CARE

The postoperative care revolves around effective anticoagulation and a multitargeted antithrombotic approach including the anticoagulants, antiplatelet, and rheological agents used.[10]

1. Heparin is routinely used in the acute phase in the absence of any contraindication.

2. Direct thrombin inhibitors (eg, argatroban and bivalirudin) are used when heparin is a contraindication.

3. Antiplatelet drugs such as aspirin, clopidogrel, and/or dipyridamole are used. Platelet function tests (eg, light transmittance aggregometry) and the thromboelastogram are used to monitor adequate platelet suppression.

4. Pentoxifylline is a rheological agent that decreases blood viscosity, platelet adhesion, and increases red blood cell deformity and appears to improve the underlying hemolysis.[11]

Long-term anticoagulation is necessary to avoid thromboembolic complications (14% of patients). Anticoagulation is initiated once adequate hemostasis has been achieved with heparin, in the absence of any contraindication for the use of heparin with a goal activated partial thromboplastin time (aPTT) of 50 to 60. Once the patient is stable and tolerating oral intake well, the patient is bridged to warfarin anticoagulation with a target international normalized ratio (INR) of 2 to 3. The mechanical nature of the device and the presence of 4 mechanical valves pose a significant risk for hemolysis due to the development of clots within the device. Careful monitoring of hemolysis should be considered by measurement of plasma lactate dehydrogenase (LDH), haptoglobin, and free hemoglobin.[12]

TOTAL ARTIFICIAL HEART CLINICAL OUTCOMES

The original safety and efficacy 2004 trial of the SynCardia TAH as a bridge to transplantation demonstrated a 70% overall 1-year survival rate versus 31% and 79% survival to transplantation as compared with 46% in the control group, respectively.[5] Although there has not been a randomized control trial with patients receiving biventricular assist devices (BiVADs) versus the TAH, more studies tend to favor the TAH group, especially after the availability of the Freedom portable driver in the clinical trials.

With more than 1400 TAHs implanted worldwide, rates for the common complications have been established. The major complications of TAH implantation based on a cumulative gathering of data from various studies include stroke, infection, bleeding, thrombosis, renal failure, and chronic anemia.

Kirsch et al conducted a retrospective analysis of 90 implants of the SynCardia t-TAH between 2000 and 2010. The survival rate on the TAH was 74%±5%, 63%±6%, and 47%±8% at 30, 60, and 180 days after implant, respectively. Complications included a stroke rate of 10%, mediastinitis of 13%, and 39% required surgical re-exploration for bleeding, hematoma, or infection, thus, supporting an acceptable survival rate with a remarkably low incidence of neurological events.[13]

In another study, Copeland et al demonstrated similar results in a 101 implant analysis from January 1993 to December 2009. Ninety-one percent of cases were Interagency Registry for Mechanically Assisted Circulatory Support (INTERMACS) Profile 1 (indicating the sickest of the sick HF patients) and the remaining 9% were failing medical therapy on multiple inotropic medications (INTERMACS Profile 2). By current standards, these patients are considered very high-risk patients for durable long-term mechanical support. Survival to transplantation was 68.3%. Causes of death included multiple organ failure, pulmonary failure, and neurological injury. Adverse events included stroke in 7.9% and reoperation for hemorrhage was 24.7%. Survival after transplantation at 1, 5, and 10 years was 76.8%, 60.5%, and 41.2%, respectively.[14] SynCardia TAH offered a real alternative for survival in these candidates who otherwise might have significant mortality and morbidity associated with their advanced HF status. In the recent Sixth INTERMACS annual report, 66 patients were implanted in 2014. The 1-year survival rate for TAH was 59%, which is comparable to continuous BiVADs (57%) and superior to results with pulsatile-flow biventricular devices (45%).[15]

More importantly, a destination-therapy application has been approved by the FDA and a smaller 50 mL pump is currently in use in smaller adults and children above a weight of 40 kg. In addition, a second-generation <13 lb portable driver and an improved 55 lb in-hospital console (replacing the washing-machine-sized "Big Blue") will be factors in wider acceptance of the TAH.[16]

The SynCardia Freedom driver (Figure 41-3) is a portable driver specially designed to enable discharge to the home of patients implanted with the TAH. It is a 13-lb piston-driven pneumatic compressor that delivers regulated pressures and vacuum to the TAH drivelines. Electric motors drive the piston and provide backup redundancy. Lithium batteries are charged in the driver when the patient plugs into normal power outlets or into a car auxiliary power plug, with a 3-hour battery life.[17]

TOTAL ARTIFICIAL HEART UNIQUE COMPLICATIONS

Renal Failure

Nearly half (42%) of all the patients implanted with TAH often have concomitant renal failure. The multifactorial etiology may include acute tubular necrosis due to low cardiac output or shock, a cardiorenal syndrome due to a failing right ventricle. The prevalence of patients on dialysis following the implantation of TAH is about 19% to 38%; it also correlates with the degree of renal insufficiency at the time of the implant. The mechanism suggestion is that, in end-stage HF, there is upregulation B type natriuretic peptide (BNP) and intracellular cyclic guanosine monophosphate (cGMP) synthesis due to the chronic stretching of the myocytes, thus inducing vasodilation, diuresis, and inhibition of the renin-aldosterone system. The resection of the native ventricles for the implantation often results in a rapid decrease of endogenous BNP production and interruption of these signaling pathways leading to a decline in renal function.[18]

Keyur et al were able to demonstrate that the estimated glomerular filtration rate (eGFR) was unchanged during infusion of nesiritide in the study group ($p = 0.4$). Despite the control group having a higher baseline eGFR prior to surgery (64 ± 11 mL/min/1.73 m^2 vs 90 ± 23 mL/min/1.73 m^2, $p = 0.05$), the eGFR at 48 hours after surgery was similar in both groups (56 ± 14 mL/min/1.73 m^2 vs 56 ± 24 mL/min/1.73 m^2, $p = 0.96$).[19]

Spiliopoulos et al studied the impact of early initiation of low-dose BNP infusion therapy on renal function and the need for renal replacement therapy and were able to demonstrate the safety and efficacy in 10 consecutive TAH implants.[20]

Chronic Anemia

Severe anemia is not uncommon after TAH implantation; although multifactorial in etiology it has been largely contributed to by hemolysis. The mechanism of the hemolysis is attributed to the sheer force exerted by the 4 mechanical valves and the diaphragms of the pneumatic pumps on the red blood cells. It also has been noted that patients with TAH implants have a more severe degree of anemia than patients with VADs. The hematocrit values between TAH versus LVADs are at 2 weeks (20 ± 2% vs 24 ± 3%), 4 weeks (22 ± 3% vs 26 ± 3%), 6 weeks (22 ± 4% vs

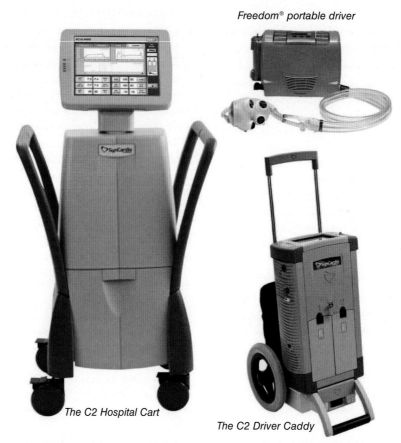

Freedom® portable driver

The C2 Hospital Cart

The C2 Driver Caddy

FIGURE 41-3 The Freedom portable driver, the C2 Driver caddy, and the Standard C2 hospital console and cart (*clockwise*). (Image courtesy www.syncardia.com.)

30 ± 4%), and 8 weeks (23 ± 4% vs 33 ± 5%; $P < 0.001$ for all). The constant hemolysis was monitored with serial LDH levels and haptoglobin, as well as clinical signs of excessive hemolysis. It was also noted that this anemia was reversible with transplantation, where the difference between the hemoglobin of the TAH patient and LVADs disappeared and returned to baseline in both groups. The hematocrit values in TAH explants versus LVADs explants were at 1 month (30 ± 4% vs 29 ± 7%; $P = 0.42$) and 3 months (35 ± 7% vs 35 ± 4%; $P = 0.98$).[21]

TOTAL ARTIFICIAL HEART: OTHER DEVICES

ABIOCOR TAH

The AbioCor (Figure 41-4A) was first implanted in humans in 2001; it consisted of both internal and external components. Its unique design featured a TET coil, making it the first device that did not require a percutaneous driveline (Figure 41-4B). The internal components included the battery, the TET coil, and the thoracic unit, which housed 2 pumps. Each blood pump was completely made of propriety polyurethane, which comprised of a flexible blood sac and 2 tricuspid valves. A hydraulic fluid filled the space between the 2 blood chambers and moved from 1 side to another, thus creating a systole and a diastole. The device had multiple issues such as the heavy weight (2 kg), the biocompatibility of the materials, and the inefficient energy transfer of the TET coils.[22,23]

THE CARMAT TAH

The CARMAT TAH (Figure 41-5A) is a bioprosthetic artificial heart that has undergone strenuous bench and animal testing; it was first implanted in humans in 2013. The device itself combines bovine pericardial tissue that lines the chambers, bioprosthetic valvses, titanium, and technology the missile-defense industry (Figure 41-5B), the European Aeronautic Defense and Space Company (EADS), and the medical expertise of professors. A unique feature of the design is the sensor technology used in guided missiles, which senses the body's activity level and adjusts accordingly. It is primarily an electrohydraulic pump that creates a systolic and diastolic phase by shifting a silicon fluid between the 2 blood chambers. The stroke volume and the beat rate of the TAH is modulated and adjusted by feedback from pressure sensors in the device that monitor the preload. A percutaneous driveline powers the devices and allows exchange of data. The company is continuing the feasibility study as of date.[24]

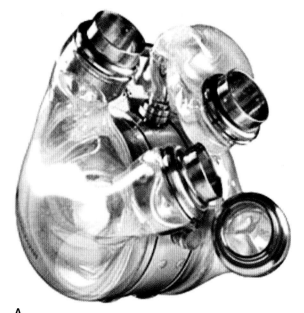

A

NEW FRONTIERS AND EVOLVING TECHNOLOGIES

The future of mechanical devices is exciting, promising pioneering days. With advancements in material sciences and technology, current research is focused on overcoming the problems we face today, such as better biomechanical interface and biocompatibility design optimization. Some of the current research advances mentioned here are prototypes and some are technology being developed for VADs.

BiVACOR (Figure 41-6) is a device being developed at Texas Heart Institute by Drs O.H. Frazier and William Cohn. The design consists of a central impeller (rotary pump) suspended by magnetic levitation technology. It can pump about 8 L/min from both right and left sides.[25,26]

The Cleveland Clinic's prototype consists of a single motor with a single rotating impeller supported by a hydrodynamic bearing. The right-sided output is based on passive axial shift of the impeller based on the left-sided output demand.[26]

ReinHeart TAH is currently being developed in Aachen, Germany. The design consists of a linear motor that alternatively compresses and releases the flexible 2 chambers with pusher plates, an implantable control unit, and a compliance chamber. The TAH is powered by a transcutaneous energy transmission system. Unlike the CARMAT and the AbioCor, it has no pumps and fewer moving parts.[27]

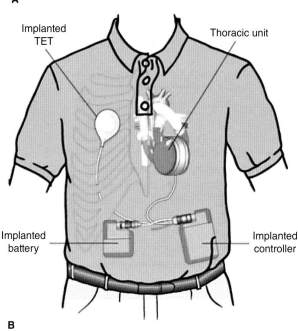

B

FIGURE 41-4 A. The AbioCor. **B.** The innovative transcutaneous energy transmission (TET) system used in AbioCor total artificial heart. (Images A and B used with permission from Abiomed.)

DEVELOPMENT OF POWER MODULES AND DELIVERY SYSTEMS

With the pioneering design of the AbioCor, TET systems[28] are currently being developed for LVAD. One example is HeartWare, a fully implantable system currently being developed in collaboration with Dualis Medtech GmbH, a company spun out of the German aerospace research organization, the DLR. Another form of emerging technology for energy transfer is the coplanar energy transfer system, which consists of internal and external components, currently being developed by Leviticus Cardio. The internal components are the receiver coil, a battery with a life up to 6 hours,

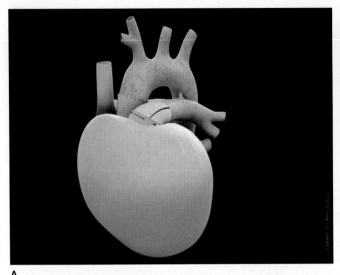

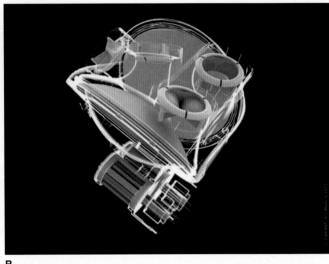

A   B

FIGURE 41-5 **A.** The CARMAT heart currently in clinical trials. **B.** A cross-sectional image showing the orientation and the placement of the bio-prosthetic valves and the bioprosthetic lining of the blood chambers. (Images A and B courtesy of http://www.carmatsa.com.)

and the LVAD. The external transmitter coil inductively transfers energy to the receiver coil, thereby eliminating the need for a percutaneous driveline.

The Free-range Resonant Electrical Energy Delivery (FREE-D) wireless power system developed by the Yale group uses magnetically coupled resonators to efficiently transfer power. The setup consists of a radiofrequency amplifier and control board, which drives the transmit resonator coil, and a receiver unit consisting of a resonant coil attached to a radiofrequency rectifier and power management module. With additional relay coils seamless wireless energy delivery was demonstrated with an efficiency of more than 80%.[29]

With advances of technologies from other industries such as alternative energy, aerospace, biomechanical, information technology, and so on, there is a promising role for translational research and its uses in the field of mechanical circulatory support, especially in pursuit of the "holy grail"—the artificial human heart.

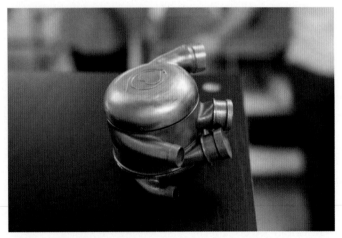

FIGURE 41-6 BiVACOR. (Image reprinted with permission from the Texas Heart Institute).

REFERENCES

1. Cooley DA. Some thoughts about the historic events that led to the first clinical implantation of a total artificial heart. *Tex Heart Inst J*. 2013;40:117-119.

2. Cooley DA. Recollections of the early years of heart transplantation and the total artificial heart. *Artif Organs*. 2011;35:353-357.

3. Cooley DA, Liotta D, Hallman GL, Bloodwell RD, Leachman RD, Milam JD. Orthotopic cardiac prosthesis for two-staged cardiac replacement. *Am J Cardiol*. 1969;24:723-730.

4. DeVries WC, Anderson JL, Joyce LD, et al. Clinical use of the total artificial heart. *N Engl J Med*. 1984;310:273-278.

5. Copeland JG, Smith RG, Arabia FA, et al. Cardiac replacement with a total artificial heart as a bridge to transplantation. *N Engl J Med*. 2004;351:859-867.

6. Frazier OH, Cohn WE. Continuous-flow total heart replacement device implanted in a 55-year-old man with end-stage heart failure and severe amyloidosis. *Tex Heart Inst J*. 2012;39:542-546.

7. Khalpey Z, Kazui T, Ferng AS, et al. First North American 50cc total artificial heart experience: conversion from a 70cc total artificial heart. *ASAIO J*. 2016;62(5):e43-e45.

8. Tang DG, Shah KB, Hess ML, Kasirajan V. Implantation of the syncardia total artificial heart. *J Vis Exp*. 2014;(89):50377.

9. Tarzia V, Buratto E, Gallo M, et al. Surgical implantation of the CardioWest total artificial heart. *Ann Cardiothorac Surg*. 2014;3:624-625.

10. Rigatelli G, Santini F, Faggian G. Past and present of cardiocirculatory assist devices: a comprehensive critical review. *J Geriatr Cardiol*. 2012;9:389-400.

11. Ensor CR, Cahoon WD, Crouch MA, et al. V. Antithrombotic therapy for the CardioWest temporary total artificial heart. *Tex Heart Inst J*. 2010;37:149-158.

12. Slaughter MS, Pagani FD, Rogers JG, et al. Clinical management of continuous-flow left ventricular assist devices in advanced heart failure. *J Heart Lung Transplant*. 2010;29:S1-S39.

13. Kirsch ME, Nguyen A, Mastroianni C, et al. SynCardia temporary total artificial heart as bridge to transplantation: current results at la pitie hospital. *Ann Thorac Surg*. 2013;95:1640-1646.

14. Copeland JG, Copeland H, Gustafson M, et al. Experience with more than 100 total artificial heart implants. *J Thorac Cardiovasc Surg*. 2012;143:727-734.

15. Kirklin JK, Naftel DC, Kormos RL, et al. The Fourth INTERMACS Annual Report: 4,000 implants and counting. *J Heart Lung Transplant*. 2012;31:117-126.

16. Copeland JG. SynCardia total artificial heart: update and future. *Tex Heart Inst J*. 2013;40:587-588.

17. Jaroszewski DE, Anderson EM, Pierce CN, Arabia FA. The SynCardia freedom driver: a portable driver for discharge home with the total artificial heart. *J Heart Lung Transplant*. 2011;30:844-845.

18. Hall C. Essential biochemistry and physiology of (NT-pro) BNP. *Eur J Heart Fail*. 2004;6:257-260.

19. Shah KB, Tang DG, Kasirajan V, Gunnerson KJ, Hess ML, Sica DA. Impact of low-dose B-type natriuretic peptide infusion on urine output after total artificial heart implantation. *J Heart Lung Transplant*. 2012;31:670-672.

20. Spiliopoulos S, Guersoy D, Koerfer R, Tenderich G. B-type natriuretic peptide therapy in total artificial heart implantation: renal effects with early initiation. *J Heart Lung Transplant*. 2014;33:662-663.

21. Mankad AK, Tang DG, Clark WB, et al. Persistent anemia after implantation of the total artificial heart. *J Card Fail*. 2012;18:433-438.

22. Dowling RD, Gray LA, Jr, Etoch SW, et al. Initial experience with the AbioCor implantable replacement heart system. *J Thorac Cardiovasc Surg*. 2004;127:131-141.

23. Samuels L. The AbioCor totally implantable replacement heart. *Am Heart Hosp J*. 2003;1:91-96.

24. Mohacsi P, Leprince P. The CARMAT total artificial heart. *Eur J Cardiothorac Surg*. 2014;46:933-934.

25. Timms D, Fraser J, Hayne M, Dunning J, McNeil K, Pearcy M. The BiVACOR rotary biventricular assist device: concept and in vitro investigation. *Artif Organs*. 2008;32:816-819.

26. Greatrex NA, Timms DL, Kurita N, Palmer EW, Masuzawa T. Axial magnetic bearing development for the BiVACOR rotary BiVAD/TAH. *IEEE Trans Biomed Eng*. 2010;57:714-721.

27. Pelletier B, Spiliopoulos S, Finocchiaro T, et al. System overview of the fully implantable destination therapy—ReinHeart-total artificial heart. *Eur J Cardiothorac Surg*. 2015;47:80-86.

28. Yanzhen W, Hu AP, Budgett D, Malpas SC, Dissanayake T. Efficient power-transfer capability analysis of the TET system using the equivalent small parameter method. *IEEE Trans Biomed Circuits Syst*. 2011;5:272-282.

29. Waters BH, Smith JR, Bonde P. Innovative Free-range Resonant Electrical Energy Delivery system (FREE-D System) for a ventricular assist device using wireless power. *ASAIO J*. 2014;60:31-37.

42 HEART-LUNG TRANSPLANTATION

Mahim Malik, MD
Ahmet Kilic, MD, FACS
Bryan A. Whitson, MD, PhD, FACS

PATIENT CASE

A 37-year-old woman is admitted to a hospital with progressive dyspnea on minimal effort, with significant worsening in the past 6 months. She states that she was diagnosed with heart murmur when she was 5 years old, but has had no treatment for it. She describes breathlessness, fatigue, and occasional presyncopal episodes. On examination she has dyspnea on exertion, 3+ bilateral lower extremity edema, ascites, and orthopnea. She has clubbing, tachypnea, mild right upper quadrant tenderness, and some bruising on her extremities. Chest x-ray demonstrates an enlarged pulmonary artery silhouette. Transthoracic echocardiogram demonstrates a large ventricular septal defect with right to left shunt, right ventricular (RV) enlargement, and an elevated estimated RV systolic pressure.

Cardiac catheterization was performed, which showed suprasystemic RV as well as pulmonary artery pressures. Pulmonary vascular resistance was measured at 8 Woods units. There was minimal change in hemodynamics with inhaled oxygen or vasodilator challenge.

INTRODUCTION

The first heart-lung transplantation (HLT) was performed in 1981 at Stanford University, for a 45-year-old woman with pulmonary hypertension.[1] According to the International Society for Heart and Lung Transplantation Registry, 3820 heart-lung transplants have been reported through June 2014 (Figure 42-1). After a spike in the late 1980s, the number of transplants performed in the last decade has plateaued to 64 to 65 transplants per year. Heart-lung transplantation remains the only viable option for patients with concomitant end-stage heart and respiratory failure.

Management of these patients is complex, and usually involves a multidisciplinary team consisting of, but not limited to, pulmonologists, cardiologists, transplant surgeons, and pharmacists. In this chapter, we will attempt to concisely elucidate the indications, management, and prognosis of this special group of patients.

PATIENT SELECTION

INDICATIONS

Combined heart-lung transplantation should be considered for patients with end-stage heart failure (HF), along with end-stage lung disease. On the basis of pathophysiology, these can be divided into 2 major subgroups, with either HF or pulmonary failure as the primary disease process. Table 42-1 summarizes the primary indications for HLT.[5]

CARDIOVASCULAR

One of the most feared complications of complex congenital heart disease is Eisenmenger syndrome, described by the triad of system-to-pulmonary communication, pulmonary artery hypertension (HTN), and cyanosis. This subset of patients may have undergone repair of a congenital heart defect in the past, so it remains crucial to obtain history of any surgeries in the past. Initial management is aimed at decreasing pulmonary vascular resistance, with special attention to avoiding systemic volume depletion, and sudden decreases in systemic vascular resistance. Transplantation is indicated in only severely symptomatic patients, because overall survival with medical management has shown good results.[3]

Previously, idiopathic pulmonary hypertension (IPAH) used to be the most common indication for HLT.[6] However, this trend has changed since it has been shown that the RV failure can be reversed after double lung transplant.[7-9] The optimal procedure for patients with IPAH is still controversial because recent single-center data have not shown any significant difference in survival.[10-12]

In patients with acquired heart disease, such as valvular pathology or cardiomyopathy, HLT is rarely performed. According to the ISHLT registry, only 5.5% of HLT reported between 1982-2014 had acquired heart disease as the primary indication. In these cases, the indication is fixed pulmonary vascular resistance (described as pulmonary vascular resistance greater than 5 Woods units [320 dynes-s/cm^5], or transpulmonary gradient >15 to 20 mm Hg). If pulmonary artery pressures can be reduced to acceptable levels with vasodilator challenge while maintaining a systolic systemic blood pressure over 88 mm Hg, an isolated heart transplant may be performed.[4]

PULMONARY

Longstanding lung parenchymal disease can lead to severe RV dysfunction, as well as left ventricular (LV) failure. Conditions such as cystic fibrosis (CF), idiopathic pulmonary fibrosis, as well as chronic obstructive pulmonary disease may be the underlying pathology. As mentioned earlier, in cases where RV failure is reversible, a single or double lung transplant may be performed. The increasing trend toward this practice is also evidenced by the decreasing numbers of HLT performed for CF.

CONTRAINDICATIONS

Absolute and relative contraindications for HLT are similar to those for isolated heart or lung transplantation (Table 42-2).

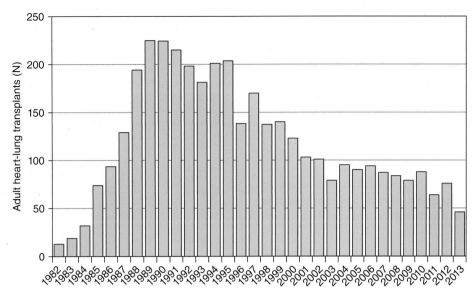

FIGURE 42-1 Number of adult heart-lung transplants by year (1982-2013). This figure includes only the adult heart-lung transplants that were reported to the International Society for Heart and Lung Transplantation Registry and does not represent the number of adult heart-lung transplants performed worldwide. (Reproduced with permission from Yusen RD, Edwards LB, Kucheryavaya AY, et al. The Registry of the International Society for Heart and Lung Transplantation: Thirty-second Official Adult Lung and Heart-Lung Transplantation Report—2015; Focus Theme: Early Graft Failure. *J Heart Lung Transplant.* 2015;34(10):1264-1277. DOI: 10.1016/j.healun.2015.08.014.)

OPERATIVE TECHNIQUE

DONOR HEART-LUNG PROCUREMENT AND PRESERVATION

The donor operation is performed via median sternotomy. The pericardium and pleural spaces are widely opened. Organs are inspected carefully but expeditiously to confirm adequacy for transplantation. The inferior pulmonary ligaments are divided. The aorta, superior vena cava, as well as inferior vena cava are mobilized. Intravenous heparin (300 U/kg) is then administered, and the aorta and pulmonary artery are cannulated. Prostaglandin E is administered prior to cross-clamp. The heart is allowed to empty and the aortic cross-clamp is applied. Cold cardioplegia and pulmoplegia solution is then administered via the aortic root cannula and the pulmonary artery, respectively. The superior vena cava (SCV), inferior vena cava (IVC) and the left atrial appendage are divided to avoid cardiac distension. The lungs are inflated to one-half to two-thirds tidal volumes prior to division on the trachea. The dissection is completed and the heart-lung block is removed. For transfer, the organs need to be immersed in ice-cold saline at 4°C.

RECIPIENT

Standard median sternotomy is performed. The patient is placed on cardiopulmonary bypass support via central aortic and bicaval cannulation. The recipient heart is excised first, followed by each of the lungs, performed in a sequential manner. The right and the

Table 42-1 Primary Indications

Cardiovascular Causes	Pulmonary Causes	Other
Congenital heart disease	Cystic fibrosis	Sarcoidosis
Idiopathic pulmonary hypertension	Chronic obstructive pulmonary disease	Obliterative bronchiolitis
Acquired heart disease	Interstitial lung disease	Retransplant

Table 42-2 Contraindications

Absolute Contraindications	Relative Contraindications
Malignancy (active, which can be worsened by immunosuppression)	Age >65 y
	Diabetes
Active infection	HIV
Active alcohol or drug use	Active hepatitis B or C
Current cigarette smoking	

left bronchi are stapled and divided. The donor heart and lung are prepared at the back table and then brought into the operative field. Our preference is to perform the anastomoses in the following order:

1. Trachea
2. IVC
3. SVC
4. Aorta
5. Pulmonary artery

The patient is weaned off cardiopulmonary bypass and hemostasis is secured. At this point, 500 mg of methylprednisone is administered to the patient. The sternotomy is closed in the usual manner.

POSTOPERATIVE MANAGEMENT

The immediate postoperative course is similar to that of other cardiac surgery patients. The most important complication in these patients is early graft dysfunction, which may be present in 10% to 15% patients.[13] This is most commonly manifested by hypercapnia and hypercarbia, and is presumed secondary to ischemic-reperfusion injury in the transplanted lung. Early treatment with initiation of pulmonary vasodilators such as inhaled nitric oxide is essential.

IMMUNOSUPPRESSION

Posttransplant immunosuppression regimens are similar to those employed for lung transplant patients. Standard protocols are as follows:[14]

Induction:

1. 500 mg methylprednisone after administration of protamine in the OR, followed by 125 mg IV every 8 hours, for 3 doses
2. Rabbit antithymocyte globulin 1.5 mg/kg IV on POD 1, up to 6 days
3. Basiliximab/daclizumab, started on POD 1 and then POD 4

Maintenance immunosuppressive therapy includes steroids, mycophenolate mofetil, and tacrolimus.

OUTCOMES

Overall, in the United States, HLT is performed at a proportion of 0.2% of all transplants (Table 42-3). Over time, since data collection in UNOS from 1988, the rate of HLT has decreased (Figure 42-2). This has paralleled the increasing success and frequency of treatment of isolated lung transplant for pulmonary disease and the improvement in treatment for primary pulmonary HTN. The typical blood types are O and A, as reflective by the U.S. population distribution (Figure 42-3). The age of patients undergoing HLT has evolved (Figure 42-4). Overall, since 1988, 1.3% of transplants have been in infants (<1 year old), 4.4% 1 to 5 years, 2.5% 6 to 10 years, 8.5% 11 to 17 years, 31.6% 18 to 34 years, 35.7% 35 to 49 years, 15.5% 50 to

Table 42-3 Transplants and Proportions of Organs Performed in the United States (Data from UNOS)

Organ	Transplants	Percent
Kidney	400,348	59.0%
Liver	145,794	21.5%
Pancreas	8291	1.2%
Kidney/pancreas	21,922	3.2%
Heart	64,890	9.6%
Lung	32,796	4.8%
Heart/lung	1192	0.2%
Intestine	2770	0.4%
Total	678,003	100.0%

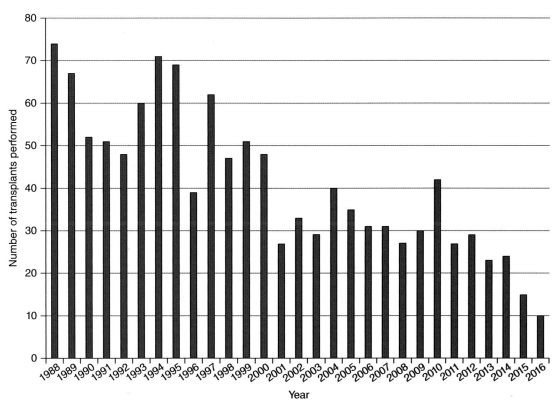

FIGURE 42-2 Number of overall heart-lung transplants by year (1988-2016). (Data from United Network for Organ Sharing Data. Accessed 5 November 2016. http://optn.transplant.hrsa.gov)

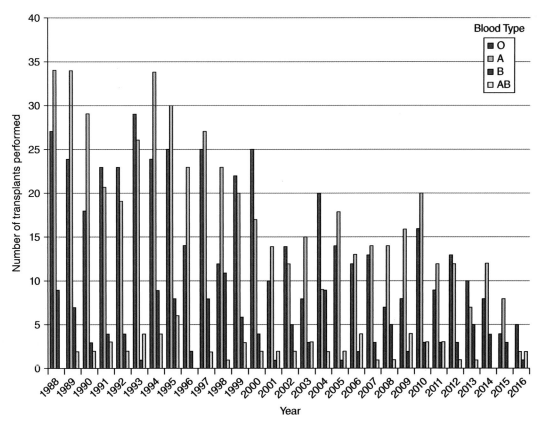

FIGURE 42-3 Number of overall heart-lung transplants by blood type of recipient by year (1988-2016). (Data from United Network for Organ Sharing Data. Accessed 5 November 2016. http://optn.transplant.hrsa.gov.)

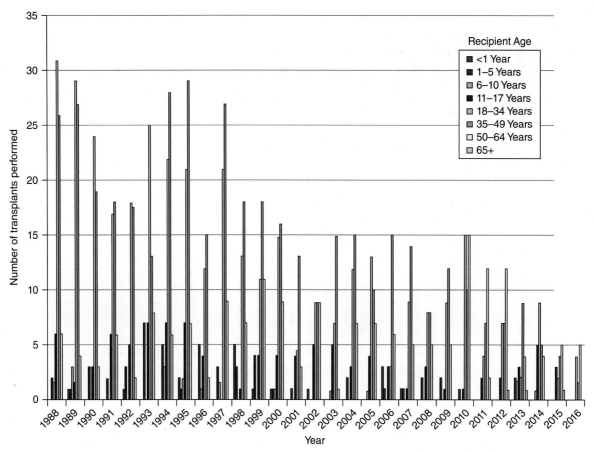

FIGURE 42-4 Number of overall heart-lung transplants by age of recipient by year (1988-2016). (Data from United Network for Organ Sharing Data. Accessed 5 November 2016. http://optn.transplant.hrsa.gov.)

64 years, and 0.4% >65 years (data, UNOS). The overall survival rate is 66% in the first year (Table 42-4).

COMPLICATIONS

As with any operation of this scope and magnitude, the potential for complications is inherent. There are associated risks with the surgical procedure and there are risks that are inherent with the transplant process (Table 42-5). The transplant risks never go away and they span the spectrum from rejection (acute to chronic), infection (bacterial, fungal, viral), and complications from the immunosuppression (eg, renal insufficiency, diabetes, hypertension, osteoporosis, wound healing).

Acute and Chronic Rejection

The majority of episodes of acute rejection occur in the first year after transplantation. Simultaneous rejection of both the heart and the lung is rare. Acute cellular rejection is usually manifested as dyspnea, chills, low-grade fevers, and an infiltrate on the chest radiograph.[15]

PROGNOSIS

According to the 2015 ISHLT registry, the overall survival rates at 3 months and 1 year were 72% and 63%, respectively. Overall, survival was 45% at 5 years and 32% at 10 years.[2] The main cause of death was varied with time after transplantation, with graft failure

Table 42-4 Survival Post-Heart/Lung Transplant (Data from UNOS)

Time	Survival Rate	95% Confidence Interval
1 year	66%	56.1%-75.9%
3 year	48%	40%-56%
5 year	38.2%	31.5%-44.9%

as the leading cause of death in the first 30 days. After the first year, bronchiolitis obliterans syndrome accounted for 21.3% to 24.4% of deaths and late graft failure for 13.3% to 17.6% of deaths.

CONCLUSION

In general, heart-lung block transplantation volume has decreased as lung transplantation quality and volume has increased. There remains a role for HLT in specialized centers for predominantly congenital heart diagnoses or pulmonary vascular diseases. There may be a role for domino transplantation on a case-by-case basis. Outcomes of these high-risk procedures are reasonable and attributed to the magnitude of the operation and the underlying disease complexity and end-organ manifestations.

Table 42-5 Complications

Rejection
Acute (<1 year)
-Cellular-mediated
-Humoral-mediated
Chronic
-Obliterative bronchitis
-Graft coronary artery disease
Infections
-Bacterial: Mediastinitis, pneumonia, line sepsis, skin infections
Gram-negative bacilli (most common)
-Viral
CMV most common
-Fungal (highest mortality)
Other
-Abdominal complications
Gastroparesis
-Airway complications

REFERENCES

1. Reitz BA, Wallwork JL, Hunt SA, et al. Heart-lung transplantation: successful therapy for patients with pulmonary vascular disease. *N Engl J Med.* 1982;306(10):557.

2. Yusen RD, Edwards LP, Kucheryavaya AY, et al. The Registry of the International Society for Heart and Lung Transplantation: Thirty-second Official Adult Lung and Heart-Lung Transplantation Report—2015; Focus Theme: Early Graft Failure. *J Heart Lung Transplant.* 2015;34(10):1264-1277.

3. Hopkins WE, Ochoa LL, Richardson GW, Trulock EP. Comparison of the hemodynamics and survival of adults with severe primary pulmonary hypertension or Eisenmenger syndrome. *J Heart Lung Transplant.* 1996;15(1 Pt 1):100.

4. Mehra MR, Kobashigawa J, Starling R, et al. Listing criteria for heart transplantation: International Society for Heart and Lung Transplantation guidelines for the care of cardiac transplant candidates—2006. *J Heart Lung Transplant.* 2006;25(9):1024-1042.

5. Hill C, Maxwell B, Boulate D, et al. Heart-lung vs. double-lung transplantation for idiopathic pulmonary arterial hypertension. *Clin Transplant.* 2015;29(12):1067-1075.

6. Yusen RD, Christie JD, Edwards LB, et al. The Registry of the International Society for Heart and Lung Transplantation: Thirtieth Adult Lung and Heart-Lung Transplant Report–2013; focus theme: age. *J Heart Lung Transplant.* 2013;32:965-978.

7. Frist WH, Lorenz CH, Walker ES, et al. MRI complements standard assessment of right ventricular function after lung transplantation. *Ann Thorac Surg.* 1995;60:268.

8. Moulton MJ, Creswell LL, Ungacta FF, Downing SW, Szabó BA, Pasque MK. Magnetic resonance imaging provides evidence for remodeling of the right ventricle after single-lung transplantation for pulmonary hypertension. *Circulation.* 1996;94: II312.

9. Globits S, Burghuber OC, Koller J, et al. Effect of lung transplantation on right and left ventricular volumes and function measured by magnetic resonance imaging. *Am J Respir Crit Care Med.* 1994;149:1000.

10. Toyoda Y, Thacker J, Santos R, et al. Long-term outcome of lung and heart-lung transplantation for idiopathic pulmonary arterial hypertension. *Ann Thorac Surg.* 2008;86:1116.

11. Fadel E, Mercier O, Mussot S, et al. Long-term outcome of double-lung and heart-lung transplantation for pulmonary hypertension: a comparative retrospective study of 219 patients. *Eur J Cardiothorac Surg.* 2010;38:277.

12. de Perrot M, Granton JT, McRae K, et al. Outcome of patients with pulmonary arterial hypertension referred for lung transplantation: a 14-year single-center experience. *J Thorac Cardiovasc Surg.* 2012;143:910.

13. Date H, Triantafillou AN, Trulock EP, et al. Inhaled nitric oxide reduces human lung allograft dysfunction. *J Thorac Cardiovasc Surg.* 1996;111:913-919.

14. Deuse T, Sista R, Weill D, et al. Review of heart-lung transplantation at Stanford. *Ann Thorac Surg.* 2010;90:329-337.

15. Hoeper MM, Hamm M, Schafers HJ, et al; Hannover Lung Transplant Group. Evaluation of lung function during pulmonary rejection and infection in heart-lung transplant patients. *Chest.* 1992;102:864-870.

43 PERIOPERATIVE HEART FAILURE

Claire Mayeur, MD
Alexandre Mebazaa, MD, PhD

PATIENT CASE

A 78-year-old man, who is treated by calcium channel blockers for arterial hypertension (HTN), has just met an anesthesiologist before hip replacement. He has no diabetes, has never smoked, and used to be a runner. Because of hip arthritis, the patient's activities are limited (barely walks, lives in a 1-floor house, does not do gardening anymore) and his wife is taking care of all the housekeeping. The patient reports a nocturnal dyspnea. The clinical examination revealed a blood pressure of 148/69 mm Hg, a heart rate of 72 beats/min, and no sign of cardiac failure. The blood chemistry reveals a normal renal function, hemoglobin levels are 14 g/dL, and brain natriuretic peptide (BNP) levels are 350 pg/mL. The anesthesiologist has advised the patient to consult a cardiologist.

This case demonstrates a situation where the anesthesiologist and cardiologist should work together, prior to surgery, to assess the status of a patient and discuss perioperative management. In fact, this patient is about to undergo a surgery that is associated with high risk of complications by major cardiac events, such as acute heart failure (HF). Although he has few cardiac risk factors, his functional activity is not assessable and nocturnal dyspnea associated with increased plasmatic BNP levels raises the suspicion of an unknown HF that must be explored. Hence, in this case, it is recommended to perform an electrocardiogram (ECG) and a transthoracic echocardiography (TTE). Additional tests, such as a stress testing, will be discussed depending on the results of the first exams. The persistent high blood pressure and the probable HF necessitate reassessing the patient's current medical treatment and considering treatment by beta blockers, if the procedure can be postponed for 3 to 6 months.

EPIDEMIOLOGY

- HF is a complex clinical syndrome that can result from a variety of lesions of the myocardium, pericardium, heart valves, or great vessels as well as metabolic abnormalities, which leads to an impairment of ventricular relaxation, ejection, or both.[1]
- HF can be classified in 4 stages, from A (patients at high risk for HF, without symptoms of HF) to D (refractory HF).[1]
- The incidence of HF increases with age. As the population is aging, and the therapeutics of HF is improving, the number of HF patients keeps raising, with an estimated 50% increase in the number of new patients with HF every year in 15 years.[2]
- Concomitantly, the number of surgical procedures performed yearly is increasing, especially in the elderly, with more than one-third of the procedures being performed in patients who are age 65 years and older.[3]
- Hence, HF is more and more often encountered in the perioperative settings.

HEART FAILURE IS A MAJOR RISK FACTOR THAT INCREASES PERIOPERATIVE MORBIDITY AND MORTALITY

- Despite improvements in perioperative care, cardiac complications are the leading cause of postoperative deaths.
- Because HF is a significant risk for perioperative morbidity and mortality, it is a component of indices that predict the risk of perioperative major cardiovascular events (MACE). MACE is defined as death from a cardiovascular cause or nonfatal myocardial infarction. The revised cardiac risk index (RCRI), which contains 6 items, is the oldest and most easily validated risk predictor (Table 43-1). Having at least 2 RCRI items classifies a patient as high risk for perioperative MACE.[4,5]
- HF is a well-established perioperative risk factor. Among patients age 65 years and older who undergo major noncardiac surgery, the perioperative mortality rate is at least doubled if they have HF. From the Medicare 5% standard analytic files, Hammill and colleagues retrospectively studied 159,327 procedures (including 13 types of major noncardiac surgery) in patients age 65 years and older. After adjustment for type of procedure, demographics, and comorbidities, patients with HF had a 63% higher mortality and a 51% higher 30-day readmission rate than patients without HF or with coronary artery disease.[6] In addition, HF was an independent risk factor for mortality, in almost all types of major noncardiac procedures (Figure 43-1).
- Among patients who have HF, those who have a more severely impaired ejection fraction (EF) have a worse outcome. In patients with HF who had a high-risk noncardiac surgical procedure, Healy and colleagues reported that severely reduced EF (<30%), but not moderately (30%-40%) or mildly (40%-50%) impaired EF was associated with more adverse perioperative events including myocardial infarction, HF exacerbation, and mortality within 30 days after surgery (Figure 43-2).[7] In this population, the 3 independent risk factors of adverse perioperative events were an age above 80 years, an EF below 30%, and diabetes.[7]
- Even in the absence of HF symptoms, isolated diastolic left ventricular (LV) dysfunction and systolic LV dysfunction are associated with increased morbidity (30-day cardiovascular events) and long-term cardiovascular mortality.[8]

- Taken together, these data suggest that prior to a major surgical procedure, patients with HF should be closely evaluated to assess their HF state. Moreover, it seems necessary to detect patients who have an asymptomatic impairment of the LV function.

EFFECTS OF ANESTHESIA AND SURGERY ON CARDIOVASCULAR FUNCTION

- During surgical procedures, injured tissues develop neuroendocrine responses. This surgical stress leads to an inflammatory state with an increase of oxygen consumption, a fluid shift, and a disruption of the balance between prothrombotic and fibrinolytic factors, the latter favoring thrombosis. Moreover, surgical stimulation activates the renin-angiotensin-aldosterone system (RAAS). Surgical factors that are associated with an increase in cardiac events are urgency, type, invasiveness, and duration of the procedure.

- During general anesthesia, anesthetic agents may impair hemodynamics via direct effects on the myocardium and the vessels, and via indirect effects through the central inhibition of the sympathetic system. The most common agents used are volatile anesthetics, propofol and morphinomimetics. Volatile anesthetics induce a dose-dependent decrease in arterial blood pressure (through a decrease in systemic vascular resistances), inhibit the baroreceptor arc, and alter the contractility as well as the relaxation of both ventricles. Propofol lowers sympathetic nerve activity and blood pressure. Morphinomimetics do not alter the cardiac function.

- General anesthesia requires mechanical ventilation. It induces an increase in intrathoracic pressure leading to a decrease of venous return and eventually cardiac output, which is more marked in cases of hypovolemia. Increased intrathoracic pressure deteriorates right ventricular (RV) function, particularly in cases of high pulmonary arterial pressure. In contrast, increased intrathoracic pressure lowers transmural pressure, which decreases the LV afterload and favors LV function.

- The magnitude of the cardiovascular effects of general anesthesia depends on the pre existing cardiovascular state of the patient. Greater effects will be observed if patients have altered systolic function of any ventricles, which will be more sensitive to a decrease of the contractility and variations of the cardiac load. In addition, long-term treatments, such as RAAS inhibitors, increase the risk of perioperative hypotension.

- Finally, depending on the surgery, general anesthesia is associated with a certain degree of fluid loss, anemia, and hypothermia, which may increase perioperative morbidity.

- Postoperative time is also a sensitive period. Factors such as withdrawal of anesthetic drugs, awakening, extubation, pain, hypothermia, and anemia contribute to activate the sympathetic system, and increase oxygen consumption. Moreover, because patients are unable to take oral drugs during the postoperative time after procedures such as major gastrointestinal tract surgery, the withdrawal of HF drugs can increase the risk of arrhythmia, HTN, and acute HF.

Table 43-1 Revised Cardiac Risk Index (RCRI) The RCRI is composed of 6 items, which are counted when at least 1 criterion that defines the item is present. Patients with 2 items or more are considered to have high risk to develop perioperative major cardiac event.

Item	Definition
Ischemic heart disease	History of myocardial infarction
	Angina pectoris
HF	History of HF
	Pulmonary edema
	Paroxysmal nocturnal dyspnea
	S^3 gallop
	Bilateral rales
Stroke	Stroke
	Transient ischemic attack
Diabetes	Requiring insulin therapy
Renal dysfunction	Serum creatinine >2 mg/dL
	Creatinine clearance <60 mL/min/1.73 m^2
High-risk procedure	Suprainguinal vascular
	Intraperitoneal
	Intrathoracic

Abbreviation: HF, heart failure.

- Taken together, surgery and anesthesia induce hemodynamic stress, fluid variations, and metabolic stress that could be compared to a stressing exercise for the myocardium and can lead to acute HF, myocardial ischemia, and death (Figure 43-3).

- The latest guidelines on perioperative cardiovascular evaluation and management of patients undergoing noncardiac surgery propose to separate the surgical procedures into 2 categories.[4] During a low-risk procedure, the combined surgical and patient characteristics predict a risk of MACE <1%. Elevated-risk surgeries are associated with a MACE ≥1% (Table 43-2).

PREOPERATIVE TIME: ASSESSMENT OF HEART FAILURE AND CARDIOVASCULAR RISKS

The preoperative assessment is the cornerstone of the care of a HF patient who has to undergo surgery. During that time, the objectives are:

- Complete a clinical examination

- Decide which additional tests should be run

- Adapt the medical treatment

- Decide when the surgery is possible

- Discuss the anesthetic and the surgical strategies

CLINICAL EXAMINATION

- Goals of the clinical examination are to assess the stability of an existing HF and search for the signs of an unknown HF. Hence, the presence of the different cardiovascular risk factors should be searched for and quantitated. Moreover, special attention should be placed on looking for signs of chronic HF (peripheral venous congestion including jugular venous distention, lower extremity edema, abdominal ascites), as well as signs of acute HF (dyspnea, weight gain, orthopnea, paroxysmal nocturnal dyspnea).

- In addition, one should assess the functional status, which is a strong predictor of perioperative and long-term cardiac events.[4,9] Patients with good functional status are at low risk to develop postoperative cardiac events whereas patients with poor functional status are at high risk to develop postoperative cardiac events. The functional capacity can be assessed by the ability to perform daily activities, expressed in terms of metabolic equivalents (METs). One MET is equivalent to the basal metabolic rate of a resting 40-year-old, 70 kg man (Figure 43-4). Functional capacity is considered poor if METs <4. In the latest recommendations on perioperative cardiovascular evaluation, before high-risk surgery, a good or very good functional status (METs ≥4) excludes the need to investigate for coronary artery disease and likely also for pulmonary and cardiac disease.

PREOPERATIVE INVESTIGATIONS

- If a patient has known HF, with symptoms that are unchanged since the last investigation (<1 year), no further test is needed.

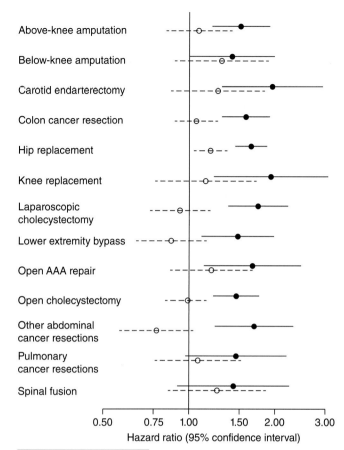

FIGURE 43-1 Effects of heart failure and coronary artery disease, compared to neither, on operative mortality by procedure. Procedure-specific models include indicators for disease group, age, sex, race, admission characteristics, comorbidities, and hospital teaching status. Abbreviation: AAA, abdominal aortic aneurysm. (Used with permission from Pr. Hernandez, MD, MHS.)

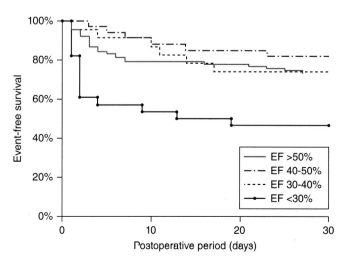

FIGURE 43-2 Perioperative outcomes, among heart failure patients undergoing noncardiac surgery, stratified by ejection fraction (EF). Subjects with a severely reduced EF (<30%) had a significantly higher risk of adverse perioperative events (myocardial infarction and HF exacerbation occurring during the incident hospitalization, and/or death occurring within 30 days) than subjects with a normal EF. (Used with permission from Dr. Maurer, MD.)

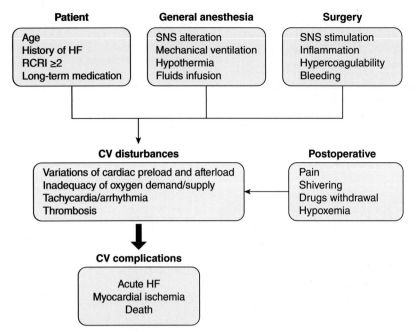

FIGURE 43-3 Perioperative heart failure. This diagram represents the risk factors of the patient, as well as physiological effects of general anesthesia, surgery, and the postoperative period that contribute to perioperative cardiovascular disturbances and eventually complications such as acute heart failure, myocardial ischemia, and death. Abbreviations: CV, cardiovascular; HF, heart failure; RCRI, revised cardiac risk index; SNS, sympathetic nervous system.

- In a patient with no history of HF but for whom the anesthesiologist suspects HF, the performance of 3 additional tests should be considered: an electrocardiogram, measurement of plasmatic natriuretic peptide levels, and a TTE.

- It is recommended to obtain a 12-lead ECG in patients who have coronary heart disease, arrhythmia, peripheral arterial disease, or cerebrovascular disease, unless they undergo a low-risk procedure, or have had an ECG within 3 months.[4]

- A TTE is recommended for patients who undergo high-risk surgery, if signs and symptoms have changed since the last investigation.[4] TTE allows the quantification of the LV systolic and diastolic functions, the assessment of filling pressures, and the search for a cause of HF, such as valvular disease. Knowledge of TTE abnormalities does not have prognostic value but allows members of the care team to adapt the perioperative management of patients.

- Natriuretic peptides (NPs) include BNP or the inactive N-terminal fragment (NT-proBNP), which are primarily synthetized by the cardiomyocytes of the ventricles, in response to an increase of cardiac wall stress. NPs are markers of ventricular dysfunction. BNP is used as a diagnostic tool during the exploration of an acute dyspnea, to attribute (if BNP >400 pg/mL) or rule out (if BNP <100 pg/mL) congestive cardiac HF. Plasmatic low levels of BNP (<100 pg/mL) or NT-proBNP (<125 pg/mL) exclude a diagnosis of chronic HF. During chronic HF, NPs are strong prognostic markers. Other factors, such as age, renal failure, sepsis, and acute coronary syndrome, can participate in increasing plasmatic NP levels.[1] In perioperative settings, increased BNP or NT-proBNP levels are powerful independent predictors of short- and long-term MACE, as well as all-cause mortality (Figure 43-5).[10,11] In noncardiac surgery, preoperative BNP levels are valuable because they have a better ability to predict cardiovascular events than the

Table 43-2 Summary of low and high risk of morbidity or mortality after surgical procedures.

Low Risk	High Risk
• Combined surgical and patient characteristics predict a risk of MACE <1% • Example: Cataracts, plastics	• Any procedure associated with a risk of MACE ≥1% • Risk could be lowered by less invasive approach • Risk is increased by the urgency of the procedure

Abbreviation: MACE, major cardiac event.

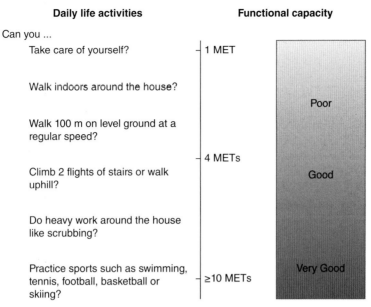

FIGURE 43-4 Equivalent between daily-life activities and metabolic equivalent (MET).

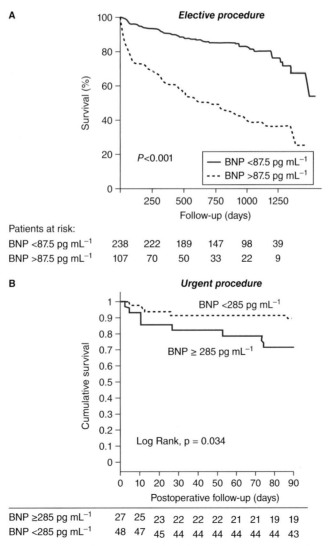

FIGURE 43-5 Increased brain natriuretic peptide (BNP) levels are associated with lower postoperative survival rates whether it is an elective procedure (A) or an urgent procedure (B). **A**. BNP levels were measured a day prior to an elective surgery. A BNP value of 87.5 pg/mL best predicted long-term mortality. (Used with permission of Oxford University Press.) **B**. Patients admitted for traumatic hip fracture had a measurement of BNP levels. A BNP value of 285 pg/mL was the most sensitive and specific value to identify major echocardiographic abnormalities. (Used with permission from Pr. Samain, MD, PhD.)

RCRI,[11] and addition of the BNP levels to the RCRI increases the RCRI's predictive value. These results suggest that measurement of BNP levels could permit a better prediction of cardiovascular risk and stratification of the patients. However, because multiple factors can influence NP levels, the threshold of NP levels that would allow a good distinction between high- and low-risk patients, remains uncertain. Although BNP-guided therapy can improve the prognosis of patients with chronic HF,[12] such therapy has not been studied in perioperative settings. However, preoperative NP levels could be used as a tool to stratify preoperative investigations. In a prospective study, patients who were about to have hip surgery had a systematic measurement of plasmatic BNP and a TTE.[13] Increased plasmatic BNP levels were associated with the discovery of a major echocardiographic abnormality (such as increased LV filling pressure, severe systolic dysfunction, pulmonary HTN, or severe valvular disease); the value of 285 pg/mL was able to discriminate patients with a major echocardiographic abnormality.

- Taken together, these results suggest that measurement of BNP could help to hierarchize the performance of preoperative investigation. We suggest a stepwise approach of HF patients (Figure 43-6).

ADAPTATION OF MEDICAL TREATMENT

- In stable HF patients, treatment by beta blockers should be continued until the day of surgery.[4,9] Treatment by beta blockers should be started when needed. However, beta blocker treatment should not be initiated within days preceding a major surgery.[14]
- Renin–angiotensin–aldosterone system (RAAS) inhibitors could be stopped the day before surgery.[4,5]
- Discontinuation of antiplatelet agents depends on the reason for the prescription (eg, primary prevention, drug-eluting stent, bare-metal stent), the time between the beginning of antiplatelet agents and surgery, and the bleeding risk of the procedure.[4]

TIMING OF THE PROCEDURE

- Decompensated HF should forbid any surgical procedure, unless life or limb is threatened if not in the operating room within 24 hours.[4]
- If possible, in the presence of signs of acute HF, surgery should be delayed by 3 months, allowing time for stabilization, and/or improvement of ventricular function prior to undergoing surgery.[15]

SURGICAL AND ANESTHETIC STRATEGIES

Surgical Strategy

The advantages of endovascular surgery are not straightforward in patients with multiple comorbidities.[4,5] The choice of endovascular surgery, over an open procedure, should be made according to the type of surgery and the patient's risks.

Compared to open procedures, endoscopic surgery presents benefits in terms of postoperative rehabilitation (bowel movements, pain, and pulmonary function). But the pneumoperitoneum created during endoscopic procedures induces a decrease in venous return and an increase in cardiac afterload that can be threatening for HF patients. Hence, the choice of endoscopic surgery should be balanced between advantages and risks.

Locoregional Anesthesia

Neuraxial anesthesia is associated with a sympathetic blockade leading to high variations of intravascular volume and arterial pressure. Hence, the beneficial effects of neuraxial anesthesia, compared to general anesthesia, are not evident. However, epidural anesthesia should be considered for postoperative pain relief.[4]

Peripheral nerve blockade does not affect the cardiovascular system as much as neuraxial or general anesthesia. Therefore, peripheral nerve blockade should be proposed to HF patients whenever it is applicable.

PEROPERATIVE TIME

During general anesthesia, the objective is to maintain homeostasis as much as possible including a sinus rhythm, as well as a control of the arterial pressure, the blood volume, the temperature, and the hemoglobin levels. To achieve these goals, attention should be placed on:

- Discuss the monitoring of invasive arterial pressure, cardiac output (by the use of esophageal Doppler or pulse contour analysis), and depth of anesthesia (using, for instance, the bispectral index).
- Dose the different anesthetic drugs to use the minimal amount of drug to obtain the intended effects with limited adverse effects.
- Avoid metabolic constrains (eg, hypercapnia, hypoxia, hypothermia, and anemia).
- Limit fluid infusions.

POSTOPERATIVE TIME

- The postoperative period remains a sensitive time and careful attention should be placed on:
  - Preventing/treating any tachycardia
  - Preventing shivering
  - Appropriate analgesia
  - Avoiding HTN
- RAAS inhibitors and beta blocker treatment should be resumed as soon as possible.[4]
- Depending on surgical procedure extent and HF severity, postoperative care could be done in intensive care.
- According to the number of cardiovascular risk factors and the perioperative events, a myocardial ischemia should be monitored via an ECG and troponin level measurements.
- Postoperative increase of NP levels is associated with an increased mortality or nonfatal myocardial infarction within 30 days or 180 days after noncardiac surgery.

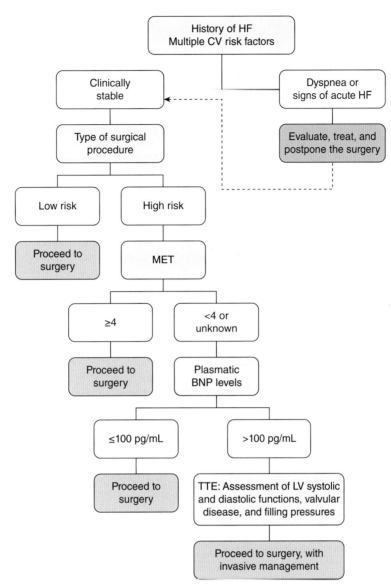

FIGURE 43-6 Approach of perioperative heart failure (HF) before an elective noncardiac surgery. If the patient presents uncompensated heart failure, a diagnostic should be done, the patient treated, and the surgery postponed until the patient is clinically stable. In order to adapt the perioperative management of a clinically stable patient with a history of (or a suspected) HF, the performance of additional tests will be discussed, depending on the type of surgical procedure (Table 43-2), the functional activity (expressed in terms of metabolic equivalent, MET), and the levels of plasmatic brain natriuretic peptide (BNP). Ultimately, if necessary, the performance of a transthoracic echocardiogram will inform about heart function and allow a more personalized anesthesia. Abbreviations: CV, cardiovascular; LV, left ventricle; TTE, transthoracic echocardiography.

TREATMENT OF POSTOPERATIVE ACUTE HEART FAILURE

The diagnosis and treatment of postoperative acute HF are not specific to that time. The principal steps are:

- Explore the mechanism, such as ischemia, hypoxia, increased systemic blood pressure, or anemia.

- Assess the severity of acute HF.

- Manage postoperative HF by way of noninvasive ventilation, together with treating the cause:

  - Restore blood pressure.

  - Give appropriate analgesia.

- In case of ischemia, discuss a treatment by antiplatelet and anticoagulant agents together with the anesthesiologist, the cardiologist, and the surgeon.

- An angiography is rarely needed within the first postoperative days.

- Discuss beta blocker therapy in case of high heart rate.

REFERENCES

1. Writing Committee Members, Yancy CW, Jessup M, et al. 2013 ACCF/AHA guideline for the management of heart failure: a report of the American College of Cardiology Foundation/American Heart Association Task Force on practice guidelines. *Circulation.* 2013;128(16):e240.

2. Braunwald E. The war against heart failure: the Lancet lecture. *Lancet.* 2015;385(9970):812-824.

3. Semel ME, Lipsitz SR, Funk LM, Bader AM, Weiser TG, Gawande AA. Rates and patterns of death after surgery in the United States, 1996 and 2006. *Surgery.* 2012;151(2):171.

4. Fleisher LA, Fleischmann KE, Auerbach AD, et al. 2014 ACC/AHA guideline on perioperative cardiovascular evaluation and management of patients undergoing noncardiac surgery: a report of the American College of Cardiology/American Heart Association Task Force on practice guidelines. *J Am Coll Cardiol.* 2014;64(22):e77-e137.

5. Kristensen SD, Knuuti J, Saraste A, et al. 2014 ESC/ESA Guidelines on non-cardiac surgery: cardiovascular assessment and management: The Joint Task Force on non-cardiac surgery: cardiovascular assessment and management of the European Society of Cardiology (ESC) and the European Society of Anaesthesiology (ESA). *Eur Heart J.* 2014;35(35):2383-2431.

6. Hammill BG, Curtis LH, Bennett-Guerrero E, et al. Impact of heart failure on patients undergoing major noncardiac surgery. *Anesthesiology.* 2008;108(4):559-567.

7. Healy KO, Waksmonski CA, Altman RK, Stetson PD, Reyentovich A, Maurer MS. Perioperative outcome and long-term mortality for heart failure patients undergoing intermediate- and high-risk noncardiac surgery: impact of left ventricular ejection fraction. *Congest Heart Fail.* 2010;16(2):45-49.

8. Flu WJ, van Kuijk JP, Hoeks SE, et al. Prognostic implications of asymptomatic left ventricular dysfunction in patients undergoing vascular surgery. *Anesthesiology.* 2010;112(6):1316-1324.

9. Hopper I, Samuel R, Hayward C, Tonkin A, Krum H. Can medications be safely withdrawn in patients with stable chronic heart failure? systematic review and meta-analysis. *J Card Fail.* 2014;20(7):522-532.

10. Rodseth RN, Biccard BM, Le Manach Y, et al. The prognostic value of pre-operative and post-operative B-type natriuretic peptides in patients undergoing noncardiac surgery: B-type natriuretic peptide and N-terminal fragment of pro-B-type natriuretic peptide: a systematic review and individual patient data meta-analysis. *J Am Coll Cardiol.* 2014;63(2):170-180.

11. Rodseth RN, Lurati Buse GA, Bolliger D, et al. The predictive ability of pre-operative B-type natriuretic peptide in vascular patients for major adverse cardiac events: an individual patient data meta-analysis. *J Am Coll Cardiol.* 2011;58(5):522-529.

12. Jang J-S, Jin H-Y, Seo J-S, Yang T-H, Kim D-K, Kim D-S. The role of brain natriuretic peptide-guided heart failure therapy: an updated meta-analysis. *J Am Coll Cardiol.* 2013;61(10):E743.

13. Pili-Floury S, Ginet M, Saunier L, et al. Preoperative plasma B-type natriuretic peptide (BNP) identifies abnormal transthoracic echocardiography in elderly patients with traumatic hip fracture. *Injury.* 2012;43(6):811-816.

14. Devereaux PJ, Yang H, Yusuf S, et al; POISE Study Group. Effects of extended-release metoprolol succinate in patients undergoing non-cardiac surgery (POISE trial): a randomised controlled trial. *Lancet.* 2008;371(9627):1839-1847.

15. Upshaw J, Kiernan MS. Preoperative cardiac risk assessment for noncardiac surgery in patients with heart failure. *Curr Heart Fail Rep.* 2013;10(2):147-156.

44 PALLIATIVE CARE IN HEART FAILURE

Christopher M. Hritz, MD
Todd A. Barrett, MD
Jillian L. Gustin, MD, FAAHPM

PATIENT CASE

Bob Hart is a 56-year-old divorced man with a history of acute on chronic systolic heart failure (HF) secondary to nonischemic cardiomyopathy, type 2 diabetes, and obesity. He was admitted to the cardiac service with multiple HF-related symptoms including shortness of breath, cough, weight gain, lightheadedness, generalized weakness, and fatigue. His HF was first diagnosed 9 years ago and a recent echo revealed a left ventricular ejection fraction (EF) of <20%. Bob underwent right heart catheterization and was found to have a low cardiac index. During the admission his condition worsened, which prompted the team to start a dobutamine infusion and begin workup for possible advanced HF therapies. In addition to HF symptoms, Bob suffers from bilateral leg pain secondary to diabetic neuropathy. Psychosocially, he is currently undergoing a divorce and lives alone, but he has an adult daughter who is very involved in his care.

Bob was evaluated by a multidisciplinary team that included a cardiologist, cardiothoracic surgeon, social worker, and palliative care team. His treatment options included a left ventricular assist device (LVAD) implant as destination therapy or continuation of inotropes with focus on comfort care. He was not a transplant candidate due to morbid obesity and complications related to diabetes. After extensive discussion with the interdisciplinary team, Bob assessed his risks and benefits and determined that home-based management without surgery was congruent with his goals of care. While in the hospital his medical therapy was optimized and he was started on low-dose oxycodone to help manage refractory dyspnea and neuropathic pain not controlled with gabapentin.

Bob was discharged home with an inotrope infusion and initiation of home hospice. The hospice team provided frequent palliative domain-focused support to Bob and his daughter. He died at home 2 months following this hospitalization, surrounded by his family with minimal symptom burden. Bereavement services were provided by hospice to the family following the patient's death.

INTRODUCTION

Heart disease is the number one cause of death in the United States, accounting for almost a quarter of all deaths in 2013.[1] HF is a chronic, terminal illness mentioned in over 11% of all death certificates in the United States.[2] Palliative care is an integral component of chronic HF care that can assist with treatment of refractory symptoms, clarify goals of care in the face of prognostic uncertainty, help with determining the appropriate location of care, and provide psychosocial support for the patient and family. This care is provided with close collaboration between a palliative care consultant and the primary cardiology team. Palliative care should be introduced early in the disease process with increasing focus as HF progresses (Figure 44-1). Early integration of palliative medicine and institutional funding for palliative care is now a recommendation by the American Heart Association.[3]

The word palliate is defined as "to alleviate (a disease or its symptoms) without effecting a cure; to relieve or ease (physical or emotional suffering) temporarily or superficially."[4] The scope of palliative care often extends beyond this, as management of disease often palliates symptoms. Palliative care utilizes a multidisciplinary team approach that often includes physicians who specialize in palliative medicine, nurse practitioners, nurses, psychologists, social workers, pharmacists, chaplains, occupational therapists, physical therapists, speech therapists, care coordinators, and nursing assistants to alleviate multiple facets of suffering and promote quality of life. It is often provided along with other disease-focused medical treatments.[5]

DIFFERENTIAL DIAGNOSIS

Symptom burden associated with HF adversely affects quality of life for patients. The differential of all symptoms evaluated in a palliative care visit is beyond the scope of this chapter, but it is important to explore reversible causes of symptoms in all patients. Symptoms are often a result of worsening HF, and optimizing HF therapy is the primary symptom management strategy. Unfortunately, despite treatment of reversible causes, there are many cases where optimal management of disease fails to alleviate symptoms.

Patients with end-stage HF experience a large symptom burden, with nearly half suffering from nausea, constipation, and anxiety. Symptoms such as pain, fatigue, and breathlessness are even more common at 77%, 82%, and 88%, respectively.[6] Tools, such as the Edmonton Symptom Assessment Scale (ESAS), assist palliative care clinicians in identifying these symptoms common in advanced illnesses including HF. Symptoms addressed include pain, tiredness (a measure of generalized weakness), nausea, depression, anxiety, drowsiness (a measure of insomnia), appetite, wellbeing, shortness of breath, and a category titled "other."[7] The Memorial Symptom Assessment Scale (MSAS) is another common symptom assessment scale that includes further detail including difficulty concentrating, cough, dry mouth, numbness/tingling in hands/feet, feeling bloated, problems with urination, diarrhea, sweats, problems with sexual interest or activity, itching, dizziness, and difficulty swallowing.[8] There are many other symptom assessment scales, some broad similar to the ESAS and MSAS, and some that deal only with a specific symptom. Systematic assessment using these tools aids the clinician in the diagnosis of symptoms along with evaluation of severity and response to therapy. In addition to clinical utility, these scales aid in research and quality improvement in palliative care.

CLINICAL FEATURES—HISTORY AND PHYSICAL

In HF, similar to other serious potentially life-limiting illnesses, suffering and distress may occur in various domains that reach beyond physical symptoms. Thus the palliative care interdisciplinary team assesses 8 different domains to provide a whole-person assessment.[9]

1. The **structure and process of care** domain includes assessing patient and family understanding of disease, prognosis, and patient preferences for type and site of care. This would also include discussion of the role of advanced HF therapies. A diagram provided to the patients can be helpful in explaining HF trajectory and prognosis (Figure 44-2).

2. **Physical aspects of care** focus on ensuring safe and timely management of pain and other physical symptoms.

3. **Psychological and psychiatric aspects** address depression, anxiety, delirium, cognitive impairment, assessment of capacity, grief, and bereavement.

4. **Social aspects of care** examine family structure, geographic location, support, living arrangements, caregiver availability, access to transportation, access to medications, and caregiver support.

5. **Spiritual, religious, and existential aspects of care** focus on life review, hopes and fears, guilt, forgiveness, life completion, and availability of leaders specific to the patient's religious traditions.

6. **Cultural aspects of care** provide a cultural needs assessment and strives for respectful communication, decision making, and communication in a language family will understand.

7. **Care of the patient at the end of life** focuses on presence, patient and family education, prognosis, symptom management, and a bereavement plan.

8. **Ethical and legal aspects of care** ensure patient preferences are followed via the patient himself or herself, a medical decision maker, or advance directives regarding administration of further treatments or withholding/withdrawing treatments.

For this chapter, we will focus more specifically on physical and psychological symptoms and possible management strategies. There are many symptoms encountered in HF patients (Table 44-1). A thorough assessment of symptoms for patients with HF may include the topics discussed in the following sections.

DYSPNEA

Dyspnea is reported in 60% to 88% of patients with HF.[6] The sensation of breathlessness is a result of the human body's perceived

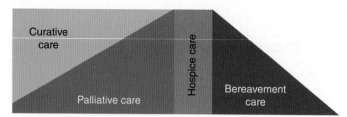

FIGURE 44-1 Role of palliative care throughout disease progression.

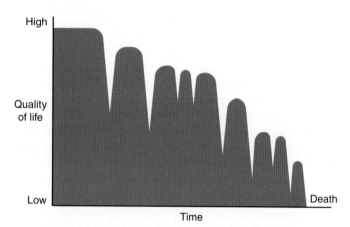

FIGURE 44-2 The trajectory of heart failure. This helps explain that though patients generally recover following exacerbations, their overall baseline quality of life declines over time.

Table 44-1[9,23] Heart Failure Symptom Prevalence

Symptom	Incidence
Dyspnea	60%-88%
Fatigue	69%-82%
Pain	41%-77%
Depression	10%-60%
Anxiety	49%
Insomnia	36%-48%
Constipation	32%-48%
Nausea	17%-48%
Lack of appetite	21%-41%
Delirium	18%-32%

inability to meet one's ventilatory demand, and it is closely tied to higher cortical processes. Subjective reporting of dyspnea is crucial as the body is extremely sensitive to ventilation inadequacies and patients may experience dyspnea in the context of normal medical test results. Laboratory studies such as blood gasses and pulse oxygenation are not reliable measures of perceived dyspnea.[10]

Nonpharmacologic management strategies often prove effective in decreasing the sensation of breathlessness. Supplemental oxygen has been found to be useful in managing dyspnea only in patients who are hypoxic. Movement of air through the nares has been shown to improve dyspnea independent of oxygenation.[11] Any method of stimulating the trigeminal nerve with cool, moving air is effective in reducing dyspnea and may be achieved with a fan blowing toward the patient's face or forced air/oxygen via nasal cannula.[12]

Pharmacologic therapies for dyspnea should always include aggressive medical management of HF such as diuretics, vasodilators, inotropes, and ultrafiltration techniques such as aquapheresis. Angiotensin-converting enzyme (ACE) inhibitors have also been found to reduce dyspnea.[13]

Opioids such as morphine are effective at minimizing shortness of breath in patients with dyspnea refractory to disease-directed therapy. Despite a common myth, opioids do not cause significant respiratory depression or sedation at appropriate doses. Opioid receptors are located throughout the central nervous system (CNS) as well as peripheral areas responsible for monitoring respiration such as the carotid bodies.[10] Even at low doses, opioids can be effective for dyspnea.[14] These doses may often be lower than what would be expected for pain management. Benzodiazepines may be appropriate in HF patients with dyspnea as a second-line agent in addition to opioid medications if anxiety is a concurrent issue.

FATIGUE

Fatigue is a hallmark symptom of heart disease and affects between 69% to 82% of patients.[6] Important factors to consider in the fatigued HF patient include deconditioning and comorbid conditions such as anemia, hypothyroidism, depression, and sleep disorders.

Regular physical exercise tailored to the patient's ability should be encouraged. Though seemingly counterintuitive, prolonged rest is thought to provide no benefit in fatigue and promotes further deconditioning. Patients may also be advised on energy conservation and taught to keep a diary to help plan for worsening fatigue and prioritizing activities.[15] Fatigue secondary to comorbid conditions should be identified and managed appropriately. If comorbidities are optimally managed, stimulants such as methylphenidate may also be helpful in reducing fatigue.[16]

PAIN

Pain is extremely common in HF patients, with a reported incidence of 63% to 80%.[6] Multiple etiologies for pain exist in HF patients. Common examples are ischemic pain, neuropathic pain, pain secondary to lower extremity or abdominal edema, and arthritic pain unrelated to cardiovascular disease. Patients may also experience pain without an easily identified etiology or other pain-causing comorbidities.[17] Pain levels tend to increase as the severity of HF increases. Special attention should be placed on pain in HF

patients as it is often undertreated and lags significantly behind the management of pain in cancer.[18]

Management of pain in patients with HF presents particular challenges. Although opioid-sparing analgesics are often first-line for pain management in chronic nonmalignant pain, such medications are often restricted in this patient population. Nonsteroidal anti-inflammatory drugs (NSAIDs) such as ibuprofen or naproxen should be avoided as they can further impair renal function affected by poor cardiac output and worsen fluid retention.[19] They are also contraindicated in patients who are on anticoagulation medications. Acetaminophen may be considered first-line for nonneuropathic pain; however, special attention must be paid to dosing when using it in the context of liver dysfunction. Given these restrictions, opioids are often required for pain management in HF patients.

Pharmacologic considerations for opioid medications must be made when patients exhibit hepatic or renal dysfunction and clinicians must monitor for opioid toxicities regardless of which opioid is chosen. In patients with renal failure, morphine should be avoided as it has active, renally excreted metabolites that cause neurotoxicity. Codeine is a prodrug of morphine and should also be avoided in renal disease. As it relies on liver metabolism, codeine is likely to be less effective in hepatic disease.[20] Hydromorphone also produces renally-excreted metabolites that may cause neurotoxicity and should be used with caution in renal impairment. Oxycodone and fentanyl do not have renally-excreted active metabolites and thus are the opiates of choice in a patient with renal failure.[21] Morphine or hydromorphone should be considered in patients with hepatic failure as they undergo glucuronidation, which is more likely to be preserved in liver disease. Hydromorphone is an acceptable option in patients with both renal and hepatic failure. Fentanyl is also commonly used in hepatorenal failure, though data supporting fentanyl use in severe hepatic failure are lacking. Methadone is also an option acceptable in both renal and hepatic failure but is challenging to dose and generally requires consultation with palliative care or pain management specialists.[22,23]

Many opioid side effects such as nausea, drowsiness, and confusion are self-limited and resolve within a week.[24] Exploring these issues with patients is important because side effects are often mistakenly listed as allergies and are not a contraindication to another trial. Unlike other transient opioid side effects, constipation is not transient and therefore needs continual monitoring and management in patients consistently taking opioids. Management of constipation is discussed later in this chapter.

The anticonvulsants gabapentin or pregabalin should be considered in patients with neuropathic pain. This class of medications is considered first-line agents, along with tricyclic antidepressants (TCAs), for neuropathy.[25] TCAs should be avoided due to risk of QT prolongation and side effects potentially compounding HF symptoms such as dry mouth and orthostatic hypotension.[26] Serotonin–norepinephrine reuptake inhibitor (SNRI) antidepressants, tramadol, topical lidocaine, and topical capsaicin are adjuvant therapies for neuropathic pain that have proven efficacy and should be considered. Opioids are considered third-line agents in neuropathic pain, though they may be necessary in refractory cases.[27]

DEPRESSION

It is well known that depression is associated with cardiovascular disease and HF. A meta-analysis consisting of 27 studies revealed rates of depression between 9% and 60%. As with pain, rates of depression increase with increased severity of HF. New York Heart Association (NYHA) functional class is correlated to incidence of depression, with greater than 40% prevalence in class IV.[28]

Depression is a challenging diagnosis in terminal illnesses such as heart failure (HF). Many symptoms of depression overlap with symptoms experienced in chronic or terminal illness. Examples of overlapping symptoms include sleep disruption, decreased appetite, and increased fatigue. Symptoms exclusive to depression include suicidality, anhedonia, and loss of hope.

Management of depression in HF is similar to management in the general population. Nonpharmacologic interventions such as cognitive behavioral therapy should be incorporated into management. Social workers can explore group support options for the patient and provide support to caregivers. Depressive symptoms in caregivers have been shown to affect a patient's likelihood to respond to depression interventions.[29]

A selective serotonin reuptake inhibitor (SSRI) should be considered. Data are limited, but sertraline has been studied and shown to be safe in HF.[30] Stimulants such as methylphenidate may also be considered, as a response will typically occur within 2 days.[31] This is helpful in situations where the 4 to 6 week onset of SSRI efficacy is unacceptable. A common example is patients with a very short life expectancy. Common risks such as arrhythmias must be taken into account when considering stimulants.[32]

ANXIETY

Anxiety has been reported to affect approximately 49% of HF patients.[6] Anxiety may arise from different etiologies including underlying psychiatric disorders, symptoms such as pain or shortness of breath, drug side effects, or as a response to the numerous concerns a patient encounters towards the end of life. Patients with implantable cardioverter defibrillators (ICDs) are more likely to experience symptoms of anxiety, especially if they have experienced a device firing.[33,34] Clinicians should remember that hyperactive delirium may be mistaken for anxiety.

Nonpharmacologic management such as supportive psychotherapy and cognitive behavior therapy are important interventions in able patients as an adjuvant to pharmacotherapy. Music therapy, art therapy, relaxation techniques, meditation, aromatherapy, and acupuncture should be considered as well.[35,36] These therapies are now available in some hospitals and are often incorporated into hospice care. A multidisciplinary approach incorporating chaplaincy and social work is also an integral component of managing a patient's anxiety.

For acute-onset anxiety, benzodiazepines are first-line drugs to provide prompt relief of symptoms. Lorazepam is a good initial choice as is it relatively short-acting and better tolerated in patients with liver dysfunction. Benzodiazepines should be used with caution as they may cause mental status changes and worsen delirium, especially in elderly or seriously ill patients. Other anxiety-provoking conditions listed earlier should be addressed as needed. If life expectancy is thought to be longer than a few weeks and exposure to the anxiety-provoking stimulus is expected to continue, management with SSRIs should be explored.

INSOMNIA

Insomnia is experienced in 36% to 48% of patients with heart disease.[6] Insomnia in HF has been correlated with increased depression, fatigue, and decreased functional performance independent of sleep-disordered breathing.[37]

Nonpharmacologic management such as cognitive behavioral therapy, which incorporates stimulus control, sleep restriction, relaxation, and sleep hygiene education has been shown to be helpful in more generalized populations and would likely be beneficial for HF patients.[38]

There are many pharmacologic options for insomnia. Melatonin receptor antagonists such as ramelteon help reduce sleep latency along with increasing total sleep time, though there is no improvement in number of awakenings or ease of falling back asleep after being woken up.[39] The supplement melatonin itself has only proven to be effective in circadian rhythm sleep disorders and sleep-onset latency.[40] Nevertheless, melatonin-related drugs have a favorable side-effect profile and are reasonable to trial for insomnia. Benzodiazepines and benzodiazepinereceptor antagonists such as zolpidem are commonly used therapies in the management of insomnia across most patient populations. These reduce sleep latency, increasing total sleep time and decreasing number of awakenings.[41] Benzodiazepines have a higher incidence of adverse effects such as paradoxical agitation, mental status changes, and paradoxical insomnia and generally have a longer half-life than benzodiazepine receptor antagonists, which are generally better tolerated. In patients with comorbid depression, antidepressants such as trazodone may be considered due to their sedative properties. Benzodiazepines, benzodiazepine receptor antagonists, and antidepressants should all be used judiciously as there is evidence for increased harm.[42] Antihistamines should generally be avoided due to anticholinergic side effects.

CONSTIPATION

Constipation is found in 32% to 48% of patients with heart disease.[6] Clinicians must be particularly cognizant of constipation when patients require opioid therapy, as it is a virtually universal side effect of opioid medications. Decreased mobility and fluid shifts associated with HF also contribute to constipation.

Constipation may cause or contribute to multiple other symptoms including nausea, abdominal pain, shortness of breath, and delirium. Identification and management of constipation is an important aspect of relieving these symptoms common to advanced illness.

There are multiple categories of medications available to manage constipation. Some act by affecting the consistency of the stool, others act as laxatives, and newer therapies target opiate receptors in the gut to alleviate opiate-induced constipation. Bulking agents such as fiber and stool softening agents such as docusate are often considered first-line therapies, but are generally ineffective if the patient is suffering from opioid-induced constipation. A stimulant laxative such as senna is often needed. Osmotic laxatives such as polyethylene glycol have the strongest evidence of efficacy, though quicker onset of action may cause more discomfort compared to stimulant laxatives.[43] In addition, relatively large volumes of liquid need to be consumed for polyethylene glycol to be effective, which may be challenging when patients are on fluid restrictions. Methylnaltrexone and naloxegol are opioid antagonists that do not cross the blood-brain barrier and therefore relieve opioid-induced constipation without reversing analgesia. These are often used as second-line due to cost and lack of long-term safety data.[44] Laxatives and opioid antagonists should be avoided in bowel obstruction due to the risk of bowel perforation.

NAUSEA

Though most research involving nausea is cancer and chemotherapy related, 17% to 48% of patients with heart disease will experience nausea.[6] The neurologic mechanisms of nausea in humans are complex and incompletely understood. Nausea involves multiple neural pathways including the cortex, vestibular system, chemoreceptor trigger zone (CTZ), and vomiting center as well as multiple receptor types including muscarinic, dopaminergic, histamine, neurokinin, and serotonin. A thorough history is helpful in determining cause and should include exacerbating and alleviating factors, vertigo, relation to meals, pain, and medication history.

Empiric management of nausea is generally effective, though special considerations should be made if the cause is clear. Dopamine antagonists such as prochlorperazine, promethazine, and haldol as well as the serotonin agonist ondansetron act on the CTZ and are effective first-line agents when using an empiric approach. Ondansetron causes constipation and thus frequency of bowel movements should be monitored. Prokinetics such as metoclopramide should be utilized in the setting of impaired gastric emptying. Common complaints related to impaired gastric emptying are early satiety and epigastric pain. Anticholinergic or antihistaminic drugs such as scopolamine, diphenhydramine, and meclizine are best suited for nausea from vestibular causes. Clinicians should be aware of side effects such as dry mouth and drowsiness with these medications.[45] Benzodiazepines are sometimes considered when controlling nausea but should be limited to anticipatory nausea and nausea clearly related to anxiety. The classic example of anticipatory nausea is nausea prior to subsequent chemotherapy, where the first chemotherapy treatment caused significant posttreatment nausea.

LACK OF APPETITE

The incidence of anorexia in patients with heart disease is reported in 21% to 41% of patients.[6] Decreased caloric intake contributes to the overall problem of cachexia in chronic disease. Cachexia is a complex, multifactorial condition where inflammation, loss of muscle mass, decreased oral intake, and alterations in metabolism lead to loss of lean muscle mass.

Evaluating a patient's caloric intake and optimizing nutrition should be performed in patients with advanced HF. Exercise will also promote conservation of muscle mass and protein biosynthesis.[46]

Pharmacotherapy for cachexia is limited and most data are from the study of cancer patients or AIDS patients. Optimal management of HF remains important in cardiac cachexia as ACE inhibitors and beta blockers will delay symptoms. Megestrol can initially increase appetite and weight gain, but patients do not report an improvement in quality of life and it can promote peripheral edema.[47] Cannabinoids such as dronabinol may promote oral intake but side effects such as ataxia, somnolence, poor concentration, and anxiety can limit the patient's ability to tolerate continued treatment. There is also no evidence that cannabinoids promote weight gain, despite increased oral intake.[48] Corticosteroids can also increase appetite, though most supportive evidence is found in cancer patients.[49]

DELIRIUM

Confusion and delirium are reported in 18% to 32% of HF patients.[6] Delirium is extremely prevalent in hospitalized patients and found in 80% of ICU patients. Delirium leads to longer hospital stays, increased complications, and worsening cognition in elderly patients.[50] Patients admitted with delirium have a 26% increase in mortality and patients who develop delirium in the hospital have a 76% increase in mortality.[51] Patients with HF are at particularly high risk of delirium or cognitive impairment, presumably from low flow due to decreased cardiac output.[52] Delirium is often multifactorial and a thorough evaluation beyond HF management is warranted. Current medications, worsening of comorbid conditions, and disruption of daily routine due to hospitalizations should all be considered in the delirious patient.

There are many ways to manage delirium with nonpharmacologic interventions. Frequent orientation, good sleep hygiene, attention to lighting to mimic day-night cycles, encouraging mobility, and consistency in caregivers is helpful in preventing and improving delirium. Ensuring patients have needed sensory aids such as glasses and hearing aids is also a useful intervention.[53] Attention should be directed toward polypharmacy and removal of potential delirium-causing medications such as anticholinergics, opioids, and benzodiazepines.

Prior to initiating pharmacotherapy, investigating underlying reversible medical causes such as infection, electrolyte disturbance, and psychoactive medications must be performed. Antipsychotics are first-line for delirium, though evidence is sparse. Haloperidol is the most commonly used antipsychotic. There is evidence that atypical antipsychotics such as risperidone, quetiapine, and olanzapine are as effective as haloperidol and may have beneficial side-effect profiles.[54] Antipsychotics contribute to QT prolongation and QT should be monitored prior to and during therapy. Revaluation of the patient's need for antipsychotic medications should occur at discharge.

Benzodiazepines may be considered in the setting of refractory-agitated delirium not responsive to antipsychotics and should not be used without antipsychotics.[55] Administration of benzodiazepines may worsen delirium and agitation, especially in elderly patients.

DYSGEUSIA

Dysgeusia, or the distortion of taste, is experienced often in HF patients, but underrecognized as patients and clinicians are unlikely to discuss it during the clinical encounter. Loss of senses such as taste is not only uncomfortable to the patient but can play a significant role in cachexia related to chronic illness. It can often be an insidious decline, further explaining the unlikelihood of patients discussing it. The screening question "Have you experienced problems with taste or smell in the past 12 months?" will help identify these patients.[56]

Hypothyroidism and thrush alter taste and should be ruled out. There are few known effective management strategies for non-cancer-related dysgeusia. Flavor enhancers such as salt, sugar, or monosodium glutamate (MSG) may be beneficial in chemotherapy patients, though these dietary modifications are likely to be limited in cardiac patients.[57] Alpha lipoic acid has produced mixed results in burning mouth syndrome, which is thought to be a neuropathy similar to idiopathic dysgeusia.[58,59] Cannabinoids may also help with taste alteration, though evidence currently exists only in advanced cancer patients.[60]

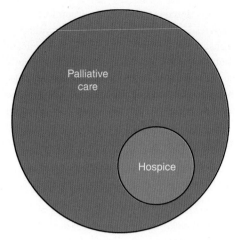

FIGURE 44-3 Hospice is a small part of what palliative care offers.

REFERRAL

PALLIATIVE MEDICINE CONSULTATION

Subspecialty palliative medicine prevalence in U.S. hospitals and health systems has increased dramatically since the year 2000, especially in hospitals with more than 50 beds. Currently over 67% of hospitals this size have a palliative care program.[61] Although palliative care services have greatly increased in the U.S. health care system in the past 20 years, they are not ubiquitous and thus it is imperative to research what services are available in your specific community/health care system. In general, subspecialty palliative care consultation should be sought in complicated situations of symptom management or delineation of goals of care. As palliative care resources are limited, it is important for all clinicians to provide primary palliative care when possible.

Outpatient palliative care clinics are becoming a valuable resource for patients with advanced HF. While data are currently limited, it is thought that outpatient palliative care can reduce symptom burden and enhance quality of life in patients with HF, similar to oncology patients utilizing palliative care.[62] Though a majority of patients treated by outpatient palliative clinics carry the diagnosis of cancer, some clinics rank HF as the most common diagnosis of their patient population.[63]

Timing of palliative care consultation can be a challenge for clinicians due to lack of guidelines. Prognostic uncertainty in HF may also make timing of consultation challenging. Clinicians may consider prognostic models such as the Seattle Heart Failure Model to identify palliative care needs in patients. Alternatively, an event-driven approach such as identifying patients with multiple hospitalizations, ICD discharge, a resuscitation event, or reaching NYHA class IV as baseline may be utilized.[64] Finally, palliative consultation should be considered for all HF patients with high symptom burden.

HOSPICE

Hospice is a Medicare benefit that offers palliative care to patients with a life expectancy of less than 6 months (Figure 44-3). Heart disease is the third leading primary diagnosis of hospice patients, accounting for 14.7% in 2014, behind cancer (36.6%) and dementia (14.8%).[65] It is offered to patients who no longer seek rehospitalization and wish to focus solely on quality of life. These patients will still have access to HF-directed therapies such as diuretics and often inotropes. Hospice care is mainly delivered in the home, though brief inpatient services are offered when needed. Hospice patients requiring 24-hour care that cannot be provided by family or friends may need to seek further support through hired care or a nursing home. Hospice services may be underutilized in the HF population given the challenges of prognostication. In general, patients with HF are eligible for hospice services if they experience NYHA class IV symptoms despite optimal treatment, though other comorbidities may be considered to support less symptomatic patients.[66]

PROGNOSIS

The 5-year mortality following the onset of HF approaches 50%.[67] Prognosis remains a challenge as the clinical course of HF tends to exhibit episodes of exacerbation and dramatic but incomplete recovery. Mortality is often underestimated in HF by both clinicians and patients. Clinical signs such as a worsening NYHA class, decline in functional status, cardiac cachexia, and depression are indicative of a worsening prognosis.[68]

Multivariate models such as the Seattle Heart Failure Model or the Enhanced Feedback for Effective Cardiac Treatment (EFFECT) model can provide more prognostic information, though may be of limited value due to differences in study populations. The Seattle Heart Failure Model can provide 1-, 2-, and 3-year survival but is limited to the outpatient setting in patients with few comorbidities. It may also be inaccurate when evaluating HF patients with a preserved ejection fraction. EFFECT can provide 30-day and 1-year risk for death and is more applicable to hospitalized patients.[68] Despite the availability of these tools, prognostication remains inexact and clinicians should be straightforward with patients about the uncertainty of HF prognostication. This emphasizes the importance of focusing on the patient's quality of life and minimal acceptable outcome, or the minimal quality of life that is acceptable to the patient that would support further pursuit of disease directed therapy.

PATIENT EDUCATION

COMMUNICATION

Patients prefer that physicians initiate discussions about prognosis at the time of diagnosis.[69] As HF is ultimately a terminal illness, advanced care planning is standard of care for primary care providers and cardiologists caring for patients with HF. Advanced care planning involves identifying a surrogate decision maker and facilitating communication between patient and surrogate, allowing the patient to express his or her desires for care when the patient's condition worsens.[70] Effective communication is achieved when discussions are initiated early and patients and families are not in crisis. Unfortunately the literature shows that resuscitation wishes are often overlooked, not elicited, or outdated.[71] This emphasizes the importance of discussing and periodically readdressing resuscitation preferences with HF patients. Sequelae of cardiac arrest, complications of mechanical circulatory support or the high likelihood of developing delirium in HF often lead to encephalopathy and loss of decision-making capacity. It is imperative that patients with advanced HF identify a surrogate decision maker. Moreover, early explicit discussions of medical treatment preferences with both the patient and the surrogate will increase the likelihood of the surrogate's accuracy when making medical decisions. In particular, patients and surrogates should discuss appropriate timing for the deactivation for ICDs, as it is unlikely for patients to have this discussion.[72] ICD deactivation is appropriate when the clinical focus has transitioned to comfort and patients have been clearly informed of the implications.[73] As pacemakers are likely to improve symptoms and will not reverse terminal events, they should not be turned off except in extremely rare events. Patient preferences and discussions with surrogates should be revisited periodically, especially following clinical status changes.

PREPAREDNESS PLANNING FOR MECHANICAL CIRCULATORY SUPPORT

Living with technology changes how a person lives and how a person dies. Due to the high morbidity and mortality associated with long-term mechanical circulatory support such as LVAD placement and mechanics of cardiac death with mechanical circulatory support, it is extremely important to explore goals and expectations with patients and their families who are considering this intervention. The complexity of care often required following implantation of mechanical circulatory support warrants planning beyond what most advanced directives can provide. Preparedness planning is a type of advanced care planning that has been developed to explore patient preferences regarding scenarios such as catastrophic LVAD-related complications, device failure, inadequate quality of life after LVAD, or debility due to comorbid conditions.[74] A successful preparedness plan addresses patient goals along with what a minimal acceptable outcome is in regard to quality of life. This acts as a guide to clinicians, family members, and the patient throughout the trajectory of illness with mechanical circulatory support.

PATIENT EDUCATION RESOURCES

- **Palliative Doctors (the American Academy of Hospice and Palliative Medicine's patient website):** http://palliativedoctors.org/
- **Advance Care Planning Packet for HF Patients through the Heart Failure Society of America:** http://www.hfsa.org/module-9/

PROVIDER RESOURCES

- **Palliative Care Fast Facts and Concepts:** http://www.mypcnow.org/fast-facts
- **National Palliative Care Research Center (includes MSAS and ESAS):** http://www.npcrc.org/content/25/Measurement-and-Evaluation-Tools.aspx

KEY POINTS

PAIN

- Opioids are often necessary as NSAIDs are contraindicated.
- Tailor opioid treatment to organ function (avoid morphine in renal failure).
- Maximize adjuvant medications (acetaminophen, neuropathic agents such as gabapentin).

DYSPNEA

- Dyspnea is subjective and cannot be measured by test results.
- Always incorporate nonpharmacologic management as cool air to face via fan or nasal cannula.
- Start low-dose opioid for refractory symptoms if patient is medically optimized.

DEPRESSION

- Differentiate between depression and symptoms of chronic illness.
- Consider nonpharmacologic management including cognitive behavioral therapy and caregiver support.
- Consider SSRI such as sertraline.

ANXIETY

- Common after ICD.
- Explore nonpharmacologic management including cognitive behavioral therapy and interdisciplinary support.
- Provide benzodiazepines for short-term relief.
- Add SSRIs for long-term management with continued anxiety-provoking stimulus.

FATIGUE

- Investigate possibility of comorbid conditions.
- Encourage prioritized physical activity.
- Consider methylphenidate in refractory cases.

LACK OF APPETITE

- Evaluate caloric intake and nutrition.
- Explore cannabinoids and corticosteroids to stimulate appetite.

NAUSEA

- Evaluate potential causes.
- Use ondansetron or haloperidol for empiric management.
- Start mirtazapine for impaired gastric emptying.
- Provide anticholinergic or antihistaminic drugs for vestibular-induced nausea.
- Use benzodiazepines only for anticipatory or anxiety-related nausea.

INSOMNIA

- Commonly found in patients with heart disease and can worsen other symptoms such as depression.
- Consider trial of nonpharmacologic options such as cognitive behavioral therapy.
- Consider melatonin or melatonin agonists as first-line therapy.
- Consider benzodiazepine receptor agonists and benzodiazepines for refractory symptoms.

DYSGEUSIA

- Screen advanced HF patients for disorders of taste.
- Rule out thrush.
- Suggest flavor enhancers consistent with a cardiac diet.
- Consider trial of alpha lipoic acid or cannabinoids in refractory cases.

CONSTIPATION

- Common in patients taking opioids.
- Constipation may contribute to other symptoms such as nausea, pain, and confusion.
- Start a scheduled stimulant laxative such as senna and have an osmotic laxative available as needed.

DELIRIUM

- Commonly found in HF patients and extremely common in ICU patients.
- Explore underlying cause and reverse if possible.
- Provide frequent orientation and natural day-night cycles.
- Consider antipsychotics such as haloperidol.

REFERENCES

1. Heron M. Deaths: leading causes for 2012. *Natl Vital Stat Rep.* 2015;64:1-93.
2. Mozaffarian D, Benjamin EJ, Go AS, et al. Heart disease and stroke statistics—2016 update: a report from the American Heart Association. *Circulation.* 2016;133:e38-e60.
3. Braun LT, Grady KL, Kutner JS, et al. Palliative care and cardiovascular disease and stroke: a policy statement from the American Heart Association/American Stroke Association. *Circulation.* 2016;134(11):e198-e225.
4. Oxford English Dictionary. "palliate, v.": Oxford University Press.
5. Palliativedoctors.org website. http://palliativedoctors.org/. Accessed 2016.
6. Solano JP, Gomes B, Higginson IJ. A comparison of symptom prevalence in far advanced cancer, AIDS, heart disease, chronic obstructive pulmonary disease and renal disease. *J Pain Symptom Manage.* 2006;31:58-69.
7. Bruera E, Kuehn N, Miller MJ, Selmser P, Macmillan K. The Edmonton Symptom Assessment System (ESAS): a simple method for the assessment of palliative care patients. *J Palliat Care.* 1991;7:6-9.

8. Portenoy RK, Thaler HT, Kornblith AB, et al. The Memorial Symptom Assessment Scale: an instrument for the evaluation of symptom prevalence, characteristics and distress. *Eur J Cancer.* 1994;30A:1326-1336.

9. Clinical Practice Guidelines for Quality Palliative Care. Pittsburgh, PA: National Consensus Project for Quality Palliative Care; 2013.

10. Hallenbeck J. Pathophysiologies of dyspnea explained: why might opioids relieve dyspnea and not hasten death? *J Palliat Med.* 2012;15:848-853.

11. Liss HP, Grant BJ. The effect of nasal flow on breathlessness in patients with chronic obstructive pulmonary disease. *Am Rev Respir Dis.* 1988;137:1285-1288.

12. Schwartzstein RM, Lahive K, Pope A, Weinberger SE, Weiss JW. Cold facial stimulation reduces breathlessness induced in normal subjects. *Am Rev Respir Dis.* 1987;136:58-61.

13. Captopril Multicenter Research Group. A placebo-controlled trial of captopril in refractory chronic congestive heart failure. *J Am Coll Cardiol.* 1983;2:755-763.

14. Johnson MJ, McDonagh TA, Harkness A, McKay SE, Dargie HJ. Morphine for the relief of breathlessness in patients with chronic heart failure—a pilot study. *Eur J Heart Fail.* 2002;4:753-756.

15. Radbruch L, Strasser F, Elsner F, et al. Fatigue in palliative care patients—an EAPC approach. *Palliat Med.* 2008;22:13-32.

16. Harris JD. Fatigue in chronically ill patients. *Curr Opin Support Palliat Care.* 2008;2:180-186.

17. Goodlin SJ. Palliative care in congestive heart failure. *J Am Coll Cardiol.* 2009;54:386-396.

18. Setoguchi S, Glynn RJ, Stedman M, Flavell CM, Levin R, Stevenson LW. Hospice, opiates, and acute care service use among the elderly before death from heart failure or cancer. *Am Heart J.* 2010;160:139-144.

19. Heerdink ER, Leufkens HG, Herings RM, Ottervanger JP, Stricker BH, Bakker A. NSAIDs associated with increased risk of congestive heart failure in elderly patients taking diuretics. *Arch Intern Med.* 1998;158:1108-1112.

20. Gasche Y, Daali Y, Fathi M, et al. Codeine intoxication associated with ultrarapid CYP2D6 metabolism. *N Engl J Med.* 2004;351:2827-2831.

21. Smith HS. Opioid metabolism. *Mayo Clin Proc.* 2009;84:613-624.

22. Novick DM, Kreek MJ, Arns PA, Lau LL, Yancovitz SR, Gelb AM. Effect of severe alcoholic liver disease on the disposition of methadone in maintenance patients. *Alcohol Clin Exp Res.* 1985;9:349-354.

23. Kreek MJ, Schecter AJ, Gutjahr CL, Hecht M. Methadone use in patients with chronic renal disease. *Drug Alcohol Depend.* 1980;5:197-205.

24. Morrison R, Goldstein N. How Should Opioids Be Started and Titrated in Routine Outpatient Settings. *Evidence-Based Practice of Palliative Medicine.* Philadelphia, PA: Elsevier Health Sciences; 2013:5.

25. Finnerup NB, Attal N, Haroutounian S, et al. Pharmacotherapy for neuropathic pain in adults: a systematic review and meta-analysis. *Lancet Neurol.* 2015;14:162-173.

26. Teply RM, Packard KA, White ND, Hilleman DE, DiNicolantonio JJ. Treatment of depression in patients with concomitant cardiac disease. *Prog Cardiovasc Dis.* 2016;58:514-528.

27. Gilron I, Baron R, Jensen T. Neuropathic pain: principles of diagnosis and treatment. *Mayo Clin Proc.* 2015;90:532-545.

28. Rutledge T, Reis VA, Linke SE, Greenberg BH, Mills PJ. Depression in heart failure a meta-analytic review of prevalence, intervention effects, and associations with clinical outcomes. *J Am Coll Cardiol.* 2006;48:1527-1537.

29. Irwin S, Block S. What treatments are effective for depression in the palliative care setting? In: Goldstein N, Morrison R, eds. *Evidence-Based Practice of Palliative Medicine.* Philadelphia, PA: Elsevier Health Sciences; 2013:183.

30. O'Connor CM, Jiang W, Kuchibhatla M, et al. Safety and efficacy of sertraline for depression in patients with heart failure: results of the SADHART-CHF (Sertraline Against Depression and Heart Disease in Chronic Heart Failure) trial. *J Am Coll Cardiol.* 2010;56:692-699.

31. Woods SW, Tesar GE, Murray GB, Cassem NH. Psychostimulant treatment of depressive disorders secondary to medical illness. *J Clin Psychiatry.* 1986;47:12-15.

32. Schelleman H, Bilker WB, Kimmel SE, et al. Methylphenidate and risk of serious cardiovascular events in adults. *Am J Psychiatry.* 2012;169:178-185.

33. Sears SF, Todaro JF, Lewis TS, Sotile W, Conti JB. Examining the psychosocial impact of implantable cardioverter defibrillators: a literature review. *Clin Cardiol.* 1999;22:481-489.

34. Bilge AK, Ozben B, Demircan S, Cinar M, Yilmaz E, Adalet K. Depression and anxiety status of patients with implantable cardioverter defibrillator and precipitating factors. *Pacing Clin Electrophysiol.* 2006;29:619-626.

35. Barraclough J. ABC of palliative care. Depression, anxiety, and confusion. *BMJ.* 1997;315:1365-1368.

36. Errington-Evans N. Acupuncture for anxiety. *CNS Neurosci Ther.* 2012;18:277-284.

37. Redeker NS, Jeon S, Muench U, Campbell D, Walsleben J, Rapoport DM. Insomnia symptoms and daytime function in stable heart failure. *Sleep.* 2010;33:1210-1216.

38. Montgomery P, Dennis J. Cognitive behavioural interventions for sleep problems in adults aged 60+. *Cochrane Database Syst Rev.* 2003:CD003161.

39. Roth T, Seiden D, Sainati S, Wang-Weigand S, Zhang J, Zee P. Effects of ramelteon on patient-reported sleep latency in older adults with chronic insomnia. *Sleep Med.* 2006;7:312-318.

40. Buscemi N, Vandermeer B, Hooton N, et al. The efficacy and safety of exogenous melatonin for primary sleep disorders. A meta-analysis. *J Gen Intern Med.* 2005;20:1151-1158.

41. Nowell PD, Mazumdar S, Buysse DJ, Dew MA, Reynolds CF, Kupfer DJ. Benzodiazepines and zolpidem for chronic insomnia: a meta-analysis of treatment efficacy. *JAMA.* 1997;278:2170-2177.

42. Buscemi N, Vandermeer B, Friesen C, et al. The efficacy and safety of drug treatments for chronic insomnia

in adults: a meta-analysis of RCTs. *J Gen Intern Med.* 2007;22:1335-1350.

43. Librach SL, Bouvette M, De Angelis C, et al. Consensus recommendations for the management of constipation in patients with advanced, progressive illness. *J Pain Symptom Manage.* 2010;40:761-773.

44. Twycross R, Sykes N, Mihalyo M, Wilcock A. Stimulant laxatives and opioid-induced constipation. *J Pain Symptom Manage.* 2012;43:306-313.

45. Wood GJ, Shega JW, Lynch B, Von Roenn JH. Management of intractable nausea and vomiting in patients at the end of life: "I was feeling nauseous all of the time . . . nothing was working." *JAMA.* 2007;298:1196-1207.

46. Goldstein N, Morrison R. *Evidence-Based Practice of Palliative Medicine.* Philadelphia, PA: Elsevier; 2013.

47. Ruiz Garcia V, López-Briz E, Carbonell Sanchis R, Gonzalvez Perales JL, Bort-Marti S. Megestrol acetate for treatment of anorexia-cachexia syndrome. *Cochrane Database Syst Rev.* 2013:CD004310.

48. von Haehling S, Lainscak M, Springer J, Anker SD. Cardiac cachexia: a systematic overview. *Pharmacol Ther.* 2009;121:227-252.

49. Miller S, McNutt L, McCann MA, McCorry N. Use of corticosteroids for anorexia in palliative medicine: a systematic review. *J Palliat Med.* 2014;17:482-485.

50. Marcantonio ER, Kiely DK, Simon SE, et al. Outcomes of older people admitted to postacute facilities with delirium. *J Am Geriatr Soc.* 2005;53:963-969.

51. Maldonado JR. Pathoetiological model of delirium: a comprehensive understanding of the neurobiology of delirium and an evidence-based approach to prevention and treatment. *Crit Care Clin.* 2008;24:789-856, ix.

52. Whellan DJ, Goodlin SJ, Dickinson MG, et al. End-of-life care in patients with heart failure. *J Card Fail.*2014;20:121-134.

53. Tabet N, Howard R. Non-pharmacological interventions in the prevention of delirium. *Age and Ageing.* 2009;38(4):374-379.

54. Lonergan E, Britton AM, Luxenberg J, Wyller T. Antipsychotics for delirium. *Cochrane Database Syst Rev.* 2007:CD005594.

55. Weckmann M, Morrison R. In: Goldstein N, Morrison R, eds. What Pharmacological Treatments Are Effective for Delirium? *Evidence-Based Practice of Palliative Medicine.* Philadelphia, PA: Elsevier Health Sciences; 2013:205-210.

56. Syed Q, Hendler KT, Koncilja K. The impact of aging and medical status on dysgeusia. *Am J Med.* 2016;129:753.e1-e6.

57. Wismer WV. Assessing alterations in taste and their impact on cancer care. *Curr Opin Support Palliat Care.* 2008;2:282-287.

58. Sun A, Wu KM, Wang YP, Lin HP, Chen HM, Chiang CP. Burning mouth syndrome: a review and update. *J Oral Pathol Med.* 2013;42:649-655.

59. Femiano F, Scully C, Gombos F. Idiopathic dysgeusia; an open trial of alpha lipoic acid (ALA) therapy. *Int J Oral Maxillofac Surg.* 2002;31:625-658.

60. Strasser F, Luftner D, Possinger K, et al. Comparison of orally administered cannabis extract and delta-9-tetrahydrocannabinol in treating patients with cancer-related anorexia-cachexia syndrome: a multicenter, phase III, randomized, double-blind, placebo-controlled clinical trial from the Cannabis-In-Cachexia-Study-Group. *J Clin Oncol.* 2006;24:3394-3400.

61. Dumanovsky T, Augustin R, Rogers M, Lettang K, Meier DE, Morrison RS. The Growth of Palliative Care in U.S. Hospitals: A Status Report. *J Palliat Med.* 2016;19:8-15.

62. Evangelista LS, Lombardo D, Malik S, Ballard-Hernandez J, Motie M, Liao S. Examining the effects of an outpatient palliative care consultation on symptom burden, depression, and quality of life in patients with symptomatic heart failure. *J Card Fail.* 2012;18:894-899.

63. Smith AK, Thai JN, Bakitas MA, et al. The diverse landscape of palliative care clinics. *J Palliat Med.* 2013;16:661-668.

64. Lemond L, Allen LA. Palliative care and hospice in advanced heart failure. *Prog Cardiovasc Dis.* 2011;54:168-178.

65. National Hospice and Palliative Care Organization. NHPCO Facts and Figures: Hospice Care in America. Alexandria, VA.

66. The National Hospice Organization. Medical guidelines for determining prognosis in selected non-cancer diseases. *Hosp J.* 1996;11:47-63.

67. Levy D, Kenchaiah S, Larson MG, et al. Long-term trends in the incidence of and survival with heart failure. *N Engl J Med.* 2002;347:1397-1402.

68. Stuart B. Palliative care and hospice in advanced heart failure. *J Palliat Med.* 2007;10:210-228.

69. Caldwell PH, Arthur HM, Demers C. Preferences of patients with heart failure for prognosis communication. *Can J Cardiol.* 2007;23:791-796.

70. NCPO advanced dirrectives. http://www.nhpco.org/advance-care-planning.

71. Krumholz HM, Phillips RS, Hamel MB, et al. Resuscitation preferences among patients with severe congestive heart failure: results from the SUPPORT project. Study to Understand Prognoses and Preferences for Outcomes and Risks of Treatments. *Circulation.* 1998;98:648-655.

72. Kelley AS, Reid MC, Miller DH, Fins JJ, Lachs MS. Implantable cardioverter-defibrillator deactivation at the end of life: a physician survey. *Am Heart J.* 2009;157:702-708.e1.

73. Mueller PS, Hook CC, Hayes DL. Ethical analysis of withdrawal of pacemaker or implantable cardioverter-defibrillator support at the end of life. *Mayo Clin Proc.* 2003;78:959-963.

74. Swetz KM, Kamal AH, Matlock DD, et al. Preparedness planning before mechanical circulatory support: a "how-to" guide for palliative medicine clinicians. *J Pain Symptom Manage.* 2014;47:926-935.e6.

45 EXERCISE AND REHABILITATION

Cemal Ozemek, PhD, CEP
Ross Arena, PhD, PT
Sam Bond, MS
Karla M. Daniels, MS

■ PATIENT CASE

A 64-year-old heart failure patient with a reduced ejection fraction complains of having to stop and rest after walking two city blocks and has difficulty carrying groceries into his house. He does not complain of feeling shortness of breath at rest or peripheral edema, his medication regimen is optimized, and he reports that he is sedentary most of the day. As a result he is referred to a phase 2 cardiac rehabilitation program, where he performs a cardiopulmonary exercise test to assess his starting functional capacity and to measure his maximal heart rate in order to optimize his exercise prescription. After regularly attending 3 cardiac rehabilitation sessions per week for 12 weeks and walking on at least one additional day on his own for 30 minutes. His maximal oxygen consumption assessed by the cardiopulmonary exercise test increased from 16.4 mL/kg/min to 20.5 mL/kg/min. The patient also reports that he is now able to walk multiple blocks without fatigue and is able to perform activities of daily living without issue. He is encouraged by the results and reports that he will continue to walk 4-5 days per week for 30-45 minutes at his local community fitness center.

INTRODUCTION

Prior to the late 1980s it was common practice to discourage heart failure (HF) patients from participating in exercise and/or physical exertion. There was a widespread belief that placing additional stress on an already weak and damaged heart would have deleterious effects and ultimately shorten the lifespan of the HF patient. However, countless investigations have subsequently demonstrated exercise to not only be a safe form of therapy, but to also minimize exacerbations of classic HF symptoms (ie, dyspnea and fatigue), thereby improving New York Heart Association (NYHA) functional class. There is also robust evidence suggesting reductions in overall mortality and hospitalizations in exercising HF patients compared to their nonexercising counterparts. Numerous mid- to small-sized studies, meta-analyses incorporating a number of those studies,[1] and a large-scale randomized clinical trial (Heart Failure—A Controlled Trial Investigative Outcomes of exercise training; HF-ACTION) consistently suggest reductions in mortality ranging from 15% to 40%.

This chapter will (1) elucidate the acute and chronic responses to aerobic exercise, (2) summarize exercise and functional testing protocols, (3) interpret the exercise testing response, and (4) utilize information garnered from points 1 to 3 to formulate an exercise prescription. Additionally, this chapter will provide an introduction to cardiac rehabilitation practices and common special exercise considerations for HF patients.

ACUTE RESPONSES TO EXERCISE

Increased myocardial oxygen demand during exercise requires coordinated adjustments and balance between the cardiovascular (CV), pulmonary, and central nervous systems to provide appropriate oxygen delivery and carbon dioxide clearance (Figure 45-1). Congestive HF is characterized by decreased left ventricular (LV) function, and an inability to meet systemic oxygen demand with exertion. These patients are frequently burdened by comorbidities such as pulmonary disease, coronary atherosclerosis, and renal dysfunction that further interfere with their exercise capacity. Depending upon a patient's classification of HF, their activities of daily living are often limited by dyspnea, chest discomfort, or general fatigue, significantly impacting their overall functional capacity and quality of life. The following section will provide an overview of the acute responses to exercise in this patient population.

CARDIOVASCULAR RESPONSE TO EXERCISE

Exercise requires adequate blood flow to the active muscles via central cardiac pump function. Increases in cardiac output (Q), determined by heart rate (HR) and stroke volume (SV) occur with exertion ($Q = HR \times SV$). Furthermore, redistribution of blood flow from inactive tissue, oxygen delivery and carbon dioxide clearance, and appropriate responses by the sympathetic and parasympathetic nervous systems all play a role in the body's ability to do work. The Fick principle quantifies both central cardiac function as well as peripheral skeletal muscle function by relating oxygen consumption (VO_2) to Q and arteriovenous oxygen (a-vO_2) difference in the following formula: $VO_2 \times Q = (a$-vO_2 diff$)$. Stress to the endothelial walls due to increased blood flow during activity promotes the release of nitric oxide (NO), causing systemic vasodilation; when coupled with increased skeletal muscle contraction during activity, this vasodilation leads to increased venous return. By means of the Frank-Starling mechanism, augmented venous return causes greater stretching of the ventricular walls, higher end-diastolic volume, increased contractility, and subsequently increased SV. Stimulation of the sympathetic nervous system and parasympathetic withdrawal lead to increases in the HR response during activity. Increased HR and systolic blood pressure augment Q up to 5 times that required at rest until a steady state or plateau is attained. Additionally, increases in Q are dependent upon HR alone at intensity levels beyond 40% to 50% maximal VO_2, due to a plateau in SV during sustained activity.

Oxygen delivery to the active muscle is enhanced by peripheral vasodilation, increased capillary flow, and coordination with the pulmonary system. Once the intensity or duration of activity

Physiological Responses to Acute Aerobic Exercise

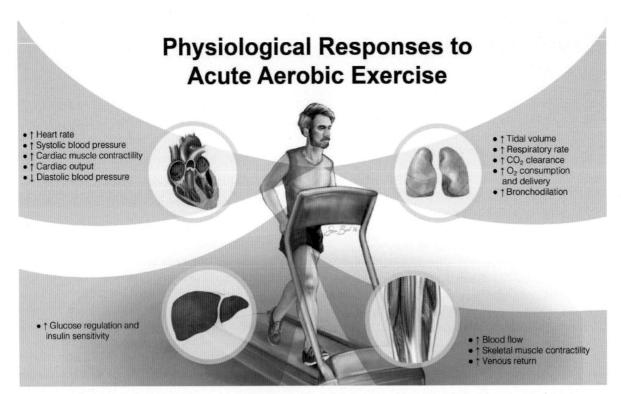

- ↑ Heart rate
- ↑ Systolic blood pressure
- ↑ Cardiac muscle contractility
- ↑ Cardiac output
- ↓ Diastolic blood pressure

- ↑ Tidal volume
- ↑ Respiratory rate
- ↑ CO_2 clearance
- ↑ O_2 consumption and delivery
- ↑ Bronchodilation

- ↑ Glucose regulation and insulin sensitivity

- ↑ Blood flow
- ↑ Skeletal muscle contractility
- ↑ Venous return

FIGURE 45-1 Cardiovascular, pulmonary, metabolic, and skeletal muscle physiological responses to acute aerobic exercise from rest.

increases beyond the CV system's ability to match oxygen demand, metabolism progressively shifts away from aerobic to anaerobic until the point of fatigue. This metabolic shift is highly dependent upon the intensity level of exercise, which can be quantified by the percentage of maximal oxygen consumption (VO_{2max}). It is also dependent upon pulmonary function (ie, the efficiency of oxygen and carbon dioxide exchange in the alveoli and subsequent oxygen delivery to the working muscle), as well as mitochondrial function and capillary oxygen and carbon dioxide exchange.

Additional factors, such as baroreceptor and chemoreceptor stimulation, thermoregulation, and levels of hydration all play a role in the body's response to activity, particularly during prolonged, submaximal exercise that frequently leads to CV drift, where HR, SV, and systolic blood pressure show an initial increase until they plateau during steady-state exercise, with a subsequent negative drift due to continued vasodilation and fluid loss.

PULMONARY RESPONSE

Pulmonary ventilation increases during exercise through increased tidal volume (depth of breath) and respiratory rate. Bronchodilation, or the expansion of the bronchial airway, leads to increased pulmonary ventilation (oxygen/carbon dioxide exchange). The difference between alveolar oxygen pressure and arterial oxygen pressure (a-vO_2 diff) increases up to 20 mm Hg during exercise due to ventilation-perfusion mismatch, oxygen-diffusing limitations with prolonged activity, and low mixed-venous oxygen. Ventilatory demand is typically dependent upon the intensity of exercise, lactic acid accumulation, and the degree of pulmonary dead space. In healthy adults, ventilation is approximately 70% of the maximum voluntary ventilation (MVV) due to a plateau in tidal breathing requiring increases in respiratory rate until the point of fatigue.

PATHOPHYSIOLOGY IN HEART FAILURE

Decreased LV function, diastolic dysfunction, ventricular hypertrophy, and general weakening of the cardiac tissue are all common traits of HF, and have a substantial effect on the CV response to exercise. Blunted or hypotensive blood pressure responses, chronotropic incompetence, and early fatigue are often seen among these patients. Due to cardiac remodeling and weakening, LV ejection fraction and therefore SV and Q can be markedly reduced in patients with HF, with downstream effects of inadequate oxygen supply to the working muscles. Patients with HF also have increased fluid retention around the lungs, interfering with the oxygen and carbon dioxide exchange in the alveoli.

More often than not, these individuals are on a cocktail of medications including diuretics, beta blockers, and angiotensin-converting enzyme (ACE) inhibitors. These medications typically result in a decreased HR and blood pressure response to exercise, causing premature muscle fatigue and dyspnea on exertion due to the body's inability to extract oxygen and clear carbon dioxide. Cachexia, or skeletal muscle weakness and atrophy, is commonly seen among the more decompensated HF patients. Cachectic HF patients frequently complain of premature muscle fatigue during activity and muscle soreness following bouts of exercise attributable to decreased venous return from low muscle tone, premature lactate accumulation, and mitochondrial dysfunction. Of note are reductions in mitochondrial fusion proteins, which are integral in mitochondrial quality control by promoting the exchange and/or cross-complementation of mitochondrial DNA between functional and dysfunctional organelles.[2] Consequently, this contributes to impairments in skeletal muscle oxidative capacity.

Furthermore, valvular disease is not uncommon in this population, and can lend to hypotensive responses in systolic blood pressure with exertion. Similarly, cardiomyopathy, also frequently seen concomitantly among HF patients, is often characterized by a small or underfilled LV, which prohibits the heart from filling adequately and therefore delivering required levels of oxygen to the peripheral and pulmonary systems. Patients with comorbid coronary artery disease can exhibit similar drops in systolic blood pressure due to ischemia, or a lack of blood flow to the coronary arteries. In an effort to maintain Q, there is often an exaggerated HR response to exercise in these patients.

PHYSIOLOGICAL ADAPTATIONS TO EXERCISE

Responses to chronic exercise at a moderate (ie, 60%-75% of peak heart rate [HR$_{peak}$] or 40%-60% of HR reserve [HRR]) intensity, 3 sessions per week, for 12 weeks, have been readily studied in HF patients. The numerous physiological adaptations to regular moderate-intensity continuous training (MCT) encompass improvements to the vascular, musculoskeletal, neurohormonal, and pulmonary systems (Figure 45-2). These adaptations collectively contribute to increases in cardiorespiratory fitness (CRF), a highly predictive marker of morbidity and mortality. It is generally thought that the positive responses to ~12 weeks of MCT in the HF population are primarily attributed to peripheral adaptations, as there are modest, if any, changes in cardiac hemodynamic variables,

such as cardiac output (Q) and stroke volume (SV). However, favorable cardiac remodeling and functional changes have been shown to occur following ≥6 months of regular, aerobic MCT.[3]

There has also been a growing interest in studying high-intensity interval training (HIIT) in HF patients. HIIT is characterized by performing intermittent bouts (1-4 minutes) of near maximal (ie, 85%-90% of HR$_{peak}$) efforts, separated by periods (~3 minutes) of active recovery (ie, 50% HR$_{peak}$). The seminal study by Wisloff et al demonstrated a 46% increase in peak VO$_2$ in HF patients who completed the HIIT protocol compared to 14% in those who completed the MCT protocol.[4] Although there are limited large-scale studies evaluating the safety of HIIT in HF patients, initial findings from a Norwegian study evaluating the safety of HIIT compared to MCT revealed CV adverse event rates of 1 per 23,182 and 1 per 129,456 patient-hours, respectively.[5] However, due to the low event rate, there was limited power to compare risks, warranting further investigation.

CARDIOVASCULAR ADAPTATIONS

Vascular

Improvements in endothelial-dependent vasodilation can be expected in response to chronic MCT in HF patients. Impairments in endothelial-dependent vasodilation observed in HF patients are partly due to reductions in NO, a key modulator of vascular function and health. One mechanism responsible for these reductions is attributed to chronically elevated levels of reactive oxygen species (ROS) that uncouple the NO-producing enzyme, endothelial NO synthase (eNOS). Shear stress along the lining of the vascular endothelium, elicited by exercise, promotes the expression of eNOS, thereby increasing NO production and improving endothelial function. Training-induced improvements in endothelial function also correlate with increased CRF in patients with HF with reduced ejection fraction (HFrEF), but this relationship in HF with preserved ejection fraction (HFpEF) is less clear due to limited studies. Further, although there have been comparatively fewer studies that have assessed endothelial function after HIIT, the available data suggest a greater improvement compared to MCT.

Cardiac

MCT, performed 3 days per week for 12 weeks, has limited positive or negative effects on cardiac remodeling or functional performance. However, longer-duration exercise interventions, particularly ≥6 months, can partially reverse cardiac chamber enlargement and reduce chamber volume at diastole. HIIT in HFrEF has been demonstrated to elicit superior cardiac structural and function improvements in only 12 weeks. Specifically, greater improvements in cardiac hemodynamics have been observed in the HIIT group with LV end-diastolic and systolic volumes declining by 18% and 25%, respectively, and ejection fraction increasing by 10 percentage points.[4] While only a few studies have performed HIIT in HFpEF patients, little to no improvements have yet been documented. A limiting factor may be the short duration (4 weeks) of studies conducting similar protocols.

SKELETAL MUSCLE ADAPTATIONS

Aerobic exercise significantly improves the skeletal muscle's ability to extract and utilize oxygen to support the increased metabolic demands of physical activity. Factors that contribute to improved

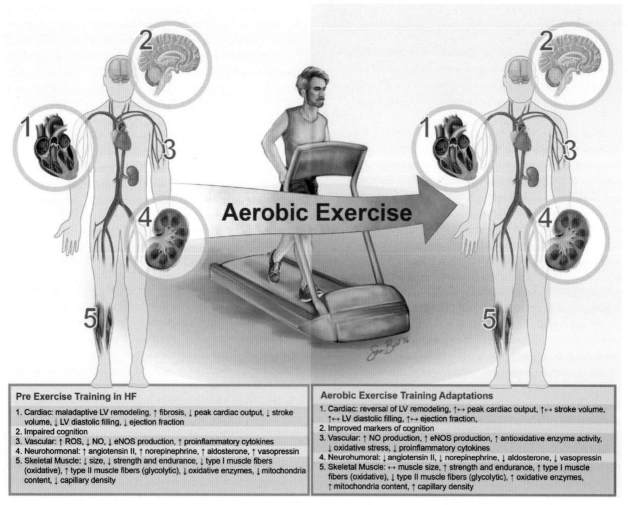

Pre Exercise Training in HF

1. Cardiac: maladaptive LV remodeling, ↑ fibrosis, ↓ peak cardiac output, ↓ stroke volume, ↓ LV diastolic filling, ↓ ejection fraction
2. Impaired cognition
3. Vascular: ↑ ROS, ↓ NO, ↓ eNOS production, ↑ proinflammatory cytokines
4. Neurohormonal: ↑ angiotensin II, ↑ norepinephrine, ↑ aldosterone, ↑ vasopressin
5. Skeletal Muscle: ↓ size, ↓ strength and endurance, ↓ type I muscle fibers (oxidative), ↑ type II muscle fibers (glycolytic), ↓ oxidative enzymes, ↓ mitochondria content, ↓ capillary density

Aerobic Exercise Training Adaptations

1. Cardiac: reversal of LV remodeling, ↑↔ peak cardiac output, ↑↔ stroke volume, ↑↔ LV diastolic filling, ↑↔ ejection fraction,
2. Improved markers of cognition
3. Vascular: ↑ NO production, ↑ eNOS production, ↑ antioxidative enzyme activity, ↓ oxidative stress, ↓ proinflammatory cytokines
4. Neurohumoral: ↓ angiotensin II, ↓ norepinephrine, ↓ aldosterone, ↓ vasopressin
5. Skeletal Muscle: ↔ muscle size, ↑ strength and endurance, ↑ type I muscle fibers (oxidative), ↓ type II muscle fibers (glycolytic), ↑ oxidative enzymes, ↑ mitochondria content, ↑ capillary density

FIGURE 45-2 System-specific, physiologic adaptations to an aerobic exercise training program in heart failure patients.

oxygen handling primarily include an increase in capillarization, mitochondrial density, and oxidative enzyme activity. Furthermore, HF patients have a preferential type II (glycolytic) muscle fiber distribution, whereas healthy age-matched individuals have a greater distribution of type I (oxidative) muscle fibers. Chronic exercise interventions in HF have induced a preferential "switch" to the more oxidative muscle fiber phenotype, which has a greater resistance to fatigue. These collective adaptations are key in limiting a pH imbalance and excessive lactate buildup, which are known to induce premature fatigue and breathlessness upon exertion.

NEUROHORMONAL ADAPTATIONS

The chronically elevated levels of circulating neurohormones, in response to inadequate cardiac function in HF patients, induce systemic abnormalities. Aerobic exercise can reverse this autonomic dysfunction and decrease plasma norepinephrine, angiotensin II, aldosterone, and vasopressin, while simultaneously increasing parasympathetic tone.[6] Reductions in these vasoconstrictive hormones reduce the afterload the heart must contract against to expel blood to the periphery, making Q more effective and efficient. Furthermore, vasorelaxation of restrictive arteries in the muscle beds enhances skeletal muscle blood flow and oxygen extraction, resulting in enhanced exercise tolerance.

Reactive Oxygen Species and Inflammation

The increased expression of ROS and inflammatory cytokines (tumor necrosis factor alpha, TNF-α and interleukin 6, IL-6) contribute to myocardial and skeletal muscle wasting and functional insufficiencies. MCT, in both HFrEF and HFpEF, attenuates ROS and inflammatory markers, while increasing free radical scavenging enzymes and antioxidants (ie, superoxide dismutase, glutathione peroxidase, glutathione, and catalase).[7]

RESPIRATORY MUSCLE ADAPTATIONS

Insufficient respiratory function and fatigue can contribute to exacerbating HF symptoms (ie, dyspnea and exercise intolerance) by initiating the respiratory muscle metaboreflex, which increases sympathetic nervous activity and vasoconstriction, thereby limiting pulmonary and peripheral gas exchange during exercise. Reduced inspiratory muscle endurance and inspiratory muscle strength are known to closely correlate with peak VO_2 and are independent predictors of mortality in HF. Inspiratory muscle training is performed using a small handheld device with adjustable inspiratory pressure threshold loads, which prohibits the subject from inhaling until a set negative pressure is overcome. Most investigations have set intensity thresholds to roughly 30% of maximal inspiratory pressure and have documented favorable results, which include increased (1) QOL, (2) balance, (3) peripheral muscle strength and blood flow, (4) peak VO_2, (5) 6-minute walk test (6MWT) distance, (6) ventilation, (7) oxygen uptake efficiency slope (OUES), and (8) circulatory power. In addition, the results include reduced (1) dyspnea with exertion, (2) peripheral muscle sympathetic nervous system activity, (3) resting HR, (4) respiratory rate, (5) minute ventilation/carbon dioxide production (VE/VCO_2) slope, and (6) recovery oxygen kinetic times.[8]

Cardiopulmonary Coupling

Inefficient ventilation, as assessed by VE/VCO_2 slope (slope >36), as well as the OUES (slope <1.4), is a robust prognostic marker in HF patients. An exaggerated ventilatory response relative to VCO_2 and/or VO_2 during exercise in HF patients occurs due to a number of systemic insufficiencies in handling exercise by-products and an associated reduced lung perfusion. Aerobic exercise training can significantly reduce the VE/VCO_2 slope by 14% to 18% and increase OUES by roughly 20%.[9,10] Additionally, exercise oscillatory ventilation (EOV), an equally, if not more sensitive prognostic marker in symptomatic HF patients, can also improve after exercise training. Presently in roughly 20% to 50% of HF patients, EOV occurs in response to cyclic changes in arterial CO_2 and O_2 tension. The periodic breathing pattern associated with EOV is initiated by a reduced cardiac output response to exercise, increasing arterial CO_2 tension, which is then detected by chemoreceptors that initiate an exaggerated ventilator response. This effectively lowers the arterial CO_2 tension, resulting in an abnormally lowered breathing rate and restarting the irregular ventilation cycle.[11] Twelve weeks of moderate intensity exercise, performed 3 times per week for 45 minutes per session, has been shown to eliminate the presence of EOV in 37 of 52 participating patients.[12] These improvements are generally thought to be attributed to increased (1) capillary density, (2) peripheral blood flow, (3) mitochondrial density, (4) alveolar-capillary membrane perfusion and capillary blood, and

(5) slow-twitch fibers. The improvements are also attributed to decreased lactic acidosis and vascular resistance.

EXERCISE ASSESSMENT

Exercise assessment is conducted in order to quantify functional capacity or identify underlying ischemic or arrhythmogenic disease responsible for symptoms such as chest pain or shortness of breath. A variety of exercise testing modalities exist, including standard treadmill testing, stress echocardiography, nuclear medicine stress tests, and cardiopulmonary exercise testing (CPX). CPX is the hallmark assessment for function, particularly in HF patients, and the only test that evaluates central cardiac, peripheral skeletal, and pulmonary parameters; therefore, CPX will be the highlight of this section. Table 45-1 describes each testing modality and the most commonly evaluated indications for testing.

CARDIOPULMONARY EXERCISE TESTING

In patients with HF, CPX has repeatedly proven to provide significant clinical prognostic value. The main objective of CPX is to obtain a direct measurement of VO_2. Various formulas taking into consideration factors such as age, height, weight, and gender provide percent predicted values of VO_2. When a functional limitation is apparent through low achievement of these predicted values, metabolic data obtained during CPX can be further delineated to determine the underlying cause of this limitation. The following section will provide an overview of testing protocols and the most commonly evaluated parameters.

Testing Procedures

During CPX, patients breathe through a mouthpiece with their nose clipped, while their electrocardiogram (ECG) and HR are continuously monitored. Manual blood pressure readings are obtained every 1 to 3 minutes during the test, and ratings of perceived exertion (RPE) are evaluated. Testing typically involves the use of a treadmill or cycle ergometer, with the workload increasing gradually until the point of fatigue, or clinically significant reasons for test termination arise, such as abnormally high blood pressure responses (systolic blood pressure >200 mm Hg or diastolic blood pressure >114 mm Hg), a drop in systolic blood pressure >10 mm Hg, moderate to severe chest pain, ischemic ECG changes, or clinically significant arrhythmias such as sustained ventricular tachycardia or high-grade atrioventricular blocks. It is important that the exercise protocol be as gradual as possible, as protocols with large changes in workload between stages, or stages that are held for several minutes, have negative effects on the linearity of the metabolic data. For example, a standard Bruce protocol that involves 3-minute stages will lead to more steady-state conditions, a potential plateau in metabolic readings, and has been demonstrated to produce inaccurate data. Ramping treadmill and cycle ergometer protocols allow for linear increases in workload and therefore metabolic readings that are more easily analyzed and provide a better depiction of underlying substrate use for energy (aerobic vs anaerobic). Cycle ergometry typically uses watts-per-minute protocols from 5 W/min up to 25 W/min, with revolutions per minute held at a constant rate (ie, 60 rpms), while ramping treadmill protocols typically change modestly in workload every 30 to 60 seconds.

Furthermore, testing protocols should be determined such that the patient is exercising for approximately 6 to 12 minutes. Research has shown that exercise duration below 6 minutes is often not sufficient enough to reach a steady state, whereas durations beyond 12 minutes often lead to submaximal exercise achievement, as the patient stops due to discomforts or even boredom rather than true fatigue.

Testing Considerations

Patients with HF frequently present with orthopedic limitations or gait instability due to skeletal muscle atrophy or cachexia, hallmarks of higher grade HF. Testing modalities should take into consideration these limitations, as well as consistency in subsequent testing; for example, elderly and frail HF patients should be tested using a cycle ergometer due to the patient's risk of fall, as well as the ease of retesting the patient in future evaluations as they may continue to functionally decline. Testing such patients on a treadmill may become unsafe over time, and it is better for annual evaluations to be able to utilize the same modality for comparative purposes. On the other hand, obese patients who may not be able to comfortably sit on a cycle ergometer, may be better suited for a treadmill protocol, and those patients with pacemaker implants that are rate-responsive should be conducted on a treadmill to avoid chronotropic incompetence on a cycle ergometer where their device may not sense motion without a heel strike.

VARIABLES OF INTEREST

As previously described, the Fick equation defines VO_2 as it relates to Q and a-vO_2 difference. This equation provides the fundamental basis of CPX, and allows for an evaluation of oxygen-carrying capacity as it relates to central cardiac, pulmonary, and peripheral function. VO_2 and VCO_2 measured at the mouth reflect the same gas exchange at a cellular level during steady-state exercise; therefore, CPX allows for gas exchange analysis and an evaluation of metabolic pathways, which provides insight regarding inadequate oxygen-carrying capacity or carbon dioxide exchange during incremental exercise. As minute ventilation (VE) increases during exercise, VO_2 continues to rise until mitochondrial oxygen saturation occurs and VO_2 plateaus. Concomitantly, while VE increases, VCO_2 also increases until the point of fatigue. Therefore, the balance between VE/VO_2 and VE/VCO_2 becomes important to evaluate during CPX, and will be further discussed in this chapter.

Patients with HF demonstrate low oxygen-carrying capacity, frequently attributable to inadequate Q due to decreased LV function. Decreased chronotropic response and stroke volume contribute to poor central cardiac function, while increased pulmonary pressures and mitochondrial dysfunction in peripheral skeletal muscle further inhibit adequate oxygen and carbon dioxide exchange. Ideally, CPX provides the ability to assess VO_{2max}; however, as tests are often terminated due to leg fatigue, shortness of breath, or various discomforts, peak VO_2 is the primary variable considered in CPX evaluation. A plateau in the VO_2 at peak incremental exercise, however, signifies that a true maximal VO_2 has been achieved. Additionally, a plateau in blood pressure or HR response near peak exercise can also indicate that a maximal effort has been achieved.

Table 45-1 Assessment Methods

Exercise Test Procedure	Test Indication
Standard ETT	Initial assessment of low-risk, symptomatic patients; precardiac rehabilitation; arrhythmia assessment; risk stratification
CPX	Decreased exercise tolerance, unexplained dyspnea, congestive heart failure, cardiomyopathy, COPD, precardiac rehabilitation, pre/post heart and lung transplant
Stress echocardiography	Lightheaded/dizziness, syncope, dyspnea, chest pain, congestive heart failure, cardiomyopathy, valvular disease
Nuclear stress test	Patients with an abnormal baseline ECG, concern for microvascular ischemia, history of CAD with or without intervention, higher-risk patients

Abbreviations: CAD, coronary artery disease; COPD, chronic obstructive pulmonary disease; CPX, cardiopulmonary exercise testing; ECG, electrocardiography; ETT, exercise tolerance test.

In addition to peak VO_2, the transition from aerobic to anaerobic metabolism can also be assessed through CPX. The anaerobic threshold (AT), also known as the lactate threshold, is the point at which lactate production overrides lactate clearance. While analyzing metabolic data from CPX, this point is often determined by looking for the crossover point between VE/VCO_2 and VE/VO_2, by a drop in the partial pressure in end-tidal CO_2 ($P_{ET}CO_2$), or by a dislinear rise in the VE/VO_2. Although a submaximal measure, AT levels below $11\ mL/kg^{-1}/min^{-1}$ have been associated with a 5-fold increase in risk of premature death.[13] Furthermore, considering the fact that most patients are not achieving their peak VO_2 on a daily basis, but are very likely to reach AT during activities of daily living, the AT is an important factor to consider. Reaching AT before ~50% of the VO_{2max} is considered early AT, and may have negative effects on activities of daily living, as this state of metabolic acidosis only allows for activity to be maintained for a brief period of time, and requires the patient to stop and rest before being able to engage in a subsequent activity. Furthermore, while peak VO_2 is often only modestly increased with exercise training, AT can be substantially affected by training, allowing the body to become more efficient in lactate clearance, subsequently resulting in longer physical performance and decreased recovery time.

The AT frequently correlates with the respiratory exchange ratio (RER), which depicts the relationship between VCO_2 and VO_2, and provides an indicator of both metabolic pathways (aerobic vs anaerobic) and patient effort. It is important to acknowledge, however, that although these 2 variables are related, they are not interchangeable. The RER is dependent upon substrate utilization during activity (fat vs carbohydrates), and is directly related to lactate accumulation in the working muscle. The peak VO_2 should always be looked at in conjunction with RER and AT to determine whether or not test sensitivity is affected by low patient effort and to rule out a premature change in metabolism. Typically, a peak RER that falls below 1.0 is considered to indicate poor patient effort, while an RER >1.1 reflects adequate effort. Patients with HF, however, may exercise to their maximal effort during CPX with the RER still not reaching values over 1.0 due to underlying pulmonary hypertension (HTN).

The $P_{ET}CO_2$ has also been shown to be abnormal in HF patients due to underlying pulmonary HTN. Normal values of $P_{ET}CO_2$ are generally between 36 and 44 mm Hg, while these values for HF patients are often below 30 mm Hg. The $P_{ET}CO_2$ during CPX should stay relatively constant, with modest decreases after AT until VO_{2max}. HF patients with underlying pulmonary HTN, however, frequently demonstrate increases in the $P_{ET}CO_2$ during incremental exercise, demonstrating ventilatory inefficiency.

The VE/VCO_2 slope is another significant variable in CPX testing that determines ventilatory efficiency. A high VE/VCO_2 slope (>34-36) is a strong prognosticator of future mortality and morbidity in HF, and has been shown to provide a functional assessment equivalent to peak VO_2.[11] As opposed to the peak VO_2, however, the VE/VCO_2 slope is valid even at submaximal levels of exertion, allowing for its value to be maintained despite the premature termination of a test due to clinical findings or patient discomfort. To further assist with the interpretation of maximal and submaximal CPX data as they relate to mortality risk, refer to Figure 45-3.

CARDIAC REHABILITATION AND EXERCISE RECOMMENDATIONS

The optimal and/or recommended exercise prescription for the HF population has gone through many iterations since the late 1980s and continues to evolve. Mounting evidence supports the implementation of exercise training on most if not all days of the week, for 30 to 60 minutes per exercise session, to improve aerobic capacity, physiological systems mentioned previously, QOL, blood lipid profile, blood glucose, and blood pressure, as well as morbidity and mortality.[14-16] This section will outline current exercise prescription practices, relating to moderate and high-intensity exercise, as well as special considerations for subgroups of HF patients.

CARDIAC REHABILITATION PHASES AND INDICATION

Patients with HF exhibit reduced physical activity levels and can be noncompliant with physical activity recommendations.[17,18] Furthermore, aversions to exercise can be enhanced by exacerbations of dyspnea and fatigue, dramatically reducing physical activity-related self-efficacy.[19] Cardiac rehabilitation (CR) programs mitigate these obstacles by offering a multidisciplinary environment that provides exercise supervision and education by appropriately trained health professionals such as exercise physiologists and nurses. In addition to receiving tailored exercise prescriptions in a closely monitored environment, contemporary CR programs provide opportunities for smoking cessation, nutritional and psychological counseling, diabetes management, and weight control counseling. All phases of CR (Figure 45-4) serve a role in the secondary prevention of cardiovascular disease (CVD), with the goal of educating patients on their specific form of cardiac disease and establishing behavioral modifications that facilitate maintenance of an active and healthy lifestyle.

Phases of Cardiac Rehabilitation

Phase I (Inpatient)

This phase is for patients who have recently been hospitalized after a cardiac event (eg, myocardial infarction [MI]) or interventional procedures (eg, cardiac valve replacement, coronary artery bypass grafting). The purpose of this phase is to remobilize patients and provide education regarding respective cardiac events and management with medication and physical activity.

Phase II (Outpatient)

Phase II is a program that delivers preventive and rehabilitative services to patients in a closely monitored (typically 1 staff to 4 patient ratio) outpatient setting early after a CVD event.

Phase III or IV (Outpatient Maintenance)

This phase provides longer-term delivery of preventive and rehabilitative services to patients requiring minimal supervision in an outpatient setting.

The placement of HF patients in respective CR programs begins with a physician referral. Unfortunately, referrals to CR have historically been low, particularly so in women, minority groups, and those

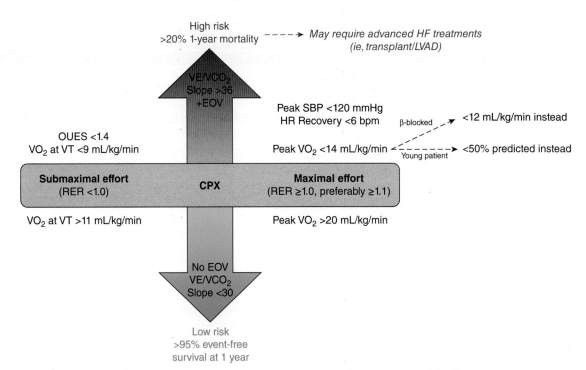

FIGURE 45-3 CPX results, independent of maximal (RER ≥ 1.0, preferably ≥ 1.1) or submaximal (RER <1.0) effort, possess potent prognostic utility in HF patients. Interpreting a HF patient's risk of mortality from a maximal CPX should begin with the evaluation of achieved VO_2. Due to the chronotropic lowering effects of beta blockers, peak VO_2 may be limited. The threshold for increased risk of mortality for patients taking a beta blocker during CPX is therefore <12 mL/kg/min. Conversely, rather than setting an absolute threshold for younger HF patients (who may have a relatively higher VO_2), 50% of age-predicted VO_2 should be considered for risk assessment. Peak hemodynamic responses are also telling prognostic markers for patients who are unable to achieve a SBP above 120, have a blunted maximal HR response, and/or have a HR recovery <6 bpm. In cases when patients are unable to put forth a maximal effort, VO_2 patterns, such as OUES and VT (or anaerobic threshold) can serve as sufficient predictors of mortality. Moreover, regardless of exercise effort, measures of ventilator efficiency such as VE/VCO_2 and EOV can be powerful markers of prognosis. Abbreviations: bpm, beats per minute; CPX, cardiopulmonary exercise test; EOV, exercise oscillatory ventilation; HF, heart failure; HR, heart rate; LVAD, left ventricular assist device; OUES, oxygen uptake efficiency slope; RER, respiratory exchange ratio; SBP, systolic blood pressure; VE, ventilation; VCO_2, carbon dioxide output; VO_2, oxygen uptake; VT, ventilator threshold. (Data from Malhotra R, Bakken K, D'Elia E, Lewis GD. Cardiopulmonary exercise testing in heart failure. *JACC Heart Fail.* 2016;4(8):607-616.)

with advanced disease severity.[20] Additional barriers to CR referral and participation include misconceptions regarding the patient's ability to tolerate exercise and poor health care provider endorsement of CR. In the United States, systolic HF is now a covered diagnosis for CR and recent data indicate a particularly poor referral pattern, with only 10% of eligible patients referred to CR after hospital discharge.[21,22] This is particularly troubling as CR programs have empirically shown to improve CV health across a wide spectrum of HF severity. Moreover, despite efforts by leading professional organizations, HFpEF is not yet recognized as a diagnosis that can be covered for CR services. A cited reason for the exclusion of the HFpEF population for CR coverage includes insufficient evidence from large-scale studies that demonstrates reduced hospital readmission rates, mortality, and improved health outcomes after exercise interventions resembling CR practices. The volume of exercise research in HFpEF pales in comparison to the vast number of small- to large-scale interventions conducted in HFrEF. Even so, evidence supporting the physiological benefits of MCT in HFpEF is growing and available data demonstrate a clear benefit in this HF subgroup.[23]

Writing an exercise prescription is similar to writing a drug prescription and titrating patients to a tolerable and efficacious dosage. The general prescription guidelines outlined in this section should serve as a template that can be tailored for the patient's needs and special considerations. The central components of any exercise

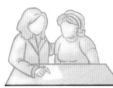

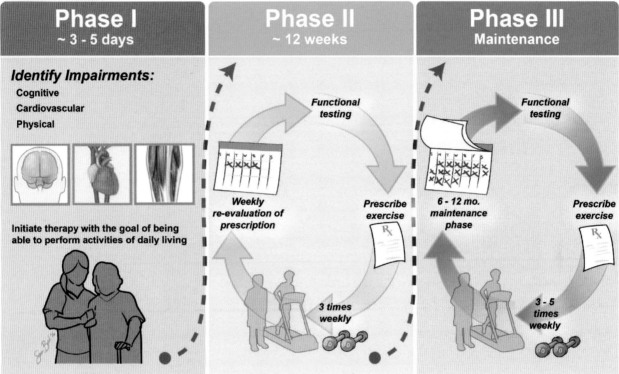

FIGURE 45-4 Progression through the 3 phases of cardiac rehabilitation.

prescription include frequency (how often), intensity (how hard), time (duration of exercise), and type (mode or type of exercise), also referred to as the FITT principle.

INPATIENT EXERCISE PRESCRIPTION

After receiving a physician referral, patients hospitalized for a cardiac event or a procedure related to coronary artery disease, cardiac valve replacement, or MI, should be evaluated by staff to determine their readiness for physical activity. The goals of inpatient or phase I CR program include:

- Identifying patients with significant CV, physical, or cognitive impairments that may influence the performance of physical activity.

- Offset the deleterious physiological and psychological effects of bedrest.

- Provide additional medical surveillance of patients and their responses to physical activity.

- Evaluate and being to enable patients to safely return to activities of daily living within the limits imposed by their CVD.

- Prepare the patient and support system at home or in a transitional setting to optimize recovery following acute-care hospital discharge.

- Facilitate physician referral and patient entry into an outpatient CR program.

Inpatient CR Phase I
Adapted from ACSM's GETP

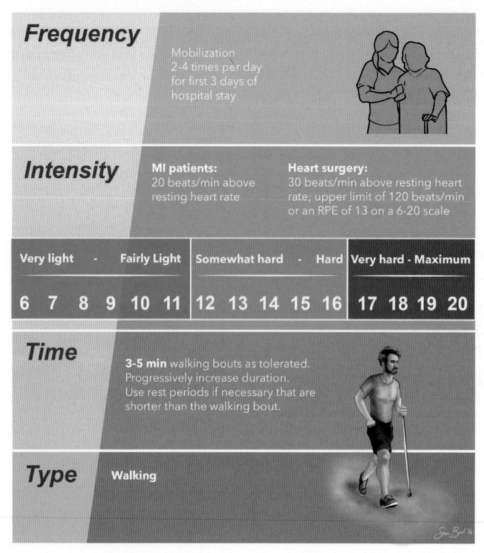

Frequency

Mobilization
2-4 times per day
for first 3 days of
hospital stay

Intensity

MI patients:
20 beats/min above
resting heart rate

Heart surgery:
30 beats/min above resting heart
rate; upper limit of 120 beats/min
or an RPE of 13 on a 6-20 scale

Very light	-	Fairly Light	Somewhat hard	-	Hard	Very hard - Maximum
6 7 8	9	10 11	12 13 14	15	16	17 18 19 20

Time

3-5 min walking bouts as tolerated.
Progressively increase duration.
Use rest periods if necessary that are
shorter than the walking bout.

Type

Walking

FIGURE 45-5 Exercise prescription recommendations for patients in phase I cardiac rehabilitation.

Strategies for accomplishing these goals will depend on the nature of the cardiac event or procedure. For example, patients undergoing percutaneous coronary interventions may only be hospitalized for 24 hours, whereas patients with coronary artery bypass graft surgery may be hospitalized for 5 days. In the case when invasive procedures are performed, activities should focus on regaining range of motion and limiting movements to intermittent sitting and standing. Then the activities may slowly progress in short- to moderate-distance walks multiple times per day until the patient is discharged from the hospital (Figure 45-5).

OUTPATIENT EXERCISE PRESCRIPTION

Outpatient exercise prescription recommendations for HF patients (Table 45-2) are similar to recommendations for healthy adults. Numerous investigations have shown these volumes of exercise to be effective in enhancing CRF, 6MWT distance, and QOL.

Table 45-2 Outpatient Cardiac Rehabilitation Exercise Prescription

	Frequency	Intensity	Time	Type
Aerobic	At least 3 d/wk	40%-80% of HRR, VO_2R, or VO_{2peak} RPE of 11-16	Warm-up and cool-down: 5-10 min Exercise session: 20-60 min	• Treadmill • Recumbent stepper • Upright and recumbent cycle • Ergometer • Arm ergometer • Elliptical
Resistance	2-3 d/wk 48 h between training sessions	30%-40% of 1-RM for upper body 50%-60% for lower body	8-10 exercises of major muscle groups 12-15 repetitions per exercise	• Hand weights • Elastic bands • Machines
Flexibility	Before and after each aerobic resistance training session	Stretch point of feeling tightness or slight discomfort	10-30 s for each major muscle group/joint	Static stretching Flexibility exercise for each major muscle group

Adapted from ACSM's GETP.

Furthermore, these levels of exercise are safe to perform, with roughly 1 cardiac arrest for every 116,905 patient hours and 1 fatality per 752,365 patient hours.[24] Due to the many health benefits and safety of exercise, patients without absolute contraindications to exercise (Table 45-3) are encouraged to initiate outpatient exercise training soon after hospital discharge. Entrance into CR should be preceded by a symptom limited exercise test (without collection of expired gases) or CPX (includes collection of expired gases) with patients taking their prescribed medications at their usual time. Variables collected from these tests provide practitioners valuable information regarding HR_{peak}, peak VO_2, blood pressure response exertion, the existence of ischemic thresholds, ECG abnormalities triggered by exercise, and/or pulmonary insufficiencies causing oxygen desaturation. This information is used to customize exercise prescriptions to the patient.

The **frequency** of exercise should be performed at least 3 days per week in a supervised setting. Patients not accustomed to regularly exercising should be encouraged to perform home-based exercises on non-CR days after demonstrating a good tolerance to exercise. A patient can typically attend up to 36 sessions of a phase II CR program. However, some insurance policies may dictate the number of sessions they are willing to cover based on the patient's relative risk stratification (Table 45-4). Low-risk patients are recommended to attend 12 to 18 sessions, moderate risk 18 to 24 sessions, and high-risk 24 to 36 sessions.

Exercise **intensity** should ideally be prescribed based on HR_{peak}, HRR (ie, HR_{peak} − resting HR), or VO_2 reserve (ie, peak VO_2 − resting VO_2). Rating of perceived exertion (RPE) can be used as a complementary marker of intensity (11-16 on a scale of 6-20). The recommended range of exercise intensity (Table 45-2) is purposefully wide, due to the broad range of functional capacities of patients in CR. High-risk patients are encouraged to begin at the lower threshold of intensity prescription while those at a low risk and previous history of exercise at the higher end of threshold. However, in all cases, starting at a lower intensity and uptitrating the intensity is a good practice to follow.

Example of Calculating an Exercise Prescription

- **METHOD:** 40% to 80% of HRR for an individual with a resting HR of 76 and HR_{peak} of 147 bpm.

  HRR = 147 bpm – 76 bpm = 71 bpm

  71 bpm × 40% = 28 bpm and 71 bpm × 80% = 57 bpm

  71 bpm + 28 bpm = 99 bpm and 71 bpm + 57 bpm = 128 bpm

  RESULT: Exercise HR range between 99 and 128 bpm.

- **METHOD:** 60% to 85% of HR_{peak}.

  147 × 65% = 96 bpm and 147 × 85% = 125

  RESULT: Exercise HR range between 96 and 125 bpm.

An example of exercise **time** is a 1-hour CR session that includes a cool-down and warm-up period of 5 to 10 minutes of light-intensity (ie, <40% HRR, <65% HR_{peak}, or <11 RPE) aerobic activities, stretching, and/or range of motion exercises. The goal of the aerobic conditioning phase is to reach 20 to 60 minutes of exercise. High-risk patients may not be able to complete the suggested duration. Instead, patients can begin with 5 to 10 minutes and gradually increase exercise time by 1 to 5 minutes with each subsequent session. Performing intermittent bouts of exercise (1-5 minutes) separated by passive rest periods can also be an effective method of reaching the targeted exercise duration in patients who do not tolerate exercise well.

The **type** or modality of exercise should incorporate weight-bearing activities (ie, walking or elliptical) with an emphasis on increased caloric expenditure. Exercise modalities that incorporate whole-body movements (ie, arm ergometers, Airdyne bikes, recumbent steppers with arm handles, and ellipticals) should also be integrated into exercise sessions to promote upper body fitness. If patients exhibit issues with walking or are at a risk of falls, seated modalities such as cycle ergometers, recumbent steppers, and/or arm ergometers should be used.

PATIENT MONITORING

Monitoring patients with an ECG during supervised exercise sessions is helpful when tracking ECG responses to exercise, documenting exercise HR responses, and adjusting exercise equipment settings to ensure patients reach their prescribed HR ranges. Objectively documenting these responses during exercise, on all session visits, can be useful in tracking a patient's progress through the program. However, continuous ECG monitoring is not required for

Table 45-3 Contraindications to Exercise

Relative Contraindications
1. 1.5-2.0 kg increase in body mass over previous 3-5 days
2. Concurrent continuous or intermittent ischemic changes
3. Abnormal increase or decrease of blood pressure with exercise
4. NYHA functional class IV
5. Complex ventricular arrhythmia at rest
6. Recent embolism or thrombophlebitis appearing with exertion
7. Supine resting HR ≥100 beats/min
8. Preexisting comorbidity or behavioral disorder
9. Implantable cardiac defibrillator with HR limit set below the target heart rate for training
10. Extensive MI resulting in LV dysfunction within previous 4 weeks

Absolute Contraindications
1. Signs or symptoms of worsening or unstable HF over previous 2-4 days
2. Abnormal blood pressure or early unexpected life-threatening arrhythmia
3. Uncontrolled metabolic disorder (ie, hypothyroidism, diabetes)
4. Acute systemic illness or fever
5. Recent embolism or thrombophlebitis
6. Active pericarditis or myocarditis
7. Third-degree heart block without pacemaker
8. Significant uncorrected valvular disease except mitral regurgitation because of HF-related LV dilation.

Abbreviations: HF, heart failure; HR, heart rate; LV, left ventricular; MI, myocardial infarction.

Table 45-4 Risk Stratification Recommendations (as outlined by the American Association of Cardiopulmonary Rehabilitation)

Low Risk

- Absence of complex ventricular dysrhythmias during exercise testing and recovery
- Absence of angina or other significant symptoms (ie, unusual shortness of breath, lightheadedness, or dizziness, during exercise testing and recovery)
- Presence of normal hemodynamics during exercise testing and recovery (ie, appropriate increases and decreases in HR and SBP with increasing workloads and recovery)
- Functional capacity ≥7 METs
- Nonexercise testing findings
  - Resting EF ≥50%
  - Uncomplicated MI or revascularization procedure
  - Absence of complicated ventricular dysrhythmias at rest
  - Absence of CHF
  - Absence of signs or symptoms of postevent/postprocedure ischemia
  - Absence of clinical depression

Moderate Risk

- Presence of angina or other significant symptoms (ie, unusual SOB, lightheadedness, or dizziness occurring only at high levels of exertion [≥7 METs])
- Mild to moderate level of silent ischemia during exercise testing or recovery (ST-segment depression <2 mm from baseline)
- Functional capacity <5 METs
- Rest EF 40%-49%

Highest Risk

- Presence of complex ventricular dysrhythmias during exercise testing or recovery
- Presence of angina or other significant symptoms (ie, unusual SOB, lightheadedness, or dizziness at low levels of exertion [<5 METs] or during recovery)
- High level of silent ischemia (ST-segment depression ≥2 mm from baseline) during exercise testing or recovery
- Presence of abnormal hemodynamics with exercise testing (ie, chronotropic incompetence or flat or decreasing SBP with increasing workloads) or recovery (ie, severe postexercise hypotension)
- Nonexercise testing findings
  - Rest EF <40%
  - History of cardiac arrest or sudden death
  - Complex dysrhythmia at rest
  - Complicated MI or revascularization procedure
  - Presence of CHF
  - Presence of signs or symptoms of postevent/postprocedure ischemia
  - Presence of clinical depression

Abbreviations: CHF, congestive heart failure; EF, ejection fraction; HR, heart rate; METs, metabolic equivalents; MI, myocardial infarction; SBP, systolic blood pressure; SOB, shortness of breath.

all exercise sessions. Instead, the following recommendations are derived based on the patient-associated risks of exercise training.[25] Low-risk HF patients may begin with continuous ECG monitoring and decrease to intermittent ECG monitoring after 6 sessions. Moderate-risk patients may begin with continuous ECG monitoring and decrease to intermittent ECG monitoring after 12 sessions or sooner, per rehabilitation staff recommendations. High-risk patients may begin with continuous ECG monitoring and decrease to intermittent ECG monitoring after 18 sessions or sooner as deemed appropriate by the rehabilitation staff.

RESISTANCE AND FLEXIBILITY TRAINING

The accelerated muscle wasting associated with HF, contributes to the debilitating decline in health. Evidence suggests that moderate resistance training can improve muscle strength by 20% to 45% and is well tolerated in stable HF patients. However, the first few weeks of a CR program should focus on introducing aerobic exercise and ensuring adherence. Once the patient has demonstrated compliance to aerobic exercise, resistance and flexibility exercises should be incorporated on at least 2 of the 3 days of CR attendance. Resistance-based exercise should focus on low weight, high repetition, for 1 to 2 sets, and targeting all of the major muscle groups (Table 45-2). Progression of load should be 5% to 10% as patients improve.

INSPIRATORY MUSCLE TRAINING

Although inspiratory muscle training (IMT) is effective in improving a CRF and physical function, it is currently a relatively underutilized form of therapy in the CR setting. Additionally, it should not be performed in place of aerobic exercise training, but rather incorporated into a CR session. A number of studies have shown favorable outcomes in response to the IMT prescription outlined in Figure 45-6. Most HF patients tolerate this form of exercise; however, patients with markedly elevated LV end-diastolic volumes, LV end-diastolic pressures, and worsening signs/symptoms of HF after IMT should discontinue IMT immediately until issues are resolved.

SPECIAL CONSIDERATIONS

BETA BLOCKER THERAPY

A majority of HF patients are prescribed beta blockers, attenuating resting and exercise HR. Prior to initiating an exercise intervention, CPX should be conducted with the HF patient following his or her daily medication regimen. This will allow for an exercise prescription to be developed for the relatively blunted HR_{peak} that is common. Additionally, the type of beta blocker (ie, long-acting vs short-acting) and the timing of CPX should also be documented as this will impact the exercise prescription. For example, patients performing an exercise test in the afternoon while on a short-acting

beta blocker taken in the morning, may achieve a higher HR compared to completing the exercise test in the morning.

STERNOTOMY

Recovery from procedures that require access to the heart typically requires 8 weeks to ensure adequate sternal stability. Patients may initiate CR therapy prior to achieving complete sternal stability; therefore, it is imperative to design an exercise prescription that limits upper body movements within the first 8 to 12 weeks postoperation. These patients should undergo routine follow-up examinations by their health care provider to evaluate progress in the healing process and readiness to introduce light upper-body movements. There are no standard weight limits; however, patients should begin with range of motion exercise, then progressively incorporate activities utilizing the thoracic musculature. Frequently checking for evidence of sternal instability indicated by movement in the sternum, pain, cracking, or popping is recommended as a standard practice.

LEFT VENTRICULAR ASSIST DEVICES

The prevalence of left ventricular assist device (LVAD) implantation as destination therapy in HF patients is exponentially growing. Although there have been few large-scale exercise intervention studies in this population, the existing evidence supports exercise to be safe and to have physiological benefits. There are however many considerations that must be made to ensure the safety of exercising patients. Patients and exercise staff must be mindful of the LVAD's drive lines, batteries, and console that can physically limit exercise. Drive lines can get caught on exercise equipment, potentially disconnecting the external components and power supply. Furthermore, patients should also avoid excessive stretching movements, as they may cause the LVAD's drive line to rotate, potentially causing skin irritation and even lead to inflammation and local infection. After patients have been deemed hemodynamically stable and require minimal assistance with activities of daily living, exercise therapy can begin at low intensities as tolerated by the patient. Much of the scientific evidence supports performing exercises at light to moderate (ie, 50% of VO_2 reserve or 12-14 RPE) intensities in LVAD patients to achieve improvements in peak VO_2.

CARDIAC TRANSPLANTATION

HF patients undergoing cardiac transplantation require much attention postoperation and may not be able to begin therapy for many weeks or months. Due to the resulting denervation, the heart may not respond appropriately to sympathetic stimulation. For this reason, patients may require longer warm-up and cool-down periods as tolerated. Initial exercise prescriptions in this population should not be based on target HR, but rather, subjective indices of effort (ie, RPE 11-16).

Deconditioned Heart Failure

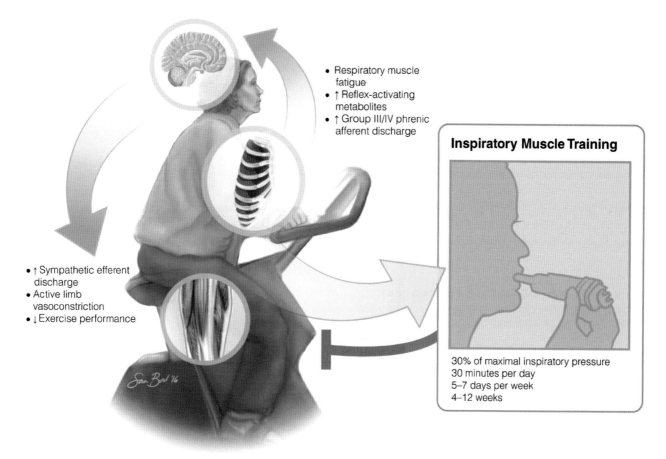

- Respiratory muscle fatigue
- ↑ Reflex-activating metabolites
- ↑ Group III/IV phrenic afferent discharge

- ↑ Sympathetic efferent discharge
- Active limb vasoconstriction
- ↓ Exercise performance

Inspiratory Muscle Training

30% of maximal inspiratory pressure
30 minutes per day
5–7 days per week
4–12 weeks

FIGURE 45-6 Respiratory muscle metaboreflex and its role in exacerbating heart failure related symptoms in response to exercise. Inspiratory muscle training can attenuate exercise-induced symptoms. (Data from Cahalin LP, Arena R, Guazzi M, et al. Inspiratory muscle training in heart disease and heart failure: a review of the literature with a focus on method of training and outcomes. *Expert Rev Cardiovasc Ther.* 2013;11(2):161-177.)

REFERENCES

1. Smart N, Marwick TH. Exercise training for patients with heart failure: a systematic review of factors that improve mortality and morbidity. *Am J Med.* 2004;116(10):693-706.

2. Molina AJ, Bharadwaj MS, Van Horn C, et al. Skeletal muscle mitochondrial content, oxidative capacity, and Mfn2 expression are reduced in older patients with heart failure and preserved ejection fraction and are related to exercise intolerance. *JACC Heart Fail.* 2016;4(8):636-645.

3. Chen YM, Li ZB, Zhu M, Cao YM. Effects of exercise training on left ventricular remodelling in heart failure patients: an updated meta-analysis of randomised controlled trials. *Int J Clin Pract.* 2012;66(8):782-791.

4. Wisloff U, Stoylen A, Loennechen JP, et al. Superior cardiovascular effect of aerobic interval training versus moderate continuous training in heart failure patients: a randomized study. *Circulation.* 2007;115(24):3086-3094.

5. Rognmo O, Moholdt T, Bakken H, et al. Cardiovascular risk of high- versus moderate-intensity aerobic exercise in coronary heart disease patients. *Circulation.* 2012;126(12):1436-1440.

6. Gademan MG, Swenne CA, Verwey HF, et al. Effect of exercise training on autonomic derangement and neurohumoral activation in chronic heart failure. *J Card Fail.* 2007;13(4):294-303.

7. Hirai DM, Musch TI, Poole DC. Exercise training in chronic heart failure: improving skeletal muscle O_2 transport and utilization. *Am J Physiol Heart Circ Physiol.* 2015;309(9):H1419-H1439.

8. Cahalin LP, Arena R, Guazzi M, et al. Inspiratory muscle training in heart disease and heart failure: a review of the literature with a focus on method of training and outcomes. *Expert Rev Cardiovasc Ther.* 2013;11(2):161-177.

9. Cipriano G, Jr., Cipriano VT, da Silva VZ, et al. Aerobic exercise effect on prognostic markers for systolic heart failure patients: a systematic review and meta-analysis. *Heart Fail Rev.* 2014;19(5):655-667.

10. Gademan MG, Swenne CA, Verwey HF, et al. Exercise training increases oxygen uptake efficiency slope in chronic heart failure. *Eur J Cardiovasc Prev Rehabil.* 2008;15(2):140-144.

11. Malhotra R, Bakken K, D'Elia E, Lewis GD. Cardiopulmonary exercise testing in heart failure. *JACC Heart Fail.* 2016;4(8):607-616.

12. Zurek M, Corra U, Piepoli MF, Binder RK, Saner H, Schmid JP. Exercise training reverses exertional oscillatory ventilation in heart failure patients. *Eur Respir J.* 2012;40(5):1238-1244.

13. Gitt AK, Wasserman K, Kilkowski C, et al. Exercise anaerobic threshold and ventilatory efficiency identify heart failure patients for high risk of early death. *Circulation.* 2002;106(24):3079-3084.

14. O'Connor CM, Whellan DJ, Lee KL, et al. Efficacy and safety of exercise training in patients with chronic heart failure: HF-ACTION randomized controlled trial. *JAMA.* 2009;301(14):1439-1450.

15. Smart NA, Larsen AI, Le Maitre JP, Ferraz AS. Effect of exercise training on interleukin-6, tumour necrosis factor alpha and functional capacity in heart failure. *Cardiol Res Pract.* 2011;2011:532620.

16. Gielen S, Adams V, Mobius-Winkler S, et al. Anti-inflammatory effects of exercise training in the skeletal muscle of patients with chronic heart failure. *J Am Coll Cardiol.* 2003;42(5):861-868.

17. van der Wal MH, Jaarsma T, Moser DK, Veeger NJ, van Gilst WH, van Veldhuisen DJ. Compliance in heart failure patients: the importance of knowledge and beliefs. *Eur Heart J.* 2006;27(4):434-440.

18. Tierney S, Mamas M, Woods S, et al. What strategies are effective for exercise adherence in heart failure? A systematic review of controlled studies. *Heart Fail Rev.* 2012;17(1):107-115.

19. Woodgate J, Brawley LR. Self-efficacy for exercise in cardiac rehabilitation: review and recommendations. *J Health Psychol.* 2008;13(3):366-387.

20. Arena R, Williams M, Forman DE, et al. Increasing referral and participation rates to outpatient cardiac rehabilitation: the valuable role of healthcare professionals in the inpatient and home health settings: a science advisory from the American Heart Association. *Circulation.* 2012;125(10):1321-1329.

21. Ades PA. Temporal trends and factors associated with cardiac rehabilitation referral among patients hospitalized with heart failure: awaiting the uptick. *J Am Coll Cardiol.* 2015;66(8):927-929.

22. Centers for Medicare & Medicaid Services. Decision Memo for Cardiac Rehabilitation (CR) Programs-Chronic Heart Failure, https://www.cms.gov/medicare-coverage-database/details/nca-decision-memo.aspx?NCAId=270

23. Dieberg G, Ismail H, Giallauria F, Smart NA. Clinical outcomes and cardiovascular responses to exercise training in heart failure patients with preserved ejection fraction: a systematic review and meta-analysis. *J Appl Physiol (1985).* 2015;119(6):726-733.

24. Thompson PD, Franklin BA, Balady GJ, et al. Exercise and acute cardiovascular events placing the risks into perspective: a scientific statement from the American Heart Association Council on Nutrition, Physical Activity, and Metabolism and the Council on Clinical Cardiology. *Circulation.* 2007;115(17):2358-2368.

25. *ACSM's Guidelines for Exercise Testing and Prescription.* 9th ed. Baltimore, MD: Lippincott Williams & Wilkins; 2013.

INDEX

Note: page numbers followed by *f* indicate figures; page numbers followed by *t* indicate tables.

Pharmacotherapy. *See also specific drugs and drug types*
adaptation of, perioperative heart failure and, 522
for autonomic modulation, 384, 384f
for bicuspid aortic valve, 204
cardiotoxicity and, 188–189
for depression, 86, 86f, 87f
outcomes of, 87, 88t
for heart failure
costs of, 3
with preserved ejection fraction, 55, 56t–57t
for hypertrophic cardiomyopathy, 106
neurohormonal. *See* Neurohormonal therapies
for peripartum cardiomyopathy, 140–141, 142–143, 142f
polypharmacy and, in elderly patients with heart failure, 152, 152f
as weight loss strategy, 28–29
Phentermine, for weight loss, 29
Physical activity. *See also* Athletic heart syndrome; Cardiac rehabilitation; Exercise
of cancer patients, 190
Polypharmacy, in elderly patients with heart failure, 152, 152f
Pomalidomide, cardiotoxicity of, 187t
Ponatinib, cardiotoxicity of, 186t
Postoperative heart failure, treatment of, 523–524
Post-thrombotic syndrome (PTS), 242, 242f
Potassium, in diet, 341t
Pregnancy
hypertrophic cardiomyopathy and, 110
peripartum cardiomyopathy and. *See* Peripartum cardiomyopathy
Preload, effect on left ventricular assist device pump function, 462
Pressure-volume relationship, left ventricular assist devices and, 459
Presyncope, hypertrophic cardiomyopathy and, 98
Primary care, 1
Primum atrial septal defect, in adults, 194, 195f
Prolactin, actions in kidney, 71t
Proliferation signal inhibitors, following heart transplantation, 488
Prostaglandins, neurohormonal regulation by, 69
Proteasome inhibitors, cardiotoxicity of, 187t
Protein, in diet, 340
Provider resources
for biomarkers, 275
for cardiac resynchronization therapy, 413–414
for cardiotoxicity, 191
for diet, 346
for economics of heart failure, 6–7
for hypertrophic cardiomyopathy, 110–111
for implantable cardioverter defibrillators, 400
for palliative care, 531
for peripartum cardiomyopathy, 144
for revascularization, 439
for venous thromboembolism, 243
Psychosocial factors
as contraindication for heart transplantation, 482
heart transplant survival and, 495–496

Psychosocial interventions, for depression, 86–87, 87f, 88f
Pulmonary angiography
computed tomography, in venous thromboembolism, 235, 236f
contrast, in venous thromboembolism, 237, 237f
magnetic resonance, in venous thromboembolism, 237
Pulmonary arterial hypertension, 335–336
cardiac magnetic resonance imaging in, 327, 328f, 329
Pulmonary artery pressure, right heart catheterization and, 334, 334f, 334t
Pulmonary artery saturation, cardiac output measurement and, 335
Pulmonary embolism (PE)
biomarkers in diagnosis of, 270
clinical prediction rules for, 237, 239t
diagnosis of, 233, 233f
prognosis of, 242
risk stratification for, 241, 241f, 241t, 242f
Pulmonary hypertension
arterial, 335–336
cardiac magnetic resonance imaging in, 327, 328f, 329
assessing for, using cardiopulmonary stress testing, 303, 303f
irreversible, as contraindication for heart transplantation, 481
Pulmonary response to exercise, 536
Pulmonary stenosis (PS), in adults, 208–212, 210f
associated defects and physiology of, 209, 211f
clinical features, diagnosis, and management of, 209–212, 211f, 212f
Pulmonary venous return, anomalous, in adults
partial, 200–202, 202f
total, 202, 203f

R
Racial minorities, heart failure in, 128–135
in African Americans, 128, 130–131
in Asians, 132–133, 133f
etiology and pathophysiology of, 128, 129t
in Hispanics, 131–132, 131f
Radiation therapy, cardiotoxicity of, 184, 185, 186t
Ranolazine, for heart failure, with preserved ejection fraction, 57t
Rastelli procedure, for dextro-transposition of the great arteries, 220
Reactive oxygen species, exercise and, 539
Rehabilitation. *See* Cardiac rehabilitation; Exercise
Rejection
following heart-lung transplantation, 514
following heart transplantation, 488–490, 489t
diagnosis of, 488–489, 489f, 490f
presentation of, 488
treatment of, 489–490
Renal artery stenosis, angioplasty or stenting for, hypertension and, 18
Renal blood flow, 63–64, 64f, 65f
Renal denervation, for heart failure, with preserved ejection fraction, 58t
Renal dysfunction, as contraindication for heart transplantation, 482